DATE DUE

THE ESSENTIALS OF RESPIRATORY CARE
Third Edition

The Essentials of Respiratory Care
Third Edition

ROBERT M. KACMAREK, PH.D., R.R.T.
Assistant Professor
Department of Anesthesia
Harvard Medical School
Director, Respiratory Care
Massachusetts General Hospital
Boston, Massachusetts

CRAIG W. MACK, M.M., R.R.T.
Director of Cardiopulmonary Services
Gottlieb Memorial Hospital
Melrose Park, Illinois

STEVEN DIMAS, R.R.T.
President, STAT Home Care
Elmhurst, Illinois

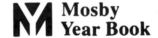
Mosby
Year Book

St. Louis   Baltimore   Boston   Chicago   London   Philadelphia   Sydney   Toronto

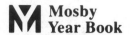

Mosby
Year Book

Dedicated to Publishing Excellence

Sponsoring Editor: Richard Lampert/David Marshall
Associate Director, Manuscript Services: Fran Perveiler
Production Project Coordinator: Carol A. Reynolds
Proofroom Supervisor: Barbara M. Kelly

1 2 3 4 5 6 7 8 9 0 CL MK 94 93 92 91 90

Library of Congress Cataloging-in-Publication Data
Kacmarek, Robert M.
   The essentials of respiratory care/Robert M. Kacmarek, Craig W.
Mack, Steven Dimas.—3rd ed.
    p. cm.
   Includes bibliographical references.
   Includes index.
   ISBN 0-8151-4956-5
   1. Respiratory therapy. 2. Respiration. I. Mack, Craig W.
II. Dimas, Steven. III. Title.
   [DNLM: 1. Respiratory Therapy. WB 342 K113e]
RC735.I5K32 1990
616.2′0046—dc20   90-12748
DNLM/DLC   CIP
for Library of Congress

With love to _____
Jan, Darla and Robert;
Karen, Brian and Justin;
Carol, Eric, Cassandra and James

CONTRIBUTORS _____

MARILYN BORKGREN, R.N., M.S.
Pulmonary Clinical Nurse Specialist
Suburban Lung Associates, S.C.
Elk Grove Village, Illinois

GAYLE PINCHCOFSKY-DEVIN, R.D.,
F.A.C.N.
Vice-President
STAT Home Care
Elmhurst, Illinois

ROBERT J. HARWOOD, R.R.T.
Assistant Professor
Department of Cardiopulmonary Sciences
Georgia State University
Atlanta, Georgia

SUSAN P. PILBEAM, M.S., R.R.T.
Program Director
Respiratory Therapy Program
Greenville Technical Educational Center
Greenville, South Carolina

JOSEPH RAU, PH.D., R.R.T.
Associate Professor
Department of Pulmonary Sciences
Georgia State University
Atlanta, Georgia

PREFACE TO THIRD EDITION _____

The profession of respiratory care is rapidly maturing. The knowledge base required of the respiratory care practitioner has expanded considerably over the last few years. This is reflected in the expansion of the third edition which contains about 33% more material than the second edition. Although no single text is capable of presenting the total scope and depth of respiratory care, we have attempted to expand on those essential aspects that we believe should be mastered by all respiratory care practitioners.

Neonatal/pediatric respiratory care is the area of the text which is most expanded. In the second edition only three chapters were devoted to this topic, whereas this edition includes five chapters covering all aspects of neonatal/pediatric respiratory care from intrauterine development to mechanical ventilation. In addition, comprehensive chapters on nutrition and pulmonary rehabilitation have been added, as well as chapters devoted to respiratory home care and high frequency ventilation.

As in previous editions, the stated goal of this text is to present what we believe is the knowledge base required of respiratory care practitioners in a logical and concise manner. The entire text is in outline form and as a result is probably best used as a secondary text, since a certain level of overall understanding is assumed. We have found that this text is best used for review and quick reference. Following each chapter is an extensive bibliography of both primary texts and periodicals to guide the practitioner to original presentations of material.

The text begins with reviews of basic sciences, and anatomy and physiology of the respiratory, cardiovascular, renal and neurological systems. Following are extensive presentations of all therapeutic aspects of neonatal, pediatric, and adult respiratory care. The text concludes with discussions of pharmacology, microbiology, sterilization, and cleaning.

We believe one of the primary uses of this text is in preparation for registration, certification, and licensure examinations.

Robert M. Kacmarek, Ph.D., R.R.T.
Craig W. Mack, M.M., R.R.T.
Steven Dimas, R.R.T.

ACKNOWLEDGMENTS

A very sincere and special thank you to all those respected colleagues whose guidance, assistance, critique and example over the years has made this text a reality:

Terry L. Alfredson, M.A., R.R.T.
Michael Aljets, R.R.T.
David Assmann, R.R.T.
Michael Callahan, R.R.T.
John Cronin, R.R.T.
Pat English, M.S., R.R.T.
Robert Goulet, M.S., R.R.T.
Ronald Harrison, M.D.
David Hauptman, R.R.T.
Dean Hess, M. Ed., R.R.T.
Fred Helmholz, M.D.
Sally Hixon, Ph.D., R.R.T.
Chris Hirsch, R.R.T.
Colleen Kigin, M.B.S., R.P.T.
Bill Kimball, M.D.
Jim Ludwig, R.R.T.
John Marini, M.D.
Neil MacIntyre, M.D.
Keith McMahon, R.R.T.
Gerry Meklaus, R.R.T.

Robert Molina, R.R.T.
Chuck Morash, R.R.T.
Norm Pucilo, R.R.T.
David Pierson, M.D.
Jane Reynolds, M.A., R.R.T.
Barry Shapiro, M.D.
Mary Simmons, R.R.T.
Bud Spearman, R.R.T.
Kevin Stanek, BSEE
Jamie Stoller, M.D.
Jeff Stout, R.R.T.
Steve Thompson, M.A., R.R.T.
Tony Torres, M.D.
John Walton, M.B.A., M.H.A., R.R.T.
Roger Wilson, M.D.
Donna Wilson, R.N., R.R.T.
Camille Woodward, R.N., R.R.T.
Paul Yinger, R.R.T.
Warren Zapol, M.D., R.R.T.

In addition, the deepest of thanks to all of our students and associates, past and present, who have continually provided the enthusiasm and dedication to inspire us to grow and repeatedly question.

Finally, we are eternally indebted to Gertrude Shaw for her understanding, skill, and everlasting patience in the preparation of this manuscript.

CONTENTS _____

Chapter 1

Basic Chemistry

I. Atomic Structure
   A. Atom: The smallest subdivision of a substance that still maintains the properties of that substance. An atom is composed of the following:
      1. Nucleus: Central portion of an atom, which contains protons and neutrons.
         a. Proton: Positively charged particle with a mass of one atomic mass unit.
         b. Neutron: Neutral particle with a mass of one atomic mass unit.
      2. Electron: Negatively charged particle that revolves around the nucleus of the atom with a mass of about 1/1,000 of an atomic mass unit.
      3. Normally, in its nonreactive state, an atom contains the same number of protons and electrons. The number of neutrons of the same substance may vary from one atom to another.
   B. Element: General term applied to each of the 106 different types of atoms.
   C. Isotope: Atom of a substance with the same number of protons but with a varying number of neutrons. All elements have at least two isotopes. The following are the three primary isotopes of oxygen:

$$0-16, \quad 8 \text{ neutrons } (99.76\% \text{ of all oxygen})$$
$$0-17, \quad 9 \text{ neutrons } (0.04\% \text{ of all oxygen})$$
$$0-18, \ 10 \text{ neutrons } (0.20\% \text{ of all oxygen})$$

   D. Atomic weight: Average weight of an atom of a particular substance based on the atomic weight of the carbon 12 isotope. The atomic weight is about equal to the sum of the weights of protons and neutrons in the nucleus of an atom and is not a whole number because of the presence of isotopes (Table 1–1).
   E. Gram atomic weight: Mass in grams of an element equal to its atomic weight (see Table 1–1).
   F. Atomic number: Number equal to the number of protons in the nucleus of an atom (see Table 1–1).
   G. Ion: Charged species of a particular atom.
II. Molecular Structure
   A. Molecule: Particle that results from chemical combination of two or more atoms and normally having a neutral charge.
   B. Compound: Molecule formed from two or more elements.
   C. Free radical: Charged compound, reacting as any other ion reacts.
   D. Molecular formula: Expression indicating the types of atoms and their numbers in the molecule. The particle that is positively charged is usually listed first.

1

TABLE 1–1.

Atomic Weights and Valences of 13 Common Elements

Element	Symbol	Atomic No.	Atomic Weight	Valence
Aluminum	Al	13	26.98	+3
Barium	Ba	56	137.34	+2
Calcium	Ca	20	40.08	+2
Carbon	C	6	12.0	±4
Chlorine	Cl	17	35.5	−1
Copper	Cu	29	63.55	+1 or +2
Fluorine	F	9	18.99	−1
Gallium	Ga	31	69.72	+3
Helium	He	2	4.00	±2
Hydrogen	H	1	1.00	+1
Iron	Fe	26	55.84	+1 or +2
Lead	Pb	82	207.19	+1 or +2
Lithium	Li	3	6.94	+1
Magnesium	Mg	12	24.31	+2
Mercury	Hg	80	200.59	+1 or +2
Oxygen	O	8	15.99	−2
Phosphorus	P	15	30.97	−3
Potassium	K	19	39.09	+1
Sodium	Na	11	22.98	+1
Sulfur	S	16	32.06	−2
Zinc	Zn	40	91.22	+1 or +2

Examples:

$NaCl$ = 1 sodium atom and 1 chloride atom contained in the molecule.

H_2SO_4 = 2 hydrogen atoms, 1 sulfur atom, and 4 oxygen atoms contained in the molecule

E. Molecular weight (MW): Sum total of all individual atomic weights of atoms that make up a molecule.

Example (H_2SO_4):

Atom	No. of Atoms		Atomic Weight	Total Contributing Weight
H	2	×	1	2
S	1	×	32	32
O	4	×	16	64
				MW 98

Example (CO_2):

Atom	No. of Atoms		Atomic Weight	Total Contributing Weight
C	1	×	12	12
O	2	×	16	32
				MW 44

F. Gram molecular weight (GMW): Mass in grams of a molecule equal to its MW.

III. Valence
    A. Valence: Number given to an atom that indicates its tendency to gain or lose electrons in a chemical reaction.
        Examples (see Table 1–1):
            Na (sodium): Valence of +1 indicates that it will react so as to lose one electron.
            Ca (calcium): Valence of +2 indicates that it will react so as to lose two electrons.
            F (fluorine): Valence of −1 indicates that it will react so as to gain one electron.
    B. Generally, valences of elements allow predictions of their reactivity with each other.

IV. Chemical Compounds
    A. Ionic compound: Compound formed as a result of the atoms in the compound gaining and losing electrons.
        Examples:
            NaCl: Na has a valence of +1, and Cl has a valence of −1. Thus, the Na atom has lost an electron, and the Cl atom has gained an electron.
            CaF_2: Ca has a valence of +2, and each F atom has a valence of −1. Thus, the Ca atom has lost 2 electrons, and each F atom has gained an electron.
      1. Properties of ionic compounds:
        a. High boiling points.
        b. High melting points.
        c. Dissolve readily in polar solvents.
        d. Strong electrolytes: Dissociate readily in polar solvents:

$$NaCl + H_2O \rightarrow Na^+ + Cl^- + H_2O$$
$$CaF_2 + H_2O \rightarrow Ca^{+2} + 2F^- + H_2O$$

    B. Covalent compound: Compound formed by the sharing of electrons between the various atoms in the compound.

$$O^{-2} + O^{-2} \rightarrow O_2$$
$$N^{-3} + N^{-3} \rightarrow N_2$$
$$Cl^- + Cl^- \rightarrow Cl_2$$

      1. Properties of covalent compounds:
        a. Exist only between atoms of the same element.
        b. Low melting points.
        c. Low boiling points.
        d. Dissolve poorly in polar solvents.
    C. Polar covalent compound: Intermediate compound between a pure covalent compound and an ionic compound characterized by incomplete sharing of electrons.
        Examples:

$$H_2O + CO_2 \rightleftharpoons H_2CO_3$$

      1. Properties of polar covalent compounds:
        a. Vary according to the particular compound.
        b. These compounds normally are weak electrolytes. Only a small percentage of ionization takes place when polar covalent compounds are added to a polar solution.

V. Volume Percent and Gram Percent
  A. Volume percent (vol%): Method of indicating the number of milliliters of a substance in 100 ml of solution.
    1. 10 vol% = 10 ml/100 ml of solution
    2. 3.5 vol% = 3.5 ml/100 ml of solution
  B. Gram percent (gm%): Method of indicating the number of grams of a substance in 100 ml of solution.
    1. 5.2 gm% = 5.2 gm/100 ml of solution
    2. 14.2 gm% = 14.2 gm/100 ml of solution
VI. Chemical Solutions
  A. Solution: Homogeneous mixture of two substances.
  B. Solute: Substance dissolved in a solution.
  C. Solvent: Substance that is the dissolving agent.
  D. Effects of a solute on the physical characteristics of water:
    1. Solutes cause an increase in the boiling point of water.
    2. Solutes cause a decrease in the freezing point of water.
    3. Osmotic pressure of a solution containing a solute is higher than that of pure water.
  E. As the temperature of the solvent increases, the volume of solute that can be dissolved in the solvent also increases.
  F. Dilute solution: A small amount of solute dissolved in each unit of solvent at a particular temperature.
  G. Saturated solution: Maximum amount of solute dissolved in each unit of solvent at a particular temperature. In a saturated solution a precipitate is seen at the bottom of the solution.
  H. Supersaturated solution: A greater amount of solute than the solvent would normally hold, dissolved at a particular temperature. However, physical disturbance of this solution causes the excess solute to precipitate.
VII. Solution Concentrations
  A. Ratio solution: Solution concentration represented as a ratio between solute and solvent in number of grams to number of mililiters.
    Examples:
      2:500 means 2 gm to 500 ml: 2 indicates the number of grams of solute, and 500 indicates the number of milliliters of solvent.
      1:1,000 means 1 gm to 1,000 ml: 1 indicates the number of grams of solute, and 1,000 indicates the number of milliliters of solvent.
    Problems:
    1. How many milligrams of solute are there in 1 ml of a 1:200 solution?

    1:200 means 1 gm to 200 ml
    1 gm = 1,000 mg, thus

    $$\frac{1,000 \text{ mg}}{200 \text{ ml}} = \frac{x}{1 \text{ ml}}$$
    $$x = 5 \text{ mg}$$

    2. How many milligrams are there in 5 ml of a 1:500 solution?

    1:500 means 1 gm to 500 ml
    1 gm = 1,000 mg, thus

    $$\frac{1,000 \text{ mg}}{500 \text{ ml}} = \frac{x}{5 \text{ ml}}$$
    $$x = 10 \text{ mg}$$

B. Percent weight/volume (W/V): Solution concentration where the actual percentage indicates the number of grams of solute per 100 ml of solution.
   Example:
       1% W/V solution means 1 gm of solute contained in 100 ml of solution.
   Problems:
   1. How many milligrams are there in 10 ml of a 3% W/V solution?

      3% W/V means 3 gm per 100 ml
         1 gm = 1,000 mg, thus
         3 gm = 3,000 mg

$$\frac{3,000\ mg}{100\ ml} = \frac{x}{10\ ml}$$
$$x = 300\ mg$$

2. How many milligrams are there in 3 ml of a 0.5% W/V solution?

      0.5% W/V means 0.5 gm per 100 ml
         1 gm = 1,000 mg, thus
         0.5 gm = 500 mg

$$\frac{500\ mg}{100\ ml} = \frac{x}{3\ ml}$$
$$x = 15\ mg$$

C. True percent solution: Solution concentration where *both* solute and solvent are expressed in either weight or volume. The solute is expressed as a true percentage of the solution.
   Examples:
       10% solution with a total solution of 100 gm means 10 gm of solute and 90 gm of solvent.
       3% solution with a total solution volume of 500 ml means 15 ml of solute and 485 ml of solvent.
   Problems:
   1. How many grams of solute are there in 250 gm of a 5% solution (5% indicates the percent by weight that the solute is of the total solution)?

$$(250)(0.05) = 12.5\ gm$$
   solution   solute
$$(250 - 12.5) = 237.5\ gm$$
              solvent

2. How many milliliters of solute are there in 500 ml of a 10% solution (10% indicates the percent by volume that the solute is of the total solution)?

$$(500)(0.10) = 50\ ml$$
   solution   solute
$$(500 - 50) = 450\ ml$$
           solvent

D. Molal solution (m): Solution concentration where the solute is expressed in moles and the solvent in kilograms, or millimoles per gram (mmoles/gm).

Example:

 2.5 m solution contains 2.5 moles of solute in 1 kg of solvent.

 1.5 m solution of KCl contains 1.5 moles, or 111.9 gm of KCl (1.5 × MW of KCl) in 1 kg of solvent.

Problems:

1. What is the molality of a solution with 117 gm of NaCl in 1,000 gm of water?

 1 m solution of NaCl   = 58.5 gm/1,000 gm of water
 117 gm/58.5 gm   = 2 moles
 2 moles of NaCl/1,000 gm of water = 2 m solution

2. How much H_2SO_4 must be dissolved in 500 gm of H_2O to make a 0.5 m solution?

$$1 \text{ mole of } H_2SO_4 = 98 \text{ gm}$$
$$1 \text{ m solution} = 98 \text{ gm}/1{,}000 \text{ gm of water}$$
$$0.5 \text{ m solution} = \frac{98}{2} \text{ or } 49 \text{ gm}/1{,}000 \text{ gm of water}$$

$$\frac{49 \text{ gm of } H_2SO_4}{1{,}000 \text{ gm of water}} = \frac{x}{500 \text{ gm of water}}$$
$$x = 24.5 \text{ gm of } H_2SO_4 \text{ needed}$$

E. Molar solution (M): Solution containing 1 mole of solute per liter of solution (or mmoles/ml).

 Examples:

 1.75 M solution contains 1.75 moles of solute per liter (L) of solution.

 2.0 M solution of NaOH contains 2 moles, or 80 gm of NaOH/L of solution (2 × MW of NaOH).

 Problems:

1. What is the molarity of 5.85 gm of NaCl in 1 L of solution?

 1 M solution   = 58.5 gm of NaCl/L
 5.85 ÷ 58.5   = 0.1 mole of NaCl
 0.1 mole of NaCl/L = 0.1 M solution

2. In what volume of solution must 149.2 gm of KCl be dissolved to make a 4 M solution?

 1 M solution = 74.6 gm/L
 4 M solution = 4 × 74.6, or 298.4 gm/L

$$\frac{298.4 \text{ gm}}{1{,}000 \text{ ml}} = \frac{149.2}{x}$$
$$x = 500 \text{ ml}$$

F. Normal solution (N): Solution concentration containing 1 gm equivalent weight (GEW; see section IX–A) of solute/L of solution (or 1 mg equivalent weight/ml).

 Examples:

 1.25 N solution contains 1.25 GEW/L of solution.

 2.00 N solution of HCl contains 2 GEWs, or 73 gm, of HCl/L of solution (1 GEW of HCl = 36.5 gm).

Problems:
1. What is the normality of a solution containing 42 gm of $NaHCO_3$?

$$1 \text{ GEW of } NaHCO_3 = 84 \text{ gm}$$
$$1 \text{ N solution} \quad\quad = 84 \text{ gm/L}$$
$$42 \text{ gm/84 gm} \quad\quad = 0.5 \text{ GEW}$$
$$42 \text{ gm/L} \quad\quad\quad = 0.5 \text{ N solution}$$

2. How many grams of NH_3Cl must be dissolved in 250 ml of solution to make a 2 N solution?

$$1 \text{ GEW of } NH_3Cl = 52.5 \text{ gm}$$
$$2 \text{ N solution} \quad\quad = 2 \text{ GEWs (105 gm)/L}$$

$$\frac{105 \text{ gm}}{1,000 \text{ ml}} = \frac{x}{250 \text{ ml}}$$
$$x = 26.25 \text{ gm}$$

VIII. Dilution Calculations
   A. The following formula is used to determine the concentration that will result when a solution is diluted:

$$V_1 \times C_1 = V_2 \times C_2 \tag{1}$$

where

V_1 is the volume before dilution
C_1 is the concentration before dilution
V_2 is the volume after dilution
C_2 is the concentration after dilution

   B. Before equation 1 can be used, three of the four variables must be known.
   Problems:
   1. What volume of water should be added to 50 ml of a 40% W/V solution of alcohol to dilute it to a 20% W/V solution?

$$V_1 \times C_1 = V_2 \times C_2$$
$$(50)(40) = (x)(20)$$
$$x = 100 \text{ ml}$$
$$100 \text{ ml} = V_2$$
$$V_2 - V_1 = \text{added volume}$$
$$100 \text{ ml} - 50 \text{ ml} = 50 \text{ ml of water to be added.}$$

   2. If 4 ml is added to 0.5 ml of a 15% W/V solution, what is the solution's final concentration?

$$V_1 \times C_1 = V_2 \times C_2$$
$$(0.5)(15\%) = (4.5)(x)$$
$$x = 1.67\% \text{ W/V}$$

IX. Gram Equivalent Weights
   A. Gram equivalent weight (GEW): Amount of a substance that will react completely with 1 mole of H^+ or OH^- or 1 mole of any monovalent substance.

B. The GEW of an element is determined by dividing the gram atomic weight of the substance by its valence. The charge of the valence is disregarded.
Examples:

$$Na^+ \text{ atomic weight 23 gm}$$
$$\frac{23 \text{ gm}}{1} = 23 \text{ gm/GEW}$$

$$Al^{+3} \text{ atomic weight 27 gm}$$
$$\frac{27 \text{ gm}}{3} = 9 \text{ gm/GEW}$$

$$S^{-2} \text{ atomic weight 32 gm}$$
$$\frac{32 \text{ gm}}{2} = 16 \text{ gm/GEW}$$

C. The GEW of an acid is determined by dividing its GMW by the number of replaceable hydrogen ions in the molecular formula. Normally all H^+ are replaceable. However, H_2CO_3 is an exception: only 1 H^+ is replaceable.
Examples:

$$H_2SO_4 \text{ GMW = 98 gm, 2 replaceable } H^+$$
$$\frac{98 \text{ gm}}{2} = 49 \text{ gm/GEW}$$

$$H_3PO_4 \text{ GMW = 98 gm, 3 replaceable } H^+$$
$$\frac{98 \text{ gm}}{3} = 32.66 \text{ gm/GEW}$$

$$H_2CO_3 \text{ GMW = 62 gm, 1 replaceable } H^+$$
$$\frac{62 \text{ gm}}{1} = 62 \text{ gm/GEW}$$

D. The GEW of a base is determined by dividing its GMW by the number of replaceable hydroxyl ions (OH^-) in the molecular formula. Normally all OH^- are replaceable.
Examples:

$$NaOH \text{ GMW = 40 gm, 1 replaceable } OH^-$$
$$\frac{40 \text{ gm}}{1} = 40 \text{ gm/GEW}$$

$$Ca(OH)_2 \text{ GMW = 74 gm, 2 replaceable } OH^-$$
$$\frac{74 \text{ gm}}{2} = 37 \text{ gm/GEW}$$

$$Al(OH)_3 \text{ GMW = 78 gm, 3 replaceable } OH^-$$
$$\frac{78 \text{ gm}}{3} = 26 \text{ gm/GEW}$$

E. The GEW of a salt is determined by dividing its GMW by the total valence of the positive ions or free radicals in the molecule.

Examples:

NaCl GMW = 58.5 gm, 1 Na$^+$ with a total valence of +1

$$\frac{58.5 \text{ gm}}{1} = 58.5 \text{ gm/GEW}$$

CaF$_2$ GMW = 78 gm, 1 Ca^{+2} with a total valence of +2

$$\frac{78 \text{ gm}}{2} = 39 \text{ gm/GEW}$$

Al$_2$(CO$_3$)$_3$ GMW = 234 gm, 2 Al^{+3} with a total valence of +6

$$\frac{234 \text{ gm}}{6} = 39 \text{ gm/GEW}$$

F. The GEW of a free radical is determined by dividing its GMW by its valence, disregarding the charge of the valence.
   Examples:

HCO$_3$$^-$ GMW = 61 gm, valence 1

$$\frac{61 \text{ gm}}{1} = 61 \text{ gm/GEW}$$

PO$_4$$^{-3}$ GMW = 95 gm, valence 3

$$\frac{95 \text{ gm}}{3} = 31.67 \text{ gm/GEW}$$

CO$_3$$^{-2}$ GMW = 60 gm, valence 2

$$\frac{60 \text{ gm}}{2} = 30 \text{ gm/GEW}$$

G. Milliequivalent weight (mEq): Weight of a substance that will react with 1 mmole of H$^+$, OH$^-$, or any monovalent substance. Numerically, the mEq of a substance is equal to its GEW.
   Examples:

NaCl 58.5 gm/GEW, 58.5 mg/mEq
H$_2$CO$_3$ 62 gm/GEW, 62 mg/mEq
Na$^+$ 23 gm/GEW, 23 mg/mEq

H. Equivalent weights are used to determine the precise quantity of a substance that reacts completely with a given quantity of another substance.
X. Temperature Scales
   A. Temperature scales (in degrees) in general use:
      1. Fahrenheit (F)
      2. Celsius or centigrade (C)
      3. Rankine (R)
      4. Kelvin (K)
   B. The Rankine and Kelvin scales are absolute zero scales, that is, zero on their scales represents the point where all molecular activity stops.
   C. Conversion formulas for temperature scales:
      1. C = 5/9 (F − 32)
      2. F = (9/5 C) + 32
      3. K = C + 273
      4. R = F + 460

Problems:

1. Convert 55°F to degrees K:

$$C = 5/9 \ (F - 32°)$$
$$C = 5/9 \ (55 - 32)$$
$$C = 12.80°$$
$$K = C + 273°$$
$$K = 12.8°C + 273°$$
$$K = 185.8°$$

2. Convert 30°C to degrees R:

$$F = 9/5 \ (C) + 32°$$
$$F = 9/5 \ (30) + 32°$$
$$F = 86°$$
$$R = F + 460°$$
$$R = 86°F + 460°$$
$$R = 546°$$

XI. Osmosis
  A. Osmosis is the movement of water from an area of high concentration of water to an area of low concentration of water.
  B. Osmosis occurs when two compartments of fluid are separated by a membrane that is selectively permeable Figs 1 and 2.
  C. Osmosis will proceed in a system until the concentration of water in the involved compartments is equal. When concentrations are equal, no net movement of fluid occurs; however, molecules still move back and forth across the system.
  D. Osmosis occurs between two solutions as a result of osmotic pressure differences in the solutions.

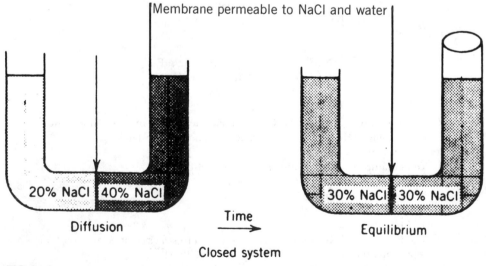

FIG 1–1.
Simple diffusion of water and NaCl across a permeable membrane. Note that the original and final volume of water is unchanged, but the concentration of NaCl equilibrated across the membrane. (From Wojciechowski WV: *Respiratory Care Sciences: An Integrated Approach.* New York, John Wiley & Sons, 1985. Used by permission.)

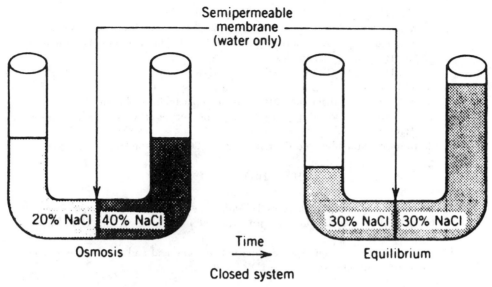

FIG 1–2.

Osmosis of water across a semipermeable membrane. Here, the membrane is permeable only to water. Sodium chloride concentrations are equilibrated but purely as a result of the movement of water. The final volume of water on each side of the membrane has markedly changed. (From Wojciechowski WV: *Respiratory Care Sciences: An Integrated Approach.* New York, John Wiley & Sons, 1985. Used by permission.)

    1. The potential pressure of the molecules of pure H_2O is about 1,073,000 mm Hg.
    2. When a solute is dissolved in H_2O, the potential pressure of the H_2O is decreased.
    3. The osmotic pressure of a solution is equal to the potential pressure of pure water minus the potential pressure of the solution.
       Example:

$$\begin{array}{rl}
\text{Pure } H_2O & 1{,}073{,}000 \text{ mm Hg} \\
\text{Solution} & 1{,}000{,}000 \text{ mm Hg} \\
\hline
\text{Osmotic pressure} & \phantom{1{,}0}73{,}000 \text{ mm Hg}
\end{array}$$

    4. Osmotic pressure is a force *drawing* water into the solution.
    5. Osmosis can be stopped by exerting a force on a solution equal to the osmotic pressure of the solution.

XII. Hydrostatic Pressure
    A. Hydrostatic pressure is the amount of force exerted by the weight of a column of water (cm H_2O).

XIII. Expressions of H^+ Ion Concentration
    A. pH: Negative log of the H^+ concentration per liter of solution, [ ] is used to symbolize molar concentration.

        1. $pH = -\log_{10} [H^+]$ or $\log_{10} \dfrac{1}{[H^+]}$
        2. pH of 7.0: Neutral
        3. pH greater than 7.0: Basic or alkalotic
        4. pH less than 7.0: Acidic or acidotic
        5. pH scale: 1 to 14, equivalent to an $[H^+]$ of 10^{-1} to 10^{-14} moles/L

    B. Nanomoles per liter (nmoles/L): H^+ concentration in number of billionths of moles of H^+ per liter.

1. The $[H^+]$ is expressed as a number multiplied by 10^{-9}.
2. A pH of 7.0 = 3.98×10^{-8} moles/L, or 39.8×10^{-9} moles/L, or 39.8 nmoles/L.
3. Nanomole expressions normally are used for $[H^+]$ in the physiologic range.
   a. pH of 6.90 = 126 nmoles/L
   b. pH of 7.70 = 20.1 nmoles/L

XIV. Acids and Bases
   A. Acid: A compound that donates H^+ ions when placed into solution.
      1. The active compound responsible for the properties of acids is the hydronium ion (H_3O^+).
      2. In solution the liberated H^+ reacts with H_2O to form the H_3O^+ ion:

$$H^+ + H_2O \rightarrow H_3O^+$$

   B. Base: A compound that accepts H^+ ions when placed into solution. The active compound responsible for the properties of most bases is the OH^- (hydroxyl ion).
   C. Neutralization reaction: The reaction between an acid and a base, where the results are a salt plus water:

$$NaOH + HCl \rightarrow NaCl + H_2O$$

XV. Oxidation and Reduction
   A. Oxidation: Process in a chemical reaction whereby a substance loses electrons.
   B. Reduction: Process in a chemical reaction whereby a substance gains electrons.

XVI. Metric System
   A. Length
      1. The basic unit of length is the meter (m). One meter is equal to 39.37 inches (in.).
      2. One meter is equal to all of the following, and they are thus equal to each other:
         a. 100 centimeters (10^2 cm)
         b. 1,000 millimeters (10^3 mm)
         c. 1,000,000 microns (10^6 μ)
         d. 10,000,000,000 angstroms (10^{10} Å)
      3. Basic factors used in converting from the metric to the British system or British to the metric system:
         a. 1 m = 39.37 in.
         b. 1 in. = 2.54 cm

Problems:
1. How many angstroms are equal to 2.2×10^2 cm?

$$1 \text{ m} = 10^2 \text{ cm}$$
$$\frac{1 \text{ m}}{10^2 \text{ cm}} = \frac{x}{2.2 \times 10^2 \text{ cm}}$$
$$x = 2.2 \text{ m}$$
$$1 \text{ m} = 10^{10} \text{ Å}$$
$$\frac{1 \text{ m}}{10^{10} \text{ Å}} = \frac{2.2 \text{ m}}{x}$$
$$x = 2.2 \times 10^{10} \text{ Å}$$

2. How many inches are equal to 5.3×10^6 mm

$$1 \text{ cm} = 2.54 \text{ cm}$$
$$10^3 \text{ mm} = 10^2 \text{ cm}$$
$$\frac{10^3 \text{ mm}}{10^2 \text{ cm}} = \frac{5.3 \times 10^6 \text{ mm}}{x}$$
$$x = 5.3 \times 10^5 \text{ cm}$$
$$\frac{1 \text{ in.}}{2.54 \text{ cm}} = \frac{x}{5.3 \times 10^5 \text{ cm}}$$
$$x = 2.09 \text{ in.}$$

B. Weight
   1. The basic unit of weight in the metric system is the kilogram (kg). One kilogram is equal to 2.2 pounds (lb).
   2. One kilogram is equal to all of the following, and they are thus equal to each other:
      a. 1,000 gm (10^3 gm)
      b. 1,000,000 mg (10^6 mg)
   3. Basic factors used in converting from metric to British system or from British to metric system:
      a. 1 kg = 2.2 lb
      b. 1 lb = 454 gm

Problems:
   1. How many milligrams are there in 1.5×10^2 kg?

$$1 \text{ kg} = 10^6 \text{ mg}$$
$$\frac{10^6 \text{ mg}}{1 \text{ kg}} = \frac{x}{1.5 \times 10^2 \text{ kg}}$$
$$x = 1.5 \times 10^8 \text{ mg}$$

   2. How many grams are equal to 0.6 lb?

$$1 \text{ kg} = 2.2 \text{ lb}$$
$$1 \text{ kg} = 10^3 \text{ gm, therefore}$$
$$10^3 \text{ gm} = 2.2 \text{ lb}$$
$$\frac{10^3 \text{ gm}}{2.2 \text{ lb}} = \frac{x}{0.61 \text{ lb}}$$
$$x = 277.2 \text{ gm}$$

C. Volume
   1. The basic unit of volume in the metric system is the liter, which is equal to 1.057 quarts (qt).
   2. One liter is equal to 1,000 ml (10^3 ml) and also to 1,000 cc (10^3 cc).
      a. The volume of 1 cc is 1 ml.
      b. 1 ml of water weighs 1 gm.
   3. One cubic meter contains 10^3 L.
   4. Basic factors used in converting from the metric to British system or from British to metric system:
      a. 1 L = 1.057 qt
      b. 1 cu ft = 28.3 L

Problems:
   1. How many liters are equal to 2.5×10^9 ml?

$$1 \text{ L} = 10^3 \text{ ml}$$
$$\frac{1 \text{ L}}{10^3 \text{ ml}} = \frac{x}{2.5 \times 10^9 \text{ ml}}$$
$$x = 2.5 \times 10^6 \text{ ml}$$

2. How many cubic feet are equal to 3.5×10^6 L?

$$1 \text{ cu ft} = 28.3 \text{ L}$$
$$\frac{1 \text{ cu ft}}{28.3 \text{ L}} = \frac{x}{3.5 \times 10^6 \text{ L}}$$
$$x = 1.3 \times 10^5 \text{ L}$$

BIBLIOGRAPHY

Beckenback EF, Drooyar I, Wooton W: *College Algebra*, ed 4, Belmont, Calif, Wadsworth Publishing Co, 1966.
Brooks SM: *Integrated Basic Sciences*, ed 4. St Louis, CV Mosby Co, 1979.
Deshpande VM, Pilbeam SP, Dixon RJ: *A Comprehensive Review of Respiratory Care*. Norwalk, Conn, Appleton & Lange, 1988.
Epstein LI, Kuzava BA: *Basic Physics in Anesthesiology: A Programmed Approach*. Chicago, Year Book Medical Publishers, 1976.
Johnson RH, Grunwald E: *Atoms, Molecules, and Chemical Change*, ed 2. Englewood Cliffs, NJ, Prentice-Hall, 1965.
Masterton WL, Slowinski E: *Chemical Principles*, ed 4. Philadelphia, WB Saunders Co, 1977.
Sackheim GI: *Chemical Calculations, Series B*, ed 8. Champaign, Ill, Stipes Publishing Co, 1962.
Sackheim GI, Schultz RM: *Chemistry for the Health Sciences*, ed 2. New York, Macmillan Publishing Co, 1973.
Shapiro BA, Harrison RA, Cane R, et al: *Clinical Application of Blood Gases*, ed 4. Chicago, Year Book Medical Publishers, 1989.
Spearman CB, Sheldon RL, Egan DF: *Egan's Fundamentals of Respiratory Therapy*, ed 4. St Louis, CV Mosby Co, 1982.
Young JA, Crocker D: *Principles and Practice of Respiratory Therapy*, ed 2. Chicago, Year Book Medical Publishers, 1976.
Wojciechowski WV: *Respiratory Care Sciences: An Integrated Approach*. New York, John Wiley & Sons, 1985.

Chapter 2

General Principles of Gas Physics

I. Basic Units and Relationships
 A. Mass: The property of matter defined as its ability to occupy space, and if in motion to stay in motion, and if at rest to stay at rest.
 B. Weight: A method of quantifying the mass of an object. The effect of gravitational attraction on the object.
 C. Velocity: The speed with which movement between two points occurs. Expressed in miles per hour or centimeters per second.
 D. Acceleration: The rate at which the velocity of an object increases. The units of acceleration are cm/sec^2 or miles/hour^2.
 E. Work is equal to the product of force and distance:

$$\text{Work} = \text{Force} \times \text{Distance} \tag{1}$$

  1. Force is defined as mass $\times$ acceleration. The units of force are:
   a. Dyne = gm $\cdot$ cm/sec
   b. Newton = kg $\cdot$ m/sec
  2. Work is not performed unless the applied force causes movement.
  3. The units of work are:
   a. ERG = dyne-centimeter
   b. Joule = Newton-meter
  4. When related to the respiratory system:
   a. Pressure replaces force
   b. Volume replaces distance
   c. Thus work can be expressed as (refer to Chapter 4 for details):

$$\text{Work} = \text{Pressure} \times \text{Volume} \tag{2}$$

   d. Respiratory work is normally expressed as (m = meter):
    (1) kg $\cdot$ m/L
    (2) joules/L (1 kg $\cdot$ m/L = 10 joules/L)
    (3) kg $\cdot$ m/min
    (4) joules/min
 F. Energy is defined as the ability to do work.
  1. Potential and kinetic energy are the two types of mechanical energy.
  2. Potential energy is the energy of position.

3. Potential energy (PE) is equal to:

$$PE = M \times g \times h \tag{3}$$

where M = mass, g = gravitational attraction of the earth, and h = height.
4. Mass times gravitational attraction is frequently represented as weight (W):

$$PE = W \times h \tag{4}$$

5. Kinetic energy is the energy of motion.
6. Kinetic energy (KE) is equal to:

$$KE = 0.5 \, MV^2 \tag{5}$$

where M = mass and V = velocity.
7. Kinetic energy of gases is normally expressed as:

$$KE = 0.5 \, DV^2 \tag{6}$$

where D = density.
G. Pressure is the force applied per unit area. The units of pressure are:
   1. Pounds per square inch (lb/in.^{2}, or PSI)
   2. Grams per square centimeter (gm/cm^2)
II. States of Matter
   A. All matter exists in one of three basic states:
      1. Solid
      2. Liquid
      3. Gas
   B. The state of a substance is determined by the relationship of two forces.
      1. Kinetic energy of the molecules.
      2. Intermolecular attractive forces among the molecules.
   C. The kinetic energy of a substance is directly related to temperature.
      1. The greater the kinetic energy of a substance, the greater its tendency to exist as a liquid or gas.
      2. Molecules of every substance are in constant motion as a result of kinetic energy.
      3. At absolute zero, the kinetic activity of a substance is theoretically zero.
   D. Intermolecular attractive forces oppose the kinetic energy of molecules and tend to force them to exist in less free (solid or liquid) states. Basically there are three types of intermolecular attractive forces: dipole, hydrogen bonding, and dispersion.
      1. Dipole forces: Forces that exist between molecules that have electrostatic polarity; the negative aspect of one molecule is lined up and attracted to the positive aspect of another molecule, as seen with NaCl. These substances frequently form crystals.
      2. Hydrogen bonding: A force that exists between molecules formed by hydrogen reacting with fluorine, oxygen, or nitrogen.
         a. As a result of the electronegative difference between hydrogen and fluorine, oxygen or nitrogen, the hydrogen atom in the molecule appears as a pure proton.
         b. The hydrogen of one molecule is thus attracted to the negative aspect of another molecule of the substance.

      c. Hydrogen bonding occurs only with compounds of fluorine, oxygen, and nitrogen because of their:
         (1) Strong electronegativity
         (2) Small atomic diameter

   3. Dispersion forces (London or van der Waals forces): Forces between molecules of relatively nonpolar substances.
      a. In nonpolar substances the electron cloud normally is distributed equally among all of the atoms in the molecule.
      b. However, at some point in time the electron cloud may be instantaneously concentrated at one end of the molecule. When this occurs, a polarity is set up on the molecule.
      c. This instantaneous polarity allows attraction between adjacent molecules.
      d. Dispersion forces are the weakest of all intermolecular forces.

E. Units of heat
   1. Calorie: Unit of heat in metric system. Essentially it is the amount of heat necessary to cause a 1°C increase in the temperature of 1 gm of water.
   2. British thermal unit (BTU): Unit of heat in the British system. Essentially it is the amount of heat necessary to cause a 1°F increase in the temperature of 1 lb of water.
   3. One BTU is equal to 252 calories of heat.
   4. Heat capacity: Number of calories needed to raise the temperature of 1 gm of a substance 1°C.
   5. Specific heat: Ratio of heat capacity of a substance compared to heat capacity of water.

F. Change of state
   1. A specific amount of heat is needed to cause the molecules of a substance to change their state.
   2. Latent heat of fusion is the amount of heat necessary to change 1 gm of a substance at its melting point from a solid to a liquid without causing a change in temperature.
      a. The melting point is the temperature (at 1 atm of pressure) at which a substance changes from a solid to a liquid.
      b. The total volume of a substance must change from a solid to a liquid before its temperature changes.
      c. Latent heats of fusion and melting points for various substances:

Substance	Heat of Fusion (Calories/gm)	Melting Point (C)
Water	80	0
Hydrogen	13.8	−259.25
Carbon dioxide	43.2	−57.6
Nitrogen	6.15	−210
Oxygen	3.3	−218.8

   3. The latent heat of vaporization is the amount of heat necessary to change 1 gm of a substance at its boiling point from a liquid to a gas without causing a change in temperature.
      a. Boiling point is the temperature at 1 atm of pressure at which a substance changes from a liquid to a gas.
      b. The total volume of a substance must change from a liquid to a gas before its temperature changes.

(1) For a substance to boil, its vapor pressure must equal the pressure of the atmosphere above it.

(2) Evaporation is a surface phenomenon whereby individual molecules of a substance gain enough heat to change their state. Boiling, on the other hand, occurs throughout the entire volume of the substance.

c. Latent heats of vaporization and boiling points for various substances:

Substance	Heat of Vaporization (Calories/gm)	Boiling Point (C)
Water	540	100
Hydrogen	40	−252.5
Carbon dioxide	83	−78.5
Nitrogen	. . .	−196
Oxygen	50	−183

G. Effects of pressure on melting and boiling points

1. In general, the greater the pressure over a substance, the higher the temperature necessary to cause the substance to change its state. Pressure has a greater effect on the boiling point of a substance than on its melting point.

2. Critical temperature: The highest temperature at which a substance can exist as a liquid, regardless of the amount of pressure applied to it (O_2 = −118.8°C).

3. Critical pressure: The lowest pressure necessary at the critical temperature of a substance to maintain it in its liquid state (O_2 = 49.7 atm pressure).

4. Critical point: Combination of critical temperature and critical pressure of a substance.

H. Triple point: Specific combination of temperature and pressure in which a substance can exist in all three states of matter in dynamic equilibrium.

I. Sublimation: Transition of a substance from a solid directly to a gas without existence in a liquid state. The heat of sublimation equals the heat of fusion plus the heat of vaporization.

III. Kinetic Theory of Gases

A. The kinetic theory normally is applied to relatively dilute gas volumes. ·

B. Principles of kinetic theory

1. Gases are composed of molecules that are in rapid continuous random motion.

2. The molecules undergo near collisions with each other and collide with the walls of their container.

3. All molecular collisions are elastic, and as long as the container is properly insulated, the temperature of the gas remains constant.

4. The kinetic energy of molecules of a gas is directly proportional to the absolute temperature.

   a. An increase in temperature causes an increase in kinetic energy of the gas.

   b. The increased kinetic energy causes an increase in the velocity of the gas molecules.

   c. The increased velocity causes an increase in the frequency of collisions.

   d. The increased frequency of collisions causes an increase in the pressure in the system.

   e. With an increase in temperature, the degree of increase in the velocity of gas molecules is indirectly related to their molecular weight (MW).

IV. Avogadro's Law
   A. One gram molecular weight (GMW), 1 gm atomic weight, 1 gm ionic weight, etc., of a substance contains 6.02×10^{23} particles of that substance.
   B. The above mass of any substance is referred to as a mole.
   C. One mole of a gas at 0°C and 760 mm Hg (standard temperature and pressure; STP) occupies a volume of about 22.4 L. (There is a small percent variation in this number for individual gases, e.g., CO_2 = 22.3 L.)
   D. An equal number or fractions of moles of different gases at a specific temperature and pressure occupy the same volume and contain the same number of particles.
V. Density
   A. Density (D) is the mass of an object per unit volume and usually is expressed as grams per liter:

$$D = \frac{M}{V} \tag{7}$$

   B. On the surface of the earth, mass in equation 7 may be replaced by weight.
   C. Calculation of densities of solids and liquids is straightforward since their volumes are relatively stable at various temperatures and pressures.
   D. The volumes of gases, on the other hand, are severely affected by temperature and pressure.
   E. For this reason, the standard density of all gases is determined at STP conditions where the volume used is 22.4 L and the weight used is the GMW of the particular gas:

$$\text{Density of gas} = \frac{GMW}{22.4\ L} = x\ gm/L \tag{8}$$

$$\text{Density of oxygen} = \frac{32\ gm\ (GMW)}{22.4\ L} = 1.43\ gm/L$$

   F. Standard densities of various substances:
      1. Oxygen: 1.43 gm/L
      2. Nitrogen: 1.25 gm/L
      3. Carbon dioxide: 1.965 gm/L
   G. The density of a mixture of gases is determined by the following equation:

$$D = \frac{(\%_A)(GMW_A) + (\%_B)(GMW_B) + (\%_C)(GMW_C)}{22.4\ L} \tag{9}$$

   Example: The density of a gas containing 40% oxygen, 55% nitrogen, and 5% carbon dioxide would be computed as follows:

$$D = \frac{(0.4)(32) + (0.55)(28) + (0.05)(44)gm}{22.4\ L}$$

$$D = \frac{(12.8) + (15.4) + (2.2)gm}{22.4\ L}$$

$$D = \frac{30.4\ gm}{22.4\ L}$$

$$D = 1.36\ gm/L$$

   H. Specific gravity: Ratio of the density of a substance to the density of a standard. The specific gravity of solids and liquids is determined using water as the standard; for gases, oxygen is used as the standard. Specific gravity is expressed purely as a ratio.

VI. Gas Pressure
   A. Pressure (P) in any sense is equal to force per unit area:

   $$P = \frac{gm}{sq\ cm}; \quad P = \frac{lb}{sq\ in.} \tag{10}$$

   B. The pressure of a gas is directly related to the kinetic energy of the gas (see section II) and to the gravitational attraction of the earth.
   C. With an increase in altitude, the gravitational attraction of the earth on molecules of gas in the atmosphere decreases.
      1. This causes a decrease in density of the atmospheric gases.
      2. Decreased density results in fewer molecular collisions.
      3. Thus, with increasing altitude there is a nonlinear decrease in the pressure of the total atmosphere and of individual gases.
      4. Even though there is a steady decrease in the pressure of the atmosphere with altitude, the concentration of gases in the atmosphere remains stable to an elevation of about 50 miles.
      5. Concentration of atmospheric gases:
         a. Oxygen: 20.95%
         b. Nitrogen: 78.08%
         c. Argon: 0.93%
         d. Carbon dioxide: 0.03%
         e. Trace elements: 0.01%
   D. The barometric pressure (P_B) of the atmosphere is equal to the height of a column of fluid times the fluid's density:

   $$P_B = (height\ of\ column\ of\ fluid)(fluid's\ density) \tag{11}$$

   If the fluid used is mercury (psi = pounds per square inch):

   $$14.7\ psi = (29.9\ in.\ Hg)(0.491\ lb/cu\ in.)$$

   E. Mercury's density in the metric system is 13.6 gm/cc; in the British system it is 0.491 lb/cu in.
   F. Gas pressure is frequently expressed as the height of a substance, that is, mm Hg, cm H_2O. These are not true pressure expressions, but they may be easily converted to the proper pressure notation by use of equation 10 if necessary.
   G. Atmospheric pressure normally is determined by a mercury or an aneroid barometer.
   H. Equivalent expressions of normal atmospheric pressure:
      1. 14.7 psi
      2. 760 mm Hg
      3. 1,034 gm/sq cm
      4. 33 ft of salt H_2O
      5. 33.9 ft of fresh H_2O
      6. 29.9 in. Hg
      7. 76 cm Hg
      8. 1,034 cm H_2O
VII. Humidity
   A. Water vapor content of the air under atmospheric conditions is variable. Temperature is the factor that most significantly affects water vapor content in the atmosphere.
   B. At a particular temperature, there is a maximum amount of water that a gas can hold.

C. Since the boiling point of water (100°C) is considerably higher than the normal temperature of the atmosphere, the maximum water vapor content of the atmosphere varies with temperature.
   1. As the temperature increases, the rate of evaporation of water accelerates, and the capacity of the atmosphere to hold water increases.
   2. All other standard gases in the atmosphere have boiling points much lower than atmospheric temperature. This causes stability in their concentrations.
   3. Water is the only standard atmospheric gas that responds to temperature changes in this manner.
D. Expressions of water vapor content
   1. Partial pressure of water vapor (P_{H_2O}), maximum P_{H_2O} at 37°C, is equal to 47 mm Hg.
   2. Maximum water vapor pressure at different temperatures:

Temperature (C)	P_{H_2O} (mm Hg)	Temperature (C)	P_{H_2O} (mm Hg)
20	17.5	29	30.0
21	18.7	30	31.8
22	19.8	31	33.7
23	21.1	32	35.7
24	22.4	33	37.7
25	23.8	34	39.9
26	25.2	35	42.2
27	26.7	36	44.6
28	28.3	37	47.0

   3. Absolute humidity is defined as the actual weight of water vapor contained in a given volume of gas.
      a. Absolute humidity may be expressed as grams per cubic meter or milligrams per liter.
      b. The maximum absolute humidity at 37°C is 43.8 gm/cu m, or 43.8 mg/L.
   4. Relative humidity (RH) is defined as a relationship between the actual weight or pressure (content) of water in air at a specific temperature and the maximum weight or pressure (capacity) of water that air can hold at that specific temperature. Relative humidity is expressed as a percentage.
      a. Expressions of actual and maximum amounts of water:
         (1) mm Hg
         (2) gm/cu m
         (3) mg/L
      b. Formula for calculating relative humidity:

$$RH = \frac{Content}{Capacity} \times 100 \tag{12}$$

Example: At 37°C, if the actual water vapor pressure is 20 mm Hg, what is the relative humidity?

$$RH = \frac{20 \text{ mm Hg}}{47 \text{ mm Hg}} \times 100 = 43\%$$

      c. If water content is kept constant and temperature is increased, relative humidity decreases because capacity of air for water increases. As temperature decreases, the opposite effect is seen.

VIII. Dalton's Law of Partial Pressure
    A. Dalton's law states that the sum of the individual partial pressures of the gases in a mixture is equal to the total barometric pressure of the system.
    B. The partial pressure (PP) of a gas is equal to the barometric pressure (PB) times the concentration of gas in the mixture:

$$(P_P) = (P_B)(Conc.) \tag{13}$$

    Example: If the P_B is 760 mm Hg and the concentration of O_2 is 21%, what is the P_{O_2}?

$$P_{O_2} = (760)(0.21) = 159.6 \text{ mm Hg}$$

    C. The concentration of a gas is equal to the partial pressure of the gas divided by the barometric pressure:

$$Conc. = \frac{P_P}{P_B} \times 100 \tag{14}$$

    Example: If the P_B is 750 mm Hg and the P_{O_2} is 200 mm Hg, what is the concentration of O_2?

$$O_2 \text{ conc.} = \frac{200 \text{ mm Hg}}{750 \text{ mm Hg}} \times 100 = 26.7\%$$

IX. Effect of Humidity on Dalton's Law
    A. Water vapor pressure does not follow Dalton's law because under normal atmospheric conditions, P_{H_2O} is dependent primarily on temperature.
    B. When the partial pressure of a gas is calculated where water vapor is present, the total barometric pressure of the system must be corrected before the partial pressure of any other gas can be calculated.
    C. Following is a modification of Dalton's law to account for the presence of water vapor:

$$(P_P) = (P_B - P_{H_2O})(Conc.) \tag{15}$$

    Example: If P_B is 770 mm Hg, P_{H_2O} is 30 mm Hg, and the concentration of O_2 is 50%, what is the P_{O_2}?

$$P_{O_2} = (770 \text{ mm Hg} - 30 \text{ mm Hg})(0.50)$$
$$P_{O_2} = 370 \text{ mm Hg}$$

    D. When the temperature is 37°C with barometric pressure at 760 mm Hg, the gas saturated with water vapor, and the oxygen concentration 21%, the P_{O_2} is 149.7 mm Hg:

$$P_{O_2} = (760 \text{ mm Hg} - 47 \text{ mm Hg})(0.21) = 149.7 \text{ mm Hg}$$

X. Ideal Gas Laws
    A. The ideal gas laws apply to dilute gases at temperatures above the gases' boiling point.
    B. The closer the temperature to the boiling point of a gas, the greater the error involved in using the gas laws.

C. The *ideal gas law* demonstrates the interrelationships among volume, pressure, temperature, and amount of gas.
  1. According to the ideal gas law, multiplying the pressure of the system by the volume of the system and dividing this by the product of the temperature (absolute) and amount of gas in any gas system yields a constant. This is referred to as *Boltzmann's constant,* which is a constant that can be applied to all gas systems.
  2. The ideal gas law is normally expressed as

$$PV = nRT \qquad (16)$$

or

$$R = \frac{PV}{nT}$$

  where P = pressure, V = volume, and n = amount of gas (expressed normally in moles), R = Boltzmann's constant, and T = temperature (expressed in degrees Kelvin).
  3. Boltzmann's constant is equal to:
    a. 82.1 ml · atm/mole · degree K when pressure is expressed in atmospheres and volume in milliliters.
    b. 62.3 L · mm Hg/mole · degree K when pressure is expressed in millimeters of mercury and volume in liters.
D. *Boyle's law* states that pressure and volume of a gas system vary inversely if the temperature and amount of gas in the system are constant.
  1. Boyle's law mathematically is

$$PV = nRT \qquad (17)$$

where nRT is equal to a constant, thus

$$PV = K \qquad (18)$$

  2. In a system where temperature and amount of gas are constant, the original pressure and volume equal the final pressure and volume:

$$P_1V_1 = P_2V_2 \qquad (19)$$

Problem:
  If a patient's exhaled volume (dry) at a barometric pressure of 760 mm Hg is 300 ml, what is the exhaled volume (dry) during air transport if the atmospheric pressure during transport is 500 mm Hg?

$$P_1 = 760 \text{ mm Hg} \qquad P_2 = 500 \text{ mm Hg}$$
$$V_1 = 300 \text{ ml} \qquad V_2 = x$$

$$P_1V_1 = P_2V_2$$
$$(760 \text{ mm Hg}) \ (300 \text{ ml}) = (500 \text{ mm Hg}) \ (x)$$

$$x = 456 \text{ ml}$$

E. *Charles' law* states that the temperature and volume of a gas system vary directly if the pressure and amount of gas in the system are constant.
   1. Charles' law mathematically is

$$\frac{V}{T} = \frac{nR}{P} \tag{20}$$

where nR/P is equal to a constant, thus

$$\frac{V}{T} = K \tag{21}$$

   2. In a system where the pressure and amount of gas are constant, the original temperature and volume equal the final temperature and volume:

$$\frac{V_1}{T_1} = \frac{V_2}{T_2} \tag{22}$$

Problem:
   A patient's exhaled volume measured at 20°C is 2.5 L. What is his actual exhaled volume at body temperature?

$$V_1 = 2.5 \text{ L} \qquad V_2 = x$$
$$T_1 = 20°C + 273° \qquad T_2 = 37°C + 273°$$
$$T_1 = 293°K \qquad T_2 = 310°K$$

$$\frac{V_1}{T_1} = \frac{V_2}{T_2}$$
$$\frac{2.5 \text{ L}}{293°K} = \frac{x}{310°K}$$
$$x = 2.65 \text{ L}$$

F. *Gay-Lussac's law* states that the pressure and temperature of a gas system vary directly if the volume and amount of gas in the system are constant.
   1. Gay-Lussac's law mathematically is

$$\frac{P}{T} = \frac{nR}{V} \tag{23}$$

where $\dfrac{nR}{V}$ is equal to a constant, thus

$$\frac{P}{T} = K \tag{24}$$

   2. In a system where the volume and amount of gas are constant, the original pressure and temperature equal the final pressure and temperature:

$$\frac{P_1}{T_1} = \frac{P_2}{T_2} \tag{25}$$

Problem:

An arterial blood gas analyzed at 37°C reveals a Po_2 of 100 mm Hg. What is the patient's actual Po_2 if his body temperature is 34°C?

$$P_1 = 100 \text{ mm Hg} \qquad P_2 = x$$
$$T_1 = 37°C + 273° \qquad T_2 = 34°C + 273°$$
$$T_1 = 310°K \qquad T_2 = 307°K$$

$$\frac{P_1}{T_1} = \frac{P_2}{T_2}$$
$$\frac{100 \text{ mm Hg}}{310°K} = \frac{x}{307°K}$$
$$x = 99.03 \text{ mm Hg}$$

G. The *combined gas law* states that pressure, temperature, and volume of gas are specifically related if the amount of gas remains constant.
   1. The combined gas law mathematically is

$$\frac{PV}{T} = nR \tag{26}$$

where nR is equal to a constant, thus

$$\frac{PV}{T} = K \tag{27}$$

   2. In a system where the amount of gas in a system is constant, the original pressure, temperature, and volume are equal to the final pressure, temperature, and volume:

$$\frac{P_1V_1}{T_1} = \frac{P_2V_2}{T_2} \tag{28}$$

Problem:

If the original pressure of system is 700 mm Hg, temperature 30°C, and volume 100 L, what will the final volume be if the pressure is increased to 750 mm Hg and temperature to 37°C?

$$P_1 = 700 \text{ mm Hg} \qquad P_2 = 750 \text{ mm Hg}$$
$$V_1 = 100 \text{ L} \qquad V_2 = x$$
$$T_1 = 30°C + 273 \qquad T_2 = 37°C + 273$$
$$T_1 = 303°K \qquad T_2 = 310°K$$

$$\frac{P_1V_1}{T_1} = \frac{P_2V_2}{T_2}$$
$$\frac{(700 \text{ mm Hg})(100 \text{ L})}{303°K} = \frac{(750 \text{ mm Hg})(x)}{310°K}$$
$$x = 95 \text{ L}$$

H. All gas law calculations must use temperature on the Kelvin scale for accurate results.

I. Water vapor does not react as an ideal gas; therefore, in a system where water vapor is present, water vapor pressure must be subtracted from total pressure before calculations are made.

J. When precision is needed, the barometric pressure reading should be corrected for expansion of mercury as affected by temperature.

XI. Diffusion

A. Diffusion is movement of gas from an area of high concentration of a gas to an area of low concentration.

B. As diffusion occurs, gases occupy the total container volume as if they were the only gas present; in other words, a gas in a container distributes itself *with time* equally throughout the whole container.

C. The rate of diffusion of a gas through another gas is affected by the following factors:

1. The concentration gradient, which is directly related to the rate of diffusion.

2. The temperature, which is directly related to the rate of diffusion.

3. The cross-sectional area available for diffusion, which is directly related to the rate of diffusion.

4. The MW, which is indirectly related to the rate of diffusion.

5. The distance the gas has to diffuse, which is indirectly related to the rate of diffusion:

$$\frac{\text{Rate of diffusion of}}{\text{a gas through a gas}} = \frac{(\text{Press.})(\text{Temp.})(\text{Cross-sectional area})}{(\text{MW})(\text{Distance})} \tag{29}$$

D. *Henry's law* states that the amount of a gas that can dissolve in a liquid is directly related to the partial pressure of the gas over the liquid and indirectly related to the temperature of the system.

1. Henry's law expresses the solubility coefficients of gases in liquids.

2. Solubility coefficients of oxygen and carbon dioxide in plasma at 37°C:

a. 0.023 ml of O_2/ml of blood/760 mm Hg P_{O_2}

b. 0.510 ml of CO_2/ml of blood/760 mm Hg P_{CO_2}

E. *Graham's law* states that the rate of diffusion of a gas through a liquid is indirectly related to the square root of the GMW of the gas.

F. If Henry's and Graham's laws are combined, the rates of diffusion of carbon dioxide to oxygen can be compared under conditions of equal pressure gradients, distances, cross-sectional areas, and temperatures.

1. When the above variables are equal, the only factors affecting the comparison would be the GMWs of the gases and their solubility coefficients.

2. The comparison may be mathematically represented as follows:
Rate of diffusion of

$$\frac{CO_2}{O_2} = \frac{(\text{sol. coef. } CO_2)(\sqrt{\text{GMW } O_2})}{(\text{sol. coef. } O_2)(\sqrt{\text{GMW } CO_2})} \tag{30}$$
$$= \frac{(0.510)(5.66)}{(0.023)(6.66)}$$
$$\approx \frac{19}{1}$$

3. Thus, under the previously mentioned conditions, carbon dioxide would diffuse about 19 times faster than oxygen.

    4. However, *at the alveolar capillary membrane, pressure gradients for oxygen and carbon dioxide are not equal.*
       a. Diffusion gradient for oxygen is 60 mm Hg.
       b. Diffusion gradient for carbon dioxide is 6 mm Hg.
       c. As a result of these pressure gradients, oxygen equilibrates across the alveolar-capillary membrane slightly faster than carbon dioxide.
       d. Oxygen equilibrates in about 0.23 second, whereas carbon dioxide equilibrates in about 0.25 second.

XII. Elastance and Compliance
  A. Elastance (E) is the ability of a distorted object to return to its original shape.
  B. Compliance (C) is the ease with which an object can be distorted.
  C. Compliance and elastance are inversely related:

$$C = \frac{1}{E} \tag{31}$$

  D. If the compliance of a system increases, the elastance of the system decreases.
  E. If the compliance of a system decreases, the elastance of the system increases.
  F. *Hook's law* defines the response of elastic bodies to distorting forces.
    1. It states that an elastic body stretches equal units of length or volume for each unit of weight or force applied to it.
    2. This relationship holds until the elastic limit of the system is reached.
    3. Beyond the elastic limit, each unit of weight or force produces smaller and smaller changes in length or volume.
    4. With a true spring, exceeding the elastic limit results in permanent distortion.
  G. Elastance can be mathematically defined as

$$E = \frac{\Delta P}{\Delta V} \tag{32}$$

    where ΔP = change in pressure and ΔV = change in volume.
  H. Compliance can be mathematically defined as

$$C = \frac{\Delta V}{\Delta P} \tag{33}$$

XIII. Surface Tension
  A. Surface tension is a force that exists at the interface between a liquid and a gas or between two liquids.
  B. The surface tension of a liquid is the result of like molecules being attracted to each other and thus moving away from the interface. This causes the liquid to occupy the smallest volume possible (Figs 2–1 and 2–2).
  C. As a result of surface tension, a force is necessary to cause a tear in the surface of the liquid.
  D. The surface tension of a liquid is expressed in dynes per linear centimeter.
  E. Surface tension is indirectly related to temperature.
  F. *LaPlace's law* is used to determine the amount of pressure generated inside a system as a result of surface tension.
    1. The law states that the pressure (P) in dynes per square centimeter as a result

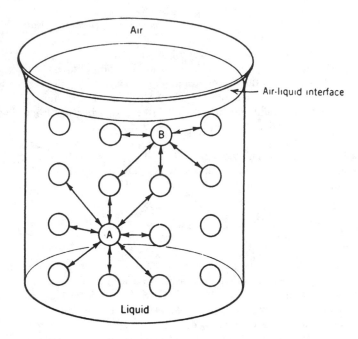

FIG 2–1.
Effect of attraction of like molecules in a beaker, resulting in the development of a surface tension at the interface of air and liquid. Molecule *A* is attracted to all molecules equally; however, molecule *B* is attracted only inward and across the top of the liquid. As a result, a barrier is created at the interface (surface tension). (From Wojciechowski WV: *Respiratory Care Sciences: An Integrated Approach.* New York. John Wiley & Sons, 1985. Used by permission.)

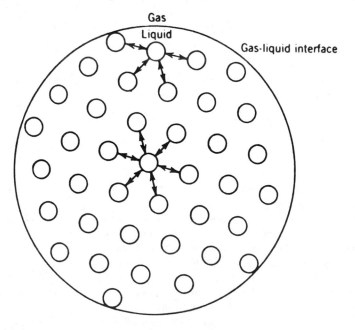

FIG 2–2.
Effect of attraction of like molecules in a drop. Molecules at the surface are attracted inward and across the surface of the liquid, establishing a gas-liquid interphase and creating a barrier at the surface (surface tension). (From Wojciechowski WV: *Respiratory Care Sciences: An Integrated Approach.* New York. John Wiley & Sons, 1985. Used by permission.)

of surface tension (ST) in dynes per centimeter is equal to the surface tension of the liquid multiplied by 1 over the radii (r) of curvature in centimeters:

$$P = ST\left(\frac{1}{r_1} + \frac{1}{r_2} + \frac{1}{r_3} + \dots \frac{1}{r_n}\right) \qquad (34)$$

    2. LaPlace's law as applied to a drop is

$$P = \frac{2\ ST}{r} \qquad (35)$$

Here reference is made to a perfect sphere that has only two radii of curvature, one in the vertical plane and one in the horizontal plane.

    3. LaPlace's law as applied to a bubble is

$$P = \frac{4\ ST}{r} \qquad (36)$$

There are two interfaces in a bubble, one on the inside of the bubble and one on the outside; thus, there is a total of four radii. All are considered equal because the film of the bubble is only angstroms in diameter.

    4. LaPlace's law as applied to a blood vessel is

$$P = \frac{ST}{r} \qquad (37)$$

When the radii of curvature of a blood vessel are considered, the only radius used in the calculation is that of the vessel's width, because the radius of length is so great. When the inverse of the radii of length is calculated, the number essentially goes to infinity and is meaningless in calculating the pressure as a result of surface tension.

    5. It is important to remember that the pressure as a result of surface tension is indirectly related to the radius. *The smaller the sphere, the greater the pressure as a result of surface tension* (Fig 2–3).

  G. *Critical volume* is a volume below which the effects of surface tension are so great that the structure collapses. Once the critical volume is reached, collapse is always imminent.

  H. The force necessary to inflate a deflated object increases significantly as the critical volume is reached but rapidly decreases once the critical volume is exceeded (Fig 2–4).

  I. The surface tension of a fluid is reduced by chemicals referred to as *surfactants*. Surfactants are surface-active agents that interfere with the molecules of the fluid at the surface, causing a reduction in the force (ST) that draws the fluid centrally. Soaps and detergents are common surfactants.

XIV. Fluid Dynamics

  A. Law of continuity

    1. The product of the cross-sectional area of a system times the velocity for a given flow rate is constant.

    2. Thus, if the flow of gas is constant, the cross-sectional area and gas velocity are inversely related.

    3. In any system with varying radii, the velocity of gas movement must change as the radius changes.

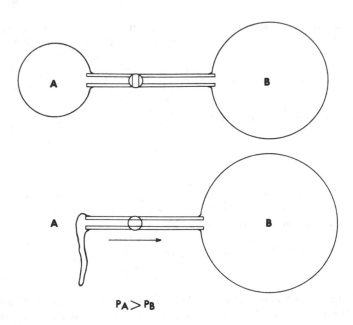

$$P_A > P_B$$

FIG 2–3.
When two bubbles of different sizes *(A and B)* but with the same surface tension are allowed to communicate, the greater pressure as a result of surface tension in the smaller bubble causes it to empty into the larger. (From Spearman CB, Sheldon RL, Egan DF: *Egan's Fundamentals of Respiratory Therapy,* ed 4. St Louis, CV Mosby Co, 1982. Used by permission.)

   B. Velocity vs. flow
       1. Velocity is the speed with which movement between two points occurs (miles/hour, cm/sec).
       2. Flow is the volume passing a single point per unit of time (L/min).
       3. The two are related and may change directly or indirectly with each other, depending on the specific changes that occur in the structure of the system.
   C. Resistance to gas flow
       1. In general, resistance is defined as the force (pressure) necessary to maintain a specific flow in a particular system.
       2. For gas movement to occur, there must be a pressure gradient. The magnitude of the pressure gradient is determined by the overall resistance of the system. In gas physics, airway resistance is equal to the change in pressure divided by flow:

$$R = \frac{\Delta P}{\dot{V}} \tag{38}$$

   where R = airway resistance, ΔP = change in pressure, and $\dot{V}$ = flow.
       3. Airway resistance is a physical property of the system.
       4. The change in pressure reflects the amount of pressure necessary to maintain a *specific flow* in the system.
       5. The resistance of a system is increased under the following situations:
           a. Decreased lumen of the system.
           b. Directional changes in the system.
           c. Branching of the system.
       6. If the resistance of a system is constant, an increase in pressure gradient results in an increase in system flow.

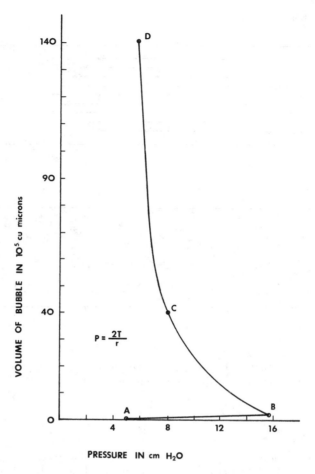

FIG 2–4.
Pressure-volume curve of a bubble as it is inflated. *A*, minimal volume providing shape. *B*, critical volume. *C* and *D*, decreased pressure is necessary to maintain a given volume as the radius of the sphere increases. See text for details.

7. An increase in resistance with a constant pressure gradient results in a decrease in flow.
8. In general, if resistance is constant, pressure gradient and system flow are directly related.

D. Conductance
   1. Conductance is the capability of a system to maintain flow.
   2. Conductance is the inverse of resistance.
   3. Mathematically:

$$\text{Conductance} = \frac{\dot{V}}{\Delta P} \qquad (39)$$

E. Types of flow
   1. *Laminar flow* is a smooth, even, nontumbling flow.
      a. Laminar flow proceeds with a cone front. The molecules of gas in the center of the system encounter the least frictional resistance and move at a greater velocity than those at the sides of the system (Fig 2–5).

LAMINAR

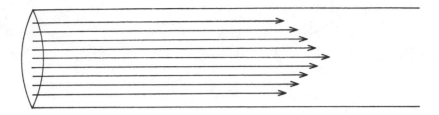

TURBULENT

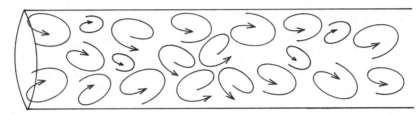

FIG 2–5.
Laminar and turbulent flow.

b. In all laminar flow situations, the pressure necessary to overcome airway resistance is directly related to flow:

$$R = \frac{\Delta P}{\dot{V}} \qquad (40)$$

2. *Turbulent flow* is a rough, tumbling, uneven flow pattern.
   a. Turbulent flow proceeds with a blunt front. Due to a tumbling effect, all of the molecules in the system encounter the walls of the vessel (see Fig 2–5).
   b. In a turbulent flow system, the pressure necessary to overcome airway resistance is directly related to the *square* of the flow:

$$R = \frac{\Delta P}{\dot{V}^2} \qquad (41)$$

   c. *The pressure gradient necessary to maintain turbulent flow is much higher than that necessary to maintain laminar flow.*
3. *Tracheobronchial flow* is a combination of areas of laminar and turbulent flow. Tracheobronchial flow is believed to be the type of flow maintained throughout the respiratory system.
F. *Reynold's number*
   1. Reynold's number (RN) is a dimensionless number that indicates whether flow through a system is laminar or turbulent.
   2. Reynold's number is calculated as follows:

$$RN = \frac{(\text{Diameter})(\text{Velocity})(\text{Density})}{(\text{Viscosity})} \qquad (42)$$

where the diameter refers to the diameter of the system and velocity, density, and viscosity refer to the gas that is flowing in the system.

3. If Reynold's number is 2,000 or greater, the flow in the system is turbulent. If it is less than 2,000, the flow is laminar.

G. *Bernoulli effect*

1. Bernoulli effect: As a gas moves through a free-flowing system, transmural pressure is inversely related to velocity of the gas; that is, as the velocity of the gas increases, the transmural pressure decreases (Fig 2–6).
2. Statement no. 1 holds true because the total energy in a free-flowing system is equal at all points.
3. In a free-flowing system of limited size functioning essentially as a non-gravity-dependent system, the total energy is equal to the sum of the kinetic energy and the transmural pressure energy.
4. Transmural pressure energy is purely a measure of the force that the gas flow exerts on the walls of the system.
5. Kinetic energy in this sense is equal to 0.5 times the gas density times the gas velocity squared:

$$\text{Kinetic energy} = 0.5 \ (D)(V^2) \tag{43}$$

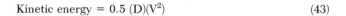

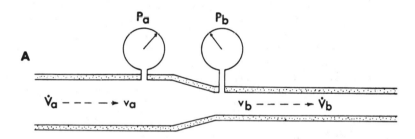

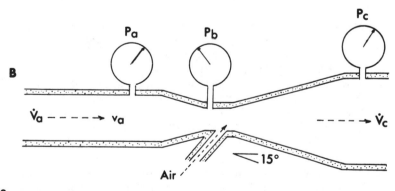

FIG 2–6.
A, the Bernoulli effect demonstrates that the pressure exerted by a steady flow of gas or liquid in a conducting tube varies inversely as the velocity of the fluid. With an abrupt narrowing of the passage since the volume of fluid per unit of time leaving (V_b) must equal the time-volume entering the tube (V_a), the linear motion of the fluid per unit of time (velocity, v) must increase as it traverses the structure $(v_b > v_a)$. Thus, there is a pressure drop distal to the restriction $(P_b < P_a)$. **B,** according to the Venturi principle, the pressure drop distal to a restriction can be closely restored to the prerestriction pressure if there is a dilation of the passage immediately distal to the stenosis, with an angle of divergence not exceeding 15 degrees. Thus, P_c approximately equals P_a. The Venturi is a widely used device to entrain a second gas to mix with the main-flow gas. The subambient pressure distal to the restriction draws in the second gas just pass the restriction, and the increased outflow $(V_c > V_a)$ is accommodated by the widened distal passage. (From Spearman CB, Sheldon RL, Egan DF: *Egan's Fundamentals of Respiratory Therapy,* ed 4. St Louis, CV Mosby Co, 1982. Used by permission.)

6. Thus, in a free-flowing system:

$$\text{Total energy} = 0.5\,(D)(V^2) + P_{transmural} \tag{44}$$

This illustrates the fact that velocity and transmural pressure are inversely related.

7. As the radius of the system decreases and velocity of the gas moving through the system increases, transmural pressure decreases, per equation 43.

8. The lower the density of a gas, the smaller the decrease in transmural pressure as the gas moves through a stenosis. This relationship demonstrates the effect of density on maintaining a more laminar flow.

9. *Venturi principle*
   a. The Venturi principle is an extension of the Bernoulli effect (see Fig 2–6).
   b. It states that distal to a stenosis in a free-flowing system, prestenotic pressure can be restored if the angle of divergence of the system from the midline does not exceed 15 degrees.
   c. Also, if the stenosis in the system is small enough, subatmospheric transmural pressure can be developed and used to entrain a second gas or liquid.
   d. Venturi systems can be designed to deliver specific oxygen concentrations.
   e. The concentration of oxygen delivered by a venturi system can be varied by:
      (1) Altering the size of the Venturi's stenosis.
      (2) Altering the size of the entrainment ports.
   f. Backpressure on a Venturi system decreases the volume of fluid or gas entrained. This causes the oxygen concentration delivered by the system to increase.

H. Jet mixing
   1. The use of a constant flow of gas (jet) to entrain a second gas.
   2. No pressure gradient exists between the jet flow and the ambient environment.
   3. Air entrainment is a result of the viscous shearing force between a dynamic fluid and a stationary fluid resulting in a change in velocities.
      a. The dynamic fluid's velocity decreases.
      b. The stationary fluid's velocity increases.
   4. Provided free access is allowed for the entrained gas, mixing at specific ratios can be maintained.
   5. Altering the *flow* of the gas from the jet alters the total volume exiting the system but does not alter entrainment ratios or $F_{I_{O_2}}$.
   6. Entrainment ratios are the same as those commonly listed for Venturi systems (see Chapter 27).
   7. Backpressure on the system decreases entrainment and increases $F_{I_{O_2}}$.
   8. Jet mixing is responsible for the function of air entrainment masks and most other systems in respiratory care commonly attributed to the Venturi effect.

I. *Poiseuille's law*
   1. Poiseuille's law is used in the determination of the viscosity of a fluid.
   2. Viscosity is defined as a fluid's resistance to deformity and, for gases, increases with increased temperature.
   3. Poiseuille's law states that viscosity (μ) is equal to the change in pressure (ΔP) times pi (π) times the radius to the fourth power (r^4) divided by eight times the length of the system (8l) times flow ($\dot{V}$):

$$n = \frac{\Delta P \pi r^4}{8l\dot{V}} \tag{45}$$

4. Rearranging equation 45 and placing on the left side of the equation those factors that would be constant when ventilating a patient and on the right side of the equation those factors that would vary, the result is

$$\frac{n8l}{\pi} = \frac{\Delta P r^4}{\dot{V}}$$

(46)

5. The right side of equation 46 indicates the relationship between pressure, flow, and radius of a gas flow system.
6. If the radius were to decrease by one half, there would be a 16-fold change in the right side of the equation.
7. To maintain the left side of the equation constant, a 16-fold change in pressure or flow or a combination of both would be necessary to minimize the effects of the decrease in radius.
8. Thus, to minimize the effects of an airway diameter decrease, it would be necessary to increase the pressure gradient and/or decrease the flow in the system.
9. Theoretically, Poiseuille's law can be applied only to homogeneous fluid flow systems that are nonpulsatile and laminar through a single cylinder.
10. Thus, Poiseuille's law cannot be directly applied to the respiratory and cardiovascular systems, but it does provide insights into the interrelationships between pressure, flow, and system radius.

BIBLIOGRAPHY

Carr HY, Weidner RT: *Physics from the Ground Up*. New York, McGraw-Hill Book Co, 1971.

Cherniack RM, Cherniack L: *Respiration in Health and Disease*, ed 3. Philadelphia, WB Saunders Co, 1983.

Comroe JH: *Physiology of Respiration*, ed 2. Chicago, Year Book Medical Publishers, 1974.

Dejours P: *Respiration*. New York, Oxford Univeristy Press, 1966.

Deshpande VM, Pilbeam SP, Dixon RJ: *A Comprehensive Review of Respiratory Care*. Norwalk, Conn, Appleton & Lange, 1988.

Epstein LI, Kuzava BA: *Basic Physics in Anesthesiology*. Chicago, Year Book Medical Publishers, 1976.

Guyton AC: *Textbook of Medical Physiology*, ed 6. Philadelphia, WB Saunders Co, 1981.

Murray JF: *The Normal Lung*. Philadelphia, WB Saunders Co, ed 2, 1987.

Nunn JF: *Applied Respiratory Physiology With Special Reference to Anesthesia*, ed 2. Stoneham, Mass, Butterworth, 1977.

Sacheim GI, Schultz RM: *Chemistry for the Health Sciences*, ed 2. New York, Macmillan Publishing Co, 1973.

Scacci R: Air entrainment masks: Jet mixing is how they work; the Bernoulli and Venturi principles is how they don't. *Respir Care* 1979; 24:928–934.

Schaim UR, et al: *College Physics*. New York, Raytheon Education Co, Physical Science Study Committee, 1968.

Shapiro BA, Harrison RA, Kacmarek RM, et al: *Clinical Application of Respiratory Care*, ed 3. Chicago, Year Book Medical Publishers, 1985.

Shapiro BA, Harrison RA, Cane R, et al: *Clinical Application of Blood Gases*, ed 4. Chicago, Year Book Medical Publishers, 1989.

Wojciechowski WV: *Respiratory Care Sciences: An Integrated Approach*. New York, John Wiley & Sons, 1985.

Young JA, Crocker D: *Principles and Practice of Respiratory Therapy*, ed 2. Chicago, Year Book Medical Publishers, 1976.

Anatomy of the Respiratory System

I. Boundaries and Functions of the Upper Airway
- Boundaries: From the anterior nares to the true vocal cords.
- Functions:
    1. Heating or cooling inspired gases to body temperature (37°C).
    2. Filtering inspired gases.
    3. Humidifying inspired gases to a relative humidity of about 100% at body temperature.
    4. Olfaction: Act of smelling.
    5. Phonation: Production of sound.
    6. Conduction passageway for ventilating gases.
  A. The nose
    1. The nose is a rigid structure of cartilage and bone, the superior one third made up of the nasal and maxilla bones, the inferior two thirds made up of five large pieces of cartilage.
    2. The two external openings are called the *nostrils, external nares,* or *anterior nares.* Their lateral borders are termed the *alae.*
    3. The nasal cavity is divided into two nasal fossae by the septal cartilage.
    4. Each nasal fossa is divided into three regions: vestibular, olfactory, and respiratory (Fig 3–1).
       a. *Vestibular region:* An area of slight dilation inside the nostril, bordered laterally by the alae and medially by the nasal septal cartilage.
          (1) Contained are coarse nasal hairs (vibrissae) that project anteriorly and inferiorly.
          (2) Sebaceous glands secrete sebum, a greasy substance that keeps the nasal hairs soft and pliable.
          (3) The nasal hairs are the first line of defense for the upper airway, acting as very gross filters of inspired air.
          (4) The vestibular region is lined with stratified squamous epithelium (Table 3–1).

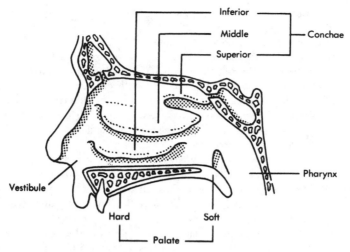

FIG 3–1.
Lateral view of the nasal cavity, representing one complete nasal fossa. (From Dail DH: Anatomy of the respiratory system, in Moser KM, Spragg RG [eds]: *Respiratory Emergencies*, ed 2. St Louis, CV Mosby Co, 1982. Used by permission.)

b. *Olfactory region:* An area in each nasal cavity defined by the superior concha laterally, nasal septal cartilage medially, and roof of the nasal cavity superiorly.

    (1) Contained is the olfactory epithelium responsible for the sense of smell.

    (2) The olfactory epithelium is yellowish brown and appears as pseudostratified columnar epithelial cells. These cells are interspersed with more deeply placed olfactory cells whose sensory filament, the olfactory hairs, protrude to the epithelial surface.

    (3) Due largely to the architecture of the nasal cavity, sniffing causes inspired gases to be drawn to the olfactory region and not much farther into the respiratory tract. This provides a protective mechanism for sampling potentially noxious environmental gases.

TABLE 3–1.

Anatomical Comparison of Epithelium in Upper Respiratory Tract

Structure	Epithelium
Vestibular region/nose	Stratified squamous
Olfactory region/nose	Pseudostratified columnar
Respiratory region/nose	Pseudostratified ciliated columnar
Paranasal sinuses	Pseudostratified ciliated columnar
Nasopharynx	Pseudostratified ciliated columnar
Oropharynx	Stratified squamous
Laryngopharynx	Stratified squamous
Larynx/above true cords	Stratified squamous

c. *Respiratory region:* An area in each nasal cavity inferior to the olfactory region and posterior to the vestibular region. The respiratory region comprises most of the surface area of the nasal fossa.

(1) Contained in the respiratory region of each nasal fossa are three bony plates called turbinates or conchae. The turbinates extend in a medial and inferior direction from the lateral walls of the nasal fossa.

(2) The three turbinates (superior, middle, and inferior) overhang and define the three corresponding passageways through each nasal cavity, respectively the superior, middle, and inferior meati.

(3) Because of the arrangement of the turbinates and folded mucous membrane covering the turbinates in the nose, it has a volume of about 20 cc and a remarkably large surface area of about 160 sq cm.

(4) Turbulent flow is created through the respective meati, which serve the three primary functions of the nose: heating, humidifying, and filtering inspired gases.

(5) Heating, humidifying, and filtering of inspired gases are accomplished by the turbulent flow, which provides a greater probability that each gas molecule will come in contact with the very large surface area of the vascular nasal mucous membrane. This large gas to nasal surface interface allows the following:

(a) The abundant underlying vasculature to heat inspired gases to body temperature.

(b) The moist nasal mucous membrane to give up 650 to 1,000 ml of H_2O per day in bringing inspired gases to a relative humidity of 80% on leaving the nose and entering the nasopharynx.

(c) Particles suspended in the inspired gas to contact the sticky mucous membrane, thus filtering out particles greater than 5 μ by inertial impaction to an efficiency of about 100%.

(6) The epithelial lining of the respiratory region of the nasal cavity is pseudostratified ciliated columnar epithelium (Fig 3–2).

(a) The cells are cylindrical and appear to be two cell layers thick due to the high lateral pressures compressing the cells. Actually, the epithelium is only one cell layer thick, each columnar cell making contact with the basement membrane.

(b) Each columnar cell has 200 to 250 cilia on its luminal surface. Each of the cilia contains two central and nine paired peripheral fibrils. It is the sliding interaction of these fibrils that is thought to cause the beating of the cilia.

(c) Goblet cells and submucosal glands are interspersed throughout the epithelium and, along with capillary seepage, are responsible for production of mucus (100 ml/day in health).

(d) Mucus exists in two layers:

(i) Sol layer: Fluid bottom layer housing the cilia.

(ii) Gel layer: A viscous layer overlying the cilia.

(e) On the forward stroke, the cilia become rigid. Their tips touch the undersurface of the gel layer and propel it toward the oropharynx. On the backward stroke, the cilia become flaccid, fold on themselves, and slide entirely through the sol layer to their resting position without producing a retrograde motion of the gel layer.

(f) The cilia of a particular cell and adjacent cells beat in a coordinated and sequential fashion that produces a motion very similar to a wave. This allows a unidirectional flow of mucus. The cilia beat about 1,000 to 1,500 times per minute and move the mucous layer at a rate of 2 cm/min.

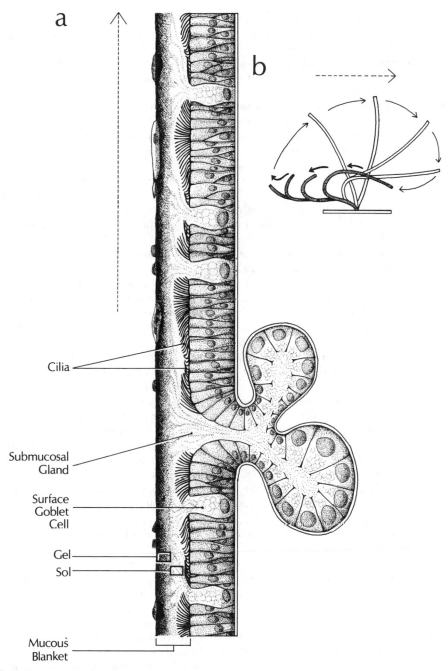

Cilia

Submucosal Gland

Surface Goblet Cell

Gel

Sol

Mucous Blanket

FIG 3-2.
Conceptual depiction of the respiratory epithelium (pseudostratified ciliated columnar epithelium). (From Shapiro BA, Harrison RA, Kacmarek RM, et al: *Clinical Application of Respiratory Care,* ed 3. Chicago, Year Book Medical Publishers, 1985. Used by permission.)

(g) Functions of the mucus and pseudostratified ciliated columnar epithelium (mucociliary blanket):
   (i) To entrap inspired particles.
   (ii) To humidify inspired gas.
   (iii) To transport debris-laden mucus out of the respiratory tract.

5. The nose is responsible for one half to two thirds of the total airway resistance during nasal breathing. It therefore is not surprising that during stress (e.g., exercise or disease) a switch is made to mouth breathing.
6. The nose ends with the outlet of the nasal cavity into the nasopharynx through the internal nares (posterior nares or choanae).

B. Paranasal sinuses (Fig 3–3)
1. Sinuses are cavities of air in the bones of the cranium.
2. The function of the sinuses is not clearly understood, but it may be twofold:
   a. To give the voice resonance (prolongation and intensification of sound).
   b. To lighten the head to some extent, the space occupied by the sinuses being filled with air rather than bone.
3. The sinuses are absent or rudimentary at birth and grow almost simultaneously with the development of the permanent teeth. Formation of the sinuses is responsible for the alteration in facial shape that occurs at this time.
4. All of the air sinuses are lined with pseudostratified ciliated columnar epithelium and produce mucus, which drains into the nasal meati.
5. If sinus drainage is blocked by nasogastric tubes or nasotracheal intubation, sinusitis and sinus infection often result.
6. Groups of paranasal sinuses: Frontal, maxillary, sphenoidal, and ethmoidal.
   a. The *frontal sinuses* appear as paired sinuses medial to the orbits of the eye and superior to the roof of the nasal cavity between the external and internal surfaces of the frontal bone. They drain into the anterior portion of the middle meati.
   b. The *maxillary sinuses* appear as paired sinuses lateral to each nasal cavity and inferior to the orbits of the eye in the body of the maxilla. These sinuses, the largest of all the air sinuses, drain into the middle meati.
   c. The *sphenoidal sinuses* appear as paired sinuses posterior and inferior to the roof of the nasal cavity and superior to the internal nares (choanae) in the body of the sphenoid bone. They drain into the superior meati.
   d. The *ethmoidal sinuses* are paired sinuses that exist in three groups: anterior, medial, and posterior ethmoidal. They exist just lateral to the superior and middle conchae, medial to the orbits of the eyes, inferior to the frontal sinuses, and superior to the maxillary sinuses in the ethmoid bone. The ethmoidal sinuses drain into the superior and middle meati.

C. Pharynx
1. The pharynx is a hollow muscular structure lined with epithelium (Fig 3–4).
2. Major functions
   a. To produce the vowel sounds (phonation) by changing its shape.
   b. To serve as a common passageway for ventilatory gases, food, and liquid.
3. The pharynx is about 5 in. long and extends from the internal nares (choanae) inferiorly to the esophagus.
4. Sections of the pharynx: Nasopharynx, oropharynx, and laryngopharynx.
   a. The *nasopharynx* is located behind the nasal cavity and extends from the internal nares superiorly to the tip of the uvula inferiorly.
      (1) The epithelium is continuous with the epithelium of the nasal cavity and is pseudostratified ciliated columnar epithelium.
      (2) The eustachian or auditory tubes open into the nasopharynx on each of its lateral walls and communicate with the tympanic cavity or middle ear (see Fig 3–3).
         (a) This allows equilibration of pressure on each side of the tympanic membrane (eardrum) with environmental pressure changes.
         (b) Nasal intubation may block the eustachian tube openings and may cause otitis media.

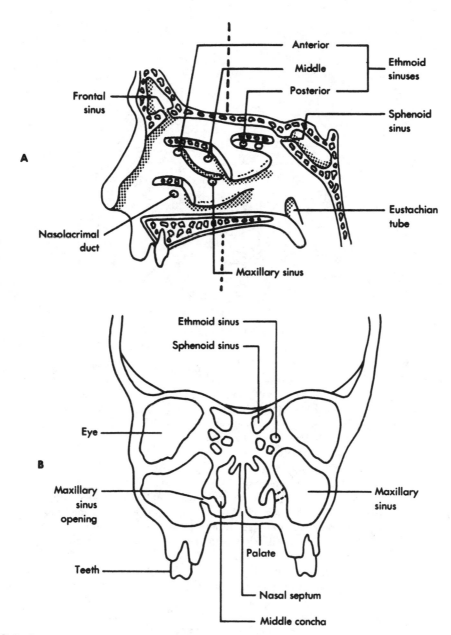

FIG 3–3.
A, lateral view of the nasal cavity, representing one complete nasal fossa with sites of sinus drainage. **B,** frontal section of the nasal cavity taken through the dotted line in **A.** (From Dail DH: Anatomy of the respiratory system, in Moser KM, Spragg RG [eds]: *Respiratory Emergencies,* ed 2. St Louis, CV Mosby Co, 1982. Used by permission.)

(3) The pharyngeal tonsil or adenoid is located in the superior and posterior wall of the nasopharynx.
    (a) The pharyngeal tonsil consists of a large concentration of lymphoid tissue comprising the superior portion of Waldeyer's ring. This ring of lymphoid tissue surrounds and guards the entrance to the respiratory and gastrointestinal tracts.

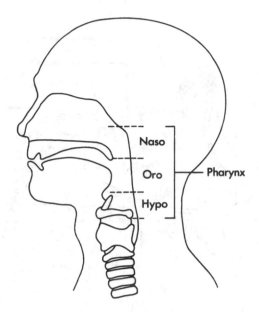

FIG 3-4.
Lateral view of the upper airway indicating the three sections of the pharynx. (From Dail DH: Anatomy of the respiratory system, in Moser KM, Spragg RG [eds]: *Respiratory Emergencies,* ed 2. St Louis, CV Mosby Co, 1982. Used by permission.)

        (4) During the process of swallowing, the uvula and soft palate move in a posterior and superior direction to protect the nasopharynx and nasal cavity from the entrance of food, liquid, or both.
        (5) Major functions of the nasopharynx:
           (a) Gas conduction
           (b) Filtration of gases
           (c) Defense mechanism of the body (tonsils)
    b. The *oropharynx* is located behind the oral or buccal cavity and extends from the tip of the uvula superiorly to the tip of the epiglottis inferiorly.
        (1) The epithelial lining is stratified squamous epithelium.
        (2) The palatine tonsils are located lateral to the uvula on the lateral and anterior aspects of the oropharynx.
        (3) The lingual tonsil is located at the base of the tongue, superior and anterior to the vallecula (the space between the epiglottis and base of the tongue).
        (4) The two palatine tonsils, one lingual and one pharyngeal (adenoid), are the major components of Waldeyer's ring.
        (5) Major functions of the oropharynx:
           (a) Gas conduction
           (b) Food and fluid conduction
           (c) Filtration of inspired gases
           (d) Defense mechanism of the body (Waldeyer's ring)
    c. The laryngopharynx or hypopharynx extends superiorly from the tip of the epiglottis to a point inferiorly where it bifurcates into larynx and esophagus.
        (1) The epithelial lining is stratified squamous epithelium.
        (2) Major functions of the laryngopharynx:
           (a) Gas conduction
           (b) Food and fluid conduction

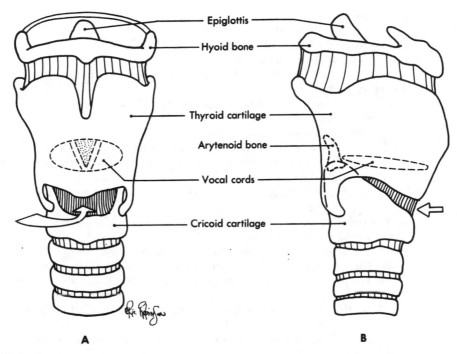

FIG 3-5.
Frontal **(A)** and lateral **(B)** views of the larynx. (From Dail DH: Anatomy of the respiratory system, in Moser KM, Spragg RG [eds]: *Respiratory Emergencies,* ed 2. St Louis, CV Mosby Co, 1982. Used by permission.)

        (3) The laryngopharynx leads anteriorly into the larynx and posteriorly into the esophagus.

        (4) The larynx* is considered the connection between the upper and lower airways, the exact division being the true vocal cords.

  II. Boundaries and Functions of the Lower Airway

    • Boundaries: From the true vocal cords to the terminal air spaces (alveoli).

    • Functions:

      1. Ventilation: To and fro movement of gas (gas conduction).

      2. External respiration: Actual gas exchange between body (pulmonary capillary blood) and external environment (alveolar gas).

      3. Sphincter or glottic mechanisms.

        a. Valsalva maneuver: Forced expiration against closed glottis.

        b. Müller maneuver: Forced inspiration against closed glottis.

        c. Cough mechanism.

        d. Protection of laryngeal inlet.

      4. Phonation: Production of sound.

    A. The larynx (Fig 3-5)

      1. The larynx is a boxlike structure made of cartilage connected by extrinsic and intrinsic muscles and ligaments. It is lined internally by a mucous membrane.

---

   *For discussion and organizational purposes, a complete description of the larynx will follow after section II on the lower airway (please note that the superior portion of the larynx is part of the upper airway and the inferior portion of the larynx is part of the lower airway).

2. Functions
   a. Gas conduction: Ventilation.
   b. Phonation: Production of sound.
   c. Sphincter or glottic mechanism.
3. The larynx extends from the third to sixth cervical vertebrae in the anterior portion of the neck.
4. Unpaired cartilages of the larynx: Epiglottis, thyroid, and cricoid.
   a. *Epiglottic cartilage*
      (1) Leaf-shaped piece of fibrocartilage.
      (2) Anteriorly attached to thyroid cartilage just inferior to the thyroid notch.
      (3) Laterally attached to folds of mucous membrane called *aryepiglottic folds.*
      (4) On swallowing, the epiglottis is squeezed between the base of the tongue and thyroid cartilage, causing the epiglottis to pivot in a posterior and inferior direction to cover the laryngeal inlet.
   b. *Thyroid cartilage*
      (1) The largest laryngeal cartilage.
      (2) The anterior aspect is called the *laryngeal prominence,* or *Adam's apple.*
      (3) Directly superior to the laryngeal prominence is the thyroid notch.
      (4) The posterior and lateral aspects of this cartilage have two superior and two inferior projections, the superior and inferior cornua.
         (a) The superior cornu articulates with the hyoid bone, which serves as a support from which the lower respiratory tract is suspended.
         (b) The inferior cornu articulates with the cricoid cartilage below.
   c. *Cricoid cartilage*
      (1) Shaped like a signet ring.
      (2) Forms the entire inferior aspect and most of the posterior aspect of the larynx.
      (3) On the posterolateral surface exist articulating surfaces for the inferior cornu of the thyroid cartilage.
      (4) On the posterosuperior surface exist articulating surfaces for the paired arytenoid cartilages.
      (5) Lies inferior to the thyroid and superior to the trachea, to which it attaches.
      (6) Lies anterior to the esophagus. Therefore, external cricoid pressure may facilitate viewing of the glottis during tracheal intubation and prevent reflux from the stomach by compressing the esophagus.
5. Paired cartilages of the larynx: Arytenoid, corniculate, and cuneiform.
   a. *Arytenoid cartilages*
      (1) Shaped like upright pyramids.
      (2) The base of each cartilage articulates with the posterosuperior surface of the cricoid cartilage.
      (3) Each arytenoid cartilage has a ventral-medial projection from its base called the vocal process, to which the vocal ligaments attach.
      (4) Arytenoid cartilages, along with the cricoid cartilage, make up the entire posterior surface of the larynx.
   b. *Corniculate cartilages*
      (1) Shaped like cones and are the smallest cartilages of the larynx.
      (2) Articulate with the arytenoid cartilages on their superior surface, to which the corniculate cartilages are sometimes fused.
      (3) When the larynx is viewed from above, the corniculate cartilages appear as two small elevations on the posteromedial aspect of the laryngeal inlet.
      (4) Housed in mucosal folds called the aryepiglottic folds.

    c. *Cuneiform cartilages*
      (1) Shaped like small, elongated clubs.
      (2) Located lateral and anterior to the corniculate cartilages.
      (3) When the larynx is viewed from above, the cuneiform cartilages appear as two small elevations just lateral and anterior to the corniculate cartilages.
      (4) Housed in the aryepiglottic folds.
      (5) The cuneiforms, along with the aryepiglottic folds, form the lateral aspect of the laryngeal inlet. The epiglottis forms the anterior aspect, the corniculates the posterior aspect of the laryngeal inlet.

6. Extrinsic ligaments of the larynx
    a. Extrinsic ligaments attach cartilages of the larynx to structures outside the larynx.
    b. The *thyrohyoid membrane* is a broad fibroelastic sheet that attaches the anterior and lateral superior aspects of the thyroid cartilage to the inferior surface of the hyoid bone (the posterior portion of the thyroid cartilage is attached to the hyoid bone by the superior cornu of the thyroid cartilage).
    c. The *hyoepiglottic ligament* is an elastic band that attaches the anterior surface of the epiglottis to the hyoid bone.
    d. The *cricotracheal ligament* connects the lower portion of the cricoid cartilage to the trachea by a very broad fibrous membrane.

7. Intrinsic ligaments of the larynx
    a. Intrinsic ligaments attach cartilages of the larynx to one another.
    b. The *thyroepiglottic ligament* attaches the inferior aspect of the epiglottis to the thyroid cartilage on its internal surface below the thyroid notch.
    c. The *aryepiglottic ligament* attaches the arytenoid cartilages to the epiglottis and acts as a point of attachment for the aryepiglottic folds.
    d. The *cricothyroid ligament* attaches the anterior portion of the thyroid cartilage to the anterior portion of the cricoid cartilage. It is through this ligament that an emergency cricothyroidotomy is performed.
    e. The *vocal ligament* is a thick band that stretches from the vocal process of the arytenoid cartilages across the cavity of the larynx to attach to the thyroid cartilage just inferior to the thyroepiglottic ligament. The lateral borders of the vocal ligament attach to the inverted free borders of the cricothyroid ligament.
    f. The *ventricular ligament* is a thick band that stretches from the arytenoid cartilage across the cavity of the larynx to the thyroid cartilage. It exists superior and lateral to the vocal ligament.

8. Cavity of the larynx (Fig 3–6)
    a. The larynx is divided into three sections by the pair of ventricular folds and vocal folds.
    b. The *upper section*, the vestibule of the larynx, extends from the laryngeal inlet to the level of the ventricular folds.
      (1) The ventricular folds are called the *false vocal cords*.
      (2) The space between the ventricular folds is the rima vestibuli.
    c. The *middle section*, the ventricle of the larynx, extends from the ventricular folds to the vocal cords.
      (1) The vocal folds are the true vocal cords.
      (2) The space between the vocal folds is the rima glottidis or glottis.
        (a) The glottis is triangular, the base being posterior, the apex anterior.
        (b) It is the smallest opening of the adult airway (important when endotracheal tube size is selected).
        (c) The dimensions of the glottis are smaller in the women than in men.
          (i) Average female transverse diameter: 7 to 8 mm.

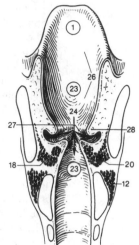

FIG 3–6.
Frontal section of larynx, posterior view, depicting laryngeal cavities. *1*, epiglottis; *18*, true vocal cords; *23*, laryngeal cavity; *24*, entrance to larynx through the rima vestibuli and rim   a glottidis; *26*, vestibule of larynx; *27*, rima vestibuli; *28*, ventricular folds. (From Feneis H: *Pocket Atlas of Human Anatomy*, ed 4. New York, Thieme-Stratton, 1976. Used by permission.)

(ii) Average male transverse diameter: 9 to 10 mm.

(iii) Average anteroposterior diameter in women: 17 mm.

(iv) Average anteroposterior diameter in men: 24 mm.

(3) The size of the rima glottidis also is variable, depending on the state of the vocal cords (Fig 3–7).

(a) Adduction is accomplished by medial rotation and approximation of the arytenoids, thus sealing the glottis.

(b) Abduction is accomplished by lateral rotation of the arytenoids, thus increasing the size of the glottis.

(4) The glottic or sphincter mechanism requires aryepiglottic folds, epiglottis, ventricular folds, and vocal folds to act in a very coordinated fashion in sealing the laryngeal inlet.

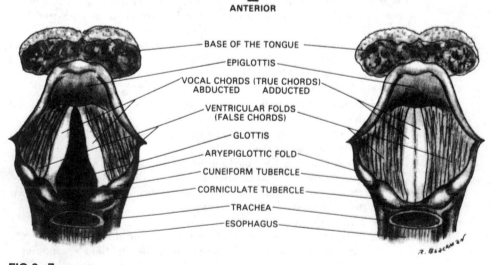

FIG 3–7.
Superior view of larynx with vocal cords closed (abduction) and opened (adduction). See text for details. (From DesJardins T: *Cardiopulmonary Anatomy ·and Physiology: Essentials for Respiratory Care*. New York, Delmar Publishers, 1988. Used by permission.)

    d. The *lower section,* subglottic cavity of the larynx, extends from vocal folds to cricoid cartilage.

    e. The epithelial lining of the larynx above the true vocal cords is continuous with the laryngopharynx and is stratified squamous epithelium (see Table 3–1).

    f. The epithelial lining of the larynx below the true vocal cords is pseudostratified ciliated columnar epithelium.

B. Tracheobronchial tree and lung parenchyma (Fig 3–8)

    1. The tracheobronchial tree functions in ventilation (to and fro movement of air) and is sometimes referred to as the *conducting airway.*

    2. The lung parenchyma functions in external respiration and is the area of the lung where actual gas exchange occurs.

    3. As the lower airway subdivides, it gives way to more and more airways (generations). Each new generation of airways is assigned a number. The numbering system below begins with assigning generation 0 to the trachea. The first branching or division of the trachea constitutes the mainstem bronchi, which are assigned generation 1. Each subsequent branching of the lower airway is assigned the subsequent generation number.

C. Trachea (generation 0)

    1. The trachea is a cartilaginous, membranous tube 10 to 13 cm in length and 2 to 2.5 cm in diameter.

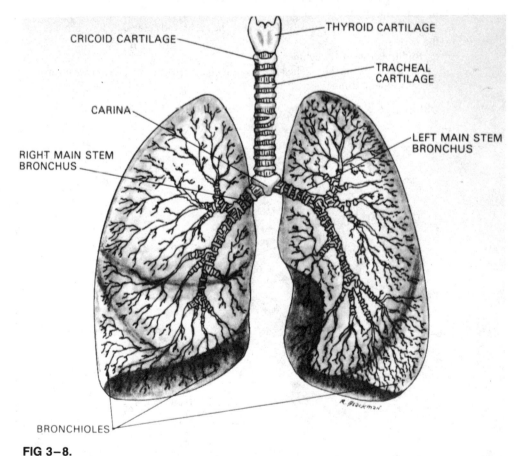

FIG 3–8.
Tracheobronchial tree. (From DesJardins T: *Cardiopulmonary Anatomy and Physiology: Essentials for Respiratory Care.* New York, Delmar Publishers, 1988. Used by permission.)

2. The trachea extends from the cricoid cartilage at the sixth cervical vertebra to its point of bifurcation (carina) at the fifth thoracic vertebra.

3. Sixteen to 20 incomplete cartilaginous rings open posteriorly and are arranged horizontally. The open ends of the cartilage and the area between individual cartilages are joined by a combination of fibrous, elastic, and smooth muscle tissue.
   a. The smooth muscle is arranged longitudinally to shorten and elongate the trachea.
   b. The smooth muscle also is arranged transversely to constrict and dilate the trachea.

4. The posterior wall of the trachea is separated from the anterior wall of the esophagus by loose connective tissue.

5. The trachea and following large airways (bronchi) contain three characteristic layers (Fig 3–9):
   a. Cartilaginous layer.
   b. Lamina propria, which contains small blood vessels, lymphatic vessels, nerve tracts, elastic fibers, smooth muscle, and submucosal glands.
   c. Epithelial, or intraluminal, layer, which is separated from the lamina propria by a noncellular basement membrane.

6. The epithelial lining of the trachea is continuous with the larynx above and consists of pseudostratified ciliated columnar epithelium (Table 3–2).

D. Mainstem bronchi (generation 1)

1. The trachea bifurcates into two airways, the right and left mainstem bronchi, at the carina.
   a. Right mainstem bronchus
      (1) Branches off the trachea at an angle of about 20 to 30 degrees with respect to the midline.

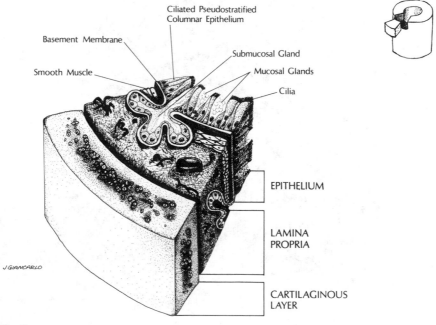

FIG 3–9.
Section of the trachea showing the three layers: epithelium, lamina propria, and cartilaginous layer. (From Shapiro BA, Harrison RA, Kacmarek RM, et al: *Clinical Application of Respiratory Care,* ed 3. Chicago, Year Book Medical Publishers, 1985. Used by permission.)

TABLE 3–2.

Anatomical Comparison of Structures in the Lower Respiratory Tract

Structure	Epithelium	Division
Larynx/below true cords	Pseudostratified ciliated columnar	X
Trachea	Pseudostratified ciliated columnar	0
Mainstem bronchi	Pseudostratified ciliated columnar	1
Lobar bronchi	Pseudostratified ciliated columnar	2
Segmental bronchi	Pseudostratified ciliated columnar	3
Subsegmental bronchi	Pseudostratified ciliated columnar	4–9
Bronchioles	Pseudostratified ciliated columnar	10–15
Terminal bronchioles	Cuboidal to simple squamous	16
Respiratory bronchioles	Simple squamous	17–19
Alveolar ducts	Simple squamous	20–24
Alveolar sacs	Simple squamous	25
Alveoli	Type I; squamous	. . .
	Type II; granular	. . .
	Type III; macrophage	. . .

   (2) Diameter: About 1.4 cm.

   (3) Length: About 2.5 cm.

  b. Left mainstem bronchus

   (1) Branches off the trachea at an angle of 40 to 60 degrees with respect to the midline.

   (2) Diameter: About 1.0 cm.

   (3) Length: About 5 cm.

 2. A portion of mainstem bronchi is extrapulmonary (exists outside the lung, in the mediastinum), but the majority of it is intrapulmonary (inside the lung proper).

 3. The structural arrangement of the mainstem bronchi is the same as that of the trachea, with C-shaped pieces of cartilage, a lamina propria, and pseudostratified ciliated columnar epithelium.

 4. The only structural difference between the mainstem bronchi and the trachea is that the intrapulmonary section of the mainstem bronchi is covered with a sheath of connective tissue, the peribronchiolar connective tissue.

  a. The function of peribronchiolar connective tissue is to encase large nerve, lymphatic, and bronchial blood vessels as they follow the branchings of the subdividing airways.

  b. The peribronchiolar connective tissue continues to follow the branching of the airways until the level of the bronchioles, where it disappears.

 5. Mainstem bronchi are sometimes referred to as primary bronchi.

E. Lobar bronchi (generation 2)

 1. Five lobar bronchi correspond, respectively, to the five lobes of the lung.

 2. The right mainstem bronchus trifurcates into right upper, middle, and lower lobar bronchi.

 3. The left mainstem bronchus bifurcates into left upper and lower lobar bronchi.

 4. The structural arrangement of lobar bronchi is the same as that of mainstem bronchi.

 5. The epithelial lining of lobar bronchi is pseudostratified ciliated columnar epithelium (see Table 3–2).

 6. Lobar bronchi are sometimes referred to as secondary bronchi.

F. Segmental bronchi (generation 3)

 1. There are 18 segmental bronchi, corresponding to the 18 segments of the lung.

  2. The structural arrangement of segmental bronchi is similar to that of lobar and mainstem bronchi except that the C-shaped pieces of cartilage become less regular in shape and volume (see Fig 3–9).
  3. The epithelial lining of segmental bronchi is pseudostratified ciliated columnar epithelium.
  4. Segmental bronchi are sometimes referred to as *tertiary bronchi.*
G. Subsegmental bronchi (generations 4–9)
  1. The diameter of subsegmental bronchi ranges from 1 to 6 mm.
  2. Cartilaginous rings give way to irregularly placed pieces of cartilage circumscribing the airway, the cartilaginous plaques (see Fig 3–9).
  3. By the ninth generation of airways, cartilage is only scantily present.
  4. As volume and regularity of cartilage have decreased from generation 0 to generation 9, so has the number of submucosal glands and goblet cells.
  5. The epithelial lining of subsegmental bronchi is pseudostratified ciliated columnar epithelium.
H. Bronchioles (generations 10–15)
  1. Diameter is characteristically 1 mm.
  2. Cartilage is totally absent (Fig 3–10).

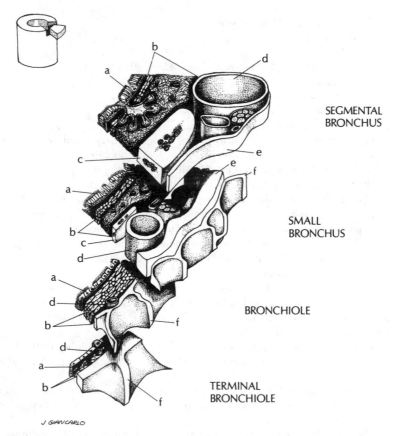

FIG 3–10.
Sections at various levels of the tracheobronchial tree: *a,* pulmonary mucosa; *b,* lamina propria; *c,* cartilage; *d,* blood vessels; *e,* peribronchial connective tissue; *f,* lung parenchyma. (From Shapiro BA, Harrison RA, Kacmarek RM, et al: *Clinical Application of Respiratory Care,* ed 3. Chicago, Year Book Medical Publishers, 1985. Used by permission.)

3. Peribronchiolar connective tissue is absent, the lamina propria of these airways being directly embedded in surrounding lung parenchyma.
4. Airway patency is dependent not on the structural rigidity of surrounding cartilage but on fibrous, elastic, and smooth muscle tissue.
5. The epithelial lining of bronchioles is pseudostratified ciliated cuboidal epithelium.
   a. This epithelium is functionally the same as pseudostratified ciliated columnar epithelium.
   b. It differs from pseudostratified ciliated columnar epithelium in three ways:
      (1) It is thinner, being constructed of cuboidal cells rather than columnar cells.
      (2) The number of goblet cells and submucosal glands gradually decreases until they are almost nonexistent by generation 15.
      (3) The number of cilia also decreases and cilia are all but gone by the end of generation 15.
I. Terminal bronchioles (generation 16)
   1. Average diameter is 0.5 mm.
   2. Goblet cells and submucosal glands disappear, although mucus is found in these airways (see Fig 3–10).
   3. Cilia are absent from the epithelium of terminal bronchioles. This epithelium serves as a transition from the cuboidal epithelium of generation 15 to the squamous epithelium of generation 17.
   4. Clara cells are located in the terminal bronchioles.
      a. Plump columnar cells that bulge into the lumen of terminal bronchioles.
      b. Probably responsible for mucus and surfactant found in terminal bronchioles.
   5. Terminal bronchioles mark the end of the conducting airways; all airway generations distal to the terminal bronchioles are considered part of the lung parenchyma.
J. Respiratory bronchioles (generations 17–19) (Fig 3–11)
   1. Average diameter is 0.5 mm.
   2. Alveoli arise from the external surface of the respiratory bronchioles, where a very small portion of external respiration takes place.
   3. The epithelial lining of respiratory bronchioles is a very low cuboidal epithelium interspersed with actual alveoli (simple squamous epithelium).
K. Alveolar ducts (generations 20–24) (see Fig 3–11)
   1. Alveolar ducts arise from respiratory bronchioles.
   2. The only difference between alveolar ducts and respiratory bronchioles is that the walls of the alveolar ducts are totally made up of alveoli.
   3. About one half of the total number of alveoli arise from alveolar ducts.
   4. Alveolar ducts give way to alveolar sacs.

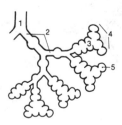

FIG 3–11.
Schematic representation of parenchymal portions of the lung: *1,* terminal bronchiole; *2,* respiratory bronchiole; *3,* alveolar ducts; *4,* alveolar sacs; *5,* alveolus. (From Feneis H: *Pocket Atlas of Human Anatomy,* ed 4. New York, Thieme-Stratton, 1976. Used by permission.)

   L. Alveolar sacs (generation 25) (see Fig 3–11)
     1. Alveolar sacs are the last generation of airways and are blind passageways.
     2. These appear functionally the same as alveolar ducts but differ in that they form grapelike clusters having common walls with other alveoli.
     3. The remaining half of alveoli rise from alveolar sacs.
  M. Alveoli (Fig 3–12)
     1. The alveoli are terminal air spaces that contain numerous capillaries in their septa, which serve as sites for gas exchange.
     2. The average number of total alveoli contained in both lungs combined is 3 million but varies directly with the height of the individual and may be as many as 6 million.
     3. The total cross-sectional area provided by the alveolar surface is about 80 sq m.
     4. The total cross-sectional area provided by the pulmonary capillaries is 70 sq m, thus constituting an alveolar gas-pulmonary blood interface of 70 sq m (the size of a tennis court).
  N. Alveolar capillary membrane (Fig 3–13)
     1. The alveolar capillary membrane has four components: surfactant layer, alveolar epithelium, interstitial space, and capillary endothelium.
       a. The surfactant is composed of a phospholipid attached to a lecithin molecule.
         (1) Surfactant lines the internal alveolar surface.
         (2) It reduces surface tension, facilitating inspiration and expiration.
       b. Alveolar epithelium (simple squamous epithelium) is a continuous layer of tissue made up of type I and II cells lying on a basement membrane (see Table 3–2).
         (1) Type I cells, or squamous pneumocytes: Very flat, thin simple squames making up 95% of alveolar surface.
         (2) Type II cells, or granular pneumocytes: Plump, highly metabolic cells credited with surfactant production and alveolar repair.

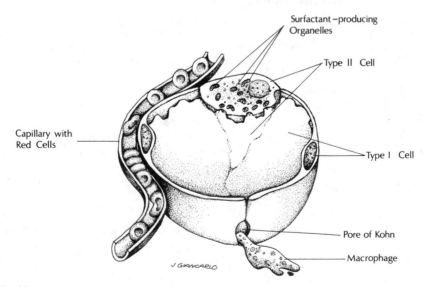

FIG 3–12.
Schematic representation of an alveoli. (From Shapiro BA, Harrison RA, Kacmarek RM, et al: *Clinical Application of Respiratory Care*, ed 3. Chicago, Year Book Medical Publishers, 1985. Used by permission.)

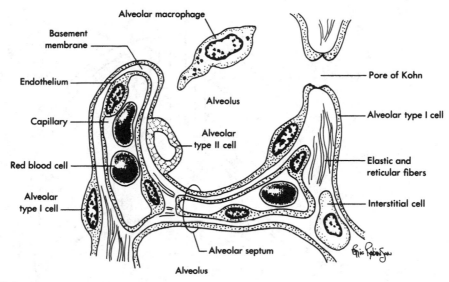

FIG 3–13.
Schematic representation of the alveolar-capillary membrane. (From Dail DH: Anatomy of the respiratory system, in Moser KM, Spragg RG [eds]: *Respiratory Emergencies,* ed 2. St Louis, CV Mosby Co, 1982. Used by permission.)

   (3) Type III cells, or alveolar macrophages: Free, wandering phagocytic cells that ingest foreign material on the alveolar surface.
c. The interstitial space is the area that separates the basement membrane of alveolar epithelium from the basement membrane of capillary endothelium.
   (1) It contains interstitial fluid.
   (2) This space may be so small, especially where diffusion is to take place, that the basement membranes appear fused.
d. Capillary endothelium is a continuous layer of tissue made up of flat, interlocking squames supported on a basement membrane.
2. Thickness of the alveolar capillary membrane varies from 0.35 to 1 μ.
III. The Lung
   A. The lung is situated in the thoracic cavity separated by a structure (mediastinum) containing the heart, great vessels, esophagus, and trachea (Fig 3–14).
      1. Each thoracic cavity is lined with a very fine serous membrane, the parietal pleura, which also covers the dome of each hemidiaphragm.
      2. The lung and each of its lobes are encased in a similar serous membrane called the *visceral pleura.*
      3. A potential space (intrapleural space) between the two pleura contains a small amount of fluid called pleural fluid.
         a. Pleural fluid allows cohesion of visceral and parietal pleura.
         b. Pleural fluid allows the two pleura to slide over each other with reduced frictional resistance.
   B. The lung is a conical-shaped organ with four surfaces: apex, base, medial surface, and costal surface (Fig 3–15).
      1. The apices are rounded superior sections of the lung. They extend 1 to 2 in. above the clavicles.
      2. The bases are concave inferior surfaces of the lung. They rest on the hemidiaphragm. The right base lies higher in the thorax than the left to accommodate the large, underlying liver.

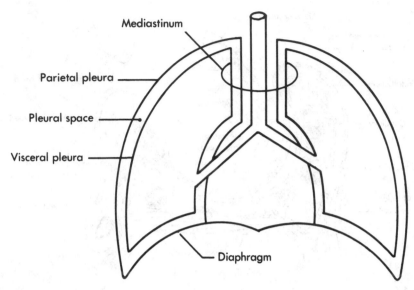

FIG 3–14.
Schematic representation of the lung and thorax. (From Dail DH: Anatomy of the respiratory system, in Moser KM, Spragg RG [eds]: *Respiratory Emergencies*, ed 2. St Louis, CV Mosby Co, 1982. Used by permission.)

3. The medial surface of each lung exhibits a deep concavity to accept the heart and great vessels. This concavity is called the *cardiac impression*. The left cardiac impression is deeper than the right because the heart projects to the left of the midline.
4. The costal surface constitutes most of the lung surface in contact with the pleura lining the thoracic cavity.
C. The root of the lung enters the lung proper at the hilum.
  1. The root of the lung consists of a mainstem bronchus, a pulmonary artery, two pulmonary veins, major lymph vessels, and nerve tracts.
  2. The hilum is the area where the root enters the lung. There the mediastinal and visceral pleura become continuous, forming the pulmonary ligament. This arrangement keeps the pleural cavity sealed and allows the root to enter the sealed lung.
D. The right lung is divided into three lobes by the horizontal and oblique fissures (Figs 3–15 and 3–16).
  1. The oblique fissure isolates the right lower lobe from the right middle and right upper lobe.
  2. The horizontal fissure divides the right upper lobe from the right middle lobe.
  3. Externally the oblique fissure courses through the following landmarks:
    a. Junction of sixth rib and midclavicular line.
    b. Junction of fifth rib and midaxillary line.
    c. Spinous process of third thoracic vertebra.
  4. Externally the horizontal fissure courses through the following landmarks:
    a. Junction of fifth rib and midaxillary line.
    b. Follows the medial course of fourth rib.
E. The left lung is divided into two lobes by the oblique fissure.
  1. The oblique fissure divides the left upper lobe from the left lower lobe.
  2. Externally the left oblique fissure courses through the same landmarks as does the right oblique fissure.

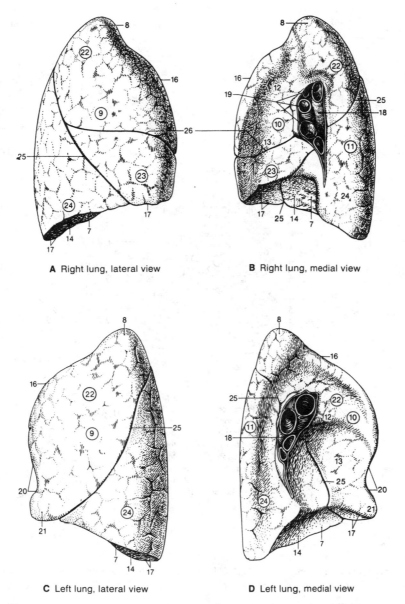

A Right lung, lateral view

B Right lung, medial view

C Left lung, lateral view

D Left lung, medial view

FIG 3–15.
Lateral and medial views of right and left lungs with fissures and hilar structures depicted. *7,* base of lung; *8,* apex of lung; *9,* costal surface; *10,* medial surface; *13,* cardiac impression; *18,* hilus of lung; *19,* root of lung; *22,* upper lobe; *23,* middle lobe; *24,* lower lobe; *25,* oblique fissure; *26,* horizontal fissure. (From Feneis H: *Pocket Atlas of Human Anatomy,* ed 4. New York, Thieme-Stratton, 1976. Used by permission.)

    F. The lobes of the lung are further subdivided into segments (see Fig 3–15).
        1. Right upper lobe
            a. Anterior segment
            b. Apical segment
            e. Posterior segment

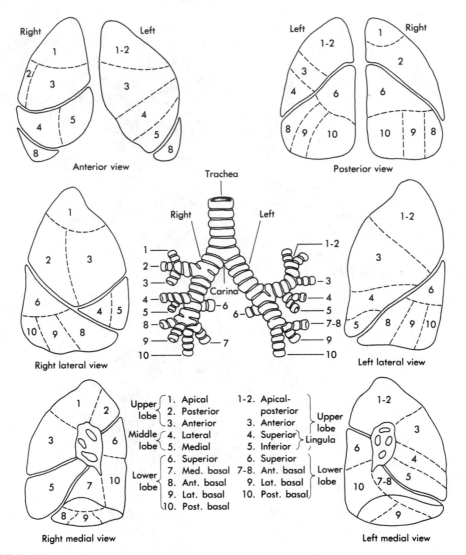

FIG 3–16.
Segmental anatomy of the lung. (From Dail DH: Anatomy of the respiratory system, in Moser KM, Spragg RG [eds]: *Respiratory Emergencies,* ed 2. St Louis, CV Mosby Co, 1982. Used by permission.)

2. Right middle lobe
   a. Lateral segment
   b. Medial segment
3. Right lower lobe
   a. Superior segment
   b. Anterior basal segment
   c. Lateral basal segment
   d. Medial basal segment
   e. Posterior basal segment
4. Left upper lobe
   a. Apical-posterior segment
   b. Anterior segment

      c. Superior segment   Lingula (anatomically corresponds to
                            right middle lobe)

      d. Inferior segment

    5. Left lower lobe

      a. Superior segment

      b. Anteromedial basal segment

      c. Lateral basal segment

      d. Posterior basal segment

    6. Knowledge of bronchopulmonary segmentation becomes important when postural drainage, auscultation, x-ray findings, and bronchoscopy are considered.

  G. The segments are further subdivided into secondary lobules.

    1. *Secondary lobules* consist of a 15th-order airway (bronchiole) associated with three to five terminal bronchioles and the distal respiratory bronchioles, alveolar ducts, and alveolar sacs.

    2. The secondary lobule is the smallest self-contained unit of the lung that is surrounded by connective tissue.

    3. Secondary lobules appear as polyhedral masses observable on the lung surface and between fissures as dark intersecting lines.

    4. Secondary lobules have their own discrete single pulmonary arteriole, venule, lymphatic, and nerve supply.

    5. Secondary lobules are the building blocks of segments and are discernible on chest x-ray film.

    6. Each secondary lobule comprises 30 to 50 primary lobules and measures 1 to 2.5 cm in diameter.

      a. Primary lobules consist of a 19th-order respiratory bronchiole and every generation distal to it.

      b. Primary lobules are not self-contained in connective tissue.

      c. There are about 23 million primary lobules in the lung.

    7. Secondary lobules may be important in isolating and maintaining disease entities locally. They also may be responsible for local matching of ventilation to perfusion.

  H. Bronchiolar and alveolar intercommunicating channels.

    1. The canals of Lambert may be important structures implicated in collateral ventilation of bronchioles (Fig 3–17).

    2. The pores of Kohn are interalveolar pores that allow collateral ventilation of alveoli. Their diameter varies from 3 to 13 μ.

IV. Bony Thorax (Fig 3–18)

  A. It is a bony and cartilaginous frame within which lie the principal organs of circulation and respiration.

  B. It is conical, narrow above and broad below.

  C. Posteriorly the thorax includes the 12 thoracic vertebrae and the posterior portion of the ribs.

  D. Laterally the thorax is convex and formed by the ribs.

  E. Anteriorly it is composed of the sternum, anterior ends of the ribs, and the costal cartilage.

  F. The superior opening into the thorax—defined by the manubrium, first rib, and first thoracic vertebra—is called the *thoracic inlet* or *operculum*.

  G. The inferior opening out of the thorax—defined by the 12th rib, costal cartilage of ribs 7 through 10, and 12th thoracic vertebra—is called the *thoracic outlet*.

  H. Functions of the bony thorax are to protect underlying organs, to aid in ventilation, and to provide a point of attachment for various bones and muscles.

  I. Sternum (see Fig 3–18)

    1. The sternum is about 17 cm long.

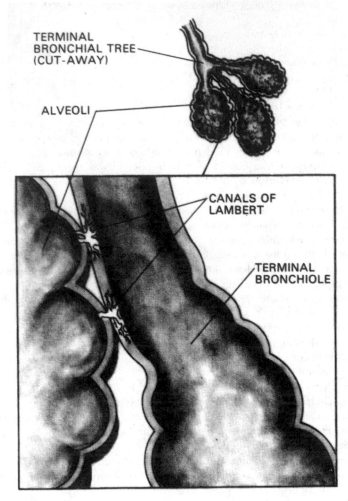

FIG 3–17.
Canals of Lambert. (From DesJardins T: *Cardiopulmonary Anatomy and Physiology: Essentials for Respiratory Care.* New York, Delmar Publishers, 1988. Used by permission.)

  2. The sternum is divided into three sections:
    a. Manubrium: Superior portion
    b. Body: Middle portion
    c. Xiphoid process: Inferior portion
  3. The manubrium articulates with the clavicle and the first and second ribs.
  4. The junction of the manubrium and the body is called the *angle of Louis.* The trachea bifurcates beneath this junction.
  5. The body of the sternum articulates with ribs 2 through 7.
  6. The xiphoid process articulates with the seventh rib.
 J. Ribs (see Fig 3–18)
  1. Twelve elastic arches of bone, posteriorly connected to vertebral column.
  2. Types of ribs: True, false, and floating.
  3. True ribs
    a. Rib pairs 1 through 7

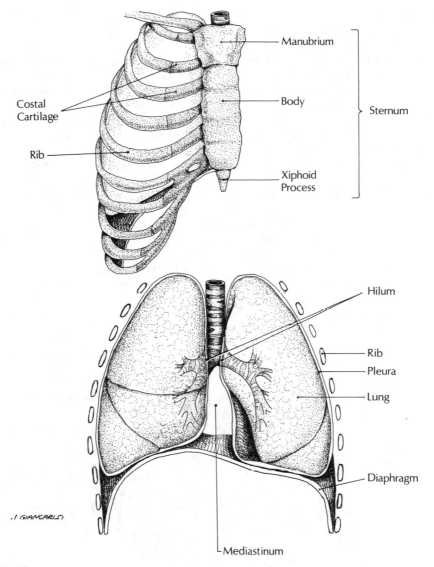

FIG 3–18.
The bony thorax and its relationship to the lung. (From Shapiro BA, Harrison RA, Kacmarek RM, et al: *Clinical Application of Respiratory Care,* ed 3. Chicago, Year Book Medical Publishers, 1985. Used by permission.)

        b. Called *vertebrosternal ribs* because they connect to the sternum via costal cartilage and the vertebrae of the spinal column.

   4. False ribs

        a. Rib pairs 8 through 10.

        b. Called *vertebrocostal ribs* because they connect to costal cartilage of superior rib and the vertebrae of the spinal column.

   5. Floating ribs

        a. Rib pairs 11 and 12.

        b. Have no anterior attachment, lying free in abdominal musculature.

      6. The space between the ribs is called the *intercostal space.*
        a. Wider anteriorly than posteriorly.
        b. Wider superiorly than inferiorly.
      7. All 12 pairs of ribs are positioned in an inferior direction. Contraction of the intercostal muscles elevates the ribs from their natural inclined position.
        a. A superoinferior motion of the ribs causes an increase in the transverse diameter of the thorax and is called the *bucket handle effect.*
        b. An anteroposterior motion of the ribs causes an increase in the anteroposterior diameter of the thorax and is called the *pump handle effect.*

V. Muscles of Inspiration (Fig 3–19)
  A. The diaphragm and external intercostal muscles are those normally used for resting inspiration.
    1. Diaphragm: Dome-shaped muscle that separates thoracic from abdominal cavity.
      a. It is the major muscle of ventilation.
      b. Origin: Thoracic outlet.
      c. Insertion: Central tendon.
      d. Action: Increases vertical diameter of thorax.
      e. Innervation: Cervical spinal motor nerves 3, 4, and 5 (phrenic nerve).
    2. External intercostals
      a. Origin: Inferior border of superior rib.
      b. Insertion: Superior border of inferior rib.

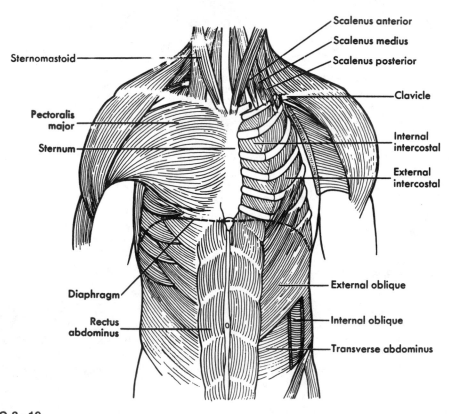

FIG 3–19.
The muscles of ventilation. (From Spearman CB, Sheldon RL, Egan DF: *Egan's Fundamentals of Respiratory Therapy,* ed 4. St Louis, CV Mosby Co, 1982. Used by permission.)

      c. Action: Elevate ribs, increasing anteroposterior and transverse diameters of thorax (pump and bucket handle effects).

      d. Innervation: Thoracic spinal motor nerves 1 through 11.

      e. Along with internal intercostals, this muscle group prevents the intercostal space from bulging and recessing with normal ventilatory efforts.

  B. Accessory muscles of inspiration

    1. Each tends to perform one of two actions, either raising the thorax or stabilizing the thorax so that other muscles can effectively raise the thorax.

      a. Sternocleidomastoid

      b. Scalenes

        (1) Anterior

        (2) Middle

        (3) Posterior

      c. Pectoralis major

      d. Pectoralis minor

      e. Trapezius

      f. Serratus anterior

      g. Levatores costarum

      h. Serratus posterior

      i. Sacrospinalis

    2. It should be noted that use of accessory muscles for resting inspiration is abnormal and that accessory muscle use should occur only with deep or forced inspiration.

VI. Accessory Muscles of Expiration (see Fig 3–19)

  A. There are no muscles of quiet resting expiration. Expiration is purely a passive process brought about by the normal elastic tendencies of the lung coupled with cessation of inspiratory muscle contraction. Therefore, any muscles used for expiration are termed accessory muscles of expiration.

  B. Any muscle usage for quiet resting expiration is abnormal.

  C. Accessory muscles of expiration are used only for forced expiration, making expiration an active process.

  D. The accessory muscles of expiration are either of the back, thorax, or abdomen and tend either to pull the thorax down or to support the thorax so that other muscle groups can effectively pull down on the thorax.

    1. Latissimus dorsi

    2. Intercostales interni

    3. Rectus abdominis

    4. Obliquus externus abdominis

    5. Obliquus internus abdominis

    6. Transversus abdominis

BIBLIOGRAPHY

Anthony CP, Kolthoff NJ: *Textbook of Anatomy and Physiology*, ed 10. St Louis, CV Mosby Co, 1981.

Comroe JH: *Physiology of Respiration*, ed 2. Chicago, Year Book Medical Publishers, 1974.

Crowley LV: *Introducing Concepts in Anatomy and Physiology.* Chicago, Year Book Medical Publishers, 1976.

DesJardins T: *Cardiopulmonary Anatomy and Physiology: Essentials for Respiratory Care.* New York, Delmar Publishers, 1988.

Feneis H: *Pocket Atlas of Human Anatomy*, ed 4. Chicago, Year Book Medical Publishers, 1976.

Fraser RG, Paré JA: *Organ Physiology: Structure and Function of the Lung.* Philadelphia, WB Saunders Co, 1977.

Grant JCB: *An Atlas of Anatomy*, ed 5. Baltimore, Williams & Wilkins Co, 1962.

Gray H, Goss CM: *Gray's Anatomy of the Human Body*, ed 30. Philadelphia, Lea & Febiger, 1979.

Guyton AC: *Textbook of Medical Physiology*, ed 6. Philadelphia, WB Saunders Co, 1981.

Jacob SW, Francone CA: *Structure and Function in Man*, ed 4. Philadelphia, WB Saunders Co, 1979.

McLaughlin AJ: *Essentials of Physiology for Advanced Respiratory Therapy*. St Louis, CV Mosby Co, 1977.

Murray JF: *The Normal Lung*. Philadelphia, WB Saunders Co, 1976.

Ruch TC, Patton HD: *Physiology and Biophysics*, ed 20. Philadelphia, WB Saunders Co, 1974.

Shapiro BA, Harrison RA, Kacmarek RM, et al: *Clinical Application of Respiratory Care*, ed 3. Chicago, Year Book Medical Publishers, 1985.

Shibel EM, Moser KM: *Respiratory Emergencies*. St Louis, CV Mosby Co, 1977.

Slonim NB, Hamilton LH: *Respiratory Physiology*, ed 2. St Louis, CV Mosby Co, 1971.

Spearman CB, Sheldon RL, Egan DF: *Egan's Fundamentals of Respiratory Therapy*, ed 4. St Louis, CV Mosby Co, 1982.

Chapter 4

Mechanics of Ventilation

I. The Lung-Thorax System
   A. As described in Chapter 3, both the lung and the thorax are lined by thin tissues; the parietal pleura on the inside of the thoracic cage and the visceral pleura on the outside of the lung and mediastinum.
   B. These two pleura are in contact with each other, being separated by only a thin film of fluid.
   C. Since the lungs have a tendency to contract inward and the thorax to expand outward, during normal breathing a negative (subatmospheric) pressure is maintained between the pleura (Fig 4–1).
   D. A convenient way of viewing the lung-thorax system is to consider it a two-springed system held together by the pleura (Fig 4–2). The thorax can be conceptualized as a band spring tending to expand outward and the lung as a coil spring tending to contract inward.'
   E. If the sternum is split, the lung and thorax move to their independent resting positions (see Fig 4–1).
      1. The lung collapses.
      2. The thorax expands.
   F. If air is allowed to enter the potential pleural space, a pneumothorax develops.
   G. Any interference with the integrity of the pleura interferes with ventilation.
II. Pulmonary Pressures and Gradients
   A. Six pressures are associated with ventilation:
      1. Mouth pressure: The pressure at the entry of the respiratory system, synonymous with end-expiratory pressure or airway opening pressure.
      2. Alveolar pressure: The pressure within the alveoli, normally assumed to be equal to end-expiratory pressure; also referred to as intrapulmonary pressure, or mouth pressure, when no gas flow exists.
      3. Pleural pressure: The pressure within the potential pleural space; also referred to as intrathoracic pressure.
      4. Esophageal pressure: The pressure at the level of the midesophagus. When the pressure is properly determined, changes in midesophageal pressure reflect changes in pleural pressure.

63

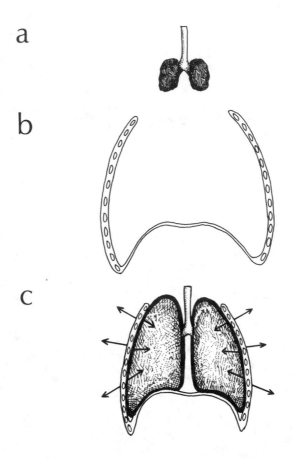

FIG 4–1.
A, resting state of normal lungs when removed from the chest cavity (i.e., elasticity causes total collapse). **B,** resting state of normal chest wall and diaphragm when apex is open to atmosphere and the thoracic contents removed. **C,** end-expiration in the normal, intact thorax. Note that elastic forces of lung and chest wall are in opposite directions. The pleural surfaces link these two opposing forces (see text). (From Shapiro BA, Harrison RA, Kacmarek RM, et al: *Clinical Application of Respiratory Care,* ed 3. Chicago, Year Book Medical Publishers, 1985. Used by permission.)

     5. Body surface pressure: Atmospheric pressure.
     6. Abdominal pressure: Pressure measured in the abdominal cavity.
  B. When the mechanics of breathing are discussed, four pressure gradients are commonly defined:
     1. Transpulmonary pressure (TPP): The pressure difference across the lung (pleural-alveolar pressure).
     2. Transthoracic pressure: The pressure difference across the thorax, including chest and diaphragm (pleural-body surface pressure).
     3. Transrespiratory pressure: The pressure difference across the lung-thorax system; also referred to as the transairway pressure (alveolar-body surface pressure).
     4. Transdiaphragmatic pressure: The pressure difference across the diaphragm (abdominal-pleural pressure).
III. Inspiration
  A. Figures 4–3 and 4–4 depict the intrapleural (intrathoracic) and intrapulmonary pressure curves during normal resting ventilation.

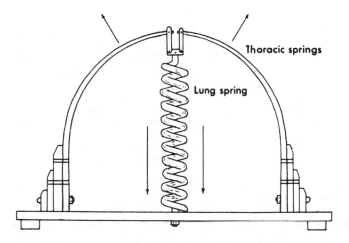

FIG 4–2.
The lung-thorax system may be conceptualized as two springs opposing the movement of each other, the thoracic band spring tending to expand and the lung coil spring tending to contract. (From Spearman CB, Sheldon RL, Egan DL: *Egan's Fundamentals of Respiratory Therapy,* ed 4. St Louis, CV Mosby Co, 1982. Used by permission.)

    B. At functional residual capacity (FRC) level or resting exhalation, the intrapleural pressure is about −5 cm H_2O, whereas the intrapulmonary pressure is zero (atmospheric).
        1. The TPP at FRC is thus equal to 5 cm H_2O.
        2. The TPP is also referred to as the alveolar distending pressure.
    C. Since the lung is a valveless pump, when gas flow stops, intrapulmonary and atmospheric pressures are equal; that is, the transrespiratory pressure gradient is zero.
        1. A negative transrespiratory pressure causes gas to enter the lung.
        2. A positive transrespiratory pressure causes gas to exit the lung.

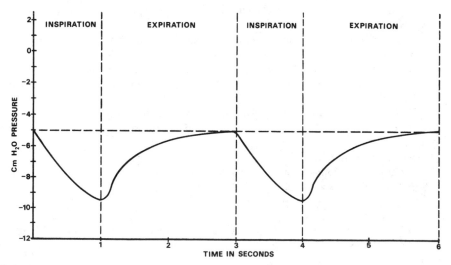

FIG 4–3.
Intrapleural (intrathoracic) pressure curve during normal spontaneous ventilation. Note that normal resting expiratory pressure is about −5 cm H_2O and decreases to −9 cm H_2O during inspiration.

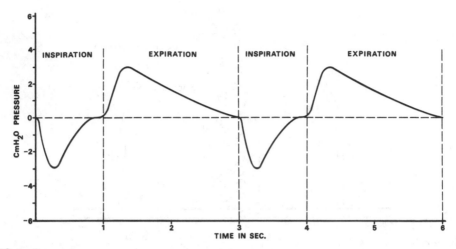

FIG 4–4.
Intrapulmonary pressure during normal spontaneous ventilation has a peak inspiratory pressure of about -3 cm H_2O and peak expiratory pressure of about $+3$ cm H_2O.

    D. This gradient is established by contraction of the diaphragm and the external inter-costal muscles.

    E. As a result, the thoracic cavity expands, causing the intrapleural pressure to become more negative (about -9 cm H_2O).

    F. This pressure drop increases the volume of the lung. Remember that because of the adherence of the pleura, the lungs must expand as the thorax expands.

    G. The expansion of the lung decreases the intrapulmonary pressure to about -3 cm H_2O.

    H. The decreased intrapulmonary pressure establishes a pressure gradient with the atmosphere, causing gas to enter the lung.

    I. Once the intrapulmonary pressure is returned to normal by gas entering the lung, inspiration stops.

    J. All of the pressure-volume changes described are explained by Boyle's law.

  IV. Exhalation

    A. Exhalation is normally a passive process. The lung-thorax system is returned to its resting state as a result of the elastic recoil of the lung.

    B. Relaxation of the muscles of inspiration allows the intrapleural pressure to return to baseline (-5 cm H_2O); as a result, the intrapulmonary pressure increases to about $+3$ cm H_2O.

    C. Since the transrespiratory pressure is positive, gas leaves the lung.

    D. Lung volume returns to the FRC level, and the transrespiratory pressure returns to zero.

  V. Resistance to Ventilation

    A. Ventilation is opposed by three major factors:

      1. Elastic resistance

      2. Nonelastic resistance

      3. Inertia

    B. Elastic resistance is a result of distention of pulmonary elastic tissue. The subdivisions of elastic resistance are:

      1. Surface tension

      2. Compliance

C. Nonelastic resistance is primarily the resistance to gas flow. It is equivalent to the frictional resistance of solids moving across each other. The subdivisions of nonelastic resistance are:
   1. Airway resistance
   2. Tissue viscous resistance
D. Inertia is the tendency of a body in motion to stay in motion and a body at rest to stay at rest.
   1. During ventilation, effort is required to move the nonelastic structures of the lung thoracic system (bone, blood, etc.).
   2. In general, inertia contributes in only a minor manner to the resistance to ventilation.
E. Total resistance to ventilation is commonly referred to as *impedance.*

VI. Surface Tension
A. Surface tension is the force occurring at the interface between a liquid and another liquid or a gas that tends to cause the liquid to occupy the smallest volume possible (see Chapter 2).
B. Surface tension causes alveoli to decrease in size and would cause collapse were it not for the presence of a pulmonary surfactant secreted by type II alveolar cells.
C. The volume of surfactant produced by the respiratory tract is relatively constant. The effect the surfactant exerts is indirectly related to the surface area it covers.
D. At FRC there is a large amount of surfactant applied per unit area. This causes a significant reduction in pressure as a result of surface tension, with the following results:
   1. Prevention of alveolar collapse on exhalation (preventing alveoli from reaching their critical volume).
   2. Reduction in pressure needed to overcome surface tension as inspiration begins.
E. At maximum inspiration, a small volume of surfactant is applied per unit area. Thus, the pressure as a result of surface tension tending to collapse the alveoli is great. This pressure assists in normal passive exhalation.
F. Pressures as a result of surface tension:
   1. At maximal inspiration: About 40 dynes/sq cm.
   2. At maximal exhalation: About 2 to 4 dynes/sq cm.
G. The effect of surface tension cannot be evaluated directly. Changes in surface tension cause a change in compliance.
H. An increase in surface tension increases elastic resistance to ventilation and is reflected in a decrease in compliance, causing an increase in the work of breathing.

VII. Compliance
A. Compliance is the ease of distention of the lung-thorax system and is inversely related to elastance (see Chapter 2).
B. Compliance is normally a static measurement so as to eliminate the effects of nonelastic resistance.
C. Compliance is determined by comparing the change in volume in a system with the pressure necessary to maintain the volume change:

$$C = \frac{\Delta V}{\Delta P} \qquad (1)$$

D. In the respiratory system, there are basically three types of compliance:
   1. Pulmonary (C_{pul})
   2. Thoracic (C_{th})
   3. Total (C_{tol})

E. In the lung-thorax system, the tendency of the lung is to collapse to its resting position, whereas the tendency of the thorax is to expand to its resting position.

F. The FRC is that volume maintained in the lung at resting expiratory position as a result of the opposing effects of pulmonary and thoracic compliance.

G. Total compliance of the lung-thorax system is a result of the interaction of pulmonary and thoracic compliance.

H. Compliance is linear only at relatively normal tidal volumes. As the lung volume exceeds or falls below tidal levels, compliance decreases. Thus, the total compliance curve is significantly distorted as lung volume approaches residual volume (RV) or total lung capacity (TLC) (Fig 4–5).

　1. As lung volume approaches TLC, the tendency of the lung to collapse far outweighs the tendency of the thorax to expand. Specifically, the thorax reaches its resting position at 70% of TLC. Beyond this level the thorax tends to collapse. Since the lung has been distorted significantly beyond its resting position, continued pulmonary expansion requires significant force. At TLC the organism cannot exert sufficient force to continue expansion (Fig 4–6).

　2. As the lung volume approaches RV, the tendency of the thorax to expand far outweighs the tendency of the lung to collapse. This occurs because the lung is now near its resting point, whereas the thorax is significantly distorted from its resting point. At RV, the tendency of the thorax to expand is so great that the individual cannot voluntarily exhale a larger volume (see Fig 4–6).

I. Total compliance is determined by dividing the tidal volume (V_T) by the static pressure necessary to maintain V_T in the lung. Pressure should be measured at the patient's mouth. In the average young adult male, total compliance is typically equal to 0.08 to 0.1 L/cm H_2O, or 80 to 100 ml/cm H_2O.

J. Pulmonary compliance is determined by dividing V_T by the static pressure necessary to maintain V_T in the lung. The pressure measured should reflect changes in intrapleural pressures. A pressure reading taken at the level of the midesophagus reflects pleural pressure changes (the patient swallows a balloon pressure transducer and its level is adjusted to a midesophageal position). In the average young man, pulmonary compliance (C_{pul}) is typically equal to 0.2 L/cm H_2O, or 200 ml/cm H_2O.

K. Thoracic compliance (C_{th}) is a calculated value based on the following equation:

$$\frac{1}{C_{total}} = \frac{1}{C_{pul}} + \frac{1}{C_{th}} \tag{2}$$

In the average young adult male, thoracic compliance is typically equal to 0.2 L/cm H_2O, or 200 ml/cm H_2O.

L. Changes in total compliance (C_{total}) reflect total elastic resistance to ventilation.

　1. Total compliance reflects surface tension and tissue elastance.

　2. A decrease in total compliance results in a decrease in FRC.

　3. An increase in total compliance results in an increase in FRC.

　4. Alterations in pulmonary or thoracic compliance result in an alteration of total compliance.

M. With an increase in total compliance, there is a corresponding decrease in elastance. This tends to increase the ease of inspiration but also increases the difficulty of expiration. In this situation a slow, deep ventilatory pattern may be assumed to minimize the work of breathing (see Chapter 18).

N. With a decrease in total compliance, there is a corresponding increase in elastance. This tends to decrease the ease of inspiration but increases the ease of exhalation. In this situation a rapid, shallow ventilatory pattern may be assumed to minimize the work of breathing (see Chapter 18).

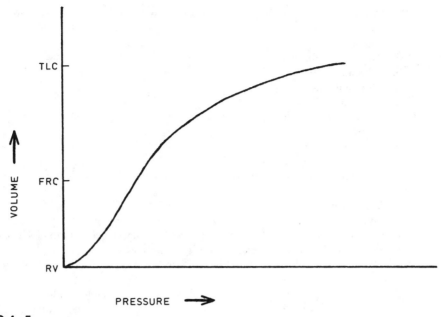

FIG 4–5.
Total compliance curve of the lung-thorax system. Compliance changes linearly about the functional residual capacity *(FRC)*. However, as lung volume nears either residual volume *(RV)* or total lung capacity *(TLC)*, the pressure needed to cause a volume change increases.

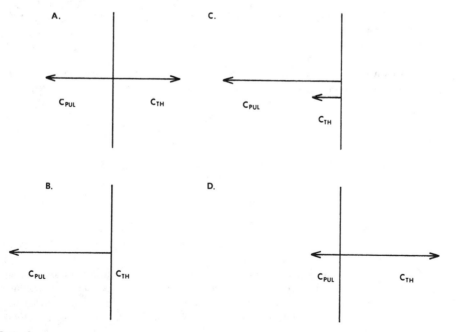

FIG 4–6.
Pulmonary *(C_{pul})* and thoracic *(C_{th})* compliance (elastance) vector forces compared at different lung volumes. **A,** at FRC, the vector forces of C_{pul} and C_{th} are equal and opposite in direction. **B,** at 70% of TLC, the thorax is at its resting position, and C_{pul} tends to cause lung volume to decrease. **C,** at TLC, the vector forces of both C_{pul} and C_{th} tend to decrease lung volume. **D,** at RV, the lung is near its resting level; therefore, its vector is decreased, whereas the vector force of the thorax tends to expand the system.

O. Total compliance is decreased by any pathophysiologic change that inhibits lung expansion:
1. Pneumonitis
2. Pulmonary consolidation
3. Pulmonary edema
4. Pneumothorax
5. Abdominal distention
6. Adult respiratory distress syndrome (ARDS)
7. Pulmonary fibrosis
8. Thoracic deformities
9. Complete airway obstruction
P. Total compliance may be increased by any factor that causes a loss of elastic lung tissue.
1. Alveolar septal destruction
2. Alveolar distention
Q. Specific compliance is a method of comparing the compliance of individuals of different sizes or different lung units in the same individual.
1. The formula for its determination takes into consideration the patient's measured FRC.
2. Specific compliance (C_s) is equal to pulmonary compliance divided by the patient's FRC and normally is equal to about 0.08 (dimensionless number):

$$C_s = \frac{C_{pul}}{FRC} = 0.08 \tag{3}$$

3. Specific compliance can be determined for a lung segment or lobe (Fig 4–7).
VIII. Airway Resistance
A. Airway resistance results from the movement of molecules of inspired gas over the surface of the airway.
B. Airway resistance accounts for about 85% of nonelastic resistance to ventilation.
C. Airway resistance (R) in laminar flow situations is equal to

$$R = \frac{\Delta P}{\dot{V}} \tag{4}$$

whereas in turbulent flow situations the relationship is:

$$R = \frac{\Delta P}{\dot{V}^2} \tag{5}$$

D. More than 60% of normal airway resistance is a result of turbulent gas flow through the nose, pharynx, and larynx.
E. Resistance to gas flow decreases as gas moves into smaller generations of the airway. Since the cross-sectional area of the respiratory tract increases dramatically with increasing generations, flow through any single airway becomes progressively smaller. The pressure necessary to maintain that flow decreases as does total airway resistance.
F. At the level of the respiratory bronchioles, flow is almost absent and gas movement basically is a result of diffusion.
G. Airway resistance is increased when the lumen of the airway is decreased. The airway lumen is primarily decreased as a result of:
1. Bronchospasm

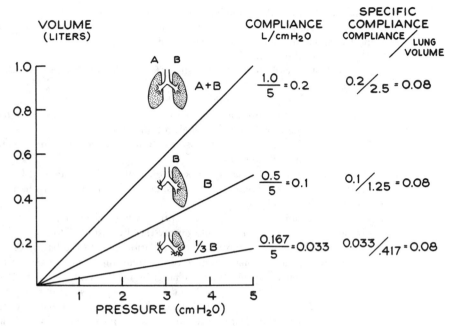

FIG 4–7.
Compliance and specific compliance for both lungs, one lung, and one lobe. Compliance decreases with decreasing lung volume; specific compliance does not. (From Comroe JR: *Physiology of Respiration*. Chicago, Year Book Medical Publishers, 1965. Used by permission.)

    2. Mucosal edema
    3. Partial airway obstruction (retained secretions)
  H. Normal airway resistance is equal to about 0.6 to 2.4 cm $H_2O/L/sec$ when measured at a standard flow rate of 0.5 L/sec.
IX. Tissue Viscous Resistance
  A. The force necessary to overcome the inertia of the nonelastic structures of the lung-thorax system (i.e., bone, pleurae sliding over each other).
  B. Tissue viscous resistance accounts for about 15% of the nonelastic resistance to ventilation.
X. Functional Residual Capacity
  A. As stated previously, the thorax tends to expand, whereas the lung tends to collapse. At the FRC level, the vector forces of pulmonary and thoracic elastance are equal in magnitude and opposite in direction.
  B. The FRC is the most stable of all lung volumes and capacities because it is the level that is assumed when complete relaxation of ventilatory muscles occurs.
  C. If the elastance of the thorax and/or the lung were to increase or decrease, the volume of FRC would be altered.
XI. Ventilation/Perfusion Relationships
  A. Distribution of ventilation is unequal because of:
    1. Variation in compliance and airway resistance within the lung.
      a. If the compliance of part of the lung is multipled by resistance of that part of the lung, a time constant is determined:

$$\text{Compliance} \times \text{Resistance} = \text{Time constant} \qquad (6)$$

      b. The time constant of a lung unit determines the amount of time it takes for that unit to fill.

2. Regional variation in TPP throughout the respiratory tract.
   a. In the vertical position, the TPP gradient is greater in the apices than in the bases. The reasons for this variation are:
      (1) Weight of the lung.
      (2) Effect of gravity on the total system, forcing blood flow to dependent areas.
      (3) Support of lung at the hilum.
   b. Transpulmonary pressure differences cause alveoli in the apices to contain a greater volume at FRC level than alveoli in the bases.
   c. As a result of TPP gradients at FRC, alveoli in the apices contain a greater volume than those in the bases.
   d. These differences in alveolar size decrease as lung volume nears TLC.
3. As a result of differing pulmonary time constants and TPP gradients when one inspires from FRC level:
   a. Alveoli in the apices fill slowly and empty slowly (slow alveoli).
   b. Alveoli in the bases fill rapidly and empty rapidly (fast alveoli).
   c. In normal tidal exchange most of the ventilation goes to the bases. Figure 4–8 illustrates the compliance curve of the total lung. The position of the apices on the curve during tidal exchange is on the flatter aspect of the curve, whereas the bases are positioned on the steeper aspect of the curve. Points *B* to *B'* indicate the volume change during normal ventilation in the bases; points *A* to *A'* indicate the volume change during normal ventilation of the apices. There is a considerably larger volume change in the bases than in the apices per unit pressure change.

B. Distribution of pulmonary blood flow normally is greater in the bases than in the apices.
   1. Perfusion of any aspect of the lung depends on the relationship between pulmonary hydrostatic pressure and the TPP gradient.

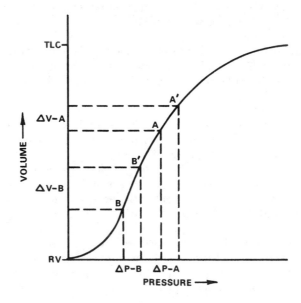

FIG 4–8.
Compliance curve of total lung at functional residual capacity. *A* to *A'* indicates volume change in the apices during tidal exchange; *B* to *B'* indicates volume change in the bases during tidal exchange. The change in volume of *B* (ΔV-B) is greater than the change in volume of *A* (ΔV A) for the same pressure change (ΔP-B is equal to P-A).

2. Since the pulmonary vascular system is a low-pressure system, in the erect individual the apices of the lung receive virtually no blood flow, whereas the bases are engorged with blood because of the effect of gravity.
3. In general, the most gravity-dependent aspect of the lung receives the majority of the blood flow, whereas the least gravity-dependent areas receive little or no blood flow.
4. Basically, in the upright lung, three zones exist (Fig 4–9):
   a. Zone 1: The extreme apex, where there is virtually no blood flow.
   b. Zone 2: The remainder of the apex and middle part of the lung, where blood flow is intermittent.
   c. Zone 3: The bases, where blood flow is constant.

C. Ventilation/perfusion ratios ($\dot{V}/\dot{Q}$ ratios).
   1. The overall $\dot{V}/\dot{Q}$ ratio for the lung is 0.8.
   2. In the apices the $\dot{V}/\dot{Q}$ ratio is about 3.3; in the bases it is about 0.6.
   3. During normal ventilation and perfusion:
      a. Bases are better perfused than apices.
      b. Bases are better ventilated than apices.
      c. Apices are better ventilated than perfused.
      d. Bases are better perfused than ventilated.

XII. Ideal Alveolar Gas Equation
   A. In addition to the effects of P_{H_2O} on the partial pressure of gases in the alveoli, the carbon dioxide diffusing from the bloodstream into the alveoli will further decrease alveolar P_{O_2}.
   B. Since carbon dioxide is leaving the bloodstream, a closed system, and entering the respiratory tract, an open system, there is an indirect relationship between the alveolar pressures of carbon dioxide and oxygen. Increases in $P_{A_{CO_2}}$ result in decreases in $P_{A_{O_2}}$.
   C. This indirect relationship basically involves only carbon dioxide and oxygen because they are the only metabolically active gases.

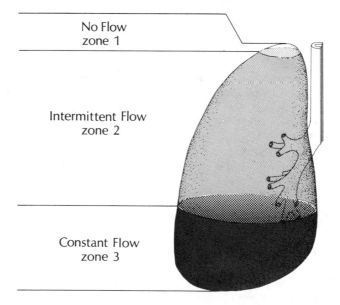

FIG 4–9.
The three-zone pulmonary blood flow model illustrating the effects of gravity on pulmonary perfusion (see text). (From Shapiro BA, Harrison RA, Kacmarek RM, et al: *Clinical Application of Respiratory Care*, ed 3. Chicago, Year Book Medical Publishers, 1985. Used by permission.)

D. In addition, the amount of oxygen and carbon dioxide moving across the alveolar capillary membrane is unequal, 200 ml of carbon dioxide being produced for every 250 ml of oxygen consumed. Thus, the respiratory exchange ratio (R) must be considered when estimating the alveolar P_{O_2}.

E. The ideal alveolar gas equation is

$$P_{A_{O_2}} = (P_B - P_{H_2O})(F_{I_{O_2}}) - (Pa_{CO_2})\left(F_{I_{O_2}} + \frac{1 - F_{I_{O_2}}}{R}\right) \qquad (7)$$

R normally equals 0.8. Pa_{CO_2} is used instead of $P_{A_{CO_2}}$ because under physiologic conditions compatible with life these are equal, and $P_{A_{CO_2}}$ is impossible to determine clinically.

F. A modification of equation (7) may be used for gross estimations of $P_{A_{O_2}}$:

$$P_{A_{O_2}} = (P_B - P_{H_2O})(F_{I_{O_2}}) - \frac{Pa_{CO_2}}{0.8} \qquad (8)$$

XIII. Work of Breathing
   A. Work associated with ventilation can be discussed from two perspectives:
      1. Mechanical principles associated with the performance of work.
      2. Total energy required for ventilatory work (cost of breathing). This topic is discussed in Chapters 11 and 19.
   B. Work (W) is defined as a force (F) applied, multiplied by a distance (D) moved:

$$W = F \times D \qquad (9)$$

   C. Thus, regardless of energy expenditure, no work is performed unless movement occurs.
   D. This relationship can be applied to the respiratory system since pressure (P) is a force per unit area and volume (V) represents a distance multiplied by an area:

$$W = P \times V \qquad (10)$$

   E. Total mechanical work is equal to lung work, plus chest wall work.
   F. Measurement of total mechanical work is illustrated in Figure 4–10.
   G. For measurement of total work, the lung-thorax system must be inflated with positive pressure in an apneic individual.
      1. During inflation, pressure change in the airway or at the mouth is measured, as is V_T, and plotted against each other (Fig 4–10).
      2. Tidal ventilation is represented by the vertical distance 1 to 3, whereas pressure required to maintain thoracic expansion is represented by the horizontal distance 3 to 2.
      3. The total mechanical work is indicated by the shaded triangle 1, 2, and 3, plus area A.
      4. Work required to overcome elastic for es is depicted by the shaded areas 1, 2, and 3.
      5. Work required to overcome nonelastic forces is depicted by area A.
      6. Work required to overcome inertial forces cannot be separated from elastic and nonelastic work by this method.
      7. The elastic and nonelastic workloads are always additive.
      8. Elastic work of inspiration is stored in the elastic structures of the thoracic cavity, whereas nonelastic work cannot be stored.
      9. Also, remember, nonelastic forces are active only during gas movement.

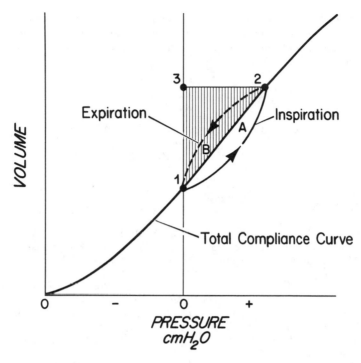

FIG 4–10.
Pressure-volume loop during tidal volume delivery via controlled positive pressure ventilation. The distance 1 to 3 equals tidal volume, and the distance 3 to 2 equals pressure change. Area *A* represents nonelastic inspiratory work, area *B* represents nonelastic expiratory work, and the shaded area represents elastic inspiratory work. (From Kacmarek RM: *Respir Care* 1988; 33:99–120. Used by permission.)

    10. Exhalation is normally passive so long as the work of exhalation does not exceed the stored elastic work. Area B is the nonelastic work required during passive exhalation. Exhalation will become active if the area of B exceeds the shaded areas 1, 2, and 3, which represent the elastic work stored during inspiration.

  H. Figure 4–10 would also represent the work of the lung if the pressure gradient used was the TPP, since the pleural pressure change represents the pressure required to move the lung, and the individual was breathing spontaneously.

  I. Chest wall work (WOB_C) is not normally directly measured. It is usually calculated from lung work (WOB_L) and total mechanical work (WOB_T):

$$WOB_T = WOB_L + WOB_C \tag{11}$$

  J. The following are normal values for total lung and chest wall work in healthy individuals:

	kg − m/L	joules/L
WOB_T	0.07–0.10	0.70–1.0
WOB_L	0.035–0.05	0.35–0.5
WOB_C	0.035–0.05	0.35–0.5

K. Workloads are also expressed over a 1-minute period. This is normally referred to as a representation of ventilatory power. If minute volume were equal to 6 L, the following values for power in kg · m/min and joules/min would be noted in normal adults:

	kg · m/min	joules/min
Total ventilatory power	0.42–0.60	4.2–6.0
Lung power	0.21–0.30	2.1–3.0
Chest wall power	0.21–0.30	2.1–3.0

BIBLIOGRAPHY

Bendixen HH, et al: *Respiratory Care.* St Louis, CV Mosby Co, 1965.

Burton GC, Hodgkin JE: *Respiratory Care,* ed 2. Philadelphia, JB Lippincott Co, 1984.

Cherniack RM, Cherniack L: *Respiration in Health and Disease,* ed 3. Philadelphia, WB Saunders Co, 1983.

Comroe JH: *Physiology of Respiration,* ed 2. Chicago, Year Book Medical Publishers, 1974.

Dejours P: *Respiration.* New York, Oxford University Press, 1966.

Forster RE, Dubois AB, Briscoe WA, et al: *The Lung-Physiologic Basis of Pulmonary Function Tests.* Chicago, Year Book Medical Publishers, 1986.

Frownfelter DL: *Chest Physical Therapy and Pulmonary Rehabilitation.* Chicago, Year Book Medical Publishers, 1979.

Guyton AC: *Textbook of Medical Physiology,* ed 6. Philadelphia, WB Saunders Co, 1980.

Hedley-Whyte J, Burgess GE, Feeley TW, et al: *Applied Physiology of Respiratory Care.* Boston, Little, Brown & Co, 1976.

Kacmarek RM: The role of pressure support ventilation in reducing work of breathing. *Respir Care* 1988; 33:99–120.

McLaughlin AJ: *Essentials of Physiology for Advanced Respiratory Therapy.* St Louis, CV Mosby Co, 1977.

Murray JF: *The Normal Lung,* ed 2. Philadelphia, WB Saunders Co, 1987.

Nunn JF: *Applied Respiratory Physiology With Special Reference to Anaesthesia,* ed 2. Stoneham, Mass, Butterworth, 1977.

Petty TL: *Intensive and Rehabilitative Respiratory Care,* ed 3. Philadelphia, Lea & Febiger, 1982.

Roussos C, Macklem PT: *The Thorax.* New York, Marcel Dekker, parts A and B, 1985.

Shapiro BA, Harrison RA, Kacmarek RM, et al: *Clinical Application of Respiratory Care,* ed 3. Chicago, Year Book Medical Publishers, 1985.

Spearman CB, Sheldon RL, Egan DF: *Egan's Fundamentals of Respiratory Therapy,* ed 4. St Louis, CV Mosby Co, 1982.

Tisi GM: *Pulmonary Physiology in Clinical Medicine,* ed 2. Baltimore, Williams & Wilkins Co, 1983.

West JB: *Ventilation/Blood Flow and Gas Exchange,* ed 3. Boston, Blackwell Scientific Publications, 1977.

West JB: *Respiratory Physiology: The Essentials,* ed 2. Baltimore, Williams & Wilkins Co, 1979.

Whitcomb ME: *The Lung Normal and Diseased.* St Louis, CV Mosby Co, 1982.

Chapter 5

Neurologic Control of Ventilation

I. The following areas located throughout the organism each play specific roles in the neurologic control of ventilation:
   A. Cerebral cortex
   B. Pons
   C. Medulla oblongata
   D. Spinal cord
   E. Upper airway reflexes
   F. Vagus (cranial X) nerve
   G. Glossopharyngeal (cranial IX) nerve
   H. Peripheral chemoreceptors
   I. Central chemoreceptors
II. Cerebral Cortex
   A. Initiates all conscious respiratory control.
   B. Mediates ventilatory changes as a result of pain, anxiety, or other emotional stimuli.
   C. Governs ventilatory control during speech.
III. Pons
   A. Two distinct centers in the pons contain afferent respiratory neurons.
      1. Pneumotaxic center
         a. Located in upper pons.
         b. Afferent impulses from pneumotaxic center "fine tune" ventilatory rhythmicity by inhibiting length of inspiration.
         c. Modulates the respiratory system's response to hypercarbia, hypoxia, and lung inflation.
         d. However, rhythmic ventilation may exist even when the pneumotaxic center is impaired.
         e. If the pneumotaxic center is destroyed, apneustic ventilation (long, sustained inspirations) occurs.
      2. Apneustic center
         a. Located in lower pons.
         b. Afferent impulses from apneustic center cause a sustained inspiratory pattern; apneustic breathing.
         c. However, normal rhythmic ventilation can exist without the apneustic center.
         d. If the apneustic and pneumotaxic centers are destroyed, a rapid, irregular, gasping respiratory pattern develops.

IV. Medulla Oblongata
   A. Located within the medulla oblongata is the respiratory control center, which receives afferent impulses from all other areas in the organism (Fig 5–1).
   B. Afferent impulses are interpreted and efferent impulses are initiated in the medulla oblongata.
   C. The medullary respiratory center maintains the normal rhythmic pattern of ventilation.
   D. Two fairly distinct areas in the medulla contain respiratory neurons.
      1. Dorsal respiratory group
         a. Functions as initial processing center of afferent impulses.
         b. Originates inspiratory efferent impulses, which travel to ventral respiratory neurons and spinal cord.
      2. Ventral respiratory group
         a. Functions primarily by sending efferent impulses to all expiratory motor neurons.
         b. Originates some inspiratory efferent impulses.
   E. Areas from which afferent impulses are sent to the medulla oblongata:
      1. Cerebral cortex
      2. Pons
      3. Upper airway reflexes
      4. Vagus (cranial X) nerve
      5. Peripheral chemoreceptors
V. Spinal Cord
   A. Axons from the higher brain centers descend into the spinal cord.
   B. These projecting axons influence phrenic intercostal and abdominal motorneuron stimulation.
   C. Ventilatory skeletal muscle is thus stimulated.

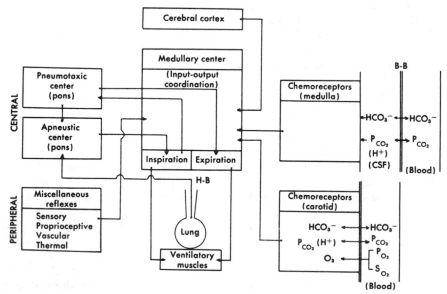

FIG 5–1.
Interrelationships among all areas responsible for ventilatory control (see text). (From Spearman CB, Sheldon RL, Egan DF: *Egan's Fundamentals of Respiratory Therapy*, ed 4. St Louis, CV Mosby Co, 1982. Used by permission.)

    D. Skeletal muscle is composed of two types of contractile fibers:
        1. Extrafusal fibers (main muscle): Contraction of these fibers is responsible for actual muscular contraction.
        2. Fusimotor fibers (muscle spindle fibers): These fibers are organs of proprioception that determine the extent of muscle contraction necessary to perform a certain workload.
    E. Ventilatory reflexes, such as cough and hiccup, are mediated by the spinal cord.
    F. Ascending spinal pathways transmit sensations of pain, touch, temperature, as well as proprioception to higher brain centers.

VI. Upper Airway Reflexes
    A. Nose
        1. Stimulation of nasal mucosa may cause exhalation.
        2. Exhalation is frequently in the form of a sneeze.
        3. Apnea and bradycardia also may result from nasal stimulation.
    B. Nasopharynx
        1. Stimulation may cause the sniff or aspiration reflex.
        2. A rapid inspiration is initiated to move the irritant from nasopharynx to oropharynx.
        3. Stimulation may also cause bronchodilation and hypertension.
    C. Larynx
        1. Stimulation may result in afferent impulses, causing:
            a. Apnea
            b. Slow, deep breathing
            c. Coughing
            d. Hypertension
            e. Bronchoconstriction
    D. Trachea
        1. Stimulation may result in afferent impulses, causing:
            a. Coughing
            b. Bronchoconstriction
            c. Hypertension

VII. Vagus Nerve
    A. Afferent impulses via the vagus nerve originate from two areas:
        1. Baroreceptors
            a. Located in the aortic arch.
            b. Stimulated by variations in blood pressure.
            c. Afferent impulses from baroreceptors cause alteration of vascular tone to maintain normal blood pressure levels.
            d. Ventilatory response is minimal.
                (1) Hyperventilation may be caused by hypotension.
                (2) Hypoventilation may be caused by hypertension.
        2. Pulmonary reflexes
            a. Pulmonary stretch receptors (Hering-Breuer reflex)
                (1) Pulmonary stretch receptors are located in the smooth muscle of conducting airways.
                (2) These receptors are stimulated by lung inflation, deflation, and increased transpulmonary pressures.
                (3) They are slowly adaptive to changes in inflating pressure.
                (4) Stimulation of these receptors may cause:
                    (a) Increased expiratory time
                    (b) Decreased respiratory rate
                    (c) Bronchodilation

        (d) Tachycardia

        (e) Vasoconstriction

     (5) Integration of information from these receptors assists in determining the rate and depth of breathing.

   b. Irritant receptors

     (1) Irritant receptors are located in the epithelium of trachea, bronchi, larynx, nose, and pharynx.

     (2) They are rapidly adaptive.

     (3) Stimulation is caused by:

        (a) Inspired irritants (histamine, ammonia)

        (b) Mechanical factors (particulate matter)

        (c) Anaphylaxis

        (d) Pneumothorax

        (e) Pulmonary congestion

     (4) Stimulation may result in:

        (a) Bronchoconstriction

        (b) Hyperpnea

        (c) Constriction of larynx (laryngospasm)

        (d) Closure of glottis

        (e) Cough

   c. Type J (juxtapulmonary-capillary) receptors

     (1) Located in the walls of pulmonary capillaries

     (2) Stimulation is caused by:

        (a) Increased interstitial fluid volume

        (b) Pulmonary congestion

        (c) Chemical irritants

        (d) Microembolism

     (3) Stimulation of these receptors may result in:

        (a) Rapid, shallow breathing

        (b) Severe expiratory constriction of larynx

        (c) Hypoventilation and bradycardia

        (d) Inhibition of spinal reflexes

VIII. Glossopharyngeal Nerve

   A. Innervates the peripheral chemoreceptor cells located in the carotid bodies.

   B. Conducts afferent impulses to the medullary respiratory center.

  IX. Peripheral Chemoreceptors

   A. Chemoreceptor cells can differentiate between concentrations or pressures of various substances.

   B. Two groups of peripheral chemoreceptor cells have been identified.

     1. *Carotid bodies*

       a. Located at the bifurcation of the common carotid artery.

       b. Innervated by the glossopharyngeal (cranial IX) nerve.

       c. Stimulated by:

         (1) Decreased Pa_{O_2}

         (2) Decreased pH

         (3) Increased Pa_{CO_2}

     2. *Aortic bodies*

       a. Located in the arch of the aorta.

       b. Innervated by the vagus (cranial X) nerve.

       c. Stimulated by

         (1) Decreased Pa_{O_2}

         (2) Decreased pH

         (3) Increased Pa_{CO_2}

C. In general, a synergistic response from these receptors is noted in the presence of hypoxemia and acidosis.

D. Effects of Pa_{O_2}
   1. Initial stimulation occurs at a Pa_{O_2} of 500 mm Hg and gradually increases as Pa_{O_2} decreases.
   2. Maximum stimulation occurs when Pa_{O_2} is between 40 and 60 mm Hg.
   3. A gradual decrease in stimulation is noted when Pa_{O_2} is less than 30 mm Hg.
   4. Additional sources of stimulation:
      a. Decreased blood flow
      b. Increased temperature
   5. These cells are primarily affected by oxygen delivery in the form of dissolved oxygen. Any pathophysiologic situation in which oxygen delivery is inadequate for the metabolic needs of these cells results in stimulation.
   6. Conditions having no stimulating effect:
      a. Carbon monoxide poisoning
      b. Anemia

E. Effects of Pa_{CO_2} and H^+ concentrations
   1. The cell membrane is permeable to both H^+ and Pa_{CO_2}.
   2. These cells are directly affected only by H^+ concentrations.
   3. Pa_{CO_2} changes cause a change in H^+ concentration, which may stimulate the receptor.
   4. Thus, Pa_{CO_2} has an indirect effect on these cells.
   5. Stimulation is primarily a result of an increase in H^+ concentration.
   6. Decreases in H^+ concentration have only a minimal effect.
   7. Stimulation of these receptors by an increase in $[H^+]$ causes:
      a. Increased respiratory rate
      b. Increased tidal volume
   8. Stimulation of these receptors by a decrease in $[H^+]$ may cause:
      a. Decreased respiratory rate
      b. Decreased tidal volume
   9. The magnitude of the response of the peripheral chemoreceptors to $[H^+]$ changes is grossly less than that of the central chemoreceptors.

F. These receptors are adaptive over time.

X. Central Chemoreceptors
   A. A poorly defined group of cells located near the ventrolateral surface of the medulla oblongata.
   B. These cells are in contact with cerebral spinal fluid (CSF) and arterial blood.
   C. Actual stimulation is caused by $[H^+]$ of CSF.
   D. The composition of the CSF differs somewhat from that of blood.
      1. Electrolytes similar in content to those in plasma
      2. Low protein content: 15 to 45 mg/100 ml
      3. Pco_2: 50.2 ± 2.6 mm Hg
      4. pH: 7.336 ± 0.012
      5. HCO_3^-: 21.5 ± 1.2 mEq/L
   E. Diffusion across blood-brain barrier
      1. The only readily diffusible substance is carbon dioxide.
      2. HCO_3^- and H^+ also move across the membrane but extremely slowly. Active transport mechanisms and diffusion are believed to be involved in the movement of these two substances.
   F. Mechanism of stimulation
      1. Changes in arterial Pco_2 alter diffusion of carbon dioxide across the blood-brain barrier, causing a change in Pco_2 of the CSF.
      2. The altered Pco_2 level will effect a change in CSF $[H^+]$.

3. The altered $[H^+]$ either stimulates or inhibits ventilation.
4. Increased P_{CO_2} (increased H^+) stimulates ventilation, whereas decreased P_{CO_2} (decreased H^+) inhibits ventilation.

G. Factors influencing CSF carbon dioxide levels:
1. Cerebral blood flow
2. CO_2 production
3. CO_2 content of venous blood
4. CO_2 content of arterial blood
5. Alveolar ventilation

XI. Medullary Adjustments in Compensated Respiratory Acidosis
A. Acute increases in Pa_{CO_2} rapidly cause an increase in CSF P_{CO_2}. This occurs because the blood-CSF barrier is very permeable to CO_2.
B. The increased P_{CO_2} in the CSF causes the CSF pH to decrease, which stimulates the central chemoreceptors.
C. If the organism is unable to increase its level of ventilation, the elevated Pa_{CO_2} and CSF P_{CO_2} levels persist.
D. As a result, the kidney will begin to retain HCO_3^-.
E. As the serum HCO_3^- level increases, active transport mechanisms and diffusion increase the CSF HCO_3^- level.
F. The CSF pH eventually returns to normal as the CSF HCO_3^- level increases.
G. When the CSF pH is returned to normal, the organism responds to changes in Pa_{CO_2} at the new elevated level.
H. Chronically elevated Pa_{CO_2} and CSF P_{CO_2} levels result in:
1. Decreased central chemoreceptor drive to ventilate.
2. Decreased sensitivity to carbon dioxide changes.
I. Because of the decreased sensitivity to carbon dioxide, the organism frequently functions on a hypoxic drive (see Chapter 20).

XII. Medullary Adjustments in Compensated Respiratory Alkalosis
A. Acute decreases in Pa_{CO_2} rapidly cause a decrease in CSF P_{CO_2}.
B. This causes the CSF pH to increase, which inhibits the central chemoreceptors.
C. If the stimulus causing hyperventilation persists, the decreased Pa_{CO_2} and CSF P_{CO_2} levels also persist.
D. As a result, the kidney will begin to excrete more HCO_3^-.
E. As the serum HCO_3^- level decreases, active transport mechanisms and diffusion decrease the CSF HCO_3^- level.
F. The CSF pH eventually returns to normal as the CSF HCO_3^- decreases.
G. When the CSF pH is returned to normal, the organism responds to changes in Pa_{CO_2} at the new decreased level.

XIII. Medullary Adjustments in Compensated Metabolic Acidosis
A. Since H^+ does not readily cross the blood-brain barrier, decreases in plasma pH stimulate the peripheral chemoreceptors.
B. This is interpreted as a rise in Pa_{CO_2}; thus, the peripheral chemoreceptors increase the level of ventilation, decreasing Pa_{CO_2}.
C. The decreased Pa_{CO_2} decreases the CSF P_{CO_2}, which increases the CSF pH, resulting in inhibition to ventilation via the central chemoreceptors.
D. As a result, the peripheral chemoreceptors stimulate ventilation, whereas the central chemoreceptors inhibit ventilation.
E. Since the effect on the peripheral chemoreceptors is the predominant stimulus, there is a stepwise readjustment (decrease) in CSF HCO_3^- levels. This allows normalization of CSF pH and a sustained increase in the drive to ventilate.
F. The maximum response of the respiratory system to a metabolic acidosis does not occur until the CSF pH is normalized.

XIV. Medullary Adjustments in Compensated Metabolic Alkalosis
  A. Since neither H^+ or HCO_3^- readily cross the blood-brain barrier and the peripheral chemoreceptors respond poorly to alkalosis, the respiratory system's response to a metabolic alkalosis is poor unless the alkalosis is significant.
  B. A significant increase in plasma pH causes inhibition of the peripheral chemoreceptors, which inhibits ventilation, resulting in increased Pa_{CO_2}.
  C. The increased Pa_{CO_2} increases the CSF P_{CO_2}, which stimulates ventilation via the central chemoreceptors.
  D. As a result, the peripheral chemoreceptors inhibit ventilation, whereas the central chemoreceptors stimulate ventilation.
  E. Since inhibition of the peripheral chemoreceptors is the predominant stimulus, there is a stepwise readjustment (increase) in the CSF HCO_3^-. This allows a normalization of the CSF pH and a sustained decrease in the drive to ventilate.
  F. It is rare that the Pa_{CO_2} rises above 50 mm Hg unless the metabolic alkalosis is severe. Remember, if the Pa_{CO_2} increases the alveolar P_{O_2} decreases, possibly resulting in hypoxemia, which stimulates ventilation via the peripheral chemoreceptors.
XV. Ventilatory Drive
  A. The drive to breathe is affected by the numerous factors presented earlier. However, many individuals have varying responses to stimuli.
  B. In general, factors that stimulate ventilation include:
    1. Hypoxemia
    2. Hypercarbia
    3. Acidosis
    4. Fever
    5. Infection, sepsis
    6. Stimulation of type J receptors
    7. Pain (somatic)
    8. Fear, anxiety
    9. Pharmacologic stimulants
  C. Those factors depressing ventilation include:
    1. Hypocarbia
    2. Alkalosis
    3. Pain (visceral)
    4. Electrolyte imbalance
    5. Pharmacologic depressants
    6. Fatigue
    7. Mechanical inability of the thoracic cage

BIBLIOGRAPHY

Berger AJ, Mitchell RA, Severinghaus JW: Regulation of respiration: Part 1. *N Engl J Med* 1977; 297:92–97.

Berger AJ, Mitchell RA, Severinghaus JW: Regulation of respiration: Part 2. *N Engl J Med* 1977; 297:138–143.

Berger AJ, Mitchell RA, Severinghaus JW: Regulation of Respiration: Part 3. *N Engl J Med* 1977; 297:194–201.

Cherniack RM, Cherniack L: *Respiration in Health and Disease*, ed 3. Philadelphia, WB Saunders Co, 1983.

Comroe JH: *Physiology of Respiration*, ed 2. Chicago, Year Book Medical Publishers, 1974.

Dejours P: *Respiration*. New York, Oxford University Press, 1966.

Fishman AP, Cherniack NS, Widdicombe JG: *Handbook of Physiology, The Respiratory System*, ed 2. Baltimore, Williams & Wilkens Co, vol II, parts 1 and 2, 1986.

84   *The Essentials of Respiratory Care*

Guyton AC: *Textbook of Medical Physiology,* ed 7. Philadelphia WB Saunders Co, 1982.

Mitchell RA, Berger AJ: Neural regulation of respiration. *Am Rev Respir Dis* 1975; 111:206.

Murray JF: *The Normal Lung,* ed 2. Philadelphia, WB Saunders Co, 1987.

Nunn JF: *Applied Respiratory Physiology,* ed 2. Stoneham, Mass, Butterworth, 1977.

Spearman CB, Sheldon RL, Egoan DF: *Egan's Fundamentals of Respiratory Therapy,* ed 4. St Louis, CV Mosby Co, 1982.

Watchko JF, Standaert TA, Mayock DE, et al: Ventilatory failure during loaded breathing: The role of central neural drive. *J Appl Physiol* 1988; 65:249–255.

West JB: *Respiratory Physiology: The Essentials,* ed 2. Baltimore, Williams & Wilkins Co, 1979.

Chapter 6

Anatomy of the Cardiovascular System

I. Blood
  A. A heterogeneous substance composed of a fluid (plasma) and a cellular component.
  B. Plasma: Whole blood minus the cellular component.
    1. It is a pale yellow (strawlike) color.
    2. Plasma, the interstitial fluid, and the intracellular fluid are the three major body fluids.
    3. Major constituents are water and chemical compounds (solutes).
      a. Water, the solvent, constitutes approximately 90% of plasma.
      b. The major solutes protein, foodstuffs, and electrolytes constitute about 10% of plasma.
    4. Plasma minus clotting factors is called *blood serum*.
  C. Cellular components: Red blood cells (RBCs), white blood cells (WBCs), and platelets (Fig 6–1).
    1. RBCs (erythrocytes): Biconcave disks with a diameter of 7 to 8 μ and a thickness of about 2 μ.
      a. Mature RBCs have no nucleus.
      b. Red blood cells are surrounded by a semipermeable membrane.
        (1) Placed in a hypotonic solution (less than 0.9% NaCl), they will swell and can rupture (hemolysis).
        (2) Placed in a hypertonic solution (greater than 0.9% NaCl), they will shrivel (crenation).
      c. Red blood cells are relatively flexible and are able to accommodate changes in shape without rupturing. This becomes important when they pass through tight spots in the circulation (e.g., capillaries or sinusoids).
      d. Red blood cells are produced in myeloid tissue (red bone marrow); a process termed *erythropoiesis*.
      e. The normal number of RBCs is higher in males than in females.
        (1) Female: 4.1 to 5.1 million RBCs/cu mm
        (2) Male: 4.8 to 6.0 million RBCs/cu mm
      f. Reticulocytes are newly released RBCs that retain a small portion of the hemoglobin-forming endoplasmic reticulum.
        (1) In 2 to 3 days, formation of hemoglobin will be complete. At this point, the endoplasmic reticulum disappears and the cell is a mature erythrocyte.

85

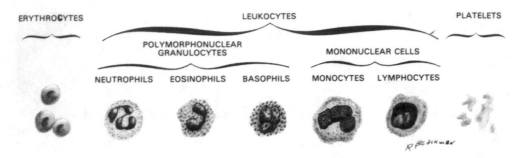

FIG 6–1.
Normal blood cell types. See text for details. (From DesJardins T: *Cardiopulmonary Anatomy and Physiology: Essentials for Respiratory Care.* New York, Delmar Publishers, 1988. Used by permission.)

    (2) The percentage of total RBCs that are reticulocytes indicates the rate of erythropoiesis.

    (3) The normal range (percentage) of reticulocytes is 0.5% to 1.5% of the total number of RBCs.

        (a) More than 1.5% usually indicates increased erythropoiesis.

        (b) Less than 0.5% usually indicates decreased erythropoiesis.

  g. Hemoglobin is the major solute contained within the RBC.

    (1) The normal amount of hemoglobin contained in the blood is higher in males than females:

        (a) Female: 12 to 14 gm of hemoglobin/100 ml of blood

        (b) Male: 13 to 16 gm of hemoglobin/100 ml of blood

  h. The hematocrit is the volume percentage of RBCs in whole blood, for example, a hematocrit equal to 45 means that 45% of whole blood is RBCs by volume.

    (1) The normal hematocrit is higher in males than females:

        (a) Females: 37 to 47

        (b) Male: 40 to 54

  i. Normally hemoglobin levels are equal to about one third of the hematocrit.

2. Types of WBCs (leukocytes): Polymorphonuclear neutrophils, eosinophils and basophils, and mononuclear monocytes and lymphocytes.

  a. Polymorphonuclear leukocytes

    (1) Are formed in myeloid tissue.

    (2) Have a multilobed nucleus.

    (3) Are collectively called *polys.*

    (4) Appear histologically to possess granulated cytoplasm and are collectively termed *granulocytes.*

    (5) All can perform phagocytosis.

    (6) Polymorphonuclear neutrophils

        (a) Have a diameter of about 10 μ.

        (b) Have a nucleus that contains one to five lobes.

        (c) Are highly phagocytic.

        (d) Make up 50% to 75% of the total number of leukocytes.

    (7) Polymorphonuclear eosinophils

        (a) Readily absorb an acid stain.

        (b) Have a bilobed nucleus.

        (c) Are implicated in parasitic as well as allergic processes.

        (d) Make up 2% to 4% of the total number of leukocytes.

        (e) Have a diameter of about 10 μ.

      (8) Polymorphonuclear basophils
- (a) Readily absorb a basic stain.
- (b) Have a three- or four-lobed nucleus.
- (c) Contain heparin, which may serve to prevent coagulation of blood at sites of inflammation.
- (d) Make up less than 0.5% of the total number of leukocytes.
- (e) Have a diameter of about 10 μ.

  b. Mononuclear leukocytes
- (1) Are formed in lymphoid tissue.
- (2) Mononuclear monocytes
    - (a) Have a diameter of 10 to 15 μ.
    - (b) Have a crescent-shaped nucleus.
    - (c) Have cytoplasm containing very fine granules.
    - (d) Are highly phagocytic cells.
    - (e) Make up 3% to 8% of the total number of leukocytes.
- (3) Mononuclear lymphocytes
    - (a) Have a diameter of about 6 to 9 μ.
    - (b) Have a round nucleus.
    - (c) Have cytoplasm that appears clear.
    - (d) Form antibodies that remain intracellular (cellular antibodies) or form antibodies that are released into the bloodstream (circulating antibodies).
    - (e) Make up 20% to 40% of the total number of leukocytes.

  c. Total WBC count has the normal range of 5,000 to 10,000 WBCs/cu mm.

  d. A differential count identifies the percentage of the total WBC count that each WBC type comprises (Table 6–1). (Note normal range [percent] in each of the WBC types previously described.)

  e. Megakaryocyte: A special type of blood cell.
- (1) Formed in myeloid tissue.
- (2) Fragments into small irregular pieces of protoplasm called *thrombocytes* or *platelets*.
    - (a) Are 2 to 4 μ in diameter.
    - (b) Have no nucleus.
    - (c) Have a granular cytoplasm.
    - (d) Normal platelet count is 200,000 to 350,000/cu mm.
    - (e) Function in clot formation (hemostasis).

D. Total blood volume of an individual
1. The total blood volume of an individual is equal to about 70 to 72 ml of blood/kg of body weight.
2. This relationship varies inversely with the amount of excess body fat; in other words, an obese individual has less blood volume per kilogram than a slender individual.

TABLE 6–1.

Normal Function and Percentage Composition of Leukocytes

Type	Function	Percentage Composition
Neutrophil	Phagocytosis	50–75
Eosinophil	Hypersensitivity reaction	2–4
Basophil	Anticoagulation	<0.5
Monocyte	Phagocytosis	3–8
Lymphocyte	Antibody formation	20–40

II. The Blood Vessels (Fig 6–2)
   A. The blood vessels consist of a closed system of connected arteries, arterioles, capillaries, venules, and veins.
   B. *Arteries* contain three characteristic layers: tunica intima, tunica media, and tunica adventitia.
      1. Tunica adventitia (external layer)
         a. It consists of connective tissue surrounding a network of collagenous and elastic fibers.
         b. It supports and protects the blood vessels.
         c. It contains vasa vasorum, very fine vessels that serve the tunica adventitia with its blood supply.
         d. It contains lymphatic vessels and nerve fibers.

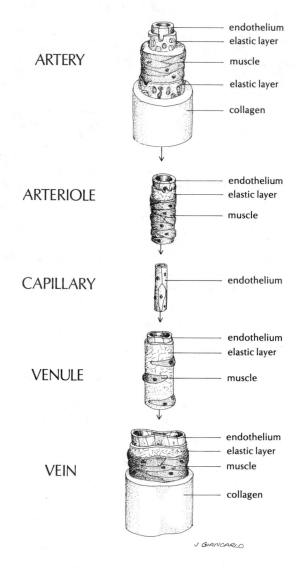

FIG 6–2.
Schematic representation of the anatomic structure of major types of blood vessels (see text). (From Shapiro BA, Harrison RA, Kacmarek RM, et al: *Clinical Application of Respiratory Care,* ed 3. Chicago, Year Book Medical Publishers, 1985. Used by permission.)

2. Tunica media (middle layer)
   a. It is the thickest layer of the artery.
   b. It is composed of circularly arranged smooth muscle and elastic fibers.
   c. Nerve fibers contained in tunica adventitia terminate in the smooth muscle layer of the tunica media.
3. Tunica intima (internal layer)
   a. It is the thinnest layer of the artery.
   b. It consists of flat layer of simple squamous cells called the *endothelium:*
      (1) The endothelium is supported by a fine layer of connective tissue.
      (2) The connective tissue is surrounded by a longitudinally placed network of elastic fibers.
   c. Common to all blood vessels, the endothelium is even continuous with the endocardium of the heart.
C. Large arteries: Termed *elastic arteries* because the tunica media has less smooth muscle and more elastic fibers.
D. Medium-sized arteries: Sometimes called *nutrient arteries* because they control the flow of blood to various areas of the body. Their ability to regulate blood flow lies in a tunica media, which is composed almost entirely of smooth muscle.
E. *Arterioles* (small arteries)
   1. The arterioles have a thin tunica intima and adventitia but have a thick, smooth muscle layer in the tunica media.
   2. The arterioles range in diameter from 20 to 50 μ.
   3. The tunica media is extensively innervated by postsynaptic sympathetic nerve fibers (Fig 6–3).
   4. Due to the extensive innervation and abundance of smooth muscle, the arterioles control regional blood flow to the capillary beds.
   5. The arterioles are frequently called the *resistance vessels.* By vasomotion, they control the rate of arterial runoff (the rate at which blood leaves the arterial tree) and thereby arterial blood volume.

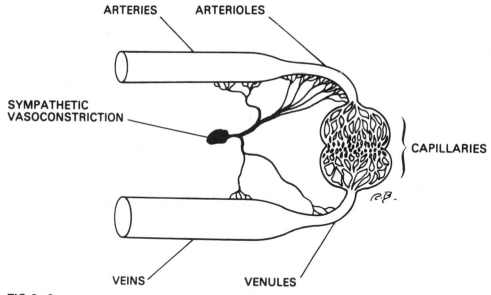

FIG 6–3.
Neural control of the vascular system. Sympathetic neural fibers to the arterioles and venules. Innervation of the arterioles are especially abundant. (From DesJardins T: *Cardiopulmonary Anatomy and Physiology: Essentials for Respiratory Care.* New York, Delmar Publishers, 1988. Used by permission.)

     6. The arterioles terminate in either metarterioles or capillaries.
       a. Metarterioles range in diameter from 10 to 20 μ.
       b. Metarterioles can bypass a capillary bed entirely by shunting blood directly to the venules.
       c. Metarterioles can also allow blood to pass from arterioles to capillaries.
  F. *Capillaries*
     1. Capillaries consist only of tunica intima.
     2. They vary in diameter from 5 to 10 μ.
     3. Where capillaries originate from arterioles or metarterioles, there frequently is a small band of smooth muscle called the *precapillary sphincter.*
       a. This sphincter controls blood flow through the distal capillary.
       b. It is responsive (vasoactive) to local P_{CO_2}, P_{O_2}, pH, and temperature.
     4. Capillaries frequently are called *exchange vessels*, because they are the site of gas, fluid, nutrient, and waste exchange.
       a. An intracellular cleft lies between the individual squames comprising the endothelium.
         (1) They are about 50 to 60 Å wide.
         (2) They act as pores through which substances can move into and out of the capillaries.
       b. The basement membrane usually is continuous in the capillaries and may limit movement of substances into and out of the capillaries.
  G. *Veins* consist of a tunica intima, media, and adventitia, but each layer is thinner than its counterpart in the arteries.
     1. Tunica adventitia
       a. Is one to five times as thick as the tunica media.
       b. Is made up of connective, elastic, and smooth muscle tissue.
     2. Tunica media
       a. Is made up of circularly arranged smooth muscle, collagenous, and elastic tissue.
       b. Is innervated by postsynaptic fibers of sympathetic nervous system (see Fig 6–3).
         (1) Veins are not as extensively innervated as arteries.
         (2) By venodilation or venoconstriction, veins can alter venous blood volume and "venous return."
     3. Tunica intima
       a. Consists of endothelial cells supported by delicate elastic fibers and connective tissue.
  H. In general, all vessels of the venous system have smaller amounts of elastic and smooth muscle tissue than their arterial counterparts.
  I. *Venules* (small veins) have the three characteristic layers, but they are very thin and almost indistinguishable.
  J. Veins are called *capacitance vessels*, or *reservoir vessels*, because 70% to 75% of the blood volume exists in the venous system.
  K. Veins contained in the periphery of the body contain one-way valves.
     1. Valves are formed by duplication of endothelial lining of veins.
     2. Valves are semilunar and prevent retrograde flow of blood.
     3. Valves are found in veins more than 2 mm in diameter and exist in areas subjected to muscular pressure (e.g., arms and legs).
     4. Valves are absent in veins less than 1 mm in diameter and in areas such as the abdominal and thoracic cavities.
III. The Lymphatic Vessels
  A. These vessels are a type of circulatory system that collects fluid and other material in the interstitial space and returns them to the venous vasculature.

B. Lymphatic vessels originate as blindly ending vessels called *lymphatic capillaries*.
   1. They have no basement membrane and consist only of loosely fitting endothelial cells.
   2. They are invested in every tissue of the body except for cartilage, bone, epithelium, and the CNS.
C. Lymphatic capillaries drain into larger lymphatic vessels, which take on three characteristic layers similar to those of the veins.
   1. Larger lymphatic channels contain smooth muscle, elastic, fibrous, and connective tissue.
   2. These vessels resemble the veins except that the three layers composing the lymphatics are much thinner.
   3. One-way semilunar valves are found about every millimeter and are more frequent in the lymphatics than in the veins.
D. The larger lymphatic vessels drain into lymph nodes (Fig 6–4).
   1. Lymph nodes are found in the neck, axilla, groin, thorax, breast, arms, and mouth.
   2. Lymph nodes are bean or oval shaped.
   3. Lymph moves into the lymph nodes via afferent lymphatic channels.
      a. The lymph is exposed to phagocytic reticular endothelial cells lining the sinus of the nodes.
      b. The lymph is filtered and exits from the lymph node via efferent lymphatic channels.
E. The large efferent lymphatic vessels join one of two major lymphatic ducts (Fig 6–5):
   1. Right lymphatic duct
      a. Drains right upper quadrant of the trunk.
      b. Drains right side of the head and neck.
      c. Drains filtered lymph into right subclavian vein.
   2. Thoracic duct
      a. Drains remainder of the body.
      b. Is the largest lymphatic vessel but is smaller than either vena cava.
         (1) The duct is 15 to 18 in. long.
         (2) It originates in the lumbar region of the abdominal cavity and ascends to the neck.
      c. Drains filtered lymph into left subclavian vein.

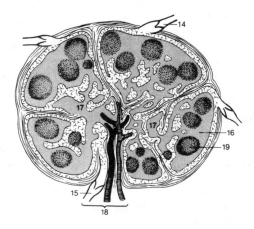

FIG 6–4.
Lymph node (transverse section). *14,* afferent lymphatic vessel; *15,* efferent lymphatic vessel (From Feneis H: *Pocket Atlas of Human Anatomy.* New York, Thieme-Stratton, 1976. Used by permission.)

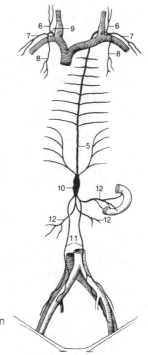

FIG 6–5.
Thoracic and right lymphatic ducts communicating with the venous system. *5,* thoracic duct, *9,* right lymphatic duct. (From Feneis H: *Pocket Atlas of Human Anatomy.* New York, Thieme-Stratton, 1976. Used by permission.)

IV. The Heart
    A. The heart is a muscular pump that maintains circulation of the blood through the vessels to all parts of the body.
    B. The heart is located between the lungs in the mediastinum (Fig 6–6).
    C. The apex is the inferior portion of the heart and is directed inferiorly, anteriorly, and to the left, with most of it left of the midline.
    D. The base is the superior aspect of the heart.
    E. The heart is about the size of the clenched fist.
    F. The heart is encased by a loose nondistensible sac called the *pericardium* (Fig-6–7).
    G. Layers of pericardium
        1. *Fibrous pericardium*
            a. Is the outermost layer of pericardium.
            b. Attaches to great vessels (major vessels entering and exiting from the heart) of the heart and loosely encases the heart proper.
            c. Is made of white fibrous tissue that protects and anchors the heart to some extent.
            d. Is externally attached to sternum, vertebral column, central tendon, and left hemidiaphragm.
        2. *Parietal serous pericardium*
            a. Lines the fibrous pericardium, to which it is closely adherent.
            b. A moist serous membrane that forms a smooth surface to reduce frictional resistances.
            c. Produces a small volume of serous fluid called *pericardial fluid.*
            d. Becomes continuous with the visceral serous pericardium.
        3. *Visceral serous pericardium*
            a. The visceral serous pericardium is directly adherent to the heart.
            b. It is commonly called *epicardium* of the heart.

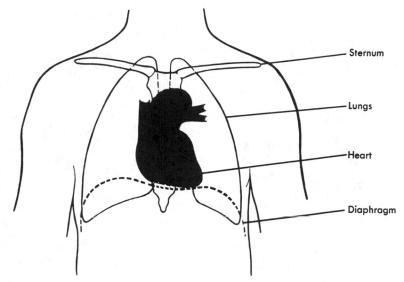

FIG 6-6.
Position of the heart in the thoracic cavity. (From Spearman CB, Sheldon RL, Egan DF: *Egan's Fundamentals of Respiratory Therapy,* ed 4. St Louis, CV Mosby Co, 1982. Used by permission.)

    c. It is a serous membrane that produces serous pericardial fluid.

    d. The small space between visceral and parietal serous pericardial layers is called the *pericardial space.*

  4. The fact that the visceral and parietal serous pericardial layers are smooth membranes with a small volume of lubricating pericardial fluid between them allows the heart to move freely in the pericardial sac opposed by reduced frictional forces.

H. The heart wall has three distinctive layers (Fig 6-8):

  1. *Epicardium,* or visceral serous pericardium

    a. Is the most superficial layer.

    b. Is a transparent serous sheet lying on a delicate network of connective tissue.

    c. Contains fat, coronary blood vessels, and coronary nerves, which are observable on cardiac surface.

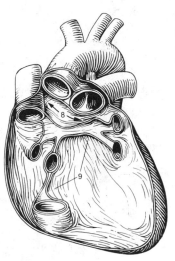

FIG 6-7.
Pericardial sac encases heart and great vessels (posterior view). (From Feneis H: *Pocket Atlas of Human Anatomy.* New York, Thieme-Stratton, 1976. Used by permission.)

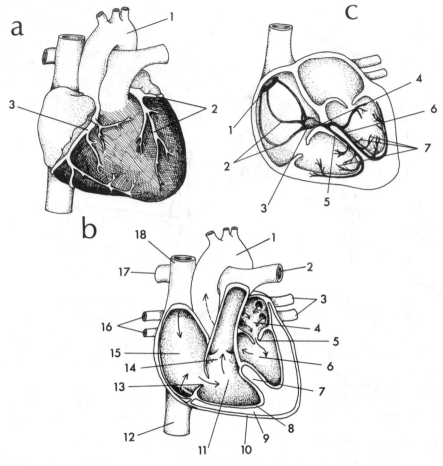

FIG 6–8.
Functional anatomy of the heart: *1*, aorta; *2*, left pulmonary artery; *3*, pulmonary veins from left lung; *4*, left atrium; *5*, mitral valve; *6*, left ventricle; *7*, intraventricular septum; *8*, endocardium; *9*, myocardium; *10*, epicardium; *11*, right ventricle; *12*, inferior vena cava; *13*, tricuspid valve; *14*, pulmonary semilunar valves; *15*, right atrium; *16*, pulmonary veins from right lung; *17*, right pulmonary artery; *18*, superior vena cava. (From Shapiro BA, Harrison RA, Kacmarek RM, et al: *Clinical Application of Respiratory Care*, ed 3. Chicago, Year Book Medical Publishers, 1985. Used by permission.)

2. *Myocardium*
   a. Is located just deep to the epicardium and is the middle layer of heart wall.
   b. Is composed almost exclusively of cardiac muscle with the exception of coronary blood vessels.
   c. Is the thickest of the three cardiac layers.
3. *Endocardium*
   a. It is the deepest cardiac layer, the internal lining of the heart.
   b. It is a smooth layer of squamous epithelium.
   c. It is continuous with endothelial lining of all blood vessels.
   d. Duplication of this layer in the heart forms the cardiac valves.
I. The heart has four chambers (Fig 6–9).
   1. It has two superior chambers, or atria.
   2. It has two inferior chambers, or ventricles.
   3. Externally the two atria are separated from the two ventricles by a groove that circumscribes the heart, the coronary sulcus.

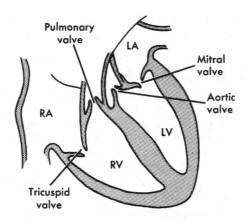

FIG 6–9.
Heart chambers and valves. *RA*, right atrium; *RV*, right ventricle; *LA*, left atrium; *LV*, left ventricle. (From Spearman CB, Sheldon RL, Egan DF: *Egan's Fundamentals of Respiratory Therapy*, ed 4. St Louis, CV Mosby Co, 1982. Used by permission.)

4. Externally the two atria are separated from each other by the roots of both the aorta and the pulmonary artery.
5. Externally the two ventricles are separated from each other by a groove, the interventricular sulcus.
6. Internally the two atria are separated from each other by a wall, the interatrial septum.
   a. The fossa ovalis, a depression in the atrial septal wall, is the remenant of the fetal foramen ovale.
7. Internally the two ventricles are separated from each other by a fibrous and muscular interventricular septum. It is continuous with the interatrial septum through its fibrous portion (see Fig 6–8).
8. Internally the atria are separated from the ventricles by a structure known as the *fibroskeleton* of the heart (Fig 6–10).
   a. The fibroskeleton consists of fibrous rings (which surround the atrioventricular [AV] cardiac valves, pulmonic semilunar valves, and aortic semilunar valves), fibrous interventricular septum, right and left trigone, and tendon of conus.
      (1) The right fibrous trigone consists of fibrous tissue that connects the two AV rings, fibrous interventricular septum, and ring of the aortic semilunar valve.
      (2) The left fibrous trigone consists of fibrous tissue that connects the fibrous ring of the left AV valve with the aortic semilunar valve.

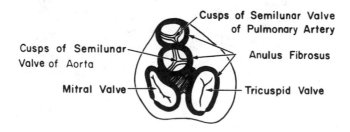

FIG 6–10.
Heart valves formed on the borders of the cardiac fibrous skeleton. View is from the base of the heart. (From Little RC: *Physiology of the Heart and Circulation*, ed 2. Chicago, Year Book Medical Publishers, 1981. Used by permission.)

(3) The tendon of conus is fibrous tissue that connects the fibrous ring of the pulmonic semilunar valve with the ring surrounding the aortic semilunar valve.

b. Functions of the fibroskeleton

   (1) Houses the four cardiac valves.

   (2) Serves as the origin of and point of insertion for atrial and ventricular bands of muscle.

   (3) Electrically isolates atrial muscle bundles from ventricular muscle bundles.

      (a) The fibroskeleton is bridged only by the common bundle branch of the electrical conduction system of the heart, called the *bundle of His*.

      (b) This arrangement allows repolarization and depolarization of the atria separate from the ventricles.

9. The *right atrium* is positioned atop the right ventricle (Fig 6–11).

a. It is anterior to the left atrium because the heart is rotated to the left.

   (1) Thus, the bulk of the anterior surface of the heart is composed of the right side of the heart (right atrium and ventricle).

   (2) Most of the posterior surface of the heart is composed of the left side of the heart (left atrium and ventricle).

b. The right atrium is larger than the left atrium and has a thinner wall.

   (1) The right atrial wall is about 2 mm thick.

   (2) The atrial musculature is divided into deep atrial muscle, which encircles each atrium individually, and superficial atrial muscle, which encircles both atria.

   (3) The deep and superficial muscle fibers run perpendicu larly to one another and originate and insert on the fibroskeleton of the heart.

   (4) Contraction of the two major groups of atrial muscle fibers tends to decrease the size of the respective atria in all dimensions.

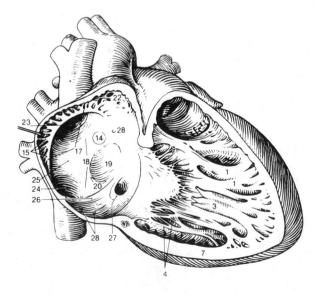

FIG 6–11.
Right atrium and systemic great veins. *1,* trabeculae carneae; *3,* papillary muscles; *4,* chordae tendineae; *14,* right atrium; *23,* opening of superior vena cava; *24,* opening of inferior vena cava; *27,* opening of coronary sinus. (From Feneis H: *Pocket Atlas of Human Anatomy*. New York, Thieme-Stratton, 1976. Used by permission.)

c. The cavity of the right atrium consists of two parts:
   (1) The major cavity of the right atrium, or sinus venarum.
   (2) The smaller cavity, which appears externally as a pouch, called the *right auricle*. (*Note:* Auricle is a term formerly used to denote the entire atrium.)
d. The right atrium accepts venous blood from the following veins:
   (1) The superior vena cava, which opens into the superior and posterior portions of the major cavity of the right atrium.
   (2) The inferior vena cava, which opens into the most inferior portion of the right atrium very near the interatrial septal wall.
   (3) The coronary sinus, which opens into the right atrium between the tricuspid valve and the opening of the inferior vena cava.

10. The *left atrium* is positioned atop the left ventricle (Fig 6–12).
    a. The left atrium is smaller than the right atrium and has a thicker wall.
       (1) The left atrial wall is about 3 mm thick.
       (2) The left atrial muscle fibers are divided into deep and superficial muscle groups and have an arrangement similar to that of the right atrium.
    b. The cavity of the left atrium consists of two parts:
       (1) The major cavity of the left atrium.
       (2) The left auricle, which appears externally as a pouchlike structure.
    c. The left atrium accepts arterial blood from the four pulmonary veins, which open into its superior and posterior aspects.

11. Right ventricle (Fig 6–13)
    a. It constitutes most of the anterior surface of heart.
    b. The right ventricular wall is one third the thickness of the left ventricular wall.
    c. The ventricular musculature classically is separated into deep and superficial muscle groups.
       (1) Both deep and superficial muscle groups appear to originate on the fibroskeleton of the heart.
       (2) Superficial fibers follow a clockwise spiral course to the apex of the heart. At the apex, these fibers turn inward and follow a spiraled course counterclockwise and upward toward the base of the heart to insert on the fibroskeleton.
       (3) Deep fibers follow a similar course to the superficial ventricular fibers, with three exceptions:
          (a) The spiraled course of the deep fibers is in a direction opposite to that of the superficial fibers.

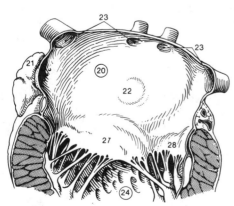

FIG 6–12.

Left atrium and pulmonary veins. *20,* left atrium; *23,* pulmonary veins; *27* and *28,* cusps of mitral valve. (From Feneis H: *Pocket Atlas of Human Anatomy.* New York, Thieme-Stratton, 1976. Used by permission.)

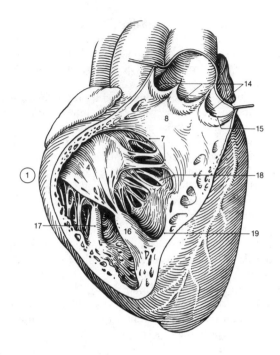

FIG 6–13.
Right ventricle with tricuspid and pulmonic semilunar valves exposed. *1*, right ventricle; *4*, tricuspid valve; *8*, outflow tract of right ventricle; *14*, cusps of pulmonic semilunar valve; *16–18*, papillary muscles. (From Feneis H: *Pocket Atlas of Human Anatomy*. New York, Thieme-Stratton, 1976. Used by permission.)

      (b) Deep fibers may not follow a course all the way to the apex of the heart before starting to ascend.

      (c) Deep fibers may insert into the cardiac fibroskeleton, papillary muscles, or trabeculae carneae.

        (i) Papillary muscles are finger-like projections of cardiac muscle located in the cavity of each ventricle.

        (ii) Trabeculae carneae are irregular bundles of muscle that form ridges along the internal wall of the ventricular cavity.

    (4) Contraction of ventricular muscle fibers tends to decrease the internal anteroposterior and transverse diameter significantly but leaves the vertical diameter virtually unchanged.

  d. The right ventricle receives venous blood from the right atrium through an opening called the *right AV orifice*.

    (1) This orifice is surrounded by a fibrous ring that is a part of the cardiac fibroskeleton.

    (2) The right AV orifice is about 4 cm in diameter.

    (3) The right AV orifice contains the tricuspid valve.

      (a) The tricuspid valve contains three cusps, each fused at its origin in the AV ring.

      (b) The cusps are formed by a duplication of the endocardial layer of the heart and are supported with fibrous tissue.

      (c) The three cusps collectively have a funnel shape that projects into the cavity of the right ventricle.

      (d) The free borders (inferior border) of each cusp have an attached fibrous cordlike structure, the chordae tendineae.

  (e) The chordae tendineae are, in turn, attached to the intraventricular papillary muscles.

  (f) The chordae tendineae commonly cross, passing from one of the cusps to a group of papillary muscles on the opposite side of the ventricle.

 e. The cavity of the right ventricle is lined with muscular ridges (trabeculae carneae) and papillary muscle covered by endocardium.

  (1) The cavity of the right ventricle has a bellows or U shape.

  (2) The muscular arrangement and shape of the right ventricle are well suited to its function of pumping blood under low pressure.

 f. Blood exits from the cavity of the right ventricle by passing through the pulmonary artery via an opening called the *orifice of the pulmonary trunk.*

  (1) This orifice is surrounded by a fibrous ring, a component of the cardiac fibroskeleton.

  (2) The pulmonary orifice is located in the superior, anterior, and medial sections of the right ventricle.

  (3) The pulmonary orifice contains the pulmonic semilunar valve.

   (a) The pulmonic semilunar valve is composed of three half-moon-shaped cusps.

   (b) This valve resembles the type found in the large veins of the periphery.

   (c) This valve, like the AV valves, is formed by duplication of the endocardial layer and is supported by fibrous tissue.

12. Left ventricle (Fig 6–14)

 a. It constitutes most of the posterior surface of the heart.

 b. The left ventricular wall is three times the thickness of the right ventricular wall.

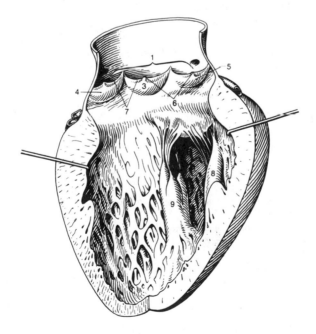

FIG 6–14.
Left ventricle with mitral and aortic semilunar valves exposed. *1,* opening of left ventricle into aorta; *3–5,* cusps of aortic semilunar valve; *8* and *9,* papillary muscles. (From Feneis H: *Pocket Atlas of Human Anatomy.* New York, Thieme-Stratton, 1976. Used by permission.)

    c. Left ventricular muscle fibers are part of the continuum of muscle circum-
scribing both ventricles and cannot be anatomically separated from right
ventricular fibers. (*Note:* The arrangement of the ventricular muscle fibers is
described in the foregoing section on the right ventricle.)

    d. The left ventricle receives arterial blood from the left atrium through the left
atrioventricular orifice (see Fig 6–8).

      (1) This orifice is surrounded by a fibrous ring, which is one of the compo-
nents of the cardiac fibroskeleton.

      (2) Contained in the left AV orifice is the bicuspid or mitral valve.

        (a) The mitral valve is composed of two cusps.

        (b) The anatomical structure is very similar to that of the previously dis-
cussed tricuspid valve except that the chordae tendineae are thicker
and stronger in the left ventricle.

    e. The cavity of the left ventricle is lined with muscular ridges (trabeculae
carneae), which appear in a more numerous and dense arrangement than in
the right ventricle. Papillary muscles with the corresponding thick chordae
tendineae, along with the trabeculae carneae, are covered by the endocardial
layer.

      (1) The cavity of the left ventricle is conical.

      (2) The arrangement of the left ventricular musculature coupled with its con-
ical shape lends well to its function of pumping blood under high pressure.

    f. Blood exits from the cavity of the left ventricle by passing through the aortic
opening.

      (1) This opening is surrounded by a fibrous ring, a component of the cardiac
fibroskeleton.

      (2) The aortic opening exists in the superior, posterior, and medial sections
of the left ventricle.

      (3) The aortic opening contains the aortic semilunar valve.

        (a) The aortic semilunar valve is anatomically similar to the pulmonic
semilunar valve except that the aortic cusps are stronger, larger, and
thicker.

BIBLIOGRAPHY

Ayres SM, Giannelli S Jr, Mueller HS: *Care of the Critically Ill*, ed 2. New York,
Appleton-Century-Crofts, 1974.

Crowley LV: *Introductory Concepts in Anatomy and Physiology*. Chicago, Year Book Medical Publishers, 1976.

DesJardins T: *Cardiopulmonary Anatomy and Physiology: Essentials for Respiratory Care*.
New York, Delmar Publishers, 1988.

Feneis H: *Pocket Atlas of Human Anatomy*. Chicago, Year Book Medical Publishers, 1976.

Gray H, Goss CM: *Gray's Anatomy of the Human Body*, ed 29. Philadelphia, Lea & Febiger, 1973.

Guyton AC: *Textbook of Medical Physiology*, ed 6. Philadelphia, Lea & Febiger, 1981.

Jacob SW, Francone CA: *Structure and Function in Man*, ed 3. Philadelphia, WB Saunders Co, 1974.

Little RC: *Physiology of the Heart and Circulation*. Chicago, Year Book Medical Publishers, 1977.

McLaughlin AJ: *Essentials of Physiology for Advanced Respiratory Therapy*. St Louis, CV
Mosby Co, 1977.

Ruch TC, Patton HD: *Physiology and Biophysics*, ed 20. Philadelphia, WB Saunders Co,
1974.

Rushmer RF: *Cardiovascular Dynamics,* ed 3. Philadelphia, WB Saunders Co, 1970.

Shapiro BA, Harrison RA, Kacmarek RM, et al: *Clinical Application of Respiratory Care,* ed 3. Chicago, Year Book Medical Publishers, 1985.

Spearman CB, Sheldon RL, Egan DF: *Egan's Fundamentals of Respiratory Therapy,* ed 4. St Louis, CV Mosby Co, 1982.

Chapter 7

Physiology of the Cardiovascular System

I. Functions of the Blood
  A. Primary vehicle of transport of substances in the body
    1. Respiratory gases (e.g., oxygen and carbon dioxide)
    2. Circulating antibodies and leukocytes involved in the body's defense mechanisms
    3. Platelets and clotting factors involved in hemostasis
    4. Cellular nutrients to all of the cells
    5. Cellular waste products away from the cells
    6. Electrolytes, proteins, water, and hormones, all of which contribute to the numerous complex functions of blood
II. Anatomic Classification of the Vascular Bed (Fig 7–1)
  A. The typical vascular bed begins with the aorta or pulmonary artery.
  B. Branches from either of these main arteries are called *large arteries*.
  C. The larger arteries continue to branch to medium arteries.
  D. The medium arteries branch further to the arterioles.
  E. The end of the arteriolar bed is marked by a thick band of smooth muscle called the *precapillary sphincter*, which marks the initial portion of the microcirculation.
  F. The arterioles branch to metarterioles or directly to capillaries.
  G. Distal to the precapillary sphincter are the capillaries.
  H. Many capillaries join to form venules.
  I. Numerous venules join to form small veins, which, in turn, join to form large veins.
  J. Large veins join the major veins of the body, either the vena cava or the pulmonary veins.
III. Functional Divisions of the Vascular Bed
  A. Distribution, resistance, exchange, and capacitance vessels
    1. Distribution vessels begin with the major arteries and include the large and medium arteries.
      a. These vessels distribute the cardiac output to the various organ systems.
      b. These vessels typically are under an elevated pressure, contain a relatively small percentage of total blood volume, and are very elastic.

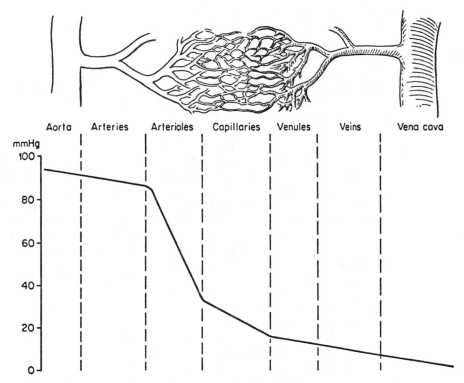

FIG 7–1.
Typical vascular bed with graphic representation of pressure drop across the systemic circulation. (From Ross G: *Essentials of Human Physiology,* ed 2. Chicago, Year Book Medical Publishers, 1982. Used by permission.)

2. Resistance vessels begin with the arterioles and end with the precapillary sphincter.
   a. These vessels have the largest proportion of smooth muscle constituting the vascular wall of any of the blood vessels.
   b. Through contraction and relaxation of the smooth muscle, the resistance vessels can regulate the distribution of blood to the various capillary beds.
   c. The resistance vessels are the major source of peripheral resistance and function in arterial blood pressure regulation.
3. The exchange vessels are the capillaries.
   a. Fluid, gas, nutrient, and waste exchange occurs in these vessels.
   b. Exchange of these substances occurs between capillary blood and interstitial fluid. Exchange then occurs from the interstitial fluid to the cells that make up the tissue.
   c. The major process underlying exchange in the capillaries is diffusion.
   d. Due to the vast distribution of capillary beds, the process of diffusion is fast enough to maintain cellular metabolism.
4. Capacitance vessels include the venules through the large veins and encompass the total venous system.
   a. Capacitance vessels serve as channels for blood return to the heart from the various capillary beds.
   b. These vessels are called *capacitance,* or *reservoir, vessels* because they contain most (70%–75%) of the total blood volume.

   c. The capacitance vessels are typically under low pressure, contain a large blood volume, and are relatively inelastic compared with their arterial counterparts.

IV. Vascular System: Systemic and Pulmonary Circulations (Fig 7–2)

  A. Systemic circulation

    1. Systemic circulation begins with the systemic pump, the left ventricle, and continues to a typical vascular bed, ending with the right atrium.

     a. Functions of systemic circulation:

      (1) To distribute left ventricular cardiac output so that each region of the body receives an adequate volume of blood per unit time.

      (2) To perfuse individual tissues so that cellular metabolism is maintained.

      (3) To return venous blood to the right side of the heart to maintain right ventricular output.

    2. Control of systemic circulation is governed by four major mechanisms: autonomic control, hormonal control, local control, and mechanical factors.

     a. The arterial portion of the systemic circulation is basically governed by three mechanisms: The autonomic nervous system, hormonal control, and local control.

      (1) Arteries and arterioles are innervated extensively and virtually exclusively by postganglionic fibers of the sympathetic nervous system.

      (2) The arterial vasculature of different tissues varies in the degree of sympathetic innervation.

       (a) The largest degree of sympathetic innervation is to the arterial vasculature perfusing the skin.

       (b) The degree of sympathetic innervation steadily decreases through the arterial vasculature perfusing spleen, mesenteric vessels, and kidneys.

       (c) A smaller degree of sympathetic innervation exists in the muscles.

       (d) The least degree of sympathetic innervation exists in the vessels perfusing the heart and brain. Furthermore, these vessels have a small degree of parasympathetic innervation.

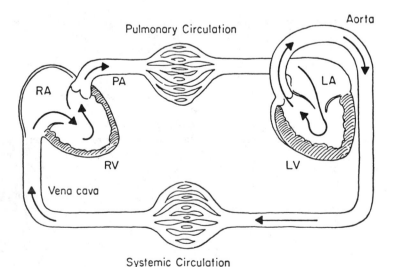

FIG 7–2.
The pulmonary and systemic circulations. (From Ross G: *Essentials of Human Physiology,* ed 2. Chicago, Year Book Medical Publishers, 1982. Used by permission.)

(3) Sympathetic stimulation of blood vessels results in smooth muscle contraction and vasoconstriction.

    (a) This principally affects the resistance vessels due to their large component of smooth muscle.

    (b) Tonic sympathetic stimulation of arterial blood vessels results in a given arteriolar caliber.

        (i) Increased sympathetic stimulation above this tonic level results in vasoconstriction and an increase in resistance to flow through these vessels.

        (ii) Decreased sympathetic stimulation below this tonic level results in vasodilation and a decrease in resistance to flow through these vessels.

        (iii) Because of differing degrees of sympathetic innervation in the different tissues, general sympathetic stimulation results in varying degrees of vasoconstriction and varying resistance to blood flow from tissue to tissue.

(4) Parasympathetic stimulation of the arterial vasculature of the brain and heart results in smooth muscle relaxation and vasodilation. This phenomenon results in a decrease in resistance to blood flow.

(5) The adrenomedullary hormones norepinephrine and epinephrine both stimulate the α (alpha) receptors and produce vasoconstriction.

(6) Acidosis, hypoxemia, hypercarbia, and increased temperature all produce local relaxation of smooth muscle in resistance vessels and resultant vasodilation.

b. The capillary bed of the systemic circulation is governed almost exclusively by local factors.

    (1) In tissues where capillary blood flow is limited by arteriolar constriction, there is local accumulation of acid and carbon dioxide as well as a deficiency of oxygen.

    (2) These local factors result in relaxation of the smooth muscle and local arteriolar dilation, which reestablishes blood flow.

    (3) Blood flow removes the local accumulation of waste products and replenishes oxygen and nutrient supply, resulting in arteriolar constriction, which, in turn, limits blood flow.

    (4) Thus, the cycle repeats itself, providing blood flow to tissues intermittently to maintain cellular metabolism.

c. The veins of the systemic circulation are governed by the autonomic nervous system, hormonal factors, and mechanical factors.

    (1) The veins are exclusively innervated by postganglionic fibers of the sympathetic nervous system.

    (2) The veins have a less extensive innervation than do their arterial counterparts. However, unlike that of the arteries, sympathetic innervation of the venous vasculature does not vary from one tissue to the next.

        (a) Thus, sympathetic stimulation causes venoconstriction of all veins of the body.

        (b) Generalized venoconstriction decreases the venous vascular space, resulting in increased venous return to the heart.

        (c) On the other hand, decreased sympathetic stimulation results in a decrease in venous tone and venodilation.

        (d) Generalized venodilation increases the venous vascular space and decreases venous return to the heart.

    (3) Adrenomedullary hormones epinephrine and norepinephrine both mimic sympathetic stimulation and produce venoconstriction.

(4) Mechanical factors that affect the veins of the systemic venous system are the thoracoabdominal pump, skeletal muscle pump, and semilunar valves.

    (a) The thoracoabdominal pump affects the veins by aiding venous return. This is accomplished by exposing the intrathoracic veins to the fluctuating subatmospheric pressure produced by spontaneous ventilation. Coupled with the fact that extrathoracic veins are surrounded by atmospheric or supra-atmospheric pressure, venous return is enhanced.

    (b) The veins in the limbs contain semilunar valves that prevent retrograde flow of blood. When skeletal muscle contracts, it compresses the veins, increasing venous pressure. Because these veins have valves, compression of vessels can squeeze blood in only one direction. This mechanism also is responsible for enhancing venous return.

B. Pulmonary circulation (see Fig 7–2)

  1. Pulmonary circulation begins with the pulmonary pump, the right ventricle, and continues to a typical vascular bed, ending with the left atrium.

    a. Functions of pulmonary circulation:

      (1) To distribute right ventricular output to pulmonary capillaries, matching the alveolar ventilation with an adequate volume of blood per unit time.

      (2) To perfuse the cells on the lung parenchyma with nutrients and rid them of waste products.

      (3) To return blood to the left side of the heart to maintain left ventricular output.

  2. Control of pulmonary circulation is governed by the same four mechanisms that affect systemic circulation.

    a. In general, the pulmonary vasculature has less smooth muscle and thinner walls than its counterpart in the systemic circulation.

    b. This makes pulmonary circulation susceptible to mechanical factors (e.g., intrathoracic and alveolar pressures) and the effects of gravity on the distribution of blood flow.

    c. Pulmonary vasculature responds to sympathetic stimulation just as does the systemic circulation but to a much lesser extent.

    d. Three local factors that have profound effects on pulmonary resistance vessels are decreased alveolar P_{O_2}, hypoxemia, and acidemia. All three cause pulmonary vasoconstriction, with increased resistance to blood flow.

    e. Adrenomedullary hormones produce pulmonary vasoconstriction but to a milder degree than in systemic circulation.

    f. Thus, most of the control of pulmonary circulation depends on passive response to mechanical factors as well as on local factors. This is in contrast to the dominance that the sympathetic nervous system displays in controlling systemic circulation.

  3. Systemic vascular resistance is normally six to ten times pulmonary vascular resistance.

V. Basic Functions of the Heart (Fig 7–3)

A. To impart sufficient energy to the blood to provide circulation through the vascular system.

  1. As has been discussed, the vascular resistance of systemic circulation is much greater than that of pulmonary circulation. Therefore, the left side of the heart must create greater pressures than the right side to bring about a given flow.

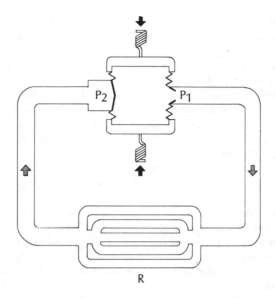

FIG 7–3.

Schematic representation of circulation depicting the heart's function of establishing the pressure gradient. (From Shapiro BA, Harrison RA, Kacmarek RM, et al: *Clinical Application of Respiratory Care,* ed 3. Chicago, Year Book Medical Publishers, 1985. Used by permission.)

   2. The major principle of circulation (blood flow) is that for circulation to exist, there must be a pressure gradient. The heart must create that pressure gradient across the respective parts of the vasculature. Therefore, for a given vascular resistance, blood flow is a direct function of the pressure gradient generated by the heart.

VI. Mechanical Events of the Cardiac Cycle (Fig 7–4)

   A. Electric events of the heart are precursors of the mechanical events of the heart.

   1. If the heart is normal, depolarization of the atria causes atrial contraction (systole).

   2. Depolarization of the ventricles causes ventricular contraction (systole).

   3. Repolarization of the atria causes atrial relaxation (diastole).

   4. Repolarization of the ventricles causes ventricular relaxation (diastole).

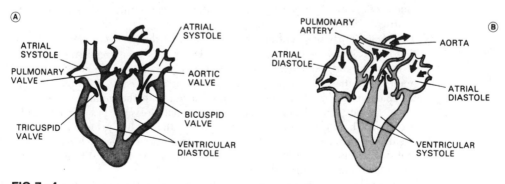

FIG 7–4.

Sequence of cardiac contraction. **A,** ventricular diastole and atrial systole. **B,** ventricular systole and atrial diastole. (From DesJardins T: *Cardiopulmonary Anatomy and Physiology: Essentials for Respiratory Care.* New York, Delmar Publishers, 1988. Used by permission.)

B. Atrial systole
   1. Mechanical left and right atrial systole begins at the peak of the P wave of the ECG.
   2. The decrease in size of the respective atria causes left atrial pressure to rise about 7 to 8 mm Hg and right atrial pressure 5 to 6 mm Hg. The pressure differential from atria to ventricles causes blood to flow from the atria through the respective atrioventricular (AV) orifices to the ventricles.
   3. Normal mean right and left atrial pressures are 0 to 8 mm Hg and 2 to 12 mm Hg, respectively.
   4. Atrial systole accounts for 20% to 40% of the total ventricular volume. This figure depends on heart rate and atrial contractility. The remaining 60% to 80% of ventricular volume is a result of passive filling by venous return.
   5. The atria are very weak pumps compared with the ventricles and should be thought of as thin-walled blood reservoirs for the respective ventricles. The 20% to 40% of ventricular volume added by atrial systole is simply a priming of the ventricles prior to ventricular systole. Atrial systole is not essential for adequate ventricular filling, as can be demonstrated by atrial fibrillation or complete heart block.
   6. Atrial systole increases the end-diastolic volume of each ventricle to about 145 ml. It also increases the end-diastolic pressure of the right and left ventricles to 2 to 8 mm Hg and 4 to 12 mm Hg, respectively. The ventricles are now prepared for their subsequent contraction.
C. Ventricular systole and atrial diastole
   1. Mechanical left and right ventricular systole begins at the peak of the R wave of the ECG and coincides with atrial diastole.
   2. Ventricular contraction increases intraventricular pressure. When pressure in the respective ventricles exceeds atrial pressure, the tricuspid and mitral valves close, producing the first, or S_1, heart sound.
   3. Aortic and pulmonic semilunar valves have been closed during ventricular diastole because pressure in the aorta and pulmonary artery has exceeded left and right ventricular pressure.
   4. With both AV and semilunar valves closed, the ventricles are functionally closed chambers. Contraction of the ventricle decreases their size and rapidly increases intraventricular pressure.
   5. The first portion of ventricular systole is called *isovolumetric contraction*. It is characterized by both the AV and semilunar valves being closed and by a rapid increase in intraventricular pressure without a concomitant change in intraventricular blood volume.
   6. The second portion of ventricular systole is called the *period of ejection*. Ejection begins when left and right intraventricular pressure exceeds the pressure in the aorta and pulmonary artery, respectively. It should be noted that this point is the diastolic pulmonary artery and aortic pressure. Previous to ventricular systole, blood has been steadily leaving both the pulmonary and systemic (aortic) arterial system, and intra-arterial pressure has been steadily dropping. The lowest intra-arterial pressure is attained just prior to actual ventricular ejection and is called *diastolic pressure* of the respective arteries. Normal diastolic pressure for the aorta and pulmonary artery is 60 to 90 mm Hg and 5 to 16 mm Hg, respectively.
   7. The period of ejection is characterized by opening of the semilunar valves.
      a. During this time intraventricular pressure steadily increases above intra-arterial pressure, causing blood to leave the ventricles.

      b. Intraventricular pressure attains its maximum value (ventricular systolic pressure), followed by an increase in intra-arterial pressure to its maximum value (arterial systolic pressure).

      c. Normal right and left ventricular systolic pressure is 15 to 28 mm Hg and 90 to 140 mm Hg, respectively.

      d. Normal pulmonary artery and aortic systolic pressure is 15 to 28 mm Hg and 90 to 140 mm Hg, respectively.

      e. When ejection is complete, intra-arterial pressure and retrograde blood flow cause closing of aortic and pulmonic semilunar valves. This produces the second, or S_2, heart sound.

   8. The total period of ejection causes a stroke volume of 70 ml to be added to each arterial system by the respective ventricles.

   9. It should be noted that the end-diastolic volume of each ventricle is 145 ml and the stroke volume 70 ml. This results in a residual blood volume of each ventricle equal to 75 ml. The residual volume is called the *end-systolic volume*. All previous blood volume values are based on the normal resting heart.

  10. Closure of aortic and pulmonic semilunar valves marks the beginning of ventricular diastole.

D. Ventricular diastole

   1. Mechanical left and right ventricular diastole begins after completion of the T wave of the ECG.

   2. Ventricular diastole begins with closure of the pulmonic and aortic semilunar valves and ends with onset of atrial systole.

   3. Tricuspid and mitral valves have remained closed all through the preceding ventricular systole and remain closed in early ventricular diastole. This is because intraventricular pressure exceeds intra-atrial pressure.

   4. The ventricles are functionally closed chambers with all cardiac valves remaining closed. Relaxation of the ventricular myocardium precipitates a large decrease in intraventricular pressure without a change in intraventricular blood volume.

   5. When right and left intraventricular pressures drop below the respective intra-atrial pressures, the tricuspid and mitral valves open. This results in a rapid filling of each ventricle by intra-atrial blood, followed by passive distention of the ventricles by blood returning from the lung and periphery.

   6. It should be noted that blood will continue to passively fill the ventricles through the AV valves, which remain open until the onset of ventricular systole. This slow but steady addition to ventricular volume is evidenced by a small increase in intra-atrial and intraventricular pressures.

   7. The ventricular filling occurring during ventricular diastole accounts for 60% to 80% of the end-diastolic volume.

   8. The entire myocardium remains relaxed until the onset of the P wave and atrial systole initiate another cardiac cycle.

E. Summary of mechanical events of the cardiac cycle

   1. After the P wave of the ECG, the atria contract, propelling blood through the open AV valves to the ventricles.

   2. During the height of the following QRS complex, the ventricles contract in unison. It is during this same time that atrial relaxation occurs.

   3. Intraventricular pressure soon rises above atrial pressure and causes the AV valves to close. This prevents retrograde flow of the blood from the ventricles to atria. Closure of the AV valves produces the S_1 heart sound.

4. Intraventricular pressure continues to rise rapidly and soon exceeds intra-arterial pressure. This causes the semilunar valves to open and provides blood flow from the ventricles to the arteries.
5. Relaxation of the ventricles occurs after completion of the T wave of the ECG.
6. As the ventricles relax, intraventricular pressure drops below the respective intra-arterial pressures. This causes the semilunar valves to close, preventing retrograde flow of blood from arteries to respective ventricles. Closure of the semilunar valves produces the S_2 heart sound.
7. Intraventricular pressure continues to drop until intraventricular pressure falls below intra-atrial pressure. This causes the respective AV valves to open and provides blood flow from atria to ventricles.
8. Blood returning from pulmonary and systemic circulations continues to flow through the atria and open AV valves passively, filling the relaxed ventricles. This passive filling continues until the onset of the subsequent atrial contraction, which begins the next cardiac cycle.

VII. Cardiac Output
   A. Cardiac output is the amount of blood pumped out of each ventricle.
   B. The cardiac output of the right and left ventricles is equal and identical over a period of time.
   C. The cardiac output (CO) is equal to the stroke volume (SV) times the heart rate (HR):

$$CO = SV \times HR \tag{1}$$

   1. The cardiac output is conventionally expressed in liters per minute.
      a. The normal range of cardiac output in a resting individual is 4 to 8 L/min.
      b. *With stress or exercise, the cardiac output can increase five to six times its normal resting value.*
   2. The stroke volume is the amount of blood ejected from the ventricle with each ventricular systole.
      a. The stroke volume is expressed in milliliters per contraction.
      b. The normal range for the stroke volume of a resting individual is 60 to 130 ml per contraction.
   3. The heart rate is the number of times the heart contracts per minute. The normal range for the heart rate of a resting individual is 60 to 100 contractions per minute.
   4. *Example:*
      An individual with a stroke volume equal to 70 ml per contraction and a heart rate of 80 contractions per minute would have a cardiac output of 5,600 ml/min, or 5.6 L/min, by the following calculation:

$$\frac{70 \text{ ml}}{\text{contraction}} \times \frac{80 \text{ contractions}}{\text{min}} = \frac{5,600 \text{ ml}}{\text{min}} \text{ or } \frac{5.6 \text{ L}}{\text{min}} \tag{2}$$

   5. It should be evident that increases in cardiac output are brought about by increases in the heart rate and/or stroke volume and that decreases in cardiac output are brought about by decreases in heart rate and/or stroke volume.
   D. Control of heart rate
   1. It should be recalled that heart rate is set by the pacemaker of the heart (SA node). The number of times per minute that the SA node depolarizes is largely governed by neural and chemical factors.

2. The neural factors that affect heart rate are mediated through the two divisions of the autonomic nervous system, namely, the parasympathetic and sympathetic nervous systems.

   a. Parasympathetic impulses are conducted to the SA node through cranial nerve X (vagus nerve).

     (1) Parasympathetic effects on the SA node are inhibitory and decrease the heart rate.

     (2) The result of decreasing the heart rate is called *negative chronotropism.* Thus, the parasympathetic nervous system exhibits negative chronotropic effects.

   b. Sympathetic impulses are conducted to the SA node through sympathetic nerve fibers originating from the upper thoracic (T1–T5) segment of the spinal cord.

     (1) Sympathetic effects on the SA node are excitatory and increase the heart rate.

     (2) The result of increasing the heart rate is called *positive chronotropism.* Thus, the sympathetic nervous system exhibits positive chronotropic effects.

   c. The sympathetic and parasympathetic nervous systems are generally considered antagonists. However, in bringing about changes in heart rate, the two divisions of the autonomic nervous system complement each other.

     (1) However, each nervous system can perform both positive and negative chronotropism. Under certain clinical conditions, heart rate is altered by selective activities of one division of the autonomic nervous system.

     (2) In general, the parasympathetic nervous system is the dominant division of the neural input into the SA node. This is evidenced by total autonomic blockade, resulting in mild tachycardia.

   d. Neural control of heart rate also is mediated through higher brain centers, such as the cerebral cortex and hypothalamus.

     (1) The cerebral cortex is responsible for changes in heart rate in response to emotional factors, such as anxiety, fear, anger, and grief.

     (2) The hypothalamus appears responsible for changes in heart rate in response to alterations in both local and environmental temperature.

3. Major chemical factors that affect heart rate: Electrolytes, exogenously administered drugs and hormones.

   a. The three major electrolytes having effects on the heart rate are potassium, sodium, and calcium.

     (1) Excess potassium and sodium have the effect of decreasing the heart rate.

     (2) Excess calcium causes an increase in the heart rate.

     (3) Potassium and sodium imbalance can alter cardiac membrane permeability and thus slow or speed the rate of electric conduction through the myocardium.

     (4) However, only electrolyte *imbalance* brings about such changes in heart rate.

   b. Classes of drugs that exert an effect on heart rate by either mimicking or inhibiting the activity of the sympathetic or parasympathetic nervous system:

     (1) Sympathomimetics such as isoproterenol or epinephrine mimic the activity of the sympathetic nervous system and cause positive chronotropism.

     (2) Sympatholytics such as dichloroisoproterenol or propranolol inhibit the activity of the sympathetic nervous system and cause negative chronotropism.

(3) Parasympathomimetics such as metacholine, pilocarpine, or neostig-mine mimic the activity of the parasympathetic nervous system and cause negative chronotropism.

(4) Parasympatholytics such as atropine inhibit the activity of the parasym-pathetic nervous system and cause positive chronotropism.

c. The major hormones that affect the heart rate are the adrenomedullary hor-mones.

(1) The adrenal medulla secretes epinephrine and norepinephrine into the circulating blood.

(2) These two naturally occurring catecholamines have direct positive chro-notropic effects on the heart.

4. *Heart rate is under many influences,* ranging from conscious control by the ce-rebral cortex to exogenously administered pharmacologic agents. The most im-portant regulatory control of heart rate is mediated through the autonomic nervous system.

E. Control of stroke volume

1. Size of stroke volume: Governed by preload, afterload, and state of contractil-ity of ventricles.

a. *Preload:* Degree of ventricular diastolic filling before ejection begins, or the presystolic ventricular loading force.

(1) The Frank-Starling law states that the more the heart is filled during diastole, the greater the subsequent force of contraction. This results in increased stroke volume (see Fig 7–5, curve A).

(2) This relationship is related primarily to presystolic myocardial fiber length.

(3) Presystolic fiber length is directly related to end-diastolic volume, be-cause it is the actual intraventricular blood volume coupled with the compliance characteristics of the ventricle that results in myocardial fi-ber stretch.

(4) Since myocardial fiber length is virtually impossible to measure in the intact heart, it would seem that end-diastolic volume is an appropriate parameter for assessing preload.

(a) The first factor affecting end-diastolic volume is the presence of a total blood volume sufficient for an effective vascular volume to vas-cular space relationship. There must be an adequate blood volume

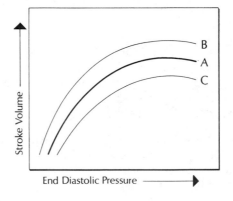

FIG 7–5.
The Frank-Starling relationship. *A,* control; *B,* positive inotropism; *C,* negative inotropism (see text). (From Shapiro BA, Harrison RA, Kacmarek RM, et al: *Clinical Application of Respiratory Care,* ed 3. Chicago, Year Book Medical Publishers, 1985. Used by permission.)

within the vascular space for the heart to circulate blood effectively. It is the *relationship* between vascular volume to vascular space that is crucial, not the absolute values of either vascular volume or vascular space.

(b) The state of the venous tone is the second factor affecting end-diastolic volume. The relationship between vascular volume and vascular space is essential to ensure adequate venous return and ventricular filling. It should be noted that 60% to 80% of ventricular filling is accomplished by passive return of blood from the veins. The state of venous tone regulates venous vascular space, and it is therefore as crucial as blood volume in determining adequacy of venous return.

(c) The third major factor that affects end-diastolic volume is force of atrial systole. As mentioned, 20% to 40% of ventricular filling is accomplished by atrial systole. This is not of critical importance in the normal heart but becomes paramount in any cardiac dysfunction where ventricular compliance is decreased (i.e., ventricular hypertrophy or myocardial infarction).

(d) The fourth major factor that affects end-diastolic volume is compliance of the ventricle. As mentioned, this factor is not of importance in the normal heart, but decreases in ventricular compliance require a greater filling pressure per unit volume change. Thus, increased filling pressure is necessary or the end-diastolic volume will have a reduced value.

(e) End-diastolic volume is an acceptable parameter for assessing preload; however, this too is difficult to measure with any accuracy in the intact heart. The most easily measured parameter that reflects preload is ventricular end-diastolic pressure.

(5) Given a constant ventricular compliance, it may be inferred that ventricular end-diastolic pressure should correlate well with ventricular end-diastolic volume. Accepting the latter as true, myocardial fiber length can be expressed as a function of end-diastolic pressure.

(a) In clinical practice, preload is assessed by measuring ventricular end-diastolic pressure.

(b) Right ventricular preload is assessed by end-diastolic pressure measurements taken from a central venous pressure (CVP) catheter as central venous pressure (see Chapter 14).

(c) Left ventricular preload is assessed by end-diastolic pressure measurements taken from a pulmonary artery catheter as pulmonary wedge pressure (see Chapter 14).

(d) In general, the higher the end-diastolic pressure (preload), the greater the subsequent ventricular contraction and resulting stroke volume.

(6) The Frank-Starling relationship is the basis for (1) matching cardiac output to venous return and (2) balancing the output of right and left ventricles. For example, if venous return to the right atrium has suddenly increased because increased venous tone has altered the vascular volume/vascular space relationship:

(a) Increased venous return to the right ventricle would increase the right ventricular end-diastolic volume.

(b) Increased end-diastolic volume would result in an increased myocardial fiber length.

(c) Increased myocardial fiber length would, in turn, result in an increased force of contraction of the right ventricle.

(d) Increased force of contraction of the right ventricle would result in an increased right ventricular stroke volume, all other factors remaining equal.

(e) It should be noted that two phenomena have occurred. First, venous blood has been mobilized back to the heart, and the increased venous return has been matched by an increase in right ventricular stroke volume. This is one of the major ways that cardiac output is increased. Second, right ventricular output now exceeds left ventricular output.

(f) Increased right ventricular output will result in increased venous return to the left atrium and left ventricle.

(g) In similar fashion, increased venous return to the left ventricle increases left ventricular end-diastolic volume.

(h) The increased end-diastolic volume would result in increasing the left ventricular myocardial fiber length. This, in turn, would result in an increase in the force of contraction of the left ventricle.

(i) The increased force of contraction of the left ventricle would result in an increased left ventricular stroke volume.

(j) At this point venous blood has been mobilized from the venous reservoirs and has resulted in increased output from both the right and left sides of the heart. Furthermore, left ventricular output is in equilibrium with right ventricular output, all in accorance with the Frank-Starling relationship.

(k) The regulatory function of the Frank-Starling mechanism is frequently referred to as *autoregulation* in that it is an intrinsic factor based on the architecture of the myocardial fibers, which automatically regulate cardiac output to equal venous return. Thus, it has led physiologists over the years to make the statement that "within the physiologic limits of the heart, it will pump out all the blood it receives without allowing a backup of blood into the venous system."

b. *Afterload:* Resistance to flow from the ventricles.

(1) The work the heart must perform to pump blood out of the ventricles and into the circulation depends on three major factors: Resistance of the semilunar valves, blood viscosity, and arterial blood pressure.

(a) As resistance of the semilunar valves (i.e., pulmonic or aortic stenosis) increases, afterload will be increased.

(b) As blood viscosity increases (i.e., hyperproteinemia or polycythemia), afterload will be increased.

(c) As arterial blood pressure increases (pulmonary or systemic hypertension), afterload will be increased.

(d) Decreases in any of these three parameters result in decreasing the afterload.

(2) Increases in afterload result in increases of ventricular work.

(a) The greater the resistance against which the ventricle must contract to eject blood, the more slowly it contracts.

(b) Increased afterload results in a decreased stroke volume, which initially increases end-systolic volume. The normal venous return will then be added to the already increased end-systolic volume and increase the end-diastolic volume above normal. This allows a more forceful contraction against an increased afterload as a result of the Frank-Starling mechanism. This enables the ventricle to pump a given stroke volume against an increased afterload. *This compensa-*

tion is at the expense of an increase in ventricular size. The larger the heart, the greater the work necessary to develop the myocardial tension required to produce a given intraventricular pressure (Laplace's law).

(c) Both the slower rate of contraction and the increased ventricular size result in greater oxygen requirements to perform a given amount of work than that of the normal heart.

(3) Thus, increases in afterload may or may not cause a decrease in stroke volume but will cause increases in myocardial work.

(4) Decreases in afterload, commonly called *afterload reduction,* may or may not cause an increase in stroke volume but will cause decreases in myocardial work.

(5) In general, the poorer the cardiac function, the more dependent is the stroke volume on afterload.

(a) Increases in afterload tend to decrease stroke volume in the patient with poor cardiac function.

(b) Increases in afterload do not cause decreases in stroke volume in the patient with normal cardiac function.

(c) Decreases in afterload tend to increase stroke volume in the patient with poor cardiac function.

(d) Decreases in afterload generally do not cause increases in stroke volume in the patient with normal cardiac function.

(6) In the absence of valvular disease, afterload is clinically assessed by measuring mean arterial blood pressure.

(a) Right ventricular afterload is assessed by mean pulmonary artery measurements taken via a pulmonary artery catheter.

(b) Left ventricular afterload is assessed by mean systemic arterial pressure measurements taken via an intra-arterial (systemic) catheter.

c. *State of ventricular contractility:* Force with which the ventricles contract.

(1) The force of contraction of the ventricles at any given preload and afterload depends on the state of contractility (Fig 7–5).

(a) An increase in the state of ventricular contractility for a given preload and afterload is termed *positive inotropism.*

(b) A decrease in the state of ventricular contractility for a given preload and afterload is termed *negative inotropism.*

(c) The net efffect of positive inotropism is generally a greater volume output per unit time.

(d) The net effect of negative inotropism is generally a smaller volume output per unit time.

(2) Ventricular contractility is altered by the sympathetic and parasympathetic nervous systems, blood gases (Po_2, Pco_2), pH, hormones, and exogenously administered drugs.

(3) The sympathetic nervous system extensively innervates the atrial and ventricular myocardium.

(a) Postganglionic nerve fibers of the sympathetic nervous system release norepinephrine to β (beta) receptor sites in the atrial and ventricular myocardium.

(b) This increases contractility of the myocardium; positive inotropism. Thus, the sympathetic nervous system displays positive inotropic effects.

(c) Alterations in sympathetic discharge to the myocardium are believed to constitute the most important regulatory control of ventricular contractility.

(4) The parasympathetic nervous system only minutely innervates the atrial myocardium, and the ventricular myocardium is innervated even more sparsely.

   (a) Postganglionic nerve fibers of the parasympathetic nervous system release acetylcholine to the muscarinic receptor sites of the atrial and ventricular myocardium.

   (b) As previously mentioned, due to the scantiness of parasympathetic innervation, the result is only a mild decrease in myocardial contractility or a slight negative inotropism. Thus, the parasympathetic nervous system displays minor negative inotropic effects.

(5) Effects of blood gases on myocardial contractility:

   (a) Mild decreases in Po_2 result in increased contractility, whereas severe drops in Po_2 result in decreased myocardial contractility.

   (b) Increases in Pco_2 result in decreased contractility, whereas decreases in Pco_2 result in increased myocardial contractility.

   (c) Metabolic or respiratory acidosis results directly in decreased contractility, whereas metabolic and respiratory alkalosis may alter contractility through electric conduction dysfunction and arrhythmia.

(6) The most important hormones affecting myocardial contractility are the adrenomedullary hormones.

   (a) As previously stated, the adrenal medulla secretes epinephrine and norepinephrine into the circulating blood.

   (b) These two naturally occurring catecholamines have direct positive inotropic effects on the myocardium.

   (c) The major differences between the effects of the catecholamines and direct sympathetic stimulation are that the effects of catecholamines take longer to establish but last longer.

   (d) This is true of the effect of catecholamines on both contractility and heart rate.

(7) The following exogenously administered drugs can alter myocardial contractility:

   (a) The sympatholytics (e.g., propranolol) produce negative inotropic effects through β-receptor blockade.

   (b) The sympathomimetics (e.g., isoproterenol or epinephrine) produce positive inotropic effects through β-receptor stimulation.

   (c) Some antiarrhythmics (e.g., quinidine or procainamide) produce negative inotropic effects.

   (d) Derivatives of digitalis produce postitive inotropic effects.

(8) Myocardial contractility is an elusive parameter to assess clinically. However, controversial attempts have been made to quantitate it.

(9) It should be remembered that the stroke volume is under a gamut of influences. However, any stroke volume is determined by the interrelation of preload, afterload, and the state of ventricular contractility.

VIII. Control of Arterial Blood Pressure

   A. Under normal circumstances, arterial blood volume exceeds arterial vascular space. This relationship results in an intravascular pressure dictated by the absolute arterial blood volume and the elastic properties of the arterial vasculature.

   B. The arterial system is continually receiving blood (inflow) from the left ventricle as cardiac output and continually allowing blood to leave the arterial system (outflow) as arterial runoff.

   C. It is the balance or imbalance between cardiac output (inflow) and arterial runoff (outflow) that results in any given arterial blood volume.

D. The relationship between arterial blood volume and arterial vascular space is the primary determinant of arterial blood pressure.

E. Thus, by the equation $P = \dot{Q} \times R$, it can be demonstrated that cardiac output ($\dot{Q}$) and peripheral resistance (R) are directly related to arterial blood pressure (P). Arterial blood pressure is dependent on alteration of the blood volume to vascular space relationship by cardiac output and/or peripheral resistance, as follows:

   1. Increases in peripheral resistance (i.e., vasoconstriction) result in decreasing the arterial runoff. If cardiac output remains the same, inflow exceeds outflow from the arterial vasculature. This results in an increase in the arterial blood volume to vascular space relationship and a concomitant increase in arterial blood pressure.

   2. Decreases in peripheral resistance (i.e., vasodilation) result in decreasing the arterial blood pressure by the exact opposite mechanism.

   3. Increases in cardiac output result in increasing the rate of inflow to the arterial system. If peripheral resistance remains the same, inflow exceeds outflow from the arterial vasculature. This results in an increase in the arterial blood volume to vascular space relationship and an increase in arterial blood pressure.

   4. Decreases in cardiac output result in decreasing arterial blood pressure by the exactly opposite mechanism.

   5. It should be noted that in the previous four examples the imbalance between inflow and outflow is only temporary. It is by these mechanisms that arterial blood pressure can be increased or decreased. Once the desired arterial pressure is attained, the balance between inflow and outflow will maintain the pressure at that level.

F. As has been described, cardiac output and peripheral resistance are, for a large part, under neural control. Therefore, it becomes apparent that regulation of arterial blood pressure is mediated through neural alterations in cardiac output and peripheral resistance.

G. Neural regulation of arterial blood pressure is mediated through autonomic fibers that originate from an area of the medulla oblongata. This area of the medulla is sometimes called the *cardiovascular center*.

H. The cardiovascular center may be functionally divided into four subcenters: The vasomotor excitatory (vasoconstrictor) center, vasomotor inhibitory (vasodilator) center, cardiac excitatory center, and cardiac inhibitory center.

   1. The vasomotor excitatory center influences the arterioles through the sympathetic nervous system. The degree of vasoconstriction or vasodilation is directly related to the amount of sympathetic stimulation.

   2. The vasomotor inhibitory center does not influence the arterioles directly but acts by inhibiting the activity of the vasomotor excitatory center.

   3. The cardiac excitatory center influences the heart through the sympathetic nervous system. Sympathetic stimulation originating from this center results in positive inotropic and chronotropic effects.

   4. The cardiac inhibitory center influences the heart through the parasympathetic nervous system. Parasympathetic stimulation originating from this center results in a negative chronotropic effect and a mild negative inotropic effect.

I. The cardiovascular center in the medulla receives sensory input from the entire body. The most important sources of sensory input are the exteroceptors, higher brain centers, local factors, peripheral chemoreceptors, and baroreceptors.

   1. Exteroceptors (e.g., proprioceptors, thermal receptors, and pain receptors) are sources of sensory input. Stimulation of the proprioceptors, pain receptors, and thermal receptors through muscular activation, pain, and heat, respec-

tively, results in an increase in heart rate. This potentially will increase arterial blood pressure. Cold and muscular inactivity slow the heart rate and potentially decrease arterial blood pressure.

2. Higher brain centers (e.g., the cerebral cortex and hypothalamus) have medullary input.
   a. Emotional factors alter blood pressure by mediation through the cerebral cortex. Fear or anger usually increases the blood pressure by stimulating the vasomotor and cardiac excitatory centers. This stimulation results in vasoconstriction and an increase in heart rate. However, decreases in blood pressure can be mediated through the cerebrum by stimulation of the vasomotor inhibitory center, as in fainting or blushing.
   b. The hypothalamus mediates its control on the vasomotor inhibitory center in response to increases in body temperature. This causes vasodilation of the vessels of the skin and loss of body heat. A decrease in body temperature will result in vasoconstriction of the vessels of the skin with heat conservation as mediated through the hypothalamus.
   c. Direct stimulation of the anterior portion of the hypothalamus produces bradycardia and a decrease in arterial blood pressure, whereas stimulation of the posterior portion of the hypothalamus produces tachycardia and an increase in arterial blood pressure.

3. The vasomotor inhibitory and excitatory centers are sensitive to local and direct effects of pH and P_{CO_2} of arterial blood perfusing these centers.
   a. Local increases in arterial pH and decreases in P_{CO_2} cause depression of the vasomotor excitatory center by the vasomotor inhibitory center. This results in vasodilation, a decrease in peripheral resistance, and a decrease in arterial blood pressure.
   b. Local decreases in arterial pH and increases in P_{CO_2} cause direct excitation of the vasomotor excitatory center. This results in vasoconstriction, an increase in peripheral resistance, and an increase in arterial blood pressure..
   c. A local drop in P_{O_2} of arterial blood potentiates the vasoconstrictor effect but alone has no local effect.

4. Peripheral chemoreceptors (aortic and carotid bodies) are responsible for initiating the vasomotor chemoreflex.
   a. Hypoxemia, hypercapnia, and acidemia all stimulate the peripheral chemoreceptors.
   b. The stimulated chemoreceptors, in turn, send an increased number of afferent impulses to the vasomotor excitatory center, with resultant vasoconstriction. This increases peripheral resistance and arterial blood pressure.
   c. When hypoxemia and hypercapnia or hypoxemia and acidemia exist, the chemoreceptors display a synergistic effect. That is, the stimulation arising from the chemoreceptors secondary to two simultaneous stimuli is greater than the mathematical sum of the two stimuli when they act alone. This results in a more profound vasoconstriction and an increase in blood pressure.

5. Baroreceptors are by far the most important short-acting regulator of arterial blood pressure.
   a. Baroreceptors (pressoreceptors) are stretch receptors located in the arch of the aorta and carotid sinus.
   b. They respond to changes in pressure, which stretch them to different degrees. The greater the pressure, the greater the number of impulses the baroreceptors will send.
   c. With a drop in arterial blood pressure, the number of impulses sent by the baroreceptors decreases. This decreased number of inhibitory impulses

causes the vasomotor excitatory and cardiac excitatory centers to become more active. This results in increased cardiac output and increased peripheral resistance, thus restoring arterial blood pressure to normal.

d. With an increase in arterial blood pressure, the number of impulses sent out by the baroreceptors increases. This increased number of inhibitory impulses causes the vasomotor excitatory center to become depressed directly and indirectly through increased activity of the vasomotor inhibitory center. In addition, the increased number of inhibitory impulses depresses the cardiac excitatory center and stimulates the cardiac inhibitory center, resulting in a decreased heart rate. Thus, peripheral resistance and cardiac output decrease, restoring normal blood pressure.

BIBLIOGRAPHY

Anthony CP, Kolthoff NJ: *Textbook of Anatomy and Physiology*, ed 8. St Louis, CV Mosby Co, 1971.

Ayres SM, Giannelli SJ, Mueller HS: *Care of the Critically Ill*, ed 2. New York, Appleton-Century-Crofts, 1974.

Crowley LV: *Introductory Concepts in Anatomy and Physiology*. Chicago, Year Book Medical Publishers, 1976.

DesJardins T: *Cardiopulmonary Anatomy and Physiology: Essentials for Respiratory Care*. New York, Delmar Publishers, 1988.

Gray H, Goss CM: *Gray's Anatomy of the Human Body*, ed 29. Philadelphia, Lea & Febiger, 1973.

Guyton AC: *Textbook of Medical Physiology*, ed 5. Philadelphia, WB Saunders Co, 1976.

Jacob SW, Francone CA: *Structure and Function in Man*, ed 3. Philadelphia, WB Saunders Co, 1974.

Little RC: *Physiology of the Heart and Circulation*. Chicago, Year Book Medical Publishers, 1977.

McLaughlin AJ: *Essentials of Physiology for Advanced Respiratory Therapy*. St Louis, CV Mosby Co, 1977.

Mountcastle VB: *Medical Physiology*, ed 14. St Louis, CV Mosby Co, 1980.

Ross G: *Essentials of Human Physiology*. Chicago, Year Book Medical Publishers, 1978.

Ruch TC, Patton HD: *Physiology and Biophysics*, ed 20. Philadelphia, WB Saunders Co, 1974.

Rushmer RF: *Cardiovascular Dynamics*, ed 3. Philadelphia, WB Saunders Co, 1970.

Schroeder JS, Daily EK: *Techniques in Bedside Hemodynamic Monitoring*. St Louis, CV Mosby Co, 1976.

Shapiro BA, Harrison RA, Kacmarek RM, et al: *Clinical Application of Respiratory Care*, ed 3. Chicago, Year Book Medical Publishers, 1985.

Chapter 8

Anatomy and Physiology of the Nervous System

I. Structure of the Nerve Fiber
   A. Each nerve fiber has three components:
      1. Cell body or soma: Primary metabolic area, site of initial synthesis of transmitter substance.
      2. Dendrite: Normally the structures that carry impulses *to* the cell body. A single neuron may contain 10,000 dendrites.
      3. Axon: Normally the structure that conducts impulses *away* from the cell body. Usually only one axon leaves a cell body; however, it may branch extensively.
II. Classification of Neurons
   A. Each neuron is classified by the direction of impulse transmission.
      1. Sensory (afferent) neurons: Transmit nerve impulses to the spinal cord or brain.
      2. Motor (efferent) neurons: Transmit nerve impulses from the brain or spinal cord to muscles or glands (effector organ).
      3. Interneurons (internuncial): Conduct impulses from sensory to motor neurons entirely within the central nervous system (CNS).
III. Nerve Cell Membrane Potential (Fig 8–1)
   A. In the resting state, the inner surface of the cell membrane is negative compared with the positive outer surface. This sets up an electric potential across the cell membrane (normal polarity).
      1. Intracellular: The primary cation, potassium (K^+), is readily diffusible across the cell membrane.
      2. Extracellular: The primary cation, sodium (Na^+), is poorly diffusible across the cell membrane.
      3. High extracellular Na^+ (142 mEq/L) and low extracellular K^+ (5 mEq/L) levels, along with high intracellular K^+ (140 mEq/L) and low intracellular Na^+ (10 mEq/L) levels, are maintained in the resting state by the Na pump (active transport).
IV. Action Potential
   A. In order for a nerve impulse to be transmitted, an alteration in the cell's resting membrane potential must be achieved.
   B. An action potential is a stimulus that is capable of significantly increasing the cell membrane's permeability to sodium.

NERVE FIBER

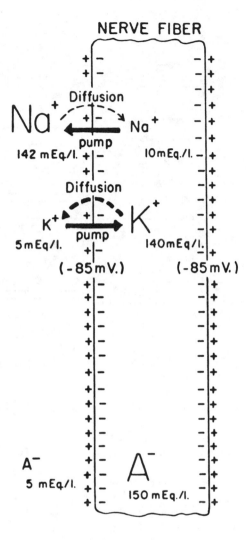

FIG 8–1.
A, establishment of a membrane resting potential as a result of active transport of sodium ions. (From Guyton AC: *Textbook of Medical Physiology,* ed 6. Philadelphia, WB Saunders Co, 1981. Used by permission.)

C. The action potential is an all-or-nothing phenomenon. That is, the stimulus must be strong enough to allow for a reversal in membrane potential; if it is not, an action potential does not occur.
D. An action potential may be caused by:
1. Electric stimulation
2. Chemicals
3. Mechanical damage to membrane
4. Heat or cold
5. Decreased serum calcium (Ca^{+2}), which increases the tendency for development of an action potential (low calcium tetany)
V. Nerve Impulse Propagation (Fig 8–2)
A. The nerve impulse is a self-propagating wave of electric charge that travels along the surface of the neuron's membrane. The nerve impulse travels in one direction only, from dendrite to cell body to axon.

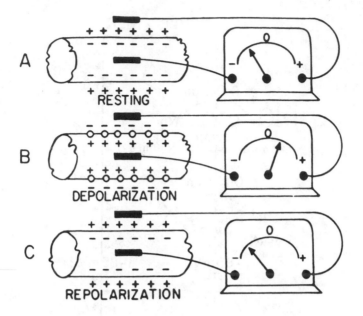

FIG 8–2.
Sequential events during the action potential showing. **A,** the normal resting potential. **B,** development of a reversal potential during depolarization. **C,** reestablishment of the normal resting potential during repolarization. (From Guyton AC: *Textbook of Medical Physiology,* ed 6. Philadelphia, WB Saunders Co, 1981. Used by permission.)

    B. Depolarization: Stage 1 of the action potential, in which an impulse travels along the nerve fiber.
       1. Sodium ions rush to the inside of the cell membrane.
       2. A positive intracellular membrane charge is set up with a negative extracellular membrane charge.
       3. There is a complete reversal of the membrane potential.
    C. Repolarization: Stage 2 of the action potential, in which the membrane returns to the normal resting membrane potential.
       1. Immediately after the impulse passes a point on the membrane, the membrane's permeability to Na^+ is again decreased.
       2. Na^+ ions are actively removed from the cell by the Na pump.
       3. The resting membrane potential is reestablished.
 VI. Nerve Synapse
    A. The nerve synapse (synaptic cleft) is the junction between one neuron and another neuron, muscle, or gland. It is an actual space between nerve fibers.
    B. Transmission of an impulse from the axon of one nerve to a dendrite, soma, or effector organ is a chemical process occurring across the synapse. The distance across the synapse is about 200 Å.
    C. Presynaptic terminals are located on the axon and contain vesicles that synthesize, store, and secrete a transmitter substance into the synapse. The transmitter substance stimulates the dendrite or soma of the next nerve, causing an action potential.
       1. Primary transmitter substances of the peripheral nervous system are:
         a. Acetylcholine
         b. Norepinephrine
    D. Postsynaptic terminals are located on dendrites, somas, or effector organs. After being stimulated, these terminals secrete a substance into the synapse to metabolize the transmitter substance.

E. Acetylcholine as the transmitter substance (Fig 8–3)
   1. Acetylcholine is synthesized, stored, and released from the presynaptic vesicles. It is formed from the reaction of acetyl coenzyme A with choline.
   2. These vesicles are formed in the cell body and migrate to the surface of the presynaptic terminal.
   3. When an action potential reaches the presynaptic terminal, acetylcholine is released into the synapse.
   4. The acetylcholine moves across the synapse and stimulates a receptor on the postsynaptic terminal.
   5. After stimulation, the acetylcholine is released back into the synapse, and the postsynaptic terminal releases cholinesterase (acetylcholinesterase and acetylcholine esterase are terms synonymous with cholinesterase), which metabolizes acetylcholine, forming choline and acetic acid.
   6. The choline is reabsorbed into the presynaptic terminal and is available to form more acetylcholine.
F. Norepinephrine as the transmitter substance (Fig 8–4)
   1. Norepinephrine is synthesized, stored, and released from the presynaptic vesicles.
   2. The synthesis of norepinephrine proceeds via three reactions:

$$Tyrosine \rightarrow Dopa$$
$$Dopa \rightarrow Dopamine$$
$$Dopamine \rightarrow Norepinephrine$$

   3. Norepinephrine is released via a mechanism identical to acetylcholine (see section VI–E).

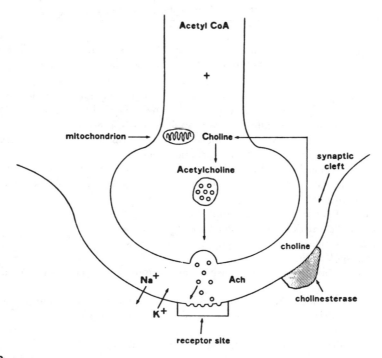

FIG 8–3.
Synthesis, storage, release, and inactivation of acetylcholine (see text). (From Rau JL: *Respiratory Therapy Pharmacology*, ed 2. Chicago, Year Book Medical Publishers, 1984. Used by permission.)

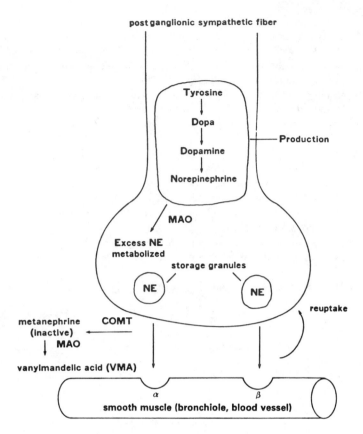

FIG 8–4.
Synthesis, storage, release, and inactivation of norepinephrine (see text). (From Rau JL: *Respiratory Therapy Pharmacology*, ed 2. Chicago, Year Book Medical Publishers, 1984. Used by permission.)

    4. After stimulation, norepinephrine has two possible immediate fates:
      a. Metabolism in the synapse by catechol-o-methyl-transferase (COMT).
      b. Reabsorption into the presynaptic terminal.
    5. Within the presynaptic terminal, norepinephrine has one of two fates:
      a. Reabsorption by the presynaptic vesicles.
      b. Metabolism in the cytoplasm by monoamine oxidase (MAO).
    6. Complete metabolism of products formed in the synapse occurs in the liver via both MAO and COMT.
VII. Alteration of Nerve Impulse Transmission
    A. Acidosis decreases transmission across the synapse.
    B. Alkalosis increases transmission across the synapse.
VIII. Neuromuscular Junction
    A. This junction is the site of transmission of impulses from nerves to skeletal muscle fibers.
    B. The axon of the nerve branches at its end to form a structure called the motor end-plate, which invaginates into muscle fiber but does not penetrate the muscle membrane.
    C. The motor end-plate's terminal aspects are referred to as *sole feet*.
    D. Sole feet provide a large area of "contact" on the muscle surface. It is from the sole feet that the transmitter substance acetylcholine is secreted.
    E. After stimulation, cholinesterase is secreted to metabolize acetylcholine.

IX. Reflex Arc or Reflex Action
   A. The reflex arc is a functional process of the nervous system. Most neuromuscular and neuroglandular mechanisms are controlled by it.
   B. The reflex arc consists of a series of neurons in which impulses are transmitted from a receptor to the CNS and then to a motor neuron to elicit a response.
   C. Most simple reflexes consist of an impulse from a sensory neuron being transmitted (normally in the spinal cord) to a motor neuron.
   D. Complex reflexes may involve many internuncial neurons.
   E. Reflex actions are involuntary, specific, predictable, and adaptive.
X. Organization of the Nervous System
   A. The nervous system is composed of the brain, spinal cord, ganglia (aggregations of nerve cell bodies), and nerves, which regulate and coordinate bodily activities.
   B. Divisions of the nervous system
     1. The CNS is composed of the brain and spinal cord, which acts as a switchboard, receiving and sending impulses to all areas of the body.
     2. The peripheral nervous system is composed of neurons that enter and leave the CNS. The peripheral nervous system has two main divisions:
       a. Somatic nervous system, which is responsible for voluntary bodily functions.
       b. Autonomic nervous system (ANS), which is responsible for involuntary bodily functions.
   C. Central nervous system
     1. The CNS is subdivided into the following structures:
       a. Cerebral cortex
       b. Diencephalon
         (1) Thalamus
         (2) Subthalamus
         (3) Hypothalamus
       c. Brain stem
         (1) Medulla
         (2) Pons
         (3) Midbrain
         (4) Cerebellum
       d. Spinal cord
     2. The cerebral cortex is primarily responsible for:
       a. All higher brain functions (memory, reasoning, sight, hearing, etc.)
       b. Integration of all sensory stimuli
       c. Voluntary control of bodily activities
     3. The diencephalon is located between the hemisphere of the cerebral cortex and the brain stem. It contains the following structures:
       a. Thalamus
         (1) Primary relay station of the brain for:
           (a) Hearing
           (b) Touch
           (c) Pressure
           (d) Position
           (e) Pain
         (2) Site of action of many psychoactive drugs.
       b. The subthalamus is responsible for the coordination of fine motor activity (extrapyramidal) with the cerebellum.
       c. Hypothalamus
         (1) It is responsible for many of the organism's vegetative functions via the ANS and hormonal control.
           (a) Eating

        (b) Drinking
        (c) Sleeping
        (d) Temperature
        (e) Sexual behavior
        (f) Fluid and electrolyte balance
      (2) The hypothalamus assists in the modulation of emotion and behavior.
      (3) Many psychoactive drugs are active at the hypothalamus.
  4. The brain stem lies within the cranium and connects the diencephalon with the spinal cord. It contains the following structures:
    a. Medulla
      (1) The medulla contains control centers for the following:
        (a) Respiration
        (b) Peripheral vasoconstriction
        (c) Gastrointestinal function
        (d) Sleeping
        (e) Walking
      (2) The ascending reticular activating system (ARAS) travels through the medulla. The ARAS helps to modulate behavior.
    b. The pons contains two centers that effect respiration (see Chapter 5):
      (1) Apneustic center
      (2) Pneumotaxic center
    c. The midbrain acts as a relay station, controlling vision and hearing.
    d. The cerebellum coordinates fine motor activity with the subthalamus.
  5. Spinal cord
    a. Channels information from the brain to the periphery.
    b. Most reflexes are coordinated via the spinal cord.
D. Somatic nervous system (Fig 8–5)
  1. The somatic nervous system is responsible for all voluntary muscular activities.
  2. It contains both sensory and motor neurons.
  3. Ganglia are located within the spinal cord.
E. Autonomic nervous system
  1. It contains only motor neurons (see Fig 8–5).
  2. It uses input via the somatic nervous system that is coordinated by the CNS.
  3. Each nerve of the ANS has a ganglion outside of the spinal cord.
  4. The ANS is responsible for all involuntary bodily activities.
  5. It is subdivided into:
    a. Parasympathetic (craniosacral) nervous system
    b. Sympathetic (thoracolumbar) nervous system (SNS)
  6. The two divisions are basically antagonistic.
  7. The ANS is activated and controlled primarily by:
    a. Spinal cord
    b. Brain stem
    c. Hypothalamus
  8. It is activated secondarily by:
    a. Cerebral cortex
    b. Visceral reflexes
  9. Sympathetic nervous system: Nerves of the SNS originate from the spinal cord at levels T–1 (thoracic) through L–2 (lumbar).
    a. Nerve fibers that transmit SNS impulses are either:
      (1) Preganglionic fibers
      (2) Postganglionic fibers

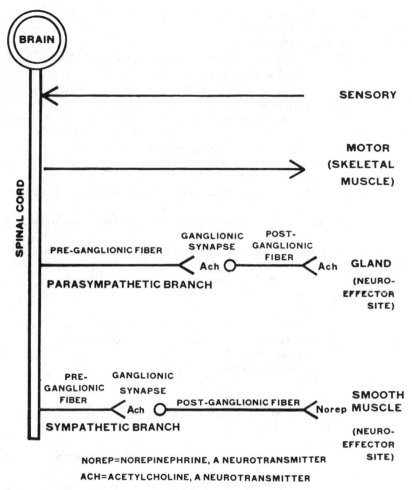

FIG 8–5.
Functional comparison of the CNS and the peripheral nervous system. (From Rau JL: *Respiratory Therapy Pharmacology,* ed 2. Chicago, Year Book Medical Publishers, 1984. Used by permission.)

    b. The SNS fibers synapse primarily at ganglia located along the spinal cord. Here they form a chain of interconnecting ganglia referred to as the *sympathetic chain.*

    c. Some SNS fibers synapse at peripheral ganglia (celiac ganglion and hypogastric plexus), bypassing the sympathetic chain.

    d. Transmitter substances of the SNS:
        (1) Preganglionic fiber: Acetylcholine
        (2) Postganglionic fiber: Norepinephrine

    e. Transmitter substance metabolism:
        (1) Acetylcholine: Metabolized by cholinesterase
        (2) Norepinephrine: Metabolized by MAO or COMT

  10. Parasympathetic nervous system (PNS): Nerves of the PNS originate from sacral nerves 1 through 4 and cranial nerves III, VII, IX, and X. Eighty percent of all PNS impulses originate from *cranial nerve X (vagus nerve).*

      a. Nerve fibers that transmit PNS impulses are either:
        (1) Preganglionic fiber
        (2) Postganglionic fiber
      b. These fibers synapse at the ganglia of the PNS, which are located very close to the organs they innervate.
      c. The transmitter substance for both preganglionic and postganglionic fibers is acetylcholine (metabolized by cholinesterase) (Table 8–1).
  F. Adrenal medulla: Secretes epinephrine (75% by volume) and norepinephrine (25% by volume) into the bloodstream, resulting in stimulation of the SNS.
    1. Innervation is via specific preganglionic fibers of the SNS.
    2. Adrenal secretions assist in maintaining normal tone of the SNS.
  G. Effects of activation of the SNS and PNS:
    1. Adrenergic effect: An effect activated or transmitted by norepinephrine or epinephrine.
    2. Adrenergic receptor: A receptor stimulated by norepinephrine or epinephrine.
    3. Cholinergic effect: An effect activated or transmitted by acetylcholine.
    4. Cholinergic receptor: A receptor stimulated by acetylcholine
    5. Effects of PNS and SNS on various organs:
      a. Lung
        (1) Bronchi
          SNS: Relaxes smooth muscles (bronchodilation)
          PNS: Contracts smooth muscles (bronchoconstriction)
        (2) Mucosal arterioles
          SNS: Vasoconstriction
          PNS: No effect
        (3) Pulmonary arterioles
          SNS: Vasoconstriction or dilation
          PNS: No effect
      b. Heart
        SNS: Increased rate (+ chronotropic effect) and force of contraction (+ inotropic effect)
        PNS: Decreased rate (− chronotropic effect) and force of contraction (− inotropic effect)
      c. Systemic blood vessels
        SNS: Vasoconstriction or dilation
        PNS: No effect

TABLE 8–1.

Comparison of the Sympathetic Nervous System and the Parasympathetic Nervous System

Feature	SNS	PNS
Origin of nerve fibers from the CNS	T-1 to L-2	S-1 to S-4; cranial nerves III, VII, IX, X
Relative length		
Preganglionic fiber	Short	Long
Postganglionic fiber	Long	Short
Transmitter substance		
Preganglionic fiber	Acetylcholine	Acetylcholine
Postganglionic fiber	Norepinephrine	Acetylcholine
Transmitter substance metabolized by		
Preganglionic fiber	Cholinesterase	Cholinesterase
Postganglionic fiber	MAO and COMT	Cholinesterase

    d. Gastrointestinal tract
       SNS: Decreased general motility
           Decreased glanular secretion
           Increased sphincter tone
       PNS: Increased general motility
           Increased glanular secretion
           Decreased sphincter tone
    e. Salivary gland
       SNS: Produces viscid secretions
       PNS: Produces profuse watery secretions
    f. Eye
       SNS: Relaxes ciliary muscle and dilates pupil
       PNS: Contracts ciliary muscle and constricts pupil

BIBLIOGRAPHY

Carrier O: *Pharmacology of the Peripheral Autonomic Nervous System.* Chicago, Year Book Medical Publishers, 1972.

Ganong WF: *Review of Medical Physiology,* ed 9. Los Altos, Calif, Lange Medical Publications, 1988.

Goodman LS, Gilman A (eds): *The Pharmacological Basis of Therapeutics,* ed 6. New York, Macmillan Publishing Co, 1984.

Guyton AC: *Textbook of Medical Pharmacology,* ed 6. Philadelphia, WB Saunders Co, 1981.

Julian RM: *A Primer of Drug Action,* ed 3. San Francisco, WH Freeman & Co Publishers, 1981.

Lehnert BE: *The Pharmacology of Respiratory Care.* St Louis, CV Mosby Co, 1980.

Rau JL: *Respiratory Therapy Pharmacology,* ed 3. Chicago, Year Book Medical Publishers, 1989.

Spearman CB, Sheldon RL, Egan DF: *Egan's Fundamentals of Respiratory Therapy,* ed 4. St Louis, CV Mosby Co, 1982.

Chapter 9

Renal Anatomy and Physiology

I. Gross Anatomy (Fig 9-1)
  A. The kidneys are located outside the peritoneal cavity on each side of the spinal column within the posterior abdominal wall.
  B. Renal vessels and nerves enter on the medial border.
  C. Exiting each kidney from the medial border is a single ureter that conducts urine to the bladder.
  D. A single urethra leaves the bladder.
  E. The renal pelvis is a continuation of the ureter and forms the control collecting area of each kidney.
   1. The outer border of the renal pelvis is divided into major calices.
   2. Each major calyx is subdivided into minor calices.
   3. Each minor calyx is cupped about a renal pyramid.
   4. Nephrons, the functional aspect of the kidney, are located within each renal pyramid (Fig 9-2).
  F. A dissection of the kidney from top to bottom demonstrates two major regions:
   1. The outer region, called the *renal cortex*
   2. The inner region, called the *renal medulla*
II. The Nephron (Fig 9-3; see also Fig 9-2)
  A. The nephron is the functional unit of the kidney.
  B. Each kidney is composed of about 1 million nephrons.
  C. Each nephron is composed of a kidney tubule and its corresponding blood supply.
  D. The site of initial formation of urine is the glomerulus. The glomerulus filters blood into Bowman's capsule, forming the glomerular filtrate.
  E. The kidney tubule itself begins with Bowman's capsule and continues sequentially with the following structures:
   1. Proximal convoluted tubule
   2. Loop of Henle
    a. Descending limb
    b. Ascending limb
   3. Distal convoluted tubule
   4. Collecting duct
  F. The circulatory supply of the nephron is provided by the arcuate artery.
   1. From this artery an afferent arteriole leads to the glomerulus.
   2. Blood exits the glomerulus via an efferent arteriole.

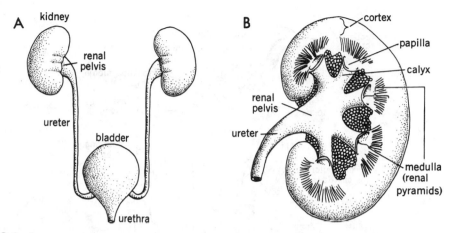

FIG 9–1.
Gross anatomy of the kidney. (From Vander AJ, et al: *Human Physiology*. New York, McGraw-Hill Book Co, 1970. Used by permission.)

3. The efferent arteriole forms the peritubular capillaries, which intertwine about the distal and proximal convoluted tubules.
4. The efferent arterioles also form the vasa recta, a long looping capillary that forms about the loop of Henle.
5. Blood leaves the peritubular capillaries and the vasa recta via the arcuate veins.

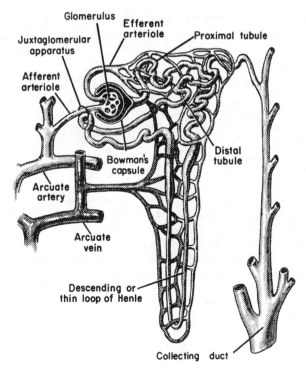

FIG 9–2.
Gross anatomy of the nephron. (From Smith: *The Kidney: Structure and Functions in Health and Disease*. New York, Oxford University Press, 1951. Used by permission.)

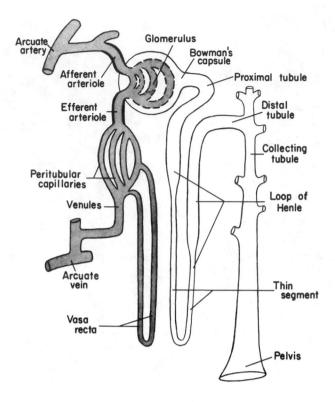

FIG 9–3.
Gross anatomy of the kidney tubular system and corresponding circulatory system. (From Guyton AC: *Textbook of Medical Physiology,* ed 6. Philadelphia, Lea & Febiger, 1981. Used by permission.)

III. Major Functions of the Kidney
    A. The primary function of the kidney is twofold:
        1. Excretion of end products of bodily metabolism
        2. Control of the concentration of constituents of the body fluids
    B. These primary functions are performed by a number of interrelated processes.
        1. Formation of the glomerular filtrate (see section IV)
        2. Tubular reabsorption (see section V)
        3. Tubular secretion (see section VI)
        4. Renin secretion (see section XI)
        5. Erythropoietic factor secretion: In the presence of hypoxemia, the kidney secretes erythropoietic factor, which stimulates red blood cell production.
        6. Activation of vitamin D: Vitamin D is necessary for appropriate absorption of calcium via the gastrointestinal tract.
        7. Gluconeogenesis, which is the formation of glucose from fats and protein during periods of significant physiologic stress.
IV. Glomerular Filtration
    A. Filtration of fluid and electrolytes at the glomerulus follows Starling's law of fluid exchange (see Chapter 15).
    B. However, since protein is poorly filterable across the glomerulus, except under pathologic conditions, only three forces normally control fluid exchange.
        1. Forces moving fluid out of the glomerulus
           a. Glomerular hydrostatic pressure   60 mm Hg
           b. Total outward force   60 mm Hg

2. Forces maintaining fluid in the glomerulus
    a. Glomerular colloid osmotic pressure   28 mm Hg
    b. Bowman's capsule hydrostatic pressure   +18 mm Hg
    c. Total inward force   46 mm Hg
3. Net filtration pressure
    a. Total outward force   60 mm Hg
    b. Total inward force   −46 mm Hg
    c. Filtration pressure   14 mm Hg

C. In the average adult about 125 ml/min of fluid is filtered across the glomerulus.
D. This filtrate is essentially protein free and has concentrations of dissolved crystalloids similar to that of plasma (see Table 9–1).
E. The kidney receives about 20% of the cardiac output, of which about 55% is fluid.
   1. If cardiac output is 5.5 L, 1.1 L perfuses the kidney each minute.
   2. Fifty-five percent of 1.1 L is 605 ml/min of fluid.
   3. From this fluid volume, 125 ml/min of glomerular filtrate is formed.
   4. The glomerular filtration fraction is the percent of the plasma volume filtered:

$$\frac{125 \text{ ml/min}}{605 \text{ ml/min}} \approx 0.20, \text{ or } 20\%$$

   5. Normally, 20% of the fluid presented to the kidney is filtered.
F. Alterations in the tone of the afferent arteriole and the efferent arteriole affect the volume of glomerular filtrate formed.
   1. Increased tone of the afferent arteriole decreases glomerular hydrostatic pressure and thus filtration volume.
   2. Increased tone of the efferent arteriole increases glomerular hydrostatic pressure and thus filtration volume.

V. Tubular Reabsorption: The movement of filtered substances back into the bloodstream.
   A. Of the 125 ml/min of glomerular filtrate formed, only 1 ml/min of urine is formed; the remainder is reabsorbed. Normally, urinary output is about 40 to 60 ml/hour.
   B. Reabsorption occurs via simple diffusion, facilitated diffusion, and active transport mechanisms (see Chapter 15).

TABLE 9–1.

Approximate Concentrations of Substances in the Glomerular Filtrate and in the Urine

Substance	Urine	Glomerular Filtrate
Glucose (mg%)	100	0
Creatinine (mEq/L)	196	1.1
Uric acid (mEq/L)	3	42
Urea (mEq/L)	26	1,820
SO_4^{-2} (mEq/L)	0.7	33
$H_2PO_4^{-1}/HPO_4^{-2}$ (mEq/L)	2	50
HCO_3^{-} (mEq/L)	28	14
Cl^{-} (mEq/L)	103	134
Mg^{+2} (mEq/L)	3	15
Ca^{+2} (mEq/L)	4	4.8
K^{+} (mEq/L)	5	60
Na^{+} (mEq/L)	142	128

    C. The vast majority of the electrolytes in the glomerular filtrate are reabsorbed. Less than 1.0% of the following filtered substances are excreted (see Table 9–1):
1. Sodium
2. Chloride
3. Potassium
4. Bicarbonate
5. Phosphate
6. Sulfate
7. Calcium
8. Magnesium
9. Albumin
    D. All filtered glucose is reabsorbed, unless the blood glucose level is more than 375 mg/dl (mg%). The threshold for the spillage of glucose in the urine is 375 mg/dl (mg%).
    E. About 50% of the urea filtered is reabsorbed.
    F. Little of the creatinine and creatine filtered is reabsorbed.

VI. Tubular Secretion
    A. Tubular secretion is the movement of substances from the blood into the kidney tubule.
    B. The following substances are secreted into the kidney tubule:
1. Potassium
2. Hydrogen
3. Urea
4. Creatinine

VII. Renal Clearance
    A. Clearance of a substance refers to the volume of plasma cleared of the substance per unit time.
    B. Every substance in the blood has its own clearance rate.
    C. Renal clearance of a substance is equal to the glomerular filtration rate (GFR) if the substance is:
1. Freely diffusible at the glomerulus.
2. Not chemically altered in the kidney.
3. Not secreted.
4. Not reabsorbed.
5. Thus, all of the substance that is filtered is excreted.
    D. Renal clearance is equal to:

$$C = \frac{(U)(V)}{P} \tag{1}$$

where C = clearance of substance X, U = urine concentration of X, V = urine volume per unit time, and P = arterial plasma concentration of X.
    E. Normally, renal clearance is determined from a 24-hour urine sample.
    F. Inulin, an inert polysaccharide, is the standard for determining the GFR because its renal clearance is equal to the GFR.
    G. Clinically, plasma creatinine and urea levels are used as indicators of GFR changes.
1. Creatinine results from the breakdown of voluntary muscle. As muscle breaks down, creatine is produced, which is converted to creatinine in the blood.
2. Urea is produced from the metabolism of amino acids.
3. Plasma creatinine levels are indirectly affected by the GFR.
4. All creatinine filtered is excreted.
5. In addition, a small quantity of creatinine is secreted.
6. Plasma concentration of creatinine is usually about 1.3 mEq/L but can increase tenfold during renal failure.

7. Plasma concentration of urea is 26 mEq/L and may increase to 200 mEq/L during renal failure.
8. Thus, as the GFR decreases, the plasma creatinine level increases.
9. Urea plasma levels are also indirectly affected by the GFR.
10. Plasma concentrations of creatinine are affected by the following:
    a. Glomerular filtration rate
    b. Breakdown of voluntary muscle
    c. Hypermetabolic states
11. Plasma concentrations of urea are affected by the following:
    a. Glomerular filtration rate
    b. Breakdown of voluntary muscle
    c. Hypermetabolic state
    d. Metabolism of sequestered (third space) blood

VIII. Counter Current Multiplier
   A. The configuration of the nephron allows for the concentrating of urine.
   B. In the descending limb of the loop of Henle, water is reabsorbed. However, Na^+ and Cl^- are not reabsorbed. Thus, the concentration of the filtrate increases toward the tip of the nephron.
   C. In the ascending limb of the loop of Henle, Na^+ and Cl^- are reabsorbed. However, water is not reabsorbed. Thus, the concentration of the filtrate decreases toward the top of the loop of Henle.
   D. This arrangement causes a variation in the osmolarity of the interstitium from the top to the bottom of the loop of Henle. This variation is maintained by the arrangement of the circulatory system.
   E. The collecting duct passes through the interstitium parallel to the loop of Henle. As a result, fluid moving through the collecting duct can be concentrated if the permeability of the collecting duct to water and Na^+ reabsorption are increased.

IX. Antidiuretic Hormone (ADH)
   A. Antidiuretic hormone affects the reabsorption of water in the distal convoluted tubule and the collecting duct.
   B. Increased ADH increases the reabsorption of water.
   C. Decreased ADH decreases the reabsorption of water.
   D. Antidiuretic hormone levels are controlled by the hypothalamus.
   E. Antidiuretic hormone is actually released by the posterior pituitary via stimulation from the hypothalamus.
   F. Antidiuretic hormone levels are controlled by:
      1. Pressure in the atria
         a. Increased atrial pressure is viewed by the body as an increased extracellular fluid volume: therefore, ADH levels are decreased.
         b. Decreased atrial pressure is viewed by the body as a decreased extracellular fluid volume; therefore, ADH levels are increased. (Positive pressure ventilation and positive end-expiratory pressure (PEEP) normally decrease atrial pressure.)
      2. Osmolarity of the extracellular fluid
         a. Decreased osmolarity is viewed by the body as an increase in extracellular fluid volume; therefore, ADH levels are decreased.
         b. Increased osmolarity is viewed by the body as a decrease in extracellular fluid volume; therefore, ADH levels are increased.
      3. Urine specific gravity provides an index of how concentrated the urine actually is.
         a. Normally, the specific gravity is about 1.020, but it may range between 1.002 and 1.045.

       b. Decreased specific gravity is associated with decreased ADH production and increased vascular volume.

       c. Increased specific gravity is associated with increased ADH production and decreased vascular volume.

X. Aldosterone

  A. Aldosterone controls the reabsorption of Na^+ and the secretion of K^+.

  B. Increased aldosterone increases the reabsorption of Na^+ and the secretion of K^+.

  C. Decreased aldosterone decreases the reabsorption of Na^+ and the secretion of K^+.

  D. Aldosterone affects Na^+ and K^+ movement at the distal convoluted tubule and the collecting duct.

  E. Aldosterone is secreted by the adrenal cortex. Its levels are increased by:

    1. Decreased serum Na^+

    2. Increased serum K^+

    3. Increased adrenocorticotropic hormone (ACTH) (see Chapter 40)

    4. Increased angiotensin II (see section XI)

XI. Renin-Angiotensin

  A. Renin is secreted by the kidney in response to a decrease in the delivery of sodium chloride to a group of cells located between the afferent and efferent arterioles, the macula densa cells.

  B. Essentially, a decrease in perfusion of the kidney increases the release of renin.

  C. Renin converts angiotensinogen formed by the liver to angiotensin I.

  D. Angiotensin I is converted to angiotensin II by the pulmonary endothelium.

  E. Figure 9–4 summarizes the effects of angiotensin II.

  F. Angiotensin II is converted to angiotensin III. Most of the effects in Figure 9–4 can also be attributed to angiotensin III.

  G. Angiotensin levels facilitate Na^+ and H_2O retention and elevate arterial blood pressure. Angiotensin is the strongest vasopressor produced by the body.

  H. Angiotensin levels increase in response to physiologic stress.

XII. Secretion of H^+ and Reabsorption of HCO_3^-

  A. Figure 9–5 illustrates the sequence of reactions maintaining normal H^+ secretion and HCO_3^- reabsorption.

  B. Carbonic anhydrase is present in kidney tubule cells, increasing the hydration of CO_2, which dissociates into H^+ and HCO_3^-.

  C. As CO_2 enters the kidney cell, H^+ and HCO_3^- are formed. The HCO_3^- formed moves into the blood, and the H^+ moves into the glomerular filtrate. As each H^+ moves into the glomerular filtrate, a Na^+ is reabsorbed into the bloodstream.

  D. In the glomerular filtrate, the H^+ is buffered by:

    1. HCO_3^-

    2. HPO_4^{-2} (dibasic phosphate)

    3. NH_3 (ammonia)

  E. Note that for every HCO_3^- reabsorbed, one H^+ is secreted.

  F. This series of reactions (see Fig 9–5) continues in the presence of normal acid-base balance.

  G. If a decrease in plasma Pa_{CO_2} occurs, there is a decrease in the amount of HCO_3^- reabsorbed and H^+ excreted.

  H. If Pa_{CO_2} levels are increased, there is an increase in the amount of HCO_3^- reabsorbed and H^+ excreted.

  I. When this occurs, the HCO_3^- in the tubular lumen is rapidly depleted; HPO_4^{-2} and NH_3 are used to buffer the excess H^+ excreted (Figs 9–6 and 9–7).

  J. The kidney can continue to buffer acid until the pH of the urine decreases to about 4.0.

  K. Normal pH of the urine is about 7.33 to 7.37.

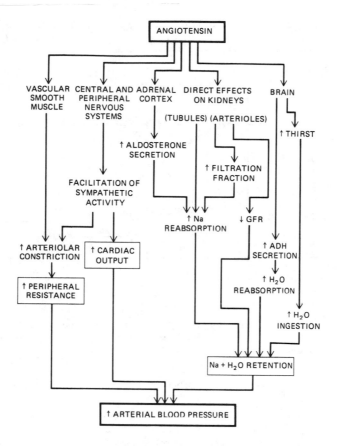

FIG 9–4.
The direct and indirect effects of an increase in angiotensin. Note that all responses are directed toward an increase in Na^+ and H_2O retention and an increase in arterial blood pressure. (From Vander AJ: *Renal Physiology,* ed 2. New York, McGraw-Hill Book Co, 1980. Used by permission.)

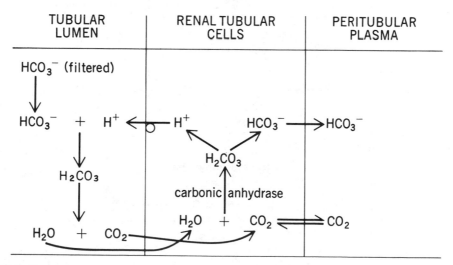

FIG 9–5.
The normal mechanism for the reabsorption of filtered HCO_3^-. For every HCO_3^- reabsorbed, one H^+ ion is secreted. *O* indicates that movement of H^+ is via an active transport mechanism. (From Vander AJ: *Renal Physiology,* ed 2. New York, McGraw-Hill Book Co, 1980. Used by permission.)

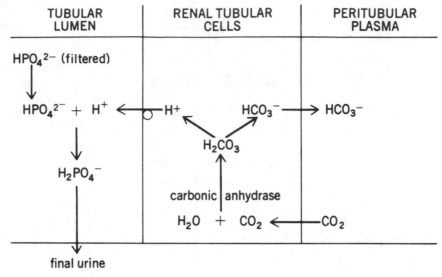

FIG 9–6.
The use of HPO_4^{-2} as a buffer of secreted H^+. This system is active primarily in the presence of excess Pa_{CO_2}, creating a larger quantity of H^+ to be secreted than normal. With each H^+ ion secreted, a HCO_3^- is reabsorbed, thus increasing total extracellular $[HCO_3^-]$. (From Vander AJ: *Renal Physiology,* ed 2. New York, McGraw-Hill Book Co, 1980. Used by permission.)

      L. The quantity of HCO_3^- reabsorbed over normal is equal to the amount of acid excreted in the form of $H_2PO_4^{-1}$ and NH_4^+.

    M. Renal compensation for respiratory acid-base imbalances:

        1. If Pco_2 level increases, more HCO_3^- is formed and moved into the blood. This normalizes the acidic pH caused by the increased Pco_2 level.

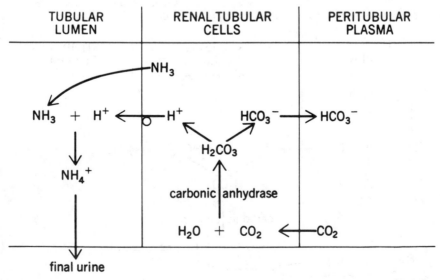

FIG 9–7.
The reaction of secreted H^+ with NH_3. This system is active primarily in the presence of excess Pa_{CO_2}. The additional H^+ formed is buffered, and HCO_3^- is reabsorbed, increasing the total extracellular $[HCO_3^-]$. (From Vander AJ: *Renal Physiology,* ed 2. New York, McGraw-Hill Book Co, 1980. Used by permission.)

2. If P_{CO_2} level decreases, less HCO_3^- is formed and moved into the blood. This normalizes the alkalotic pH caused by the decreased P_{CO_2} level.
3. Compensation by the kidney is relatively complete, but the mechanism may take hours to normalize the pH (24–48 hours).

BIBLIOGRAPHY

Ellerbe S: *Fluid and Blood Component Therapy in the Critically Ill and Injured.* New York, Churchill Livingstone, 1981.

Gabow PA: *Fluids and Electrolytes: Clinical Problems and Their Solution.* Boston, Little, Brown & Co, 1983.

Guyton AC: *Textbook of Medical Physiology,* ed 7. Philadelphia, Lea & Febiger, 1988.

Rose BD: *Clinical Physiology of Acid-Base and Electrolyte Disorders.* New York, McGraw-Hill Book Co, 1977.

Schrier RW (ed.): *Renal and Electrolyte Disorders,* ed 2. Boston, Little, Brown & Co, 1980.

Smith K: *Fluids and Electrolytes: A Conceptual Approach.* New York, Churchill Livingstone, 1980.

Sullivan LP: *Physiology of the Kidney.* Philadelphia, Lea & Febiger, 1975.

Tepperman J: *Metabolic and Endocrine Physiology: An Introductory Text,* ed 3. Chicago, Year Book Medical Publishers, 1973.

Vanatta JC, Fogelman MJ: *Moyers Fluid Balance: A Clinical Manual,* ed 2. Chicago, Year Book Medical Publishers, 1976.

Vander AJ: *Renal Physiology,* ed 2. New York, McGraw-Hill Book Co, 1980.

Weldy NJ: *Body Fluids and Electrolytes: A Programmed Presentation,* ed 3. St Louis, CV Mosby Co, 1980.

Chapter 10

Intrauterine Development and Comparative Respiratory Anatomy

I. General Developmental Periods
   A. Fertilization period (weeks 1–3)
      1. Egg is fertilized by the sperm.
      2. Blood vessels first appear.
      3. Heart tubes form that will develop into the heart.
      4. Blood cells form from endothelial cells within the yolk sac.
   B. Embryonic period (weeks 4–7)
      1. Embryo forms a C-shaped appearance.
      2. Primitive gut is formed.
      3. Umbilical cord develops.
      4. Three primary germ layers differentiate into various organs and tissues.
      5. The brain, heart, eyes, ears, nose, and mouth are developing, giving the embryo human characteristics.
   C. Fetal period (week 8–birth)
      1. The embryo is now called a *fetus*.
      2. Rapid body growth and organ system maturation occur.
II. Respiratory System Development
   A. Upper airway
      1. By the fourth week, branchial arches form and develop the maxillary (upper) and mandibular (lower) jaw.
      2. The brachial arches also form the pharynx, mouth, oropharyngeal airway, and laryngeal cartilages.
      3. The tongue develops within weeks 4 to 7.
      4. The palate starts to develop in the fifth week and is complete by the 17th week of gestation.
      5. A cleft lip may develop as a result of the lip not completely forming and extending into the nostril. A cleft palate occurs from malformation of the palate and may be unilateral or bilateral.
      6. The nasal cavity with nasal concha develop when the oronasal membrane ruptures, allowing the oral and nasal cavities to develop. This occurs about the seventh week.
      7. Nasal sinuses develop during the latter part of fetal development, with further development of the ethmoid, maxillary, frontal, and sphenoidal sinuses continuing into puberty.

B. Lower airway
1. An epithelial groove will give rise to the larynx, trachea, br
    epithelium, and assorted glands.
2. The tracheoesophageal septum divides into the esophagu
    cheal tube.
3. The first lung bud develops from the laryngotracheal tube by 24 to 26 days of
    fertilization.
4. The laryngotracheal tube, along with the surrounding tissue, develops into
    the larynx, trachea, bronchi, and lungs.
5. Visceral and parietal pleura develop from the lung buds (bronchopulmonary
    buds).
6. The phrenic nerve innervates the diaphragm within the fourth week, and the
    diaphragm is completely formed by the seventh week.
7. By the tenth week, true and false vocal cords are formed.
8. Further growth of the lung buds develop into secondary buds, two on the
    right and one on the left.
9. This branching continues, with 24 orders of branches present at 16 weeks.
C. Periods of lung maturation
1. Embryonic period (fertilization–5 weeks)
    a. The laryngotracheal groove forms.
    b. The lung bud first appears.
    c. The lung bud divides into left and right mainstem bronchi.
2. Pseudoglandular period (5–13 weeks)
    a. The conducting airways develop and are complete up to and including the
        terminal bronchiole.
    b. Mucous glands and goblet cells appear.
    c. Bronchi and bronchioles are lined with cuboidal epithelium.
3. Canalicular period (13–24 weeks)
    a. Enlargement of the conducting airways continues, with proliferation of
        pulmonary blood vessels.
    b. Gas exchange units develop from respiratory bronchioles.
    c. Cilia appear at 13 weeks.
    d. Meconium is present at 16 weeks.
    e. Breathing movements can be detected between 18 and 20 weeks.
    f. Elastic tissue develops beginning at 20 weeks.
    g. Type I and II alveolar pneumocytes develop, with synthesis and produc-
        tion of surfactant starting by weeks 22 to 24.
4. Terminal sac period (24 weeks–birth)
    a. Primitive alveoli develop from alveolar ducts.
    b. Further development of the pulmonary vasculature occurs, as does lym-
        phatic proliferation.
    c. The fetus weighs approximately 1,000 gm at 26 to 28 weeks.
    d. The fetal lungs represent 2% to 3% of the total body weight. This percentage
        decreases as the weight of the fetus increases toward the end of gestation.
    e. The air sacs change from a cuboidal cellular configuration to a squamous
        epithelium, allowing greater diffusion of gases.
    f. As the lung matures, the number of alveoli increase, and the thickness of
        the alveoli wall decreases.
    g. At birth the number of alveoli range from 24 to 75 million.
    h. The number of alveoli continues to increase until there are approximately
        300 to 400 million alveoli in adulthood.
    i. The size of the lung increases from approximately 1 to 2 sq m at 32 weeks'
        gestation to adult size of 70 sq m.
    j. Extrauterine life is first possible in this period.

III. Fetal Lung Fluid
   A. The lung begins secreting fluid by the 70th day of gestation.
   B. This fluid is composed of a combination of sodium, potassium, chloride, bicarbonate, and a small percentage of protein in water.
   C. The presence of lung fluid assists lung growth and the development of the functional residual capacity (FRC).
   D. Fetal breathing helps secrete lung fluid and mixes lung fluid with amniotic fluid.
   E. Because of this process, amniotic fluid can be analyzed to determine lung maturation (see section V).
   F. Amniocentesis is the procedure in which amniotic fluid is removed from the uterus.

IV. Surfactant
   A. Surfactant is synthesized and secreted by type II alveolar pneumocytes.
   B. Surfactant first appears between 22 and 24 weeks' gestation.
   C. Surfactant reduces surface tension, maintaining alveolar stability and preventing atelectasis.
   D. Protein makes up 10% to 20% of the surfactant, and 80% to 90% of the protein is phospholipids. A very small percentage of cholesterol is also present.
   E. Two important phospholipids, lecithin and sphingomyelin, are present in surfactant.
   F. Sphingomyelin is present early in gestation and remains constant from 18 weeks to approximately 34 weeks before decreasing in concentration.
   G. Lecithin, the major phospholipid of adult surfactant, abruptly increases between 32 and 34 weeks' gestation.
   H. The increased concentration of lecithin denotes lung maturation. The increase of lecithin in surfactant reduces the incidence of respiratory distress syndrome (RDS).
   I. Without appropriate surfactant production, newborns will have a reduced lung compliance, a decreased FRC, an increased work of breathing, and a greater oxygen consumption.
   J. Inadequate surfactant levels can occur in a newborn as a result of:
      1. Prematurity
      2. Hypoxia
      3. Malnutrition
      4. Maternal diabetes
      5. Hypothermia
      6. Acidosis

V. Amniotic Fluid
   A. Amniotic fluid is composed of amniotic cells, maternal blood, and fetal urine.
   B. There is approximately 30 ml of amniotic fluid at 10 weeks, which increases to 1 L by term.
   C. The fetus swallows amniotic fluid, which is absorbed by the gastrointestinal tract. Every 3 hours, amniotic fluid is exchanged by the placenta.
   D. Amniotic fluid protects the fetus and acts as a cushion surrounding the fetus. It also allows growth and development, movement, and maintenance of a thermoneutral environment.
   E. Amniocentesis can determine sex, lung maturity, biochemical abnormalities, and chromosomal defects.
   F. Lung maturity is determined by the concentration of lecithin and sphingomyelin.
   G. The ratio of lecithin to sphingomyelin (L/S) determines the incidence of RDS.
   H. An L/S ratio of 2.0 or greater indicates a very low incidence.
   I. An L/S ratio of 1.5 to 1.0 indicates a transitional lung with a moderate incidence of RDS.

J. An L/S ratio of less than 1.0 indicates a high incidence of RDS.

K. Another test that determines lung maturity is the shake test.

  a. A mixture of amniotic fluid, saline and alcohol is placed in a test tube, shaken for 15 minutes, and then allowed to stand.

  b. A complete ring of bubbles around the tube indicates appropriate fetal production of surfactant.

  c. These results can be compared with an L/S ratio of greater than 2.0.

  d. Absence of bubbles indicate that surfactant maturity is incomplete.

VI. Placenta

  A. Major activities of the placenta include metabolism, transfer of nutrients and wastes, and endocrine secretion.

  B. It provides exchange of oxygen, carbon dioxide, and metabolic nutrients between fetal and maternal blood supplies.

  C. Blood supplies of the mother and fetus are in close proximity to one another but are not in actual contact.

  D. Fetal blood enters the placenta by way of two umbilical arteries and leaves by one umbilical vein.

  E. During birth, contractions of the uterus slow blood flow to the placenta, and gas exchange may be reduced.

VII. Fetal Circulation (Fig 10–1)

  A. After oxygenated blood leaves the placenta, a portion of the blood enters the portal sinus to perfuse the kidney. The remainder enters the ductus venosus, bypassing the liver and entering the inferior vena cava (see Fig 10–1).

  B. The oxygen saturation of the blood (Sa_{O_2}) coming from the placenta is approximately 80%. The Pa_{O_2} is 27 to 29 mm Hg.

  C. Blood coming from the inferior vena cava has perfused lower body tissues and has reduced Sa_{O_2} and Pa_{O_2}. Thus, as the oxygenated blood from the ductus venosus enters the inferior vena cava and mixes, the Sa_{O_2} drops to about 67%.

  D. The blood enters the right atrium from the inferior vena cava, where it mixes with blood returning from the upper part of the body and head. This further reduces the saturation to approximately 62%.

  E. The blood flow entering the right atrium is divided into two streams, with the larger stream entering the left atrium by way of the foramen ovale.

  F. The foramen ovale is an opening of the interatrial septum between the right and left atria.

  G. This opening remains patent due to the increase in blood pressure in the right side of the heart relative to that of the left.

  H. The blood enters the left atrium, then mixes with a small amount of deoxygenated blood returning from the lungs by way of the pulmonary veins. This blood enters the left ventricle and is pumped out the aorta.

  I. A portion of this blood is directed up to the head and upper extremities. This flow of blood has a higher oxygen content and Sa_{O_2} than the flow that is pumped out of the right ventricle.

  J. The second stream of blood in the right atrium is pumped to the right ventricle and out the pulmonary artery. This blood has mixed with blood coming in from the superior vena cava.

  K. About 10% of the cardiac output from the right side of the heart enters the pulmonary arteries and the lung. Very little blood is needed by the lungs at this time, because gas exchange occurs within the placenta.

  L. The pulmonary arteries are constricted from the low Pa_{O_2} and lung fluid compressing the vessels within the lung. In general, the pulmonary vascular resistance is high, with the peripheral vascular resistance low.

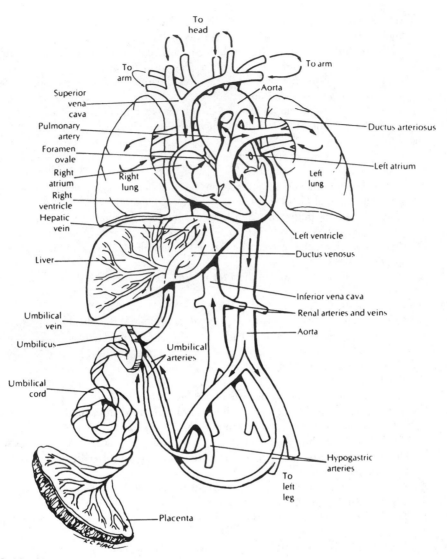

FIG 10–1.
Fetal circulation as it leaves the placenta and enters the heart. (From Eubanks D, Bone R: *Comprehensive Respiratory Care*. St Louis, CV Mosby Co, 1985. Used by permission.)

  M. The greater volume of blood from the right side of the heart enters the arch of the aorta by way of the ductus arteriosus. This ductus connects the pulmonary arteries and aorta and creates a right-to-left shunt. The saturation of this blood is approximately 50%.

  N. Blood flow moves out of the heart through the ductus arteriosus to the arch of the aorta, descending aorta, and thoracic aorta. Here blood is directed to the kidney, gut, and lower part of the body.

  O. A major portion of the blood (about 50% of the cardiac output) enters the placenta for oxygenation.

 VIII. Transfer of Oxygen From Maternal to Fetal Blood (Fig 10–2)

  A. Maternal blood enters the placenta through spiral arteries. The Pa_{O_2} of the maternal blood is 100 mm Hg.

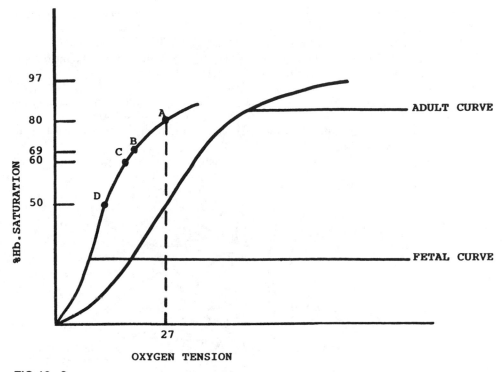

FIG 10–2.
Adult and fetal dissociation curve. Point *A* is saturation level in the umbilical artery. Point *B* is saturation in inferior vena cava prior to entering the right atrium. Point *C* is the Sa_{O_2} within the right atrium, and point *D* is Sa_{O_2} of the blood returning to the placenta and lower extremities.

B. Fetal blood enters the placenta through two umbilical arteries, which divide to form a vascular network. The Pa_{O_2} of the fetal blood entering the placenta is approximately 17 mm Hg.

C. As both circulations come into proximity of one another, maternal blood releases oxygen to fetal circulation while at the same time accepting metabolic waste from fetal circulation.

D. The metabolic components alter the pH of maternal blood, shifting the oxyhemoglobin curve to the right, which reduces the affinity of hemoglobin for oxygen. This allows more oxygen to be released to fetal blood.

E. The fetal oxyhemoglobin curve is shifted to the left from the release of metabolic waste as well as fetal hemoglobin (HbF).

F. Oxygen is able to combine with HbF to a greater extent than adult hemoglobin (HbA) because 2,3-diphosphoglycerate (2,3-DPG) does not affect HbF.

G. One of the primary mechanisms regulating the release of oxygen from HbA is the binding of 2,3-DPG to β (beta) chains of hemoglobin. Fetal hemoglobin has no β chains, so 2,3-DPG cannot attach to it.

H. As a result, the oxyhemoglobin curve is shifted further to the left than that seen in the adult. Therefore, even with a low maternal Pa_{O_2}, HbF is able to maintain a higher Sa_{O_2} than seen in maternal circulation. However, since the curve is shifted to the left, release of oxygen at the tissue level is impeded (see Fig 10–2).

I. Maternal blood flow leaving the placenta and returning to the mother has a Pa_{O_2} of approximately 38 to 40 mm Hg.

J. The fetal blood flow leaving the placenta has an umbilical artery Pa_{O_2} of approximately 29 mm Hg. The Sa_{O_2} is 80%.

K. In contrast, an adult with a Pa_{O_2} of 27 mm Hg would have an Sa_{O_2} of 50%.

L. At birth, approximately 77% of the total hemoglobin is HbF. Within 8 to 11 months, only 1% to 2% of the total hemoglobin will be HbF.

IX. Transition From Fetal to Newborn Circulation (Fig 10–3)

A. By the end of the normal gestational period of 38 to 40 weeks, the fetus has completely developed and is able to assume extrauterine life (see Fig 10–3).

B. Following birth, inflation of the lungs and transition of fetal circulation to newborn circulation occurs.

C. Vaginal birth of the fetus is initiated by contraction of the uterus.

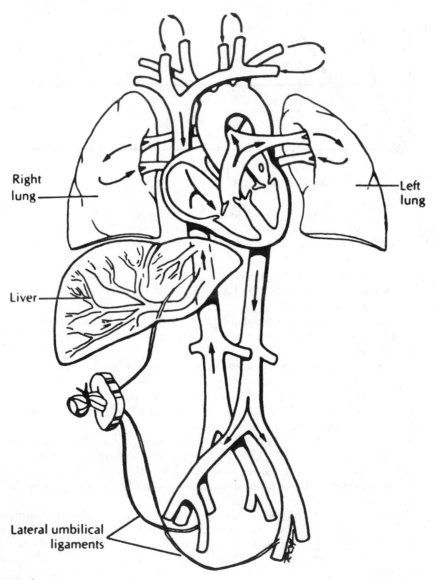

FIG 10–3.
Newborn circulation. (From Eubanks D, Bone R: *Comprehensive Respiratory Care*. St Louis, CV Mosby Co, 1985. Used by permission.)

D. The fetus moves head first through the birth canal, where the chest is compressed. Intrathoracic pressures of 30 to 160 cm H_2O develop, which forces lung fluid from the airways.

E. Further presentation of the fetus allows passive recoil and the first introduction of air into the lungs.

F. A greater flow of blood enters the pulmonary vasculature as a result of vasodilation from the increase in Pa_{O_2} and partial removal of lung fluid. Additional lung fluid is removed by lymphatic drainage.

G. For a short period of time, a small left-to-right shunt exists as pulmonary artery pressure falls while the ductus arteriosus remains patent.

H. The ductus arteriosus constricts from the increased Pa_{O_2}. This diverts more blood into the pulmonary vasculature. The ductus arteriosus remains partially open after birth but closes within 3 weeks.

I. If the newborn develops hypoxia following birth, the ductus arteriosus remains open and continues to shunt blood. This reduces the pulmonary blood flow and further reduces the Pa_{O_2}.

J. The ductus arteriosus responds by constricting to increased Pa_{O_2} with the administration of supplemental oxygen.

K. Prostaglandin synthetase inhibitor such as indomethacin (Indocin) is used to constrict the ductus arteriosus.

L. During fetal development, prostaglandin E_1 and E_2, along with the decreased Pa_{O_2}, maintain the opening of the ductus arteriosus, thus providing the higher saturated blood to be routed to the brain.

M. Following complete presentation of the fetus, the umbilical cord is clamped and cut, which discontinues umbilical circulation and placental function.

N. The umbilical arteries and vein constrict.

O. The ductus venosus closes within 3 to 7 days and forms the ligamentum venosum.

P. Blood flow now follows the normal circulatory pathway through the liver.

Q. Left atrial pressure increases as a result of greater return of blood from the pulmonary veins. This pressure change functionally closes the foramen ovale. Anatomic closure from proliferation of fibrous and endothelial tissue occurs within a few weeks of birth. Changes in pressures in the left and right sides of the heart can reopen the foramen ovale.

R. A number of factors contribute to the first and subsequent breaths of the newborn. These include:
1. Neuronal activity from the central and peripheral chemoreceptors
2. Hypoxia
3. Hypercapnea
4. Acidosis
5. Light and noise
6. Cooling of the body surface
7. Tactile stimulation

X. Laboratory Values of the Newborn
A. Blood gas values of a normal term newborn:

	Umbilical Vein	Umbilical Artery	Within 5 min After Birth	24 hr–7 days
pH	7.32	7.24	7.20–7.34	7.37
Pco_2 (mm Hg)	38	49	35–46	33–35
Po_2 (mm Hg)	27	16	49–73	72–73
HCO_3 (mEq/L)	20	11	16–19	20
Sa_{O_2} (%)	80	60	>80	>90

B. Blood pressure (first 12 hours of life):

	1,000–2,000 gm	2,001–3,000 gm	>3,000 gm
Systolic	45–59	59–64	65–70
Diastolic	26–30	32–37	39–44
Mean	35–40	41–44	50–54

C. Blood volume: 80 to 90 ml/kg of birth weight
D. Blood chemistry on the first day of life (cord):

Na	147	mEq/L (126–159)
K$^+$	6.5	mEq/L (5.6–8.9)
Cl$^-$	104	mEq/L (98–114)
Total CO_2	20	mEq/L (19–20)

E. Glucose levels
   1. Normal newborn: 30–85 mg/dl
   2. Preterm: 20–75 mg/dl
F. Fetal hemoglobin
   1. Newborn: 72% of total hemoglobin.
   2. 6 months: 4.7% of total hemoglobin.
   3. 8 to 11 months: 1% to 2% of total hemoglobin.
   4. Newborn P_{50} is lower than that of the adult; however, it does approximate the adult P_{50} by 4 to 6 months.
G. Pulmonary function values in the normal newborn
   1. Respiratory rate: 30 to 60 breaths per minute (bpm), mean of 40 bpm
   2. Tidal volume: 5 to 7 ml/kg of body weight
   3. Vital capacity: 35 ml/kg of birth weight
   4. Functional residual capacity: 25 ml/kg of birth weight
   5. Total lung capacity: 60 ml/kg of birthweight
   6. Total lung compliance: 2.6 ml/cm H_2O
   7. Dead space volume: 2.0 to 2.2 ml/kg of birth weight
   8. Oxygen consumption: 7 mg/kg/min
   9. Dead space/tidal volume ratio: 0.30 to 0.35
   10. A-aDO$_2$: 24 mm Hg
   11. A-aDCO$_2$: 1 mm Hg
XI. Comparative Neonatal Respiratory Anatomy (Table 10–1)
   A. Neonatal head: Very large, about one fourth of total body length, in contrast to the adult head, which is about one eighth of body height.
   B. Neonatal tongue
      1. The neonatal tongue is very large in relation to size of oral cavity.
      2. Size is the primary factor forcing neonates to be obligate nose breathers. Normally only during crying will an infant actively ventilate through the mouth.
      3. Because of tongue size, nasal continuous positive airway pressure (CPAP) without use of endotracheal intubation can be accomplished.
      4. Positive end-expiratory pressure (PEEP) levels up to about 8 to 10 cm H_2O can be used; PEEP levels above this usually cause an oral leak and are difficult to maintain nasally.

TABLE 10–1.

Comparison of Neonatal and Adult Respiratory Anatomy

Structure	Neonate	Adult
Head/body size ratio	1:4	1:8
Tongue size	Large	Proportional
Laryngeal shape	Funnel-shaped	Rectangular
Narrowest portion of upper airway	Cricoid cartilage	Rima glottidis
Shape and location of epiglottis	Long, C1	Flat, C4
Level of tracheal bifurcation	T3–4	T5
Compliance of trachea	Compliant, flexible	Noncompliant
Angle of mainstem bronchi	10 degrees right, 30 degrees left	30 degrees right, 50 degrees left
Anteroposterior transverse diameter ratio	1:1	1:2
Thoracic shape	Bullet-shaped	Conical
Resting position of diaphragm	Higher than adult	Normal
Location of heart	Center of chest, midline	Lower portion of chest, left of midline
Body surface area/body size ratio	9 times adult	Normal

C. Neonatal neck: Very short and normally is creased.
D. Neonatal larynx
   1. The length is about 2 cm compared with 5 to 6 cm in the adult.
   2. The neonatal larynx is funnel shaped, whereas the diameter of the adult larynx is more or less constant.
   3. The narrowest portion of the neonate's upper airway is the cricoid cartilage; in the adult, the rima glottidis is the narrowest point. The normal anteroposterior diameter of the neonatal glottis is about 7 to 9 mm, the anteroposterior diameter of the cricoid cartilage about 4 to 6 mm.
     a. Endotracheal tube size must be based on the diameter of cricoid cartilage.
     b. The larynx is much higher in relation to the oral pharynx, and the opening of the larynx is more in a straight line that in the adult.
     c. Therefore, an infant frequently extends the neck when in respiratory distress, whereas the adult will thrust the head forward.
E. Neonatal epiglottis
   1. Stiffer, relatively longer, and U or V shaped compared with a flatter and much more flexible epiglottis in the adult.
   2. Located at the level of the first cervical vertebra; located in the adult at the fourth cervical vertebra.
F. Neonatal trachea
   1. The neonatal trachea is about 4 cm long compared with 10 to 13 cm in the adult.
   2. The anteroposterior diameter is about 3.5 mm and the lateral diameter about 5 mm.
   3. Normally it is located to the right of the midline.
   4. Bifurcation of the trachea is at the third or fourth thoracic vertebra in the neonate and at the fifth thoracic vertebra in the adult.

     5. The angle of right and left mainstem bronchi widens with age. At birth the angles from the midline are 10 degrees for the right and 30 degrees for the left; in adulthood the angles are about 30 and 50 degrees, respectively.

     6. Cartilage of the trachea may not be fully formed and often is more flexible than in the adult.

        a. As a result, hyperextension of the head may cause compression of the trachea and result in airway obstruction.

        b. Thus, during artifical ventilation without an endotracheal tube, the neonate's head should be maintained in a neutral position.

  G. Neonatal mainstem bronchi

     1. Short and relatively wide compared with those of the adult.

  H. Neonatal thoracic cage

     1. The neonatal thoracic cage has nearly equal anteroposterior and transverse diameters, and in general appearance is bullet shaped.

     2. Range of movement is limited, and the ribs are basically fixed in a horizontal position.

     3. The diaphragm is much higher than in the adult because of the relative size of the abdominal viscera. The diaphragm shows minimal movement during ventilation.

     4. The heart is located in the center of the chest and slightly higher than in the adult. When external cardiac massage is performed, compression should be applied over the middle of the body of the sternum.

XII. Body Surface Area

  A. The neonate's body surface area in relation to its size is about nine times that of the adult.

  B. Maintenance of body heat is thus a significant problem in the neonate and is even more so in the premature infant.

  C. The skin of the neonate plays a much greater role in water and heat balance than does that of the adult. This is a result of the large body surface area, which allows significant evaporation of water. In the neonate, 80% of body weight is water; in the adult, only 55% to 60% is water.

BIBLIOGRAPHY

Aloan C: *Respiratory Care of the Newborn: A Clinical Manual.* Philadelphia, JB Lippincott Co, 1987.

Avery G: *Neonatology, Pathophysiology and Management of the Newborn,* ed 2. Philadelphia, JB Lippincott Co, 1981.

Beard R, Nathaneilsz P: *Fetal Physiology and Medicine: The Basis of Perinatology.* Philadelphia, WB Saunders Co, 1976.

Berhardt T, Hehre D, Feller R, et al: Pulmonary mechanics in normal infants and young children during first 5 years of life. *Pediatr Pulmonol* 1987; 3:309–316.

Fallon M, Merisalo RL, Kennedy JL Jr: The frequency of apnea and bradycardia in a population of healthy, normal newborns. *Neuropediatrics* 1983; 14:73–75.

Gentz J, Persson B, Westin B, et al: *Perinatal Medicine.* Praeger Special Studies. New York, Praeger Publishers, 1984.

Korones S: *High-Risk Newborn Infants: The Basis for Intensive Nursing Care.* St Louis, CV Mosby Co, 1986.

Lough M, Doershuk C, Stern R: *Pediatric Respiratory Care.* Chicago, Year Book Medical Publishers, 1985.

Martin D: *Respiratory Anatomy and Physiology,* St Louis, CV Mosby Co, 1988.

Moore K: *The Developing Human Clinically Oriented Embryology.* Philadelphia, WB Saunders Co, 1973.

Murray J: *The Normal Lung,* ed 2. Philadelphia, WB Saunders Co, 1986.

Pawlak R, Herfect L: *Drug Administration in the NICU: A Handbook for Nurses.* Neonatal Network.
Sibal BM, Shaver DC, Anderson GD: Inaccuracy of Dubowitz gestational age in low birth weight infants. *Obstet Gynecol* 1984; 63:491–495.
Thibeault D, Gregory G: *Neonatal Pulmonary Care.* New York, Appleton-Century-Crofts, 1986.
Walters DV, Strang LB, Geubelle F: *Physiology of the Fetal and Neonatal Lung.* MTP Press, 1987.
Warshaw J: *The Biological Basis of Reproductive and Developmental Medicine.* New York, Elsevier North-Holland, 1983.

Chapter 11 _____

Oxygen and Carbon Dioxide Transport

I. Oxygen Cascade
   A. The partial pressure of oxygen (Po_2) decreases significantly from 159.6 mm Hg in dry air at sea level to less than 3 to 23 mm Hg in the mitochondria of the cell (see Table 11–1).
   B. Four body systems are responsible for the movement of oxygen from the atmosphere to the mitochondria:
      1. Lungs
      2. Blood
      3. Circulation
      4. Body tissue
   C. Specifics regarding movement of oxygen from the atmosphere into the blood are detailed in Chapter 2.

II. Role of Oxygen in the Cell
   A. About 90% of the oxygen consumed is a result of oxygen being the final electron acceptor of the electron transport chain in the mitochondria of the cell.
   B. The actual reaction produces H_2O:

$$\tfrac{1}{2}\,O_2 + 2\,H^+ \rightarrow H_2O \tag{1}$$

   C. Without the presence of O_2, aerobic metabolism is stopped while anaerobic metabolism continues, resulting in the production of lactic acid.
   D. The reaction of O_2 with H^+ to form H_2O allows the formation of the high-energy phosphate group adenosine triphosphate (ATP).
   E. The yield of ATP molecules from aerobic metabolism significantly exceeds that from anaerobic metabolism:

Aerobic Metabolism	Anaerobic Metabolism
Glucose	Glucose
↓	↓
Pyruvic acid	Pyruvic acid
↓	↓
CO_2 + H_2O + 38 moles of ATP	Lactic acid + 2 moles of ATP

F. Mitochondrial Po_2 values of less than 2 mm Hg inhibit aerobic metabolism.

III. Carriage of Oxygen in the Blood

    A. Oxygen is carried in two distinct compartments in the blood:

        1. Physically dissolved in plasma

        2. Chemically attached to hemoglobin molecules

    B. Volume physically dissolved in plasma

        1. According to the Bunsen solubility coefficient for oxygen, 0.023 ml of oxygen can be dissolved in 1 ml of plasma for every 760 mm Hg of Po_2.

        2. Simplifying this factor to the number of milliliters of oxygen per milliliter of plasma per mm Hg of Po_2:

$$0.023 \text{ ml } O_2/760 \text{ mm Hg} = 0.00003 \text{ ml } O_2/1 \text{ ml plasma/mm Hg } Po_2 \quad (2)$$

        3. Since the oxygen content normally is expressed in volumes percent, multiplying 0.00003 ml of oxygen per milliliter of plasma by 100 gives the factor:

$$(0.00003 \text{ ml } O_2/\text{ml of plasma})(100)/1 \text{ mm Hg of } Po_2 = 0.003 \text{ ml } O_2/100 \text{ ml of plasma/1 mm Hg of } Po_2 \quad (3)$$

        4. Thus, multiplying the Po_2 of blood by 0.003 will yield the number of milliliters of oxygen physically dissolved in every 100 ml of blood (vol%):

$$(Po_2)(0.003) = \text{ml of oxygen physically dissolved} \quad (4)$$

    C. Hemoglobin: Structure and carrying capacity

        1. Composition of the normal hemoglobin molecule:

          a. Four porphyrin rings, called *hemes*, each with a central iron atom.

          b. Four polypeptide chains: two α (alpha) chains and two β (beta) chains, called the *globin portion* of the molecule.

          c. Each chain is twisted and folded into a basket in which a heme is located.

          d. Each iron atom of the heme is bonded via four covalent bonds to the porphyrin ring and via one covalent bond to the globin portion. One bond is available to combine with oxygen.

          e. The four chains are held together by chemical bonds between unlike chains (α to β, β to α).

          f. The hemoglobin molecule undergoes structural changes when it reacts with oxygen.

          g. The total molecule contracts when it combines with oxygen and expands when oxygen is released.

TABLE 11–1.

The Oxygen Cascade

Location	Partial Pressure (mm Hg)	Reason for Change
Dry atmospheric air	159.6	
Conducting airways	149.6	Addition of H_2O vapor
End-expiratory gas	114	Mixing of deadspace gas with alveolar gas
Ideal alveolar gas	101	Addition of CO_2
Arterial blood	97	Intrapulmonary shunting
Mean systemic capillary	40	O_2 diffusion into cell
Cellular cytoplasm	<40	O_2 diffusion into mitochondria
Mitochondria	3–23	Metabolic rate

      h. The site of carbon dioxide attachment is the amino groups ($R\text{-}NH_2$) on the porphyrin rings.

      i. Also, the terminal imidazole (R-NH) groups are available to buffer H^+ (see Chapter 13).

          (1) The importance of hemoglobin as a buffer is second only to that of the HCO_3^-/H_2CO_3 buffer system.

          (2) The buffering capacity of the hemoglobin molecule depends on attachment of oxygen to the iron portion of the molecule.

          (3) Oxygenated hemoglobin (oxyhemoglobin) is a stronger acid but weaker buffer than unoxygenated hemoglobin (deoxyhemoglobin).

          (4) Thus, the buffering capacity of venous blood is greater than that of arterial blood.

  2. The molecular weight of hemoglobin is about 64,500 gm.

  3. Since oxygen attaches to each of the four iron atoms in the hemoglobin molecule, 4 gram molecular weights (GMWs) of oxygen combine with 64,500 gm of hemoglobin (1 mole).

$$\frac{64,500 \text{ gm/mole of Hb}}{4 \text{ gm/mole of } O_2} = 16,125 \text{ gm of Hb/mole of } O_2 \tag{5}$$

  4. That is, 1 mole of oxygen can combine maximally with 16,126 gm of hemoglobin.

  5. Since 1 GMW of oxygen at STP will occupy 22.4 L:

$$\frac{22,400 \text{ ml of } O_2}{16,125 \text{ gm of Hb}} = 1.34 \text{ ml of } O_2/\text{gm of Hb} \tag{6}$$

  6. Thus, at 100% saturation, 1.34 ml of oxygen can combine with each gram of hemoglobin.

  7. The actual volume of oxygen carried attached to hemoglobin is equal to:

$$(\text{Hb content})(1.34)(\text{HbO}_2\% \text{ sat.}) = \text{vol\% of } O_2 \text{ carried attached to Hb} \tag{7}$$

  8. As hemoglobin combines with oxygen to form HbO_2, the complex takes on a negative charge and as a result it forms a salt with K^+, $KHbO_2$.

  9. When O_2 is released at the tissue level, the K^+ is also released and the Hb buffers H^+, forming HHb (reduced hemoglobin).

D. Oxygen content

  1. The total oxygen content of blood is equal to the volume of oxygen physically dissolved in plasma plus the amount chemically combined with hemoglobin (Fig 11–1).

  2. Mathematically, this statement is equal to

$$O_2 \text{ content in vol\%} = (\text{Po}_2)(0.003) + (\text{Hb content})(1.34)(\text{HbO}_2\% \text{ sat.}) \tag{8}$$

E. Oxyhemoglobin dissociation curve (Fig 11–2)

  1. The overall sigmoidal shape of the curve is a result of the varied affinities of the four oxygen-bonding sites on the hemoglobin molecule.

    a. In general, the affinity of the last site bound is considerably less than the other three sites.

    b. In addition, the affinity of the first site is less than that of the second or third sites.

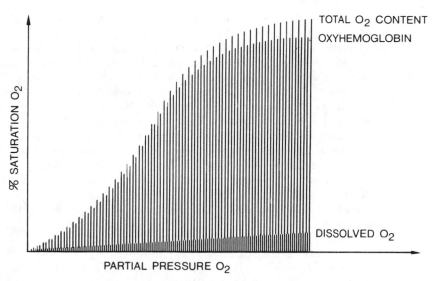

FIG 11–1.
Volume of oxygen dissolved, as oxyhemoglobin, and total oxygen content are indicated. The overall sigmoidal shape of the curve demonstrates varying bonding affinities for oxygen molecules as oxyhemoglobin saturation is increased. (From Shapiro BA, Harrison RA, Walton JR: *Clinical Application of Blood Gases,* ed 3. Chicago, Year Book Medical Publishers, 1982. Used by permission.)

    2. The steep aspect of the curve is that portion where minimal changes in Po_2 normally result in significant increases in HbO_2% saturation and therefore oxygen content.

        a. Increasing the saturation from 50% to 75% normally necessitates only a 13 mm Hg Po_2 increase, whereas increasing the saturation from 75% to 100% normally necessitates well over a 100 mg Hg Po_2 increase.

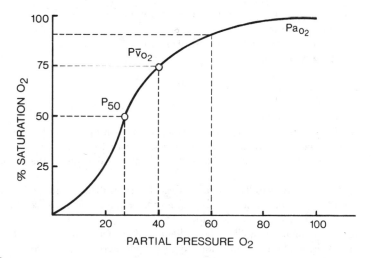

FIG 11–2.
The partial pressure at which hemoglobin is 50% saturated is 27 mm Hg. This is referred to as P_{50}. Normal venous Po_2 of 40 mm Hg and 75% oxyhemoglobin saturation are also indicated. A Po_2 of 60 mm Hg results in 90% saturation of the hemoglobin, whereas the normal arterial Po_2 of 97 mm Hg results in 97% saturation of the hemoglobin. (From Shapiro BA, Harrison RA, Walton JR: *Clinical Application of Blood Gases,* ed 3. Chicago, Year Book Medical Publishers, 1982. Used by permission.)

3. P_{50} is defined as that Po_2 at which the hemoglobin is 50% saturated with oxygen. Normally the P_{50} is equal to 27 mm Hg (see Fig 11–2).
   a. An increased P_{50} indicates a shift of the oxyhemoglobin dissociation curve to the right, resulting in a decreased hemoglobin affinity for oxygen (greater unloading of oxygen at the tissue and decreased loading at the alveoli).
   b. A decreased P_{50} indicates a shift of the oxyhemoglobin dissociation curve to the left, resulting in an increased hemoglobin affinity for oxygen (decreased unloading of oxygen at the tissue and increased loading at the alveoli).
   c. Hemoglobin is considered an allosteric enzyme because of the two conformational structures it assumes (deoxyhemoglobin and oxyhemoglobin). Allosteric enzymes are substances with two binding sites, one active site and one secondary site. The binding of substances at the secondary site can affect the affinity of binding at the active site.
   d. The following alter the affinity of hemoglobin for oxygen by affecting the secondary site:
      (1) Pco_2
      (2) H^+ or pH
      (3) Temperature
      (4) 2,3-Diphosphoglycerate (2,3-DPG)
      (5) Carbon monoxide
      (6) Abnormal forms of hemoglobin
4. The shape of the oxyhemoglobin dissociation curve is affected by various substances. Shifting the position of the curve alters the binding capabilities of hemoglobin. A shift to the right decreases the affinity of hemoglobin for oxygen, whereas a shift to the left increases affinity of hemoglobin for oxygen.
5. The oxyhemoglobin curve is shifted to the right by:
   a. Increased Pco_2
   b. Increased $[H^+]$ or decreased pH
   c. Increased temperature
   d. Increased 2,3-DPG
6. The oxyhemoglobin curve is shifted to the left by:
   a. Decreased Pco_2
   b. Decreased $[H^+]$ or increased pH
   c. Decreased temperature
   d. Decreased 2,3-DPG
   e. Increased carbon monoxide (CO)
   f. Fetal hemoglobin
   g. Methemoglobin
F. *Bohr effect:* The effect of carbon dioxide or $[H^+]$ on uptake and release of oxygen from the hemoglobin molecule. The effect is relatively mild.
   1. As seen earlier, carbon dioxide and $[H^+]$ will cause a shift in the oxyhemoglobin dissociation curve.
   2. At the systemic capillary bed, increased carbon dioxide and $[H^+]$ moving into the blood decreases hemoglobin affinity for oxygen and increases the volume of oxygen released at the tissue level.
   3. At the pulmonary capillary bed, decreased carbon dioxide and $[H^+]$ levels increase hemoglobin affinity for oxygen, thus increasing the volume of oxygen picked up at the pulmonary level.
G. Carbon monoxide
   1. Carbon monoxide attaches to hemoglobin at the same site as O_2.
   2. The affinity of hemoglobin for carbon monoxide is 200 times greater than its affinity for O_2.

3. In addition, carboxyhemoglobin (HbCO) shifts the oxyhemoglobin dissociation curve to the left, decreasing the ability of hemoglobin to unload oxygen.

H. Abnormal hemoglobins
   1. There are more than 100 abnormal forms of hemoglobins.
   2. Twelve of these have an effect on the affinity of hemoglobin for oxygen.
   3. Fetal hemoglobin has two γ (gamma) chains instead of β chains, which results in a decreased P_{50} (shift to the left).
   4. Methemoglobin is formed by Fe atoms being oxidized from the ferrous to the ferric state; this also results in a decreased P_{50} (shift to the left).

IV. Oxygen Availability
   A. The quantity of oxygen available to the tissue is dependent on oxygen content and cardiac output.
   B. The amount of oxygen transported to tissue is equal to

   $$(O_2 \text{ content in vol\%})(10)(\text{Cardiac output in L/min}) \qquad (9)$$

   C. In the normal healthy adult, oxygen content equals about 20 vol% and cardiac output is about 5 L/min. Thus:

   $$O_2 \text{ transport} = (20 \text{ vol\%})(10)(5 \text{ L/min}) = 1,000 \text{ ml/min}$$

   D. Oxygen availability is most significantly affected by the hemoglobin level and cardiac output.
   E. Normal oxygen transport ranges from about 900 to 1,200 ml/min at rest.
   F. Oxygen transport may be decreased by any of the following:
      1. Decreased cardiac output
      2. Decreased oxygen content
         a. Decreased P_{O_2}
         b. Decreased hemoglobin
         c. Rightward shift of the oxyhemoglobin dissociation curve

V. Oxygen Consumption
   A. The normal arterial oxygen content is 20 vol%.
   B. The normal mixed venous oxygen content is about 15 vol%.
   C. Thus, $Ca_{O_2} - C\bar{v}_{O_2}$ is 5 vol%.
   D. If the cardiac output is 5 L/min, the organism consumes 250 ml/min of oxygen.
   E. Oxygen consumption in the adult varies from about 150 to 350 ml/min (basal metabolic level), depending on body size and metabolic rate.
   F. Oxygen consumption is altered by:
      1. Physical activity (metabolic rate)
      2. Physiologic stress
      3. Temperature
      4. Alterations in microcirculation
   G. In the adequately perfused normothermic patient who is not shivering or seizing, oxygen consumption is equal to about 3.0 ml/kg/min of body weight.

VI. Production of Carbon Dioxide
   A. Carbon dioxide is produced by the metabolism of all food.
   B. In addition, carbon dioxide is produced in the conversion of glucose to fatty acids.
   C. Normal carbon dioxide production is about 120 to 280 ml/min, depending on body size and metabolic rate, or about 2.4 ml/kg/min.

VII. Carriage of Carbon Dioxide in the Blood
   A. Carriage in plasma occurs in three distinct ways (Fig 11–3):
      1. Carbon dioxide is dissolved in plasma as P_{CO_2}, which is in equilibrium with the P_{CO_2} in red blood cells (RBCs).

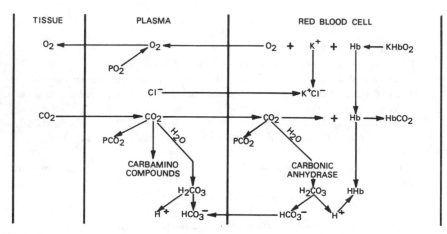

FIG 11–3.
Overall scheme of O_2 and CO_2 transport in blood (see text).

2. Carbon dioxide is carried predominantly as bicarbonate (HCO_3^-) formed in the RBCs and by the kidney. The HCO_3^- levels in plasma are in equilibrium with the HCO_3^- in RBCs.
   a. Plasma carbon dioxide reacts minimally with water, forming carbonic acid, which dissociates into H^+ and HCO_3^-:

$$CO_2 + H_2O \leftrightarrows H_2CO_3 \rightleftarrows H^+ + HCO_3^- \qquad (10)$$

   b. The H^+ formed is buffered in the plasma and therefore causes a mild decrease in pH (venous blood).
   c. The previous reaction's point of equilibrium is shifted to the left in the plasma, therefore favoring formation of reactants.
   d. The mathematical relationship between dissolved CO_2 and H_2CO_3 is

$$(P_{CO_2} \text{ mm Hg})(0.0301) = H_2CO_3 \text{ mEq/L, or mmoles/L} \qquad (11)$$

3. Carbon dioxide is attached to plasma proteins, forming carbamino compounds.
   a. Carbon dioxide reacts with the terminal amino groups on the plasma proteins ($R\text{-}NH_2$):

$$R\text{—}N \begin{matrix} H \\ \diagup \\ \diagdown \\ H \end{matrix} + CO_2 \rightleftarrows R\text{—}N \begin{matrix} H \\ \diagup \\ \diagdown \\ COO^- \end{matrix} + H^+ \qquad (12)$$

   (R— indicates the remainder of the plasma protein)
   b. Most of the H^+ liberated is buffered and therefore causes a mild decrease in the pH (venous blood).
   c. The ionization state of the amino groups affects their ability to bond with carbon dioxide. If the NH_2 groups are oxidized to NH_3^+, their ability to combine with carbon dioxide is significantly decreased.
B. Carriage of carbon dioxide in RBCs occurs in three distinct ways (see Fig 11–3):
   1. As dissolved P_{CO_2} in equilibrium with plasma P_{CO_2}.

2. As HCO_3^- formed in the RBC.
   a. The reaction shown in equation 10 is significantly increased as a result of the presence of the enzyme carbonic anhydrase (CA). The point of equilibrium is shifted to the right, favoring formation of the products:

$$\overset{\text{CA}}{CO_2 + H_2O \rightleftarrows H_2CO_3 \rightleftarrows H^+ + HCO_3^-} \tag{13}$$

   b. As increasing levels of HCO_3^- are formed in the RBC, HCO_3^- diffuses into the plasma. As HCO_3^- diffuses, there is an imbalance of electric charges inside the RBC, causing Cl^- to move into the RBC. This process is referred to as the *chloride shift,* or *Hamburger phenomenon.* The Cl^- diffusing into the RBC associates with the K^+ released as the hemoglobin molecule gives up O_2 and buffers H^+.
3. As carbon dioxide attached to the terminal amino ($R-NH_2$) groups of the hemoglobin molecule. This reaction is the same as that shown in equation 12. Again, the H^+ released from the formation of HCO_3^- must be buffered.
   a. In RBCs, the primary buffer is the imidazole groups on the hemoglobin molecule.
   b. The ability of the imidazole groups to buffer is affected by oxyhemoglobin saturation. With oxygen bound to the heme, the imidazole groups are poor buffers. Without oxygen attached to the heme, the imidazole groups are good buffers.
   c. As oxygen attaches to the heme, more $R-NH_2$ groups will exist in the $R-N-H_3^+$ form. The tendency for carbon dioxide to attach to the $R-NH_3^+$ form is less than to the $R-NH_2$ form.
VIII. Haldane Effect
   A. Figure 11–4 illustrates the Haldane effect, which is defined as the effect of oxygen on carbon dioxide uptake and release.

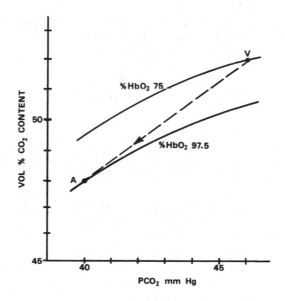

FIG 11–4.
Effect of oxyhemoglobin saturation on volume of CO_2 carried in blood. The carrying capacity of blood for CO_2 is decreased as oxyhemoglobin saturation is increased (Haldane effect). The arrow from *V* to *A* depicts change of CO_2 content from venous to arterial blood.

B. As P_{O_2} increases at the pulmonary capillary bed, the ability of hemoglobin to carry carbon dioxide is decreased because more amino groups exist in the oxidized $R\text{-}NH_3^+$ state. This allows large volumes of carbon dioxide to be released at the pulmonary capillary bed.

C. As the P_{O_2} decreases at the tissue level, the ability of hemoglobin to carry carbon dioxide is increased because more amino groups exist in the reduced $R\text{-}NH_2$ form. This allows large volumes of carbon dioxide to be picked up at the systemic capillary bed (see Fig 11–4).

D. The Haldane effect facilitates carriage of the normal 4 vol% (200 ml/min) of carbon dioxide picked up from the tissue and released at the lung.

IX. Quantitative Distribution of Carbon Dioxide
A. Percentage of carbon dioxide carried in each compartment:
1. Ninety percent of carbon dioxide in blood exists as HCO_3^-.
2. Five percent of carbon dioxide in blood exists as carbamino compounds.
3. Five percent of carbon dioxide in blood exists as dissolved P_{CO_2}.
B. Percentage of carbon dioxide exhaled from various compartments:
1. Sixty percent of the carbon dioxide exhaled is carried as HCO_3^-.
2. Thirty percent of the carbon dioxide exhaled is carried as carbamino compounds.
3. Ten percent of the carbon dioxide exhaled is carried as dissolved P_{CO_2}.

X. Total Carbon Dioxide
A. Total carbon dioxide is an expression of the sum of HCO_3^- plus dissolved CO_2.
B. Total carbon dioxide may be expressed in millimoles per liter (mmoles/L), milliequivalents per liter (mEq/L), or vol%.
C. $(P_{CO_2})(0.0301) = $ mmoles/L, or mEq/L, of H_2CO_3
D. Vol% of $CO_2 = $ (mEq/L)(2.23), or (mmoles/L)(2.23)
E. mmoles/L or mEq/L of $CO_2 = $ vol%/2.23
F. In arterial blood:
1. Total $CO_2 = [HCO_3^-] + [\text{dissolved } P_{CO_2}]$
2. 25.2 mmoles/L = 24 mmoles/L + 1.2 mmoles/L
3. 56.2 vol% = 53.52 vol% + 2.68 vol%

XI. Respiratory Quotient, Respiratory Exchange Ratio, and Ventilation/Perfusion Ratio
A. The respiratory quotient (RQ) is defined as the volume of carbon dioxide produced divided by the volume of oxygen consumed per minute:

$$RQ = \frac{4 \text{ vol\% } CO_2}{5 \text{ vol\% } O_2} \text{ or } \frac{200 \text{ ml } CO_2}{250 \text{ ml } O_2} = 0.8 \tag{13}$$

B. The RQ is an expression of *internal* respiration.
C. The respiratory exchange ratio (R) is defined as the volume of carbon dioxide moving from the pulmonary capillaries to the lung divided by the volume of oxygen moving from the lung into the pulmonary capillaries:

$$R = \frac{4 \text{ vol\% } CO_2}{5 \text{ vol\% } O_2} = \frac{200 \text{ ml } CO_2}{250 \text{ ml } O_2} = 0.8 \tag{14}$$

D. The R is an expression of *external* respiration.
E. Under normal circumstances RQ and R are equal, with a mean value of about 0.8.
F. The ventilation/perfusion ($\dot{V}/\dot{Q}$) ratio is equal to the minute alveolar ventilation divided by the minute cardiac output:

$$\dot{V}/\dot{Q} = \frac{4 \text{ L alveolar minute volume}}{5 \text{ L minute cardiac output}} = 0.8 \tag{15}$$

G. $\dot{V}/\dot{Q}$ is equal to RQ and R under normal circumstances.
H. It is the alveolar ventilation and the cardiac output that maintain the RQ and R equal.

BIBLIOGRAPHY

Bendixen HH, et al: *Respiratory Care.* St Louis, CV Mosby Co, 1965.
Cherniack RM, Cherniack L: *Respiration in Health and Disease,* ed 3. Philadelphia, WB Saunders Co, 1983.
Comroe JH: *Physiology of Respiration,* ed 2. Chicago, Year Book Medical Publishers, 1974.
Deshpande VM, Pilbeam SP, Dixon RJ: *A Comprehensive Review in Respiratory Care.* Norwalk, Mass, Appleton & Lange, 1988.
Des Jardins TR: *Clinical Manifestations of Respiratory Disease.* Chicago, Year Book Medical Publishers, 1984.
Guyton AC: *Textbook of Medical Physiology,* ed 6. Philadelphia, WB Saunders Co, 1981.
Murray JF: *The Normal Lung.* Philadelphia, WB Saunders Co, 1976.
Nunn JF: *Applied Respiratory Physiology,* ed 2. Stoneham, Mass, Butterworth, 1977.
Shapiro BA, Harrison RA, Kacmarek RM, et al: *Clinical Application of Respiratory Care,* ed 3. Chicago, Year Book Medical Publishers, 1985.
Shapiro BA, Harrison RA, Cane R, et al: *Clinical Application of Blood Gases,* ed 4. Chicago, Year Book Medical Publishers, 1989.
Snyder JV, Pinsky MR: *Oxygen Transport in the Critically Ill.* Chicago, Year Book Medical Publishers, 1987.
Spearman CB, Sheldon RL, Egan DF: *Egan's Fundamentals of Respiratory Therapy,* ed 4. St Louis, CV Mosby Co, 1982.
West JB: *Respiratory Physiology: The Essentials.* Baltimore, Williams & Wilkins Co, 1981.
Young JA, Crocker D: *Principles and Practice of Respiratory Therapy,* ed 2. Chicago, Year Book Medical Publishers, 1976.

Chapter 12

Acid-Base Balance and Blood Gas Interpretation

I. Electrolytes
   A. An electrolyte is a substance that is capable of conducting an electrical current when placed into solution.
   B. When an electrolyte dissolves in solution, it dissociates, producing ions. For example, sodium chloride (NaCl) dissociates into sodium (Na^+) and chloride (Cl^-) ions.

$$NaCl \rightarrow Na^+ + Cl^- \tag{1}$$

   C. Strong electrolytes dissociate completely when dissolved in solution.
   D. Weak electrolytes only partially dissociate, with the majority of electrolyte remaining dissolved but undissociated.
   E. A weak acid electrolyte produces H^+ when dissolved.
   F. A weak basic electrolyte produces OH^- when dissolved.
II. Law of Mass Action
   A. The basic chemical and mathematical relationships involved in blood gas interpretation are based on the law of mass action (also referred to as the *law of electrolyte dissociation* and *law of chemical equilibrium*).
   B. *The law of mass action* states that when a weak electrolyte is placed into solution, only a small percentage of it dissociates, the vast majority remaining undissociated. Determining the product of the molar concentrations of the dissociated species and dividing that by the molar concentration of the undissociated weak electrolyte yields a dissociation constant for that weak electrolyte. This constant is true for the particular electrolyte at the temperature it was originally determined.
   C. If the weak acid HA is placed into solution, it will reversibly dissociate to H^+ and A^- (the negative ion formed whenever H^+ dissociates from an acid):

$$HA \rightleftharpoons H^+ + A^- \tag{2}$$

D. If 0.01 moles/L of HA were added to solution and 5% of HA dissociated, the following quantities of all three species would exist in solution:

$$HA \quad 95\% \text{ of } 0.01, \text{ or } 0.0095 \text{ moles/L}$$
$$H^+ \quad 5\% \text{ of } 0.01, \text{ or } 0.0005 \text{ moles/L}$$
$$A^- \quad 5\% \text{ of } 0.01, \text{ or } 0.0005 \text{ moles/L}$$

Note: One H^+ and one A^- are formed as every HA molecule dissociates.

E. According to the law of mass action:

$$K = \frac{[H^+][A^-]}{[HA]} \tag{3}$$

where K = the dissociation constant.

F. Inserting the molar concentrations of the individual species and calculating the dissociation constant yields the following:

$$0.0000263 = \frac{[0.0005][0.0005]}{[0.0095]}$$

Thus, $K = 2.63 \times 10^{-5}$.

G. As explained in sections II and IV, the dissociation constant indicates the pH at which a buffer functions most efficiently.

H. The law of mass action applied to water is the basis for the pH scale.

   1. Water (H_2O) dissociates into H^+ plus OH^-:

$$H_2O \rightleftharpoons H^+ + OH^- \tag{4}$$

   2. The molar concentration of both H^+ and OH^- is 10^{-7} moles/L.

   3. Since the concentration of the undissociated water is so large compared with the $[H^+]$ and $[OH^-]$, it is considered a constant:

$$\frac{[H^+][OH^-]}{K_{H_2O}} = K \tag{5}$$

   4. This relationship is frequently written as

$$[H^+][OH^-] = K_w \tag{6}$$

where K_w = the dissociation constant for H_2O.

   5. The value of K_w is

$$[10^{-7}][10^{-7}] = 10^{-14}$$

   6. Thus, a neutral solution is one with 10^{-7} moles of H^+ per liter.

   7. Since the H^+ concentration can vary from 10^{-1} to 10^{-14} in this relationship, the limits of the pH scale are defined.

   8. pH is equal to $-\log [H^+]$.

   9. The pH scale therefore goes from a pH of 1.0 ($[H^+] = 10^{-1}$ moles/L) to a pH of 14.0 ($[H^+] = 10^{-14}$ moles/L).

  10. Remember the product of $[H^+]$ and $[OH^-]$ must equal 10^{-14}. As a result, as the $[H^+]$ increases, the $[OH^-]$ decreases, and vice versa.

I. The law of mass action when applied to carbonic acid (H_2CO_3) dissolved in plasma at 37°C yields the following:

   1. Carbonic acid (H_2CO_3) dissociates into $H^+ + HCO_3^-$ (bicarbonate ion):

$$H_2CO_3 \rightleftarrows H^+ + HCO_3^- \tag{7}$$

   2. If the molar concentration of H^+ is multiplied by the molar concentration of HCO_3^-, and the answer is divided by the molar concentration of H_2CO_3, the dissociation constant for H_2CO_3 in plasma is calculated:

$$\frac{[H^+][HCO_3^-]}{[H_2CO_3]} = K \tag{8}$$

   3. K for reaction 8 in blood is equal to 7.85×10^{-7}.

J. The mathematical manipulation of the law of mass action results in the development of the Henderson-Hasselbalch equation.

III. Henderson-Hasselbalch Equation (Standard Buffer Equation)

  A. Derivation of the Henderson-Hasselbalch equation from equation 8:

   1. Rearranging equation 8 and solving for $[H^+]$ results in the following:

$$[H^+] = \frac{K[H_2CO_3]}{[HCO_3^-]} \tag{9}$$

   2. Taking the log to the base of 10 of each side of equation 9 yields the following:

$$\log [H^+] = \log K + \log \frac{[H_2CO_3]}{[HCO_3^-]} \tag{10}$$

   3. Multiplying each side of equation 10 by -1 yields the following:

$$-\log [H^+] = -\log K - \log \frac{[H_2CO_3]}{[HCO_3^-]} \tag{11}$$

   4. Rearranging $-\log \frac{[H_2CO_3]}{[HCO_3^-]}$ in equation 11 yields the following:

$$\begin{aligned} -\log [H_2CO_3]\,(-)\, &-\log [HCO_3^-] \\ = -\log [H_2CO_3] &+ \log [HCO_3^-] \\ = +\log [HCO_3^-] &- \log [H_2CO_3] \\ = +\log \frac{[HCO_3^-]}{[H_2CO_3]} \end{aligned} \tag{12}$$

   5. Inserting equation 12 in equation 11 yields the following:

$$-\log H^+ = -\log K + \log \frac{[HCO_3^-]}{[H_2CO_3]} \tag{13}$$

   6. $-\log H^+ = pH$ and $-\log K$ is termed the pK (refer to section IV). Equation 13 is rewritten as:

$$pH = pK + \log \frac{[HCO_3^-]}{[H_2CO_3]} \tag{14}$$

7. Equation 14 is the classic buffer equation (see section V) as applied to the HCO_3^-/H_2CO_3 buffer system.

8. A universal representation of the classic buffer equation as applied to a weak acid electrolyte is

$$pH = pKa + \log \frac{[\text{Conjugate base}]}{[\text{Undissociated acid}]} \tag{15}$$

where pKa is the pK of a weak acid electrolyte.

9. If the derivation were carried out for a weak basic electrolyte, the standard equation would be:

$$pOH = pKb + \log \frac{[\text{Conjugate acid}]}{[\text{Undissociated base}]} \tag{16}$$

10. However, the type of buffer systems used in describing pulmonary physiology are all weak acid electrolytes.

IV. pK ($-$Log of the Dissociation Constant)

A. This value represents the pH at which a buffer functions most efficiently.

B. When the pH of a solution equals the pK, 50% of the buffer exists in the form of the conjugate base and 50% as the undissociated acid.

C. All buffers have a narrow pH range, identifying where they function appropriately.

D. In general, if the pH of a solution is above its pK, the solution will buffer acid more effectively than base.

E. If the pH of a solution is below its pK, the solution will buffer base more effectively than acid.

F. The further away a solution's pH moves from its pK, the poorer its buffering capabilities.

G. If the pH of a buffered solution is outside the 1 to 1.5 pH range about the buffer's pK, the system's buffering capabilities are lost.

V. Buffers

A. A buffer is a weak acidic or basic electrolyte that has the capability of determining the pH of a solution.

B. Buffers are used to prevent significant changes in a solution pH.

C. One should always choose a buffer whose pK is numerically near the pH of the solution to be buffered.

D. Chemical functioning of buffers:

1. If the buffer HA from section II is titrated into solution until the pH of the solution is equal to the pK of the buffer, an ideally buffered solution is established. The pK of this system is 4.58 ($-$log of 2.63×10^{-5}, see section II-F.).

2. After titration, the final concentrations of HA and A^- are equal to 0.01. Thus, the classic buffer equation would be

$$pH = pK + \log \frac{[A^-]}{[HA]} \tag{17}$$

or

$$4.58 = 4.58 + \log \frac{0.01}{0.01}$$

Note: The log of $\frac{0.01}{0.01}$ is 0.

3. If acid is added to this buffer, it reacts with the conjugate base (A^-) and forms more undissociated acid (HA):

$$A^- + H^+ \rightarrow HA \tag{18}$$

This should result in only a minimal change in the pH.

a. If 0.001 mole/L of H^+ is added to the buffer, the H^+ would react with 0.001 mole/L of A^-:

$$A^- + H^+ \rightarrow HA$$
$$0.001 + 0.001 \rightarrow 0.001$$

Note: 100% efficiency is assumed.

b. As a result, the concentration of A^- would decrease by 0.001, and the concentration of HA would increase by 0.001:

$$pH = 4.58 + \log \frac{0.01 - 0.001}{0.01 + 0.001} \text{ or } \frac{0.009}{0.011}$$

c. The resulting pH of this solution would be 4.49, or a 0.09 pH unit change.

d. By comparison, if 0.001 mole/L of H^+ were added to water with a pH of 7.0, the resulting pH would be about 2.99, more than a 4.0 pH unit change.

4. If base is added to a buffer, it reacts with free H^+, allowing more HA to dissociate:

$$H^+ + OH^- \rightarrow H_2O \tag{19}$$

causing the following:

$$HA \rightarrow H^+ + A^-$$

resulting in a minimal change in the pH.

a. If 0.001 mole/L of OH^- is added to the buffer in equation 17, the OH^- would react with 0.001 mole/L of H^+, causing 0.001 mole/L of HA to dissociate:

$$H^+ + OH^- \rightarrow H_2O$$
$$0.001 + 0.001 \rightarrow 0.001$$

causing the following:

$$HA \rightarrow H^+ + A^-$$
$$0.001 \rightarrow 0.001 + 0.001$$

b. As a result, the concentration of HA is decreased by 0.001, and the concentration of A^- is increased by 0.001.

$$pH = 4.58 + \log \frac{0.01 + 0.001}{0.01 - 0.001} \text{ or } \frac{0.011}{0.009}$$

    c. The resulting pH of the solution would be 4.67, a 0.09 pH unit change.

    d. By comparison, if 0.001 mole/L of OH^- were added to water with a pH of 7.0, the resulting pH would be about 10.99, almost a 4.0 pH unit change.

VI. The HCO_3^-/H_2CO_3 Buffer System

  A. The most important buffer system in the body is the HCO_3^-/H_2CO_3 system:

$$pH = pK + \log \frac{HCO_3^-}{H_2CO_3} \tag{20}$$

  B. The pK of this system is 6.1 ($K = 7.85 \times 10^{-7}$).

  C. Arterial HCO_3^- levels are about 24 mEq/L.

  D. Arterial H_2CO_3 levels are about 1.2 mEq/L.

  E. Thus, arterial pH is about 7.4:

$$7.4 = 6.1 + \log \frac{24 \text{ mEq/L}}{1.2 \text{ mEq/L}}$$

  F. The ratio of HCO_3^- to H_2CO_3 is 20:1:

$$\frac{HCO_3^-}{H_2CO_3} = \frac{24}{1.2} = \frac{20}{1}$$

  G. If this ratio increases (30:1), the arterial pH increases.

  H. If this ratio decreases (10:1), the arterial pH decreases.

  I. Clinically, HCO_3^- and H_2CO_3 concentrations are extremely time consuming and costly to determine.

    1. Since the $(P_{CO_2}) \times (0.0301)$ is equivalent to the H_2CO_3 concentration, this value can be substituted into equation 20 for H_2CO_3:

$$pH = 6.10 + \log \frac{[HCO_3^-]}{(P_{CO_2})(0.0301)} \tag{21}$$

    2. Clinically the pH of the blood is easily measured, as is the P_{CO_2} (see Chapter 34).

    3. $[HCO_3^-]$ is always the calculated value when blood gas results are reported.

  J. In this buffer system, $[HCO_3^-]$ is regulated and controlled by the kidney, and P_{CO_2} is regulated and controlled by the lung with the pH a result of the $[HCO_3^-]$ and P_{CO_2}.

  K. The HCO_3^-/H_2CO_3 buffer system in blood is a poor chemical buffer.

    1. This is true because of the pK (6.1) of the buffer in relation to the pH (7.4) of the blood.

    2. The pH of blood is outside the chemical buffering range of the HCO_3^-/H_2CO_3 system.

    3. However, this system is considered an essential *physiologic* buffer. That is, the lungs can control the excretion or retention of large quantities of acid in the form of CO_2.

    4. The following reversible reaction illustrates the relationship:

$$CO_2 + H_2O \rightleftharpoons H_2CO_3 \rightleftharpoons H^+ + HCO_3^- \tag{22}$$

    5. If there is an increase in H^+, the reaction is shifted to the left, increasing plasma CO_2 levels, which are exhaled.

6. If there is a decrease in H^+, the reaction is shifted to the right, decreasing plasma CO_2 levels.
7. The effectiveness of HCO_3^- administration in the face of a metabolic acidosis is based on equation 22 shifting to the left, allowing acid to be exhaled as CO_2. If ventilation cannot eliminate the increased CO_2 produced, the acidosis changes from metabolic to respiratory.

VII. Actual Versus Standard HCO_3^-
   A. Actual HCO_3^-: Value calculated from actual, measured P_{CO_2} and pH of arterial blood.
      1. Value normally given with arterial blood gas results.
      2. Indicative of nonrespiratory acid-base imbalances.
   B. Standard HCO_3^-: Value calculated from measured pH and P_{CO_2} of venous blood after P_{CO_2} of blood has been equilibrated to 40 mm Hg.
      1. Value usually reported with electrolyte studies by clinical laboratory.
      2. Indicative of a change in acid-base balance but not precise as to magnitude when compared with arterial pH and P_{CO_2}.
      3. Arterial pH and P_{CO_2} most closely correlate with actual HCO_3^-.

VIII. Base Excess/Base Deficit
   A. The total buffering capacity of the body can be broken down approximately as follows:
      1. Sixty percent by the HCO_3^-/H_2CO_3 system
      2. Thirty percent by hemoglobin buffering system
      3. Ten percent by all other blood buffers (e.g., phosphates, plasma proteins, ammonia)
   B. Of the total body buffers, HCO_3^- and all proteins (including hemoglobin) are the most important.
   C. These two systems may be chemically depicted as follows:

$$CO_2 + H_2O \rightleftharpoons H_2CO_3 \rightleftharpoons HCO_3^- + H^+ \qquad (23)$$

$$H\ Prot \rightleftharpoons H^+ + Prot^- \qquad (24)$$

   D. If a respiratory acidosis were to develop, the reaction shown in equation 23 would be driven to the right, causing an equal shift of the reaction shown in equation 24 to the left. As a result, the total amount of base in the body would remain unchanged.
   E. If a respiratory alkalosis were to develop, the reaction shown in equation 23 would be driven to the left, causing an equal shift of the reaction shown in equation 24 to the right. As a result, the total amount of base in the body would remain unchanged.
   F. The sum of $[HCO_3^-]$ + $[Prot^-]$ is the buffer base, which (as demonstrated in sections VIII–D and VIII–E) remains unchanged in all pure acute respiratory acid-base disturbances.
   G. However, if metabolic acid is added to the body, the reactions shown in equations 23 and 24 would both be driven to the left, and the quantity of buffer base would decrease and if metabolic base were added to the body, both reactions (23 and 24) would be driven to the right and the quantity of buffer base would increase.
   H. Base excess/base deficit (BE/BD) is defined as the actual buffer base (BB) minus the normal BB:

$$BE/BD = actual\ BB - normal\ BB \qquad (25)$$

   I. In all pure acute respiratory acid-base disturbances, the BE/BD is normal. However, once compensation occurs, the BE/BD becomes positive or negative.

    J. All metabolic acid-base disturbances are accompanied by a change in the BE/BD.

    K. The BE/BD is the most reliable index of metabolic acid base disorders.

    L. The normal BE/BD is zero, with a range of ± 2 mEq/L. The normal total buffer base is 54 mEq/L.

IX. Normal Ranges for Blood Gases

    A. *Absolute normals: Arterial blood* (mean population values):

        1. pH: 7.40

        2. P_{CO_2}: 40 mm Hg

        3. P_{O_2}: 100 mm Hg

        4. HCO_3^-: 24 mEq/L

        5. Base excess: 0

        6. Hemoglobin content: 14 gm%

        7. Oxyhemoglobin saturation: 97.5%

        8. Oxygen content: 19.8 vol%

        9. Carboxyhemoglobin saturation: 0%

    B. *Normal ranges: Arterial blood* (± 2 standard deviations from the population mean):

        1. pH: 7.35 to 7.45

        2. P_{CO_2}: 35 to 45 mm Hg

        3. P_{O_2}: 80 to 100 mm Hg

        4. HCO_3^-: 22 to 27 mEq/L

        5. Base excess: ± 2

        6. Hemoglobin content: 12 to 15 gm%

        7. Oxyhemoglobin saturation: 95% or more

        8. Oxygen content: more than 16 vol%

        9. Carboxyhemoglobin saturation: less than 2%

    C. *Absolute normals: Venous blood* (mean population values):

        1. pH: 7.35

        2. P_{CO_2}: 46 mm Hg

        3. P_{O_2}: 40 mm Hg

        4. HCO_3^-: 27 mEq/L

        5. Oxyhemoglobin saturation: 75%

    D. *Clinical ranges: Arterial blood* (± 3 standard deviations from the population mean):

        1. pH: 7.30 to 7.50

        2. P_{CO_2}: 30 to 50 mm Hg

        3. The ranges for arterial blood values given in section IX–B indicate the "normal" variation in arterial pH and P_{CO_2}. Slight variations outside these normal ranges may not indicate a clinically significant change.

        4. These clinical ranges indicate an acceptable pH and P_{CO_2} from a *patient management* point of view. Results outside these ranges normally indicate situations requiring clinical intervention.

X. Mathematical Interrelationships Between pH, P_{CO_2}, and HCO_3^-

    A. If the constants and log relationship are eliminated in the HCO_3^-/H_2CO_3 buffer equation, the equation may be simplified to:

$$pH \approx \frac{HCO_3^-}{P_{CO_2}} \tag{26}$$

This relationship demonstrates the mathematical interrelationship between these variables.

    B. In general, under all clinical circumstances the pH will be a result of the HCO_3^- and P_{CO_2} levels.

C. In a pure respiratory abnormality where the HCO_3^- remains essentially constant, the P_{CO_2} and pH are indirectly related:

$$HCO_3^- \approx (pH)(P_{CO_2}) \tag{27}$$

D. In a pure metabolic abnormality where the P_{CO_2} remains essentially constant, the HCO_3^- and pH are directly related:

$$P_{CO_2} \approx \frac{HCO_3^-}{pH} \tag{28}$$

E. These interrelationships provide the basis for blood gas interpretation.

XI. Compensation for Primary Acid-Base Abnormalities
   A. Compensation involves the various mechanisms used by the body to normalize the pH after a primary acid-base abnormality. Compensation does not imply correction of the primary abnormalities.
   B. Compensation for primary respiratory acid-base imbalances is via the kidney (see Chapter 9).
   C. Compensation for primary metabolic acid-base abnormalities is via the respiratory system (see Chapter 5).

XII. Estimation of pH Changes Based Purely on P_{CO_2} Changes
   A. Since the pK of the HCO_3^-/H_2CO_3 system is 6.10 and the quantity of HCO_3^- is 20 times greater than the quantity of H_2CO_3, the body buffers acid more efficiently than base.
   B. If, starting at a baseline pH of 7.40 and a P_{CO_2} of 40 mm Hg, for every 10 mm Hg P_{CO_2} increase there is an approximate 0.05 pH unit decrease:
      1. P_{CO_2} 50: pH 7.35: HCO_3^- 25
      2. P_{CO_2} 60: pH 7.30: HCO_3^- 26
      3. P_{CO_2} 70: pH 7.25: HCO_3^- 27
      4. P_{CO_2} 80: pH 7.20: HCO_3^- 28
      This relationship holds if *no* compensation by the kidney has occurred. The HCO_3^- increases as a result of a shifting of the components of the buffer base (see section VIII).
   C. If, starting at a baseline pH of 7.40 and a P_{CO_2} of 40, for every 10 mm Hg P_{CO_2} decrease there is an approximate 0.10 pH unit increase:
      1. P_{CO_2} 35: pH 7.45: HCO_3^- 23
      2. P_{CO_2} 30: pH 7.50: HCO_3^- 22
      3. P_{CO_2} 25: pH 7.55: HCO_3^- 21
      4. P_{CO_2} 20: pH 7.60: HCO_3^- 20
      This relationship holds if no compensation by the kidney has occurred. The HCO_3^- decreases as a result of a shifting of the components of the buffer base (see section VIII).

XIII. Interpretation of Arterial Blood Gases
   Blood gas interpretation is performed in three steps:
   A. Interpretation of acid-base status
   B. Assessment of level of hypoxemia
   C. Assessment of tissue hypoxia

XIV. Interpretation of Acid-Base Status
   A. Tables 12–1 and 12–2 list ranges for interpretation of blood gases using the classic and clinical methods.
   B. The classic method uses the terminology uncompensated, partially compensated, and compensated, along with the normal ranges for P_{CO_2} and pH.

TABLE 12–1.

Classic Textbook Method of Blood Gas Interpretation

Status	pH	P_{CO_2}	HCO_3^-	BE
Respiratory acidosis				
Uncompensated	↓ 7.35	↑ 45	Normal	Normal
Partially compensated	↓ 7.35	↑ 45	↑ 27	↑ +2
Compensated	7.35–7.45	↑ 45	↑ 27	↑ +2
Respiratory alkalosis				
Uncompensated	↑ 7.45	↓ 35	Normal	Normal
Partially compensated	↑ 7.45	↓ 35	↓ 22	↓ −2
Compensated	7.40–7.45	↓ 35	↓ 22	↓ −2
Metabolic acidosis				
Uncompensated	↓ 7.35	Normal	↓ 22	↓ −2
Partially compensated	↓ 7.35	↓ 35	↓ 22	↓ −2
Compensated	7.35–7.40	↓ 35	↓ 22	↓ −2
Metabolic alkalosis				
Uncompensated	↑ 7.45	Normal	↑ 27	↑ +2
Partially compensated*	↑ 7.45	↑ 45	↑ 27	↑ +2
Compensated*	7.40–7.45	↑ 45	↑ 27	↑ +2
Combined respiratory and metabolic acidosis	↓ 7.35	↑ 45	↓ 22	↓ −2
Combined respiratory and metabolic alkalosis	↑ 7.45	↓ 35	↑ 27	↑ +2

*In general, partially compensated or compensated metabolic alkalosis is rarely seen clinically because of the body's mechanism to prevent hypoventilation, as outlined in Chapter 5.

TABLE 12–2.

Clinical Method of Blood Gas Interpretation

Status	pH	P_{CO_2}	HCO_3^-	BE
Ventilatory failure (respiratory acidosis)				
Acute	↓ 7.30	↑ 50	Normal	Normal
Chronic	7.30–7.45	↑ 50	↑ 27	↑ +2
Alveolar hyperventilation (respiratory alkalosis)				
Acute	↑ 7.50	↓ 30	Normal	Normal
Chronic	7.40–7.50	↓ 30	↓ 22	↓ −2
Metabolic acidosis				
Uncompensated	↓ 7.30	Normal	↓ 22	↓ −2
Partially compensated	↓ 7.30	↓ 30	↓ 22	↓ −2
Compensated	7.30–7.40	↓ 30	↓ 22	↓ −2
Metabolic alkalosis				
Uncompensated	↑ 7.50	Normal	↑ 27	↑ +2
Partially compensated*	↑ 7.50	↑ 50	↑ 27	↑ +2
Compensated*	7.40–7.50	↑ 50	↑ 27	↑ +2
Combined ventilatory failure and metabolic acidosis	↓ 7.30	↑ 50	↓ 22	↓ −2
Combined alveolar hyperventilation and metabolic alkalosis	↑ 7.50	↓ 30	↑ 27	↑ +2

*In general, partially compensated or compensated metabolic alkalosis is rarely seen clinically because of the body's mechanism to prevent hypoventilation, as outlined in Chapter 5.

C. The clinical method, developed by Shapiro, uses the classic terminology only for metabolic disturbances and acute or chronic alveolar hyperventilation and ventilatory failure for respiratory acid-base imbalances. In addition, the clinical ranges for pH and Pco_2 are used.

D. Approach to blood gas interpretation (classic method; see Table 12–1)

1. Determine if the pH is within the normal range

   a. If normal, the blood gas is normal or compensated.

   b. If it is outside the normal range, it is uncompensated or partially compensated.

2. Determine if the Pco_2 is normal or abnormal

   a. If the Pco_2 is normal and:

      (1) The pH is normal, the blood gas is normal.

      (2) The pH is decreased, an uncompensated metabolic acidosis exists.

      (3) The pH is increased, an uncompensated metabolic alkalosis exists.

   b. If the Pco_2 is higher than normal and:

      (1) The pH is decreased and the HCO_3^- is normal, an uncompensated respiratory acidosis exists.

      (2) The pH is decreased and the HCO_3^- is above normal, a partially compensated respiratory acidosis exists.

      (3) The pH is between 7.35 and 7.40 and the HCO_3^- is elevated, it is a compensated respiratory acidosis.

      (4) The pH is 7.40 to 7.45 and the HCO_3^- is elevated, it *may be* a compensated metabolic alkalosis; however this acid-base state is rare, and usually a compensated respiratory acidosis with a mild metabolic alkalosis actually exists.

      (5) The pH is increased with an elevated HCO_3^-, a partially compensated metabolic alkalosis exists.

   c. If the Pco_2 is lower than normal and:

      (1) The pH is increased and the HCO_3^- is normal, an uncompensated respiratory alkalosis exists.

      (2) The pH is between 7.35 and 7.40 and the HCO_3^- is decreased, a compensated metabolic acidosis exists.

      (3) The pH is between 7.40 and 7.45 and the HCO_3^- is decreased, a compensated respiratory alkalosis exists.

      (4) The pH is increased and the HCO_3^- is decreased, a partially compensated respiratory alkalosis exists.

      (5) The pH is decreased and the HCO_3^- is decreased, a partially compensated metabolic acidosis exists.

   d. In addition, combined respiratory and metabolic acidosis or combined respiratory and metabolic alkalosis can occur.

      (1) If the pH is markedly decreased, the Pco_2 is increased, and the HCO_3^- is decreased, an uncompensated respiratory and metabolic acidosis exists.

      (2) If the pH is markedly increased, the Pco_2 is decreased, and the HCO_3^- is increased, an uncompensated respiratory and metabolic alkalosis exists.

   e. The same guidelines can be used for the clinical method of interpretation, with the following variations:

      (1) The acceptable pH range is 7.30 to 7.50.

      (2) The acceptable Pco_2 range is 30 to 50 mm Hg.

      (3) Replace "uncompensated" and "partially compensated" respiratory acidosis with "acute ventilatory failure."

(4) Replace "compensated" respiratory acidosis with "chronic ventilatory failure."

(5) Replace "uncompensated" and "partially compensated" respiratory alkalosis with "acute alveolar hyperventilation."

(6) Replace "compensated" respiratory alkalosis with "chronic alveolar hyperventilation."

XV. Assessment of Level of Hypoxemia

A. For patients who are breathing room air and who are less than 60 years of age:

1. Mild hypoxemia: Arterial P_{O_2} 60 to 79 mm Hg
2. Moderate hypoxemia: Arterial P_{O_2} 40 to 59 mm Hg
3. Severe hypoxemia: Arterial P_{O_2} less than 40 mm Hg

B. For individuals over age 60, 1 mm Hg should be subtracted from the lower limits of mild and moderate hypoxemia for each year over 60. At any age a P_{O_2} less than 40 mm Hg indicates severe hypoxemia, and a P_{O_2} of less than 60 to 65 is always considered hypoxemic.

C. More precisely, acceptable lower limits for P_{O_2} can be determined by the following (at sea level):

1. For patients in the supine position: $P_{O_2} = 103.5 - (0.42 \times age) \pm 4$ mm Hg.
2. For patients in the sitting position: $P_{O_2} = 104.2 - (0.27 \times age)$ mm Hg.

D. Patients on $F_{I_{O_2}}$ greater than 0.21

1. Uncorrected hypoxemia: Arterial P_{O_2} less than room air acceptable limit.
2. Corrected hypoxemia: Arterial P_{O_2} between minimal acceptable room air limit and 100 mm Hg.
3. Excessively corrected hypoxemia: Arterial P_{O_2} greater than 100 mm Hg.

XVI. Assessment of Tissue Hypoxia

A. At present there is no direct method of assessing tissue hypoxia; it must be clinically assessed indirectly.

B. Normally, adequate tissue oxygenation requires:

1. Normal volume of oxygen must be carried by arterial blood
2. Acid-base status must be relatively normal
3. Tissue perfusion must be adequate

C. The likelihood of tissue hypoxia existing is increased in the presence of the following:

1. Severe hypoxemia
2. Metabolic acidosis
3. Decreased cardiac output or poor perfusion

D. If tissue hypoxia has occurred, blood lactate levels are increased (see Chapter 11).

XVII. Clinical Causes of Acid-Base Abnormalities

A. Ventilatory failure (respiratory acidosis): Primary causes:

1. Cardiopulmonary disease, particularly end-stage chronic obstructive pulmonary disease (COPD) or chronic restrictive pulmonary disease.
2. Central nervous system depression by drugs, trauma, or lesion.
3. Neurologic or neuromuscular disease resulting in profound weakness of ventilatory muscles.
4. Fatigue following any acute pulmonary disease.

B. Alveolar hyperventilation (respiratory alkalosis): Primary causes:

1. Hypoxemia: Its primary effect on the respiratory system is hyperventilation.
2. Compensation for primary metabolic acidosis.
3. Central nervous system stimulation by drugs, trauma, or lesion.
4. Emotional disorders (e.g., pain, anxiety, or fear).

C. Metabolic acidosis
1. Primary causes
a. Lactic acidosis
(1) In the absence of oxygen as final electron acceptor in the electron transport chain, aerobic metabolism is decreased.
(2) An increase in anaerobic metabolism results, which increases formation of lactic acid, a nonvolatile organic acid.
(3) If the oxygenation state of the patient is improved, lactic acidosis is reversed.
(4) Normal lactate levels
(a) 0.5 to 2.5 mmoles/L
b. Ketoacidosis
(1) Primary causes
(a) Uncontrolled diabetes mellitus
(b) Starvation
(c) High fat content in the diet for extended periods
(2) In all cases insufficient volumes of glucose enter the cell, resulting in an increase in metabolism of body fats.
(3) The metabolic end products of fat metabolism are ketoacids (acetone and β-hydroxybutyric acid).
(4) The patient in a diabetic acidosis is generally hyperventilating significantly and his or her breath has a sweet, acetone odor.
(5) The patient needs glucose and insulin.
c. Renal failure (see Chapter 9)
(1) Decreased renal function inhibits the body's primary mechanism for maintaining blood HCO_3^- levels and excretion of H^+.
(2) Thus, free $[H^+]$ increases and free $[HCO_3^-]$ decreases.
d. Ingestion of base-depleting drugs or acids
(1) Aspirin
(2) Alcohol
(3) Ethylene glycol
(4) Paraldehyde
D. Metabolic alkalosis
1. Primary causes
a. Hypokalemia (see Chapter 15)
b. Hypochloremia (see Chapter 15)
c. Gastric suction or vomiting
(1) Since gastric contents are very acidic (pH 1.0–2.0), excessive loss of gastric fluid results in alkalosis.
d. Massive doses of steroids
(1) Steroids increase reabsorption of Na^+ and accelerate excretion of H^+ and K^+.
e. Diuretics
(1) Diuretics cause an increase in the amount of K^+ excreted.
(2) With excessive or uncontrolled use, hypokalemia may result.
f. Ingestion of acid-depleting drugs or bases
(1) $NaHCO_3$ (sodium bicarbonate)
XVIII. Mixed Venous Blood Gases
A. $P\bar{v}_{O_2}$, $\%Hb\bar{v}_{O_2}$ and $Ca_{O_2} - C\bar{v}_{O_2}$ levels are reflective of the adequacy of O_2 delivery to peripheral tissue.
B. Alterations in these values may be caused by:
1. Decreased O_2 content
2. Decreased cardiac output (CO)

      3. Increased tissue metabolism

      4. Altered peripheral microcirculation (i.e., sepsis)

  C. All are predictive of alterations in cardiac output if O_2 content, tissue metabolism, and peripheral distribution of CO are unaltered.

  D. A decrease in $P\bar{v}_{O_2}$ and $\%Hb\bar{v}_{O_2}$ and an increase in $Ca_{O_2} - C\bar{v}_{O_2}$ are indicative of a decrease in CO relative to tissue demands and may be used as a reflection of cardiovascular reserve (Table 12–3).

      1. If cardiac output decreases, the tissue must extract a greater quantity of O_2 per unit of blood.

      2. As a result, $P\bar{v}_{O_2}$ and $\%Hb\bar{v}_{O_2}$ must decrease, whereas the difference between arterial and venous O_2 contents $(Ca_{O_2} - C\bar{v}_{O_2})$ must increase.

  E. For maximum accuracy, these values must be obtained from a pulmonary artery catheter. This is necessary since peripheral venous blood is reflective of only local events, whereas pulmonary artery values reflect means of all tissue beds.

  F. Many pulmonary artery catheters employ oximetry to continuously monitor $\%Hb\bar{v}_{O_2}$. Some believe the $\%Hb\bar{v}_{O_2}$ is best used as an early indicator of a cardiovascular incident resulting in altered O_2 delivery.

XIX. Estimation of Base Excess/Base Deficit

  A. Determine the pH predicted by an acute change in the P_{CO_2}.

      1. For every 10 mm Hg P_{CO_2} increase, the pH decreases by 0.05.

      2. For every 10 mm Hg P_{CO_2} decrease, the pH increases by 0.10.

  B. Determine the difference between the actual and predicted pH.

    Example:

Actual pH	7.50
Predicted pH	7.35
Difference	0.15

  C. Eliminate the decimal and multiply by $\frac{2}{3}$ to obtain BE/BD in milliequivalents per liter.

    Example:

      $\frac{2}{3}$ of 15 = 10 mEq/L

  D. If the actual pH is less than the predicted pH, this is a base deficit.

  E. If the actual pH is greater than the predicted pH, this is a base excess.

    Example:

Actual pH	7.50
Predicted pH	7.35
Base excess of 10 mEq/L	

  F. This is an excess of 10 mEq/L of base in all extracellular fluid.

XX. Calculation of Bicarbonate Administration

  A. Normally HCO_3^- is administered only in the case of severe metabolic acidosis.

TABLE 12–3.

Mixed Venous Blood Gas Values During Various Levels of Cardiovascular Stress

Status	$Ca_{O_2} - C\bar{v}_{O_2}$ (vol%)		$P\bar{v}_{O_2}$ (mm Hg)		$\%Hb\bar{v}_{O_2}$	
	Avg	Range	Avg	Range	Avg	Range
Normal	5.0	3.4–6.0	40	37–43	75	70–76
Critically ill but stable	3.5	2.5–4.5	37	35–40	70	68–75
Critically ill with limited reserve	5.0	4.5–6.0	32	30–35	60	56–68
Cardiovascularly decompensated	>6.0	>6.0	<30	<30	<56	<56

B. Severe metabolic acidosis is defined as a base deficit of at least 10 mEq/L and one of the following:
   1. A pH of less than 7.20
   2. A pH between 7.20 and 7.25 with an unstable cardiovascular system.
C. If the pH is greater than 7.25, HCO_3^- is normally not administered, even if the base deficit is 10 mEq/L.
D. Extracellular fluid volume in liters can be estimated by taking one fourth the body weight in kilograms.
E. The total body deficit in base is determined by multiplying the extracellular fluid volume by the base deficit in milliequivalents per liter.
F. One-half this estimated amount is normally administered.
   Example:

Base deficit	15 mEq/L
Weight	80 kg
Extracellular fluid volume	80/4 = 20 L

   20 L × 15 mEq/L = 300 mEq total body deficit
   ½ of 300 mEq = 150 mEq administered

XXI. Calculation of Ammonium Chloride (NH_3Cl) or Dilute Hydrochloric Acid (HCl) Administration
A. In severe metabolic alkalosis, NH_3Cl or HCl can be administered to correct an acute base excess.
B. The same calculations outlined in section XX are used.

XXII. Typical Blood Gas Contaminants
A. Heparin
   1. Sodium heparin is commonly used to prevent coagulation of arterial blood to be used for blood gas analysis.
   2. Ammonium heparin may affect pH even in small quantities.
   3. Normal pH of sodium heparin is 6.0 to 7.0.
   4. Concentration used is 1,000 units/cc.
   5. P_{CO_2} of sodium heparin is less than 2 mm Hg.
   6. P_{O_2} of sodium heparin is approximately 159 mm Hg.
   7. Normally 0.05 ml of heparin/ml of blood should be used for anticoagulation.
   8. If the concentration or volume of heparin used is above this level:
      a. The pH level of the blood may decrease or remain the same.
      b. The P_{CO_2} of the blood will decrease.
      c. The P_{O_2} may be altered, depending on the blood's original P_{O_2} in relation to heparin's P_{O_2}.
      d. The HbO_2% sat may be altered, depending on the blood's original P_{O_2} and HbO_2% sat.
      e. The HbCO% sat will not be altered.
      f. Hemoglobin content will decrease.
      g. The HCO_3^- level will decrease.
      h. Base excess will decrease.
      i. Oxygen content may be altered.
   9. If insufficient heparin levels are used:
      a. Machine clotting is very likely.
      b. Results are questionable.
B. Saline and other intravenous solutions alter blood gas values in a manner similar to that of heparin except that the pH may also increase.
C. Air bubbles
   1. The pH level of the blood normally will increase.
   2. The P_{CO_2} of the blood normally will decrease.

3. The Po_2 of the blood may be altered, depending on the blood's original Po_2 compared to atmospheric Po_2.
4. The $HbO_2\%$ sat may be altered, depending on the blood's original Po_2 and $HbO_2\%$ sat.
5. The $HbCO\%$ sat may increase.
6. Hemoglobin content is unaltered.
7. The HCO_3^- level may decrease.
8. Base excess may decrease.
9. Oxygen content may be altered.

BIBLIOGRAPHY

Bartlett RH, Whitehouse WM Jr, Turcotte JC, et al: *Life Support Systems in Intensive Care.* Chicago, Year Book Medical Publishers, 1984.

Bendixen HH, et al: *Respiratory Care.* St Louis, CV Mosby Co, 1965.

Burton GC, Hodgkin JE: *Respiratory Care: A Guide to Clinical Practice,* ed 2. Philadelphia, JB Lippincott Co, 1984.

Cane RD, Shapiro BA: *Case Studies in Critical Care Medicine.* Chicago, Year Book Medical Publishers, 1985.

Carvelli ML, Schriver AJ, Peterson WE, et al: Acid-base assessment without journal peripheral venous blood. *Heart Lung* 1984; 13:48–54.

Clank LC, Noyes LK, Grooms TA, et al: Rapid micromeasurements of lactate in whole blood. *Crit Care Med* 1984; 12:461–464.

Cohen JJ, Kassier JP: *Acid-Base.* Boston, Little, Brown & Co, 1982.

Comroe JH: *Physiology of Respiration,* ed 2. Chicago, Year Book Medical Publishers, 1974.

Davenport HW: *The ABC's of Acid-Base Chemistry,* ed 6. Chicago, University of Chicago Press, 1977.

Deshpande VM, Pilbeam SP, Dixon RJ: *A Comprehensive Review in Respiratory Care.* Norwalk, Mass, Appleton & Lange, 1988.

Filey GF: *Acid-Base and Blood Gas Regulation.* Philadelphia, Lea & Febiger, 1972.

Guyton AC: *Textbook of Medical Physiology,* ed 6. Philadelphia, WB Saunders Co, 1981.

Hodgkins JE, Soeprono FF, Chan DM: Incidence of metabolic alkalemia in hospitalized patients. *Crit Care Med* 1980; 8:725–728.

Jones NL: *Blood Gases and Acid-Base Physiology.* New York, Marcel Dekker, 1980.

Kirby RR, Smith RA, Desautels DA: *Mechanical Ventilation.* New York, Churchill Livingstone, 1985.

Levesque PR: Acid-base disorders: Application of total body carbon dioxide titration in anesthesia. *Anesth Analg* 1975; 54:299–307.

Masoro EJ, Siegel PD: *Acid-Base Regulation: Its Physiology, Pathophysiology and the Interpretation of Blood Gas Analysis,* ed 2. Philadelphia, WB Saunders Co, 1977.

Masterton WL, Slowinski EJ: *Chemical Principles,* ed 4. Philadelphia, WB Saunders Co, 1977.

Olszowka AJ, et al: *Blood Gases, Hemoglobin, Base Excess and Maldistribution.* Philadelphia, Lea & Febiger, 1973.

Rooth G: *Acid-Base and Electrolyte Balance.* Chicago, Year Book Medical Publishers, 1974.

Rose BD: *Clinical Physiology of Acid-Base and Electrolyte Disorders.* New York, McGraw-Hill Book Co, 1977.

Ryder KW, Jay SJ: Comparison of measured and calculated arterial bicarbonate concentrations: Potential application for prevention of random errors in blood gas results. *Respir Care* 1983; 28:1268–1272.

Shapiro BA, Harrison RA, Cane R, et al: *Clinical Application of Blood Gases,* ed 4. Chicago, Year Book Medical Publishers, 1989.

Snyder JV, Pinsky MR: *Oxygen Transport in the Critically Ill.* Chicago, Year Book Medical Publishers, 1987.

Spearman CB, Sheldon RL, Egan DF: *Egan's Fundamentals of Respiratory Therapy*, ed 4. St Louis, CV Mosby Co, 1982.

Walter RM, Warsaw T: Diabetic ketoacidosis: A treatment appraisal. *Heart Lung* 1981; 10:112–113.

Winters RW, Dell RB: *Acid-Base Physiology in Medicine*, ed 3. Boston, Little, Brown & Co, 1982.

Chapter 13

Intrapulmonary Shunting and Deadspace

I. Spectrum of Ventilation/Perfusion ($\dot{V}/\dot{Q}$) Abnormalities (Fig 13–1)
  A. Ideal alveolar-capillary unit: An alveolar-capillary unit in which perfusion and ventilation are normal; theoretically, a unit with a $\dot{V}/\dot{Q}$ ratio of 1.0.
  B. Deadspace unit: An alveolar-capillary unit in which ventilation is normal but perfusion is diminished or absent; a unit with a $\dot{V}/\dot{Q}$ ratio greater than 1.0.
  C. Shunt unit: An alveolar-capillary unit in which perfusion is normal but ventilation is diminished or absent; a unit with a $\dot{V}/\dot{Q}$ ratio less than 1.0.
  D. Silent unit: An alveolar-capillary unit without perfusion or ventilation and therefore a $\dot{V}/\dot{Q}$ ratio of 0.0.
  E. For greater detail on ventilation/perfusion relationships, see Chapter 4.
II. Intrapulmonary Shunting
  A. A pathophysiologic process in which blood enters the left side of the heart without having been oxygenated by the lungs. The mixing of venous blood with oxygenated blood from the pulmonary capillaries to form arterial blood.
  B. The total quantity of shunted blood is the *physiologic shunt*, which is composed of three subdivisions (Fig 13–2).
    1. Anatomic shunt: That portion of the total cardiac output that bypasses the pulmonary capillary bed.
      a. Normally about 2% to 5% of the cardiac output bypasses the pulmonary capillaries because the following veins empty into the left side of the heart:
        (1) Bronchial
        (2) Pleural
        (3) Thebesian
      b. Increases in anatomic shunt may occur as a result of:
        (1) Vascular pulmonary tumors
        (2) Arterial venous anastomosis
        (3) Congenital cardiac anomalies (see Chapter 25)
        (4) Severe liver disease
    2. Capillary shunt: That portion of the total cardiac output that perfuses nonventilated alveoli.
      a. Normally, capillary shunting does not exist.
      b. Capillary shunting is caused by:
        (1) Atelectasis
        (2) Consolidating pneumonia

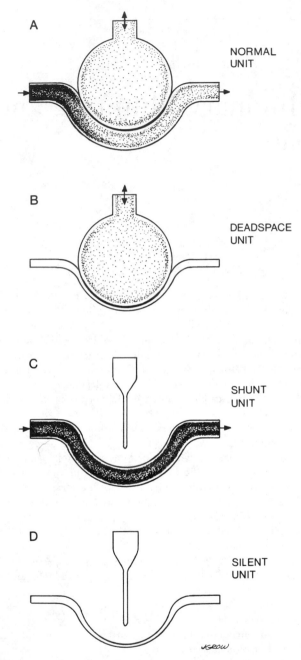

FIG 13-1.
The theoretical respiratory unit. **A,** normal ventilation, normal perfusion; **B,** normal ventilation, no perfusion; **C,** no ventilation, normal perfusion; **D,** no ventilation, no perfusion. (From Shapiro BA, Harrison RA, Walton JR: *Clinical Application of Arterial Blood Gases,* ed 3. Chicago, Year Book Medical Publishers, 1982. Used by permission.)

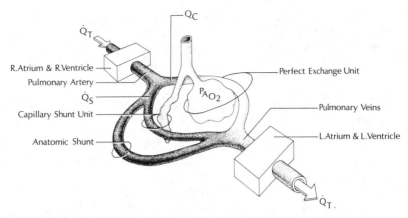

FIG 13–2.
Concept of physiologic shunting (see text). $\dot{Q}t$ is cardiac output per unit time; $\dot{Q}c$ is the portion of the cardiac output that exchanges perfectly with alveolar air; $\dot{Q}s$ is the portion of the cardiac output that does not exchange with alveolar air; $P_{A_{O_2}}$ is the alveolar oxygen tension. (From Shapiro BA, Harrison RA, Walton JR: *Clinical Application of Arterial Blood Gases,* ed 3. Chicago, Year Book Medical Publishers, 1982. Used by permission.)

      (3) Complete airway obstruction
      (4) Pneumothorax
      (5) Any pathophysiologic process that eliminates ventilation to perfused alveoli
   3. Shunt effect (ventilation/perfusion inequality, venous admixture): Any pathophysiologic process in which perfusion is in excess of ventilation; however, some ventilation is still present.
     a. Under normal conditions, shunt effect occurs in the bases of the lung where $\dot{V}/\dot{Q}$ ratios are less than 1.0.
     b. Shunt effect may be increased by:
       (1) Retained secretions
       (2) Bronchospasm
       (3) Partial airway obstruction
       (4) Regional increases in fibrotic tissue
       (5) Decreased tidal volumes
       (6) Mucosal edema at the bronchiolar level
 III. Derivation of Classic Shunt Equation
   A. Definition of abbreviations
     1. $\dot{V}_{O_2}$: Volume of oxygen consumed per minute
     2. $\dot{Q}s$: Shunted cardiac output
     3. $\dot{Q}c$: Capillary cardiac output
     4. $\dot{Q}t$: Total cardiac output
     5. Cc_{O_2}: Capillary oxygen content
     6. Ca_{O_2}: Arterial oxygen content
     7. $C\bar{v}_{O_2}$: Mixed venous oxygen content
     8. $P_{A_{O_2}}$: Alveolar oxygen partial pressure
     9. Pa_{O_2}: Arterial oxygen partial pressure
   B. The shunt equation is based on the Fick equation, which normally is used to calculate oxygen consumption or cardiac output:

$$\dot{V}_{O_2} = \dot{Q}t(Ca_{O_2} - C\bar{v}_{O_2}). \tag{1}$$

C. Since $\dot{Q}c$ represents that portion of the cardiac output that actually perfuses ventilated alveoli and Cc_{O_2} is the oxygen content of blood leaving those perfused and ventilated alveoli, this equation may be rewritten as:

$$\dot{V}o_2 = \dot{Q}c(Cc_{O_2} - C\bar{v}_{O_2}) \tag{2}$$

D. Thus, total cardiac output is equal to shunted cardiac output plus capillary cardiac output:

$$\dot{Q}t = \dot{Q}s + \dot{Q}c \tag{3}$$

E. Solving equation 3 for $\dot{Q}c$:

$$\dot{Q}c = \dot{Q}t - \dot{Q}s \tag{4}$$

F. Substituting into equation 2 the equivalent of $\dot{V}o_2$ from equation 1:

$$\dot{Q}t(Ca_{O_2} - C\bar{v}_{O_2}) = \dot{Q}c(Cc_{O_2} - C\bar{v}_{O_2}) \tag{5}$$

G. Substituting into equation 5 the equivalent of $\dot{Q}c$ from equation 4:

$$\dot{Q}t(Ca_{O_2} - C\bar{v}_{O_2}) = (\dot{Q}t - \dot{Q}s)(Cc_{O_2} - C\bar{v}_{O_2}) \tag{6}$$

H. Rearranging equation 6:

$$\dot{Q}tCa_{O_2} - \dot{Q}tC\bar{v}_{O_2} = \dot{Q}tCc_{O_2} - \dot{Q}tC\bar{v}_{O_2} - \dot{Q}sCc_{O_2} + \dot{Q}sC\bar{v}_{O_2} \tag{7}$$

I. Eliminating $-\dot{Q}tC\bar{v}_{O_2}$ from both sides of equation 7:

$$\dot{Q}tCa_{O_2} = \dot{Q}tCc_{O_2} - \dot{Q}sCc_{O_2} + \dot{Q}sC\bar{v}_{O_2} \tag{8}$$

J. Rearranging equation 8:

$$\dot{Q}sCc_{O_2} - \dot{Q}sC\bar{v}_{O_2} = \dot{Q}tCc_{O_2} - \dot{Q}tCa_{O_2} \tag{9}$$

K. Simplifying equation 9:

$$\dot{Q}s(Cc_{O_2} - C\bar{v}_{O_2}) = \dot{Q}t(Cc_{O_2} - Ca_{O_2}) \tag{10}$$

L. Rearranging equation 10:

$$\dot{Q}s/\dot{Q}t = \frac{Cc_{O_2} - Ca_{O_2}}{Cc_{O_2} - C\bar{v}_{O_2}} \tag{11}$$

M. Equation 11 is the classic shunt equation, which states that the difference between the capillary oxygen content and arterial oxygen content divided by the difference between the capillary oxygen content and the mixed venous oxygen content equals the intrapulmonary shunt fraction.

N. This equation is used to calculate the total physiologic shunt.

IV. Calculation of the Total Physiologic Shunt

A. The intrapulmonary shunt is calculated by calculating the capillary oxygen content, arterial oxygen content, and mixed venous oxygen content.

B. All oxygen content determinations are based on the following equation (see Chapter 11 for details):

$$O_2 \text{ content (vol\%)} = (\text{Hb cont})(\text{HbO}_2\% \text{ sat})(1.34) + (0.003)(P_{O_2}) \tag{12}$$

C. Calculation of the arterial oxygen content requires data from an arterial blood gas.

D. Calculation of the mixed venous oxygen content requires data from a pulmonary artery blood gas.

E. Capillary oxygen content
   1. Since a blood sample from an *ideally functioning alveolar-capillary* unit is impossible to obtain, this calculation is based on the assumption that the end pulmonary capillary oxygen tension ($P_{c_{O_2}}$) is equal to the alveolar oxygen tension ($P_{A_{O_2}}$) in an ideally ventilated and perfused alveolar-capillary unit.
   2. The $P_{A_{O_2}}$ is obtained by calculation, using the ideal alveolar gas equation (see Chapter 4 for details):

$$P_{A_{O_2}} = (P_B - P_{H_2O})(F_{I_{O_2}}) - (P_{a_{CO_2}})\left(F_{I_{O_2}} + \frac{1 - F_{I_{O_2}}}{R}\right) \tag{13}$$

   3. Hemoglobin content is the same as that measured in arterial blood or mixed venous blood.
   4. Oxyhemoglobin percent saturation ($\text{HbO}_2\%$ sat)
      a. If the $P_{A_{O_2}}$ is 150 mm Hg or greater, it is assumed that the $\text{HbO}_2\%$ sat is 100%.
      b. For $P_{A_{O_2}}$ values of less than 150 mm Hg, an oxyhemoglobin dissociation curve is used to estimate the $\text{HbO}_2\%$ sat.
      c. The capillary $\text{HbO}_2\%$ sat is also corrected for the $\text{HbCO}\%$ sat present in the arterial blood.

F. *Example:*

$$C_{a_{O_2}} = 17.5 \text{ vol\%}$$
$$C_{c_{O_2}} = 19.5 \text{ vol\%}$$
$$C\bar{v}_{O_2} = 13.0 \text{ vol\%}$$

$$\frac{\dot{Q}s}{\dot{Q}t} = \frac{C_{c_{O_2}} - C_{a_{O_2}}}{C_{c_{O_2}} - C\bar{v}_{O_2}}$$

$$\frac{\dot{Q}s}{\dot{Q}t} = \frac{19.5 - 17.5}{19.5 - 13.0} = 0.31$$

or 31% intrapulmonary shunt.

V. Estimated Intrapulmonary Shunt Calculation
   A. In patients without a pulmonary artery catheter, it is impossible to measure the $C\bar{v}_{O_2}$.
   B. However, in the majority of critically ill patients with cardiovascular stability, it has been determined that the $C_{a_{O_2}} - C\bar{v}_{O_2}$ is approximately 3.5 vol%.
   C. Thus, in these patients 3.5 vol% may be used as an estimate of $C_{a_{O_2}} - C\bar{v}_{O_2}$.
   D. The denominator of the classic shunt equation may be expressed as follows:

$$C_{c_{O_2}} - C\bar{v}_{O_2} = (C_{c_{O_2}} - C_{a_{O_2}}) + (C_{a_{O_2}} - C\bar{v}_{O_2}) \tag{14}$$

E. Since $Ca_{O_2} - C\bar{v}_{O_2}$ is estimated at 3.5 vol%, the denominator in equation 11 can be expressed as:

$$(Cc_{O_2} - Ca_{O_2}) + 3.5 \tag{15}$$

F. The modified shunt equation used to estimate intrapulmonary shunt is:

$$\frac{\dot{Q}s}{\dot{Q}t} = \frac{Cc_{O_2} - Ca_{O_2}}{(Cc_{O_2} - Ca_{O_2}) + 3.5} \tag{16}$$

G. Equation 16 should be used only if pulmonary artery blood is unavailable and the patient is cardiovascularly stable.

VI. $F_{I_{O_2}}$ Used to Calculate Percent Intrapulmonary Shunt
   A. Historically, shunt fractions were determined at an $F_{I_{O_2}}$ of 1.0.
   B. However, it has been demonstrated that the shunt fraction is increased at an $F_{I_{O_2}}$ of 1.0.
   C. This occurs secondary to:
      1. Nitrogen washout atelectasis
         a. Areas of the lung that are ventilated poorly tend to collapse if the nitrogen is removed.
         b. Nitrogen normally maintains alveolar stability. When nitrogen is removed and replaced by oxygen, the oxygen is absorbed by the blood faster than it can be replaced because of the poor ventilation.
         c. As a result, alveolar size decreases, eventually falling below its critical volume, and collapse occurs (Fig 13–3).
      2. Redistribution of pulmonary blood flow
         a. If an area of lung is poorly ventilated or not ventilated at all, the decreased Po_2 in the area causes the pulmonary vasculature surrounding the alveoli to constrict.
         b. This decreases blood flow to poorly ventilated areas and increases blood flow to areas more appropriately ventilated.
         c. When a high $F_{I_{O_2}}$ is administered, this autoregulatory mechanism is abated, because the Po_2 throughout the lung is elevated, and capillaries that were previously constricted are now dilated.
         d. This results in increased blood being shunted past nonventilated and poorly ventilated alveoli.
   D. Figure 13–4 represents the relationship between $F_{I_{O_2}}$ and percent shunt. Clinically it appears that the lowest measured shunt occurs at about 50% oxygen.
      1. The percent shunt increases as the $F_{I_{O_2}}$ decreases below 0.5 because of the effect of venous admixture.
      2. The percent shunt increases as the $F_{I_{O_2}}$ increases above 0.5 because of nitrogen washout atelectasis and redistribution of pulmonary blood flow.
   E. Percent intrapulmonary shunts should be calculated at the $F_{I_{O_2}}$ at which the patient is maintained.
   F. If a determination at a comparable $F_{I_{O_2}}$ is desired, an $F_{I_{O_2}}$ of 0.5 is recommended.
VII. Clinical Use of the Shunt Calculation
   A. Differentiating causes of hypoxemia
      1. Hypoxemia is caused by:
         a. True shunting: A combination of anatomic and capillary shunting.
         b. Shunt effect: A decrease in alveolar oxygen tension.
         c. Decreased mixed venous oxygen content.
            (1) This causes hypoxemia or an increase in hypoxemia only if intrapulmonary shunting also exists.

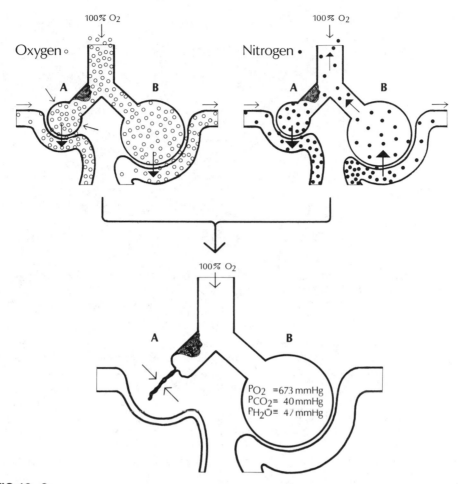

FIG 13–3.
Schematic representation of primary mechanisms causing denitrogenation absorption atelectasis. *Top drawings* represent aveolar capillary units shortly after administration of 100% inspired oxygen. *White circles* represent oxygen molecules that have increased in concentration in both units *A* and *B*. The ablation of alveolar hypoxia in unit *A* results in loss of vasoconstriction with considerably increased blood flow. The increased blood flow to this still poorly ventilated alveolus results in significantly increased oxygen extraction, which results in diminished gas volume. *Black circles* represent nitrogen, which is rapidly depleted from all units secondary to the fact that inspired nitrogen concentration is now zero. Initially, more nitrogen leaves the blood and the body via unit *B* because it is better ventilated. However, as the blood P_{N_2} level progressively decreases, nitrogen will start to leave alveolus *A* via the blood. This results in further loss of gas volume from alveolus *A* since it remains poorly ventilated but well perfused. Thus, nitrogen is depleted from all units within 5 to 15 min. *Bottom drawing* represents the final steady state, in which increased oxygen and nitrogen extraction has caused the alveolus to collapse. Thus, a poorly ventilated poorly perfused unit *A* becomes a nonventilated, poorly perfused unit after administration of 100% inspired oxygen. (From Shapiro BA, Harrison RA, Walton JR: *Clinical Application of Blood Gases,* ed 3. Chicago, Year Book Medical Publishers, 1982. Used by permission.)

    (2) Essentially it accentuates the effect of a preexisting shunt, because the blood that is shunted is now more deoxygenated than normal.

  2. The numerator of the shunt equation, $Cc_{O_2} - Ca_{O_2}$, can be considered a reflection of intrapulmonary pathology. That is, hypoxemia of pulmonary origin will increase the $Cc_{O_2} - Ca_{O_2}$ value, increasing the calculated shunt fraction.

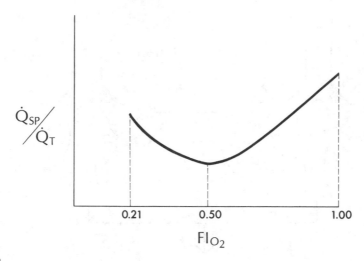

FIG 13–4.
Schematic representation of intrapulmonary shunt calculations *(Qs/Qt)* vs. inspired oxygen concentration *(F$_{IO_2}$)* in both normal and diseased lungs. (From Shapiro BA, Harrison RA, Walton JR: *Clinical Application of Blood Gases,* ed 3. Chicago, Year Book Medical Publishers, 1982. Used by permission.)

    3. The denominator in the shunt equation, $Cc_{O_2} - C\bar{v}_{O_2}$ can be considered a reflection of the relationship of cardiac output to oxygen demand.
      a. This is true because $Ca_{O_2} - C\bar{v}_{O_2}$ is contained in the denominator.
      b. If hypoxemia is a result of cardiovascular pathology, it is primarily reflected in a widening of the $Cc_{O_2} - C\bar{v}_{O_2}$ but may not be accompanied by a proportional widening of the numerator.
    4. Hypoxemia accompanied by an increased shunt measurement generally denotes an increase in intrapulmonary pathology.
    5. Hypoxemia without a major increase in shunt fraction usually denotes cardiovascular causes of hypoxemia.
  B. Assessment of spontaneous ventilatory capabilities in patients being mechanically ventilated
    1. An intrapulmonary shunt determination of less than 10% during mechanical ventilation is clinically comparable to normal lungs.
    2. An intrapulmonary shunt determination of 10% to 19% should not represent sufficient pulmonary disease to interfere with spontaneous ventilation.
    3. An intrapulmonary shunt of 20% to 30% may result in ventilatory failure in patients with central nervous system or cardiovascular dysfunction if spontaneous ventilation is attempted. However, many patients are able to sustain spontaneous ventilation with this level of shunt.
    4. An intrapulmonary shunt of greater than 30% represents a degree of pulmonary disease that normally requires aggressive cardiopulmonary support.
  C. Assessment of specific cardiopulmonary abnormalities
    1. Performance of intrapulmonary shunt studies while a patient is in different positions may delineate the locale and extent of certain pulmonary pathology.
      a. This is true because of the effects of gravity on pulmonary blood flow.
      b. If the diseased area is gravity dependent, the percent intrapulmonary shunt is increased.
    2. In the neonate the extent of right-to-left shunting in the presence of the following congenital anomalies can be determined:
      a. Ventricular septal defects

   b. Atrial septal defects
   c. Patent ductus arteriosus
D. Monitoring of oxygen and positive end-expiratory pressure (PEEP) therapy
   1. If the hypoxemia is of pulmonary origin and caused primarily by shunt effect, the appropriate application of oxygen therapy should demonstrate a decrease in intrapulmonary shunt (see Chapter 28).
   2. If the hypoxemia is of pulmonary origin and caused primarily by capillary shunting of a generalized diffuse nature (e.g., adult respiratory distress syndrome [ARDS]), PEEP therapy is primarily indicated (see Chapter 37), along with appropriate adjustment of F_{IO_2}.
   3. However, the greater the $\dot{Q}s/\dot{Q}T$, the less effect increasing F_{IO_2} has on Pa_{O_2} (Fig 13–5).

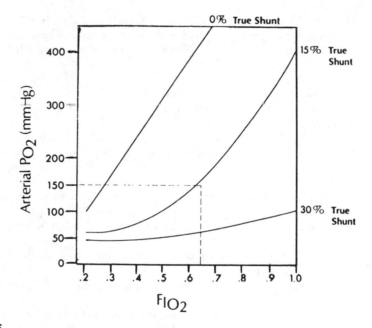

FIG 13–5.

Comparison of the theoretical F_{IO_2}-Pa_{O_2} relationships in 0%, 15%, and 30% true shunts. These relationships were calculated assuming normal lung ventilation, a hemoglobin of 15 gm%, arteriovenous oxygen content difference of 5 vol%, as well as normal cardiac output, metabolic rate, pH, and P_{CO_2}. This schema assumes that only true shunting exists; that is, no shunt effect is present. The 0% true shunt line reveals a Pa_{O_2} of 100 mm Hg at room air. There is a predictable increase in Pa_{O_2} for incremental increases in F_{IO_2}, because the arterial hemoglobin is nearly fully saturated at room air. Because all the blood exchanges with alveolar gas, incremental increases in alveolar oxygen tensions produce similar increases in arterial oxygen tensions. Note that with 15% true shunt, the arterial P_{O_2} is approximately 60 mm Hg (90% saturation) because 15% of the cardiac output enters the left side of the heart with approximately a 75% hemoglobin saturation. Incremental increases in alveolar P_{O_2} result in small increases in oxygen content (dissolved oxygen) in 85% of the cardiac output, whereas 15% of the cardiac output continues to enter the left side of the heart with a hemoglobin saturation of approximately 75%. Note that the arterial blood does not approach 100 mm Hg (near complete hemoglobin saturation) until the F_{IO_2} approaches 0.5. With incremental F_{IO_2} increases above 0.5, near linear increases in Pa_{O_2} occur but at a slightly lesser slope than with 0% true shunt. Thirty percent true shunt produces an arterial P_{O_2} of approximately 45 mm Hg at room air. This degree of true shunt does not allow an arterial P_{O_2} of 100 mm Hg, even at 100% inspired oxygen concentration. (From Shapiro BA, Harrison RA, Walton JR: *Clinical Application of Blood Gases*, ed 3. Chicago, Year Book Medical Publishers. Used by permission.)

4. In patients with more than 30% $\dot{Q}s/\dot{Q}T$, $F_{I_{O_2}}$ of 1.0 may not raise the P_{O_2} to a clinically acceptable level.

VIII. Other Methods of Estimating Shunting and Oxygenation Status

    A. Alveolar-arterial P_{O_2} difference: $P(A - a)_{O_2}$

        1. The $P(A - a)$ gradient has been used to estimate the percent intrapulmonary shunt.

        2. The normal $P(A - a)_{O_2}$ when room air is breathed is 7 to 14 mm Hg.

        3. However, at an $F_{I_{O_2}}$ of 1.0, it increases to 31 to 56 mm Hg.

        4. During 100% oxygen breathing, some estimate the shunt fraction as 1% for every 10 to 15 mm Hg of $P(A - a)_{O_2}$.

        5. The fact that $P(A - a)_{O_2}$ exhibits variability with changes in $F_{I_{O_2}}$ limits its usefulness as an indicator of overall cardiopulmonary function.

    B. Arterial-alveolar ratio: Pa_{O_2}/PA_{O_2}

        1. The lower limit of normal for Pa_{O_2}/PA_{O_2}, regardless of $F_{I_{O_2}}$, is 0.75 or greater.

        2. The lower the Pa_{O_2}/PA_{O_2}, the greater the cardiopulmonary abnormality.

        3. Since Pa_{O_2}/PA_{O_2} is not affected by changes in $F_{I_{O_2}}$, it is a more reliable index of abnormality than $P(A - a)_{O_2}$

    C. Arterial-$F_{I_{O_2}}$ ratio: $Pa_{O_2}/F_{I_{O_2}}$

        1. The normal $Pa_{O_2}/F_{I_{O_2}}$ is about 450 to 500.

        2. A $Pa_{O_2}/F_{I_{O_2}}$ less than 200 has been associated with a shunt fraction of greater than 20%.

        3. The $Pa_{O_2}/F_{I_{O_2}}$ is inversely affected by Pa_{CO_2}, as well as increasing $F_{I_{O_2}}$.

        4. As a result, it is a much cruder index of cardiopulmonary dysfunction than $P(A - a)_{O_2}$ or Pa_{O_2}/PA_{O_2}.

IX. Pulmonary Deadspace

    A. Pulmonary deadspace is that portion of the total ventilation that does not undergo external respiration.

    B. The total quantity of pulmonary deadspace is the *physiologic deadspace* and is composed of three subdivisions:

        1. Anatomic deadspace: That portion of the total ventilation that does not contact the alveolar epithelium.

           a. Normally the anatomic deadspace is equal to about 1.0 ml/lb of ideal body weight.

           b. The relationship between anatomic deadspace and tidal volume is increased by small tidal volumes and rapid rates.

           c. The absolute quantity of anatomic deadspace is increased by:

               (1) Positive pressure ventilation

               (2) The use of mechanical deadspace

           d. Anatomic deadspace is decreased by:

               (1) Tracheostomy/endotracheal tubes

               (2) Pneumothorax

         2. Alveolar deadspace: That portion of the total ventilation that contacts the alveolar epithelium but does not participate in gas exchange due to a lack of pulmonary capillary blood flow.

           a. Alveolar deadspace accounts for a very small amount of the total physiologic deadspace in the healthy individual.

           b. Alveolar deadspace is increased by:

               (1) Pulmonary emboli

               (2) Vascular tumors

         3. Deadspace effect (ventilation/perfusion inequality): Any pathophysiologic process in which ventilation is in excess of perfusion but some perfusion does exist (i.e., $\dot{V}/\dot{Q}$ ratio greater than 1.0).

           a. In the standing individual, deadspace effect occurs in the apices of the lungs since blood flow to this region is greatly diminished.

   b. Deadspace effect is increased by:
    (1) Positive pressure ventilation
    (2) Decreased cardiac output
    (3) Alveolar septal wall destruction
X. Derivation of the Deadspace Equation
 A. Definition of abbreviations
   1. V_T: Tidal volume
   2. V_D: Deadspace volume
   3. V_A: Alveolar volume
   4. $F_{A_{CO_2}}$: Fractional concentration of CO_2 in alveolar gas
   5. $F\bar{E}_{CO_2}$: Mean fractional concentration of CO_2 in mixed expired gas
   6. Pa_{CO_2}: Partial pressure of arterial CO_2
   7. $P\bar{E}_{CO_2}$: Partial pressure of mean expired CO_2
   8. $F_{D_{CO_2}}$: Fractional concentration of deadspace CO_2
 B. Tidal volume is equal to deadspace volume plus alveolar volume.

$$V_T = V_D + V_A \tag{17}$$

 C. The total volume of CO_2 in exhaled gas is equal to V_T times the fractional concentration of CO_2 in the exhaled gas.

$$(V_T)(F\bar{E}_{CO_2}) = \text{total } CO_2 \text{ exhaled} \tag{18}$$

 D. This volume can be subdivided into the amount of CO_2 exhaled from deadspace and alveoli:

$$(V_T)(F\bar{E}_{CO_2}) = (V_A)(F_{A_{CO_2}}) + (V_D)(F_{D_{CO_2}}) \tag{19}$$

 E. Since the concentration of CO_2 in exhaled deadspace gas is about zero, equation 19 can be rewritten as:

$$(V_T)(F\bar{E}_{CO_2}) = (V_A)(F_{A_{CO_2}}) \tag{20}$$

 F. Since $V_A = V_T - V_D$, equation 20 may be rewritten as:

$$(V_T)(F\bar{E}_{CO_2}) = (V_T)(F_{A_{CO_2}}) - (V_D)(F_{A_{CO_2}}) \tag{21}$$

 G. By rearrangement of and simplification of equation 21, the Bohr equation for the determination of the deadspace/tidal volume ratio (V_D/V_T ratio) is generated.

$$V_D/V_T = \frac{F_{A_{CO_2}} - F\bar{E}_{CO_2}}{F_{A_{CO_2}}} \tag{22}$$

 H. Since the concentration of CO_2 in the alveoli is equal to the concentration of CO_2 in the arterial blood and since the partial pressures of gases are proportional to their concentration, equation 22 may be rewritten as the Enghoff modification of the Bohr equation:

$$V_D/V_T = \frac{Pa_{CO_2} - P\bar{E}_{CO_2}}{Pa_{CO_2}} \tag{23}$$

 I. In all circumstances, as the deadspace increases, there is a widening of the $Pa_{CO_2} - P\bar{E}_{CO_2}$ gradient.
 J. Normal V_D/V_T ratios are about 20% to 40%.

XI. Calculation of the Deadspace/Tidal Volume Ratio
   A. A *simultaneous* sampling of arterial blood and exhaled gas is obtained.
      1. The exhaled gas sample must be large enough to reflect a mean exhaled P_{CO_2} value.
      2. In spontaneously breathing patients, about 40 L of exhaled gas is collected. This is done to compensate for tidal volume variations.
      3. If a patient is being ventilated in the control mode with consistent tidal volumes, a 5-L sample is sufficient.
   B. The patient should be stable and quiet at the time the sample is obtained.
      Example:

$$V_D/V_T = \frac{Pa_{CO_2} - P\overline{E}_{CO_2}}{Pa_{CO_2}}$$
$$0.52 = \frac{42 - 20}{42}$$

XII. Minute Volume–Pa_{CO_2} Relationship
   A. Since the physiologic adequacy of ventilation is clinically defined by the arterial Pa_{CO_2} level, a relationship between total minute volume and arterial Pa_{CO_2} must exist.
   B. In the average adult, a minute volume of 4 to 6 L maintains a Pa_{CO_2} of 40 mm Hg.
   C. If the minute volume increases, the Pa_{CO_2} should decrease, and if the minute volume decreases, the Pa_{CO_2} should increase.
   D. It is generally accepted that with each doubling of the minute volume, the Pa_{CO_2} decreases by 10 mm Hg (Table 13–1).
   E. If there is a disparity between the minute volume and the expected Pa_{CO_2}, deadspace is increased.
      Example:
      If the Pa_{CO_2} is 42 mm Hg and the minute volume is 20 L, deadspace ventilation is increased. A Pa_{CO_2} of about 20 mm Hg would be expected with a minute ventilation of 20 L.
XIII. Clinical Use of the Deadspace/Tidal Volume Ratios
   A. Assessment of spontaneous ventilatory capabilities in patients being mechanically ventilated
      1. The V_D/V_T ratio is typically increased during mechanical ventilation and is considered normal up to 0.50.
      2. A V_D/V_T ratio less than 0.60 normally does not represent pulmonary pathology of sufficient magnitude to interfere with spontaneous ventilation.
      3. A V_D/V_T ratio of 0.60 to 0.80 represents significant disease and frequently interferes with an individual's ability to maintain prolonged spontaneous ventilation.

TABLE 13–1.

Normal Minute Volume-Pa_{CO_2} Relationships

V_A (L/min)	Pa_{CO_2} (mm Hg)
1.25	60
2.50	50
5.00	40
10.00	30
20.00	20

4. A V$_D$/V$_T$ ratio greater than 0.80 normally requires mechanical ventilatory support.
   B. Evaluation of the presence of pulmonary embolism
      1. An increase in deadspace supports the diagnosis of pulmonary embolism.
      2. However, a definitive diagnosis cannot be made by deadspace studies alone.
   C. Because of the difficulty in securing an ideal sample of exhaled gas, the determination of V$_D$/V$_T$ ratio is infrequently performed outside of the pulmonary function laboratory.
XIV. Guidelines for Differentiating Shunt-Producing From Deadspace-Producing Diseases
   A. Deadspace-producing diseases
      1. Minute volume greatly increased with little or no decrease in Pa$_{CO_2}$.
      2. Even though hypoxemia is present and correctable by oxygen therapy, minute ventilation changes are minimal when hypoxemia is corrected.
   B. Shunt-producing diseases
      1. Pa$_{CO_2}$ decreases as minute volume increases.
      2. Assuming the hypoxemia is responsive, oxygen therapy will decrease myocardial and ventilatory work and relieve hypoxemia. Thus, minute volume and Pa$_{CO_2}$ return to normal.
      3. If hypoxemia is refractory, the application of PEEP is necessary to reverse the hypoxemia.

BIBLIOGRAPHY

Burton GG, Hodgkin JE: *Respiratory Care: A Guide to Clinical Practice,* ed 2. Philadelphia, JB Lippincott Co, 1984.
Cane RD, Shapiro BA, Harrison RA, et al: Minimizing errors in intrapulmonary shunt calculation. *Crit Care Med* 1980; 8:294–297.
Cohen JJ, Kassirer JP: *Acid/Base.* Boston, Little, Brown & Co, 1982.
Comroe JH: *Physiology of Respiration,* ed 2. Chicago, Year Book Medical Publishers, 1974.
Comroe JH, Forster RE II, Dubois AB, et al: *The Lung: Clinical Physiology and Pulmonary Function Tests,* ed 2. Chicago, Year Book Medical Publishers, 1962.
Deshpande VM, Pilbeam SP, Dixon RJ: *A Comprehensive Review in Respiratory Care.* Norwalk, Mass, Appleton & Lange, 1988.
Dimas S, Kacmarek RM: Intrapulmonary shunting: Part I. Basic concepts and derivation of equation. *Curr Rev Respir Ther* 1981; 1:35–39.
Dimas S, Kacmarek RM: Intrapulmonary shunting: Part II. Clinical application. *Curr Rev Respir Ther* 1981; 1:43–47.
Duranceau A, et al: Ventilatory deadspace in diagnosis of acute pulmonary embolism. *Surg Forum* 1974; 25:229–233.
Fisher SR, et al: Comparative changes in ventilatory deadspace following micro and massive pulmonary emboli. *J Surg Res* 1976; 29:195–199.
Gilbert R, Auchinloss JH Jr, Kuppinger M, et al: Stability of the arterial-alveolar oxygen partial pressure ratio. *Crit Care Med* 1979; 7:267–272.
Gilbert R, Keighley JF: The arterial/alveolar oxygen tension ratio. An index of gas exchange applicable to varying inspired oxygen concentrations. *Am Rev Respir Dis* 1974; 109:142–145.
Hoffstein V, Duguid N, Zamel N, et al: Estimation of changes in alveolar-arterial oxygen gradient induced by hypoxia. *J Lab Clin Med* 1984; 104:685–692.
Kacmarek RM, Dimas S: Pulmonary deadspace: Concepts and clinical application. *Curr Rev Respir Ther* 1981; 1:147–150.
Maxwell C, Hess D, Shefet D: Use of the arterial/alveolar oxygen tension ratio to predict the inspired oxygen concentration needed for a desired arterial oxygen tension. *Respir Care* 1984; 29:1135–1139.
Murray JF: *The Normal Lung: The Basis for Diagnosis and Treatment of Pulmonary Disease.* Philadelphia, WB Saunders Co, 1976.

Peris LV, Boix JH, Salom JV, et al: Clinical use of the arterial/alveolar oxygen tension ratio. *Crit Care Med* 1983; 11:888–891.

Shapiro BA, Cane RD, Harrison RA, et al: Changes in intrapulmonary shunting with administration of 100 percent oxygen. *Chest* 1980; 77:138–141.

Shapiro BA, Harrison RA, Cane R, et al: *Clinical Application of Blood Gases,* ed 4. Chicago, Year Book Medical Publishers, 1989.

Shapiro BA, Harrison RA, Kacmarek RM, et al: *Clinical Application of Respiratory Care,* ed 3. Chicago, Year Book Medical Publishers, 1985.

Spearman CB, Sheldon RL, Egan DF: *Egan's Fundamentals of Respiratory Therapy,* ed 4. St Louis, CV Mosby Co, 1982.

Snyder JV, Pinshy MR: *Oxygen Transport in the Critically Ill.* Chicago, Year Book Medical Publishers, 1987.

Chapter 14

Hemodynamic Monitoring

I. Systemic Arterial Blood Pressure

Systemic arterial blood pressure is expressed as a systolic pressure divided by a diastolic pressure (Fig 14–1).

  A. Systolic pressure is the highest pressure attained in the artery and is determined by three major factors:
  1. Stroke volume
     a. Increased stroke volume generally causes an increased systolic pressure.
     b. Decreased stroke volume generally causes a decreased systolic pressure.
  2. Rate of blood ejection from left ventricle
     a. An increased rate of left ventricular ejection generally results in increased systolic pressure.
     b. A decrease in the rate of ejection generally results in decreased systolic pressure.
  3. Elasticity of the arterial tree
     a. Increased arterial elasticity generally results in an increased systolic pressure.
     b. Decreased arterial elasticity generally results in a decreased systolic pressure.

  B. Diastolic pressure is the lowest pressure attained in the artery and is determined by three major factors:
  1. Magnitude of preceding systolic pressure
     a. In general, the higher the preceding systolic pressure, the higher the resulting diastolic pressure.
     b. The lower the preceding systolic pressure, the lower the resulting diastolic pressure.
  2. Length of ventricular diastolic interval
     a. The longer the diastolic interval, the greater the time available for blood to leave the arterial system and the lower the resultant diastolic pressure.
     b. The shorter the diastolic interval, the higher the diastolic pressure by the opposite mechanism.
  3. State of peripheral resistance
     a. The greater the peripheral resistance, the lower the rate of arterial runoff and the higher the resultant diastolic pressure.
     b. The lower the peripheral resistance, the higher the rate of arterial runoff and the lower the resultant diastolic pressure.

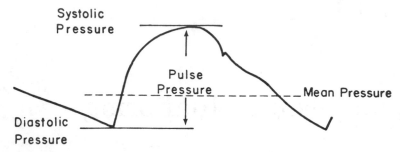

FIG 14–1.
Graphic representation of arterial pressure tracing depicting systolic, diastolic, mean, and pulse
pressures (see text). (From Little RC: *Physiology of the Heart and Circulation,* ed 2. Chicago, Year
Book Medical Publishers, 1981. Used by permission.)

C. In general, measurement of arterial blood pressure assesses left ventricular function by systolic pressure and peripheral resistance by diastolic pressure. It should
be recalled that one factor responsible for systolic pressure is stroke volume, and a
factor responsible for diastolic pressure is the state of peripheral resistance.

D. Thus, it is assumed that the greater the difference between systolic and diastolic
pressures, the greater the resultant flow. The difference between systolic and diastolic pressures is called the *pulse pressure.*

1. By the equation

$$\dot{Q} = P \times \frac{1}{R} \tag{1}$$

increases in systolic pressure indicate increases in the pressure gradient (P)
across the systemic circulation, and decreases in diastolic pressure indicate decreases in peripheral resistance (R).

2. Therefore, widening of pulse pressure is generally thought to indicate increased
blood flow ($\dot{Q}$).

3. By the opposite mechanism, narrowing of pulse pressure is generally thought to
indicate decreased flow.

4. It should be noted that a widening of pulse pressure can occur without increased blood flow. Also, normal blood flow can exist with a narrow pulse pressure. These phenomena occur by alterations in the other factors (i.e., diastolic
interval, arterial elasticity) that determine systolic and diastolic pressure.
Therefore, it is imperative to assess all factors responsible for systolic and diastolic pressure before blindly stating that an increased or decreased pulse pressure represents increased or decreased blood flow in a given patient.

E. The mean arterial pressure (MAP) represents the average pressure over one complete systolic and diastolic interval.

1. The MAP can be directly measured or estimated by the following formula:

$$MAP = \frac{(2 \times \text{diastolic pressure}) + (\text{systolic pressure})}{3} \tag{2}$$

2. The MAP is the average pressure in the arterial tree over a given time and
therefore generally is used as an assessment of the average pressure to which
the arterial system is exposed.

3. The pressure gradient across the systemic circulation is generally expressed as
MAP − CVP, where CVP equals central venous pressure (see section II).

4. The MAP is also commonly used as an indicator of left ventricular afterload, thus representing the resistance (in terms of pressure) that the left ventricle must pump against.

F. Both arterial blood pressure and mean arterial blood pressure can be directly measured by an intra-arterial line (catheter). Arterial blood pressure can be indirectly measured by use of a sphygmomanometer and the MAP calculated from the obtained values.

G. Normal values for arterial blood pressure in the adult are as follows:

> Systolic: 140 to 90 mm Hg
> Diastolic: 90 to 60 mm Hg
> Mean: 70 to 105 mm Hg

II. Central Venous Pressure (CVP)

The CVP usually is expressed as a single number representing the mean right atrial pressure ($\overline{RAP}$).

A. The numerical pressure value of CVP will be the result of the following factors:
   1. The pump capabilities of the right side of the heart in part determine the CVP. If the right ventricle pumps what it receives, blood will not back up in the atrium, and the CVP should be normal. If the right side of the heart is not pumping adequately, there will be a backup of blood in the atrium that will be reflected in an elevated CVP.
   2. The venous tone determines CVP in that venous tone is responsible for determining the venous vascular space. It thus has major implications in venous return and filling pressure of the right atrium.
   3. Blood volume, which in part determines CVP, must be adequate to fill the venous vascular space, or venous return to the heart will be impeded.
   4. If the pump capabilities of the right side of the heart are adequate, the CVP will directly reflect the venous vascular volume (blood volume) to venous vascular space relationship. Fluid therapy and diuresis are frequently gauged in terms of the CVP's reflection of this relationship.

B. The CVP is commonly used as an indicator of right ventricular preload when measured as the right ventricular end-diastolic pressure (RVEDP).
   1. The RVEDP represents compliance of the right ventricle.
   2. The RVEDP also represents the filling pressure necessary for adequate right ventricular function.

C. The CVP is measured directly through a catheter inserted in a peripheral vein, its tip resting in the right atrium (Fig 14–2).

D. Normal values for CVP in the adult are 0 to 8 mm Hg.

III. Pulmonary Artery Pressure (PAP)

The PAP is expressed as a systolic pressure divided by a diastolic pressure.

A. Systolic pressure is the highest pressure attained in the pulmonary artery and is determined by the same three factors that determine systolic pressure in the systemic arterial system:
   1. Size of stroke volume
   2. Rate of blood ejection from right ventricle
   3. Elasticity of pulmonary arterial tree

B. Diastolic pressure is the lowest pressure attained in the pulmonary artery and is determined by the same three factors that determine diastolic pressure in the systemic arterial system:
   1. Magnitude of preceding systolic pressure
   2. Length of right ventricular diastolic interval
   3. State of peripheral resistance of pulmonary arterial tree

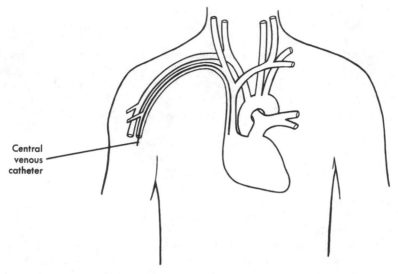

FIG 14–2.
Location of a central venous catheter. (From Spearman CB, Sheldon RL, Egan DF: *Egan's Funda-mentals of Respiratory Therapy,* ed 4. St Louis, CV Mosby Co, 1982. Used by permission.)

    C. In general, measurement of PAP assesses right ventricular function by systolic pressure and pulmonary arterial resistance by diastolic pressure. Thus, PAP is used in precisely the same fashion as systemic arterial pressure. In this light, it should be noted that all factors contributing to systolic and diastolic PAP should be fully assessed before inferences concerning blood flow are made from these values.

    D. The mean pulmonary artery pressure ($\overline{\text{PAP}}$) represents the average pressure over one complete systolic and diastolic interval.

        1. The $\overline{\text{PAP}}$ is the average pressure in the pulmonary artery over a given time and is used as an assessment of the average pressure head (or front) that the pulmonary arterial system is exposed to.

        2. Thus, the pressure gradient across the pulmonary circulation is generally represented by the expression $\overline{\text{PAP}}$ − PWP, where PWP equals the mean left atrial or pulmonary wedge pressure (see section IV).

        3. The $\overline{\text{PAP}}$ is commonly used as an assessment of right ventricular afterload, thus representing the resistance (in terms of pressure) that the right ventricle must pump against.

    E. Both the PAP and $\overline{\text{PAP}}$ are directly measured by use of a pulmonary artery catheter. The pulmonary artery catheter is inserted through a peripheral vein and traverses the right atrium and ventricle, its tip resting in the pulmonary artery (Fig 14–3).

    F. Normal values for pulmonary arterial blood pressure in the adult are as follows:

Systolic:	15 to 28 mm Hg
Diastolic:	5 to 16 mm Hg
Mean:	10 to 22 mm Hg

  IV. Pulmonary Wedge Pressure

      Pulmonary wedge pressure (PWP) is expressed as a single number representing the mean left atrial pressure ($\overline{\text{LAP}}$).

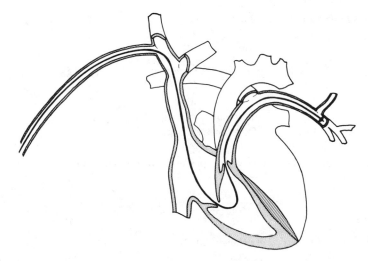

FIG 14–3.
Location of a pulmonary artery catheter. (From Spearman CB, Sheldon RL, Egan DF: *Egan's Fundamentals of Respiratory Therapy,* ed 4. St Louis, CV Mosby Co, 1982. Used by permission.)

    A. The numerical pressure value of the PWP will be the result of the following factors:

        1. The pump capabilities of the left side of the heart in part determine the PWP. If the left ventricle pumps what it receives, blood will not back up into the atrium, and the PWP should be normal. If the left ventricle is not pumping adequately, there will be a backup of blood into the atrium that will be reflected as an elevated PWP.

        2. Blood return to the left atrium is due largely to an adequate blood volume to pulmonary venous (venomotor tone) vascular space relationship.

        3. If the left ventricle is pumping adequately, the PWP is dependent on the forementioned vascular volume to vascular space relationship.

    B. The PWP is commonly used as an indicator of left ventricular preload when measured as the left ventricular end-diastolic pressure (LVEDP).

        1. The LVEDP represents compliance of the left ventricle.

        2. The LVEDP also represents the filling pressure necessary for adequate left ventricular function.

    C. The PWP is measured directly through a pulmonary artery catheter by inflation of a balloon that occludes that branch of the pulmonary artery. Pressure readings are taken from the tip of the catheter, which is distal to the balloon. The pressure reflects backpressure from the left atrium.

    D. Normal values for the PWP in the adult are 2 to 12 mm Hg.

 V. Calculation and Comparison of Systemic and Pulmonary Vascular Resistance

    A.

$$R = \frac{\Delta P}{\dot{Q}} \qquad (3)$$

where R = vascular resistance expressed in mm Hg/L/min
ΔP = change in pressure across the circulation or pressure gradient, expressed in mm Hg
$\dot{Q}$ = cardiac output or flow expressed in L/min

B. Systemic vascular resistance equals:
   1.

$$R = \frac{MAP - \overline{RAP}}{\dot{Q}} \tag{4}$$

where MAP = mean arterial pressure
$\overline{RAP}$ = mean right atrial pressure (CVP)
$\dot{Q}$ = cardiac output

   2. Replacing the factors with representative normal values results in

$$R = \frac{(90 - 5) \text{ mm Hg}}{5 \text{ L/min}} = 17 \text{ mm Hg/L/min} \tag{5}$$

C. Pulmonary vascular resistance equals:
   1.

$$R = \frac{\overline{PAP} - \overline{LAP}}{\dot{Q}} \tag{6}$$

where $\overline{PAP}$ = mean pulmonary arterial pressure
$\overline{LAP}$ = mean left atrial pressure (PWP)
$\dot{Q}$ = cardiac output

   2. Replacing the factors with representative normal values results in

$$R = \frac{(16 - 6) \text{ mm Hg}}{5 \text{ L/min}} = 2 \text{ mm Hg/L/min} \tag{7}$$

D. By these calculations, systemic vascular resistance equals 17 mm Hg/L/min and pulmonary vascular resistance equals 2 mm Hg/L/min. This relationship results in systemic vascular resistance being about 8½ times the pulmonary vascular resistance.

VI. Techniques of Measuring Cardiac Output
   A. Fick method
      1. The total amount of oxygen available for tissue utilization must be equal to arterial oxygen content (Ca_{O_2}), expressed in vol%, times the volume of blood presented to the tissues per unit time ($\dot{Q}$ or cardiac output), expressed in L/min:

$$\text{Total O}_2 \text{ available} = (\dot{Q}) \times (Ca_{O_2}) \tag{8}$$

      2. The total amount of oxygen returned to the lung from the tissues must be equal to the mixed venous oxygen content ($C\overline{v}_{O_2}$) times the volume of blood presented to the lung per unit time ($\dot{Q}$ or cardiac output):

$$\text{Total O}_2 \text{ returned} = (\dot{Q}) \times (C\overline{v}_{O_2}) \tag{9}$$

      3. Therefore, total tissue extraction of oxygen per unit time ($\dot{V}_{O_2}$) must be equal to the total oxygen available minus the total oxygen returned:

$$\dot{V}_{O_2} = [(\dot{Q}) \times (Ca_{O_2})] - [(\dot{Q}) \times (C\overline{v}_{O_2})] \tag{10}$$

4. Equation 10 may be simplified by extracting the common factor of $(\dot{Q})$ and rewriting it as follows:

$$\dot{V}_{O_2} = (\dot{Q}) \times (Ca_{O_2} - C\bar{v}_{O_2}) \tag{11}$$

5. Equation 11 is called the *Fick equation,* and by solving for cardiac output $(\dot{Q})$, it becomes

$$\dot{Q} = \frac{\dot{V}_{O_2}}{Ca_{O_2} - C\bar{v}_{O_2}} \tag{12}$$

6. Thus, by measuring total oxygen consumption per minute and arterial and mixed venous oxygen content in vol%, the cardiac output can be easily calculated by equation 12.
   (1) Total oxygen consumption generally is calculated by analysis of exhaled gases.
   (2) Arterial oxygen content requires systemic arterial blood sampling.
   (3) Mixed venous oxygen content requires pulmonary arterial blood sampling.
7. *Example:* Given the following values:

$$\dot{V}_{O_2} = \frac{280 \text{ cc of } O_2}{\text{min}}$$

$$Ca_{O_2} = \frac{20 \text{ cc of } O_2}{100 \text{ cc of blood}} \text{ or } 20 \text{ vol\%}$$

$$C\bar{v}_{O_2} = \frac{15 \text{ cc of } O_2}{100 \text{ cc of blood}} \text{ or } 15 \text{ vol\%}$$

the cardiac output must equal 5.6 L/min by the following calculation:

$$\dot{Q} = \frac{\dfrac{280 \text{ cc of } O_2}{\text{min}}}{\dfrac{20 \text{ cc of } O_2}{100 \text{ cc of blood}} - \dfrac{15 \text{ cc of } O_2}{100 \text{ cc of blood}}}$$

$$\dot{Q} = \frac{5,600 \text{ cc of blood}}{\text{min}} \text{ or } \frac{5.6 \text{ L of blood}}{\text{min}}$$

8. The cardiac output determination obtained by using the Fick equation is considered the most accurate. The Fick method is therefore the standard by which other methods of cardiac output determinations are compared for accuracy.
B. Dye dilution method
   1. A dye (typically indocyanine green) that can be analyzed by a spectrophotometer is used as an indicator.
   2. A known amount (milligrams) of dye is injected rapidly into the right atrium or pulmonary artery.
   3. The dye is allowed to mix in the pulmonary circulation, and a continuous representative sampling of blood is drawn from the sampling catheter located in a major systemic artery.

4. Blood samples are analyzed by spectrophotometry for concentration of dye, and the concentrations are plotted on a graph against time.
5. Knowing the number of milligrams of dye injected and plotting the measured concentrations against time allow calculation of the cardiac output ($\dot{Q}$) by the following equation:

$$\dot{Q} = \frac{d_o}{\overline{d}_c \times t} \tag{13}$$

where $\dot{Q}$ = cardiac output
    d_o = mg of dye injected
    $\overline{d}_c$ = mean concentration of dye
    t = time from appearance to disappearance of dye at sampling site

C. Thermal dilution method
1. This technique uses a four-lumen pulmonary artery catheter (Swan-Ganz catheter) with a port about 30 cm proximal from the end of the catheter (Fig 14–4).
2. This proximal port usually lies in the right atrium and is used for injection of a known volume (usually 10 cc) of fluid (D_5W) at a known temperature (usually 0°C).
3. At the distal end of the catheter is a device, a thermistor, which senses changes in temperature. This device normally resides in a branch of the pulmonary artery.
4. The bolus of cold solution is injected into the right atrium. The right ventricle is used as the mixing chamber, and the blood is continually sampled by the thermistor for changes in temperature.
5. The changes in blood temperature can be plotted on a graph against time.
6. The principle underlying cardiac output determination by thermal dilution is identical to that previously described for dye dilution.

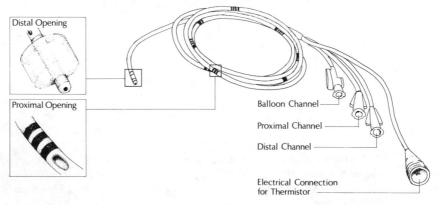

FIG 14–4.
The four-channel pulmonary artery catheter. The distal channel and balloon channel comprise the basic two-channel catheter. Addition of the proximal channel that opens in the right atrium results in the triple-channel catheter, usually 7 French in diameter. Addition of the thermistor channel results in the four-channel catheter used for thermodilution cardiac output measurements, usually 7 French in diameter. (From Shapiro BA, Harrison RA, Walton JR: *Clinical Application of Blood Gases*, ed 3. Chicago, Year Book Medical Publishers, 1982. Used by permission.)

7. Knowing the volume of the injected solution and the blood and solution temperatures and plotting the changes in blood temperature against time allow calculation of the cardiac output by the following equation:

$$\dot{Q} = \frac{V \times (T_b - T_s)}{\overline{T_b} \times t} \tag{14}$$

where $\dot{Q}$ = cardiac output
V = volume of solution injected
T_b = temperature of blood
T_s = temperature of solution injected
$\overline{T_b}$ = mean change in temperature of blood
t = time from appearance to disappearance of temperature change at sampling site

    D. The cardiac output of different individuals varies greatly according to body size. Therefore, cardiac output is frequently expressed in terms of body size and is then called the *cardiac index* (CI).
      1. The CI is equal to the cardiac output in liters per minute per body surface area in square meters.
      2. The CI becomes a more meaningful value when comparing cardiac outputs of different individuals.
      3. Since the CI is a more consistent value among different individuals, it has a narrow normal range of 2.5 to 4 L/min/sq m.

VII. Data Obtained From Arterial and Venous Lines
    A. Arterial line measurements
      1. Systemic systolic pressure
      2. Systemic diastolic pressure
      3. Systemic mean arterial blood pressure
      4. Arterial blood gases
    B. Central venous line measurements
      1. Central venous pressure
      2. Venous blood sample
    C. Pulmonary arterial line (catheter) measurements
      1. Pulmonary systolic pressure
      2. Pulmonary diastolic pressure
      3. Mean pulmonary arterial pressure
      4. Pulmonary wedge pressure
      5. Mixed venous blood gases
      6. Cardiac output
      7. Central venous pressure (on catheters so equipped)
VIII. Complications of Arterial and Venous Lines
    A. Arterial lines
      1. Thrombosis
      2. Embolism
      3. Hemorrhage
      4. Infection
    B. Central venous line
      1. Thrombosis
      2. Thromboembolism and/or air embolism
      3. Infection/sepsis

    C. Pulmonary arterial line
      1. Thrombosis
      2. Thromboembolism and/or catheter embolism
      3. Pulmonary hemorrhage
      4. Knotting of line in the cardiac chambers
      5. Cardiac dysrhythmias
      6. Endocarditis
      7. Infection/sepsis
IX. Effects of Ventilation on Intrathoracic Hemodynamic Pressure Values
    A. Alterations during spontaneous ventilation
      1. Pulmonary and central venous pressures follow intrathoracic pressure changes.
      2. During spontaneous inspiration, intrathoracic pressure decreases and thereby decreases all pulmonary arterial and central venous pressures.
        a. This phenomenon is exaggerated by deep inspiratory efforts and in patients who are experiencing increased work of breathing.
      3. During spontaneous exhalation, intrathoracic pressure increases and thereby increases all pulmonary arterial and central venous pressures.
        a. This phenomenon is exaggerated by forced expiratory efforts (i.e., Valsalva's maneuver) and in patients who are experiencing increased work of breathing.
    B. Alterations during positive pressure ventilation
      1. As in spontaneous ventilation, pulmonary arterial and central venous pressures follow intrathoracic pressure changes; however, they are influenced to a greater degree.
        a. The extent of the influence is dependent on the combination of transmitted intrathoracic and intra-airway pressures resulting from the following factors:
          (1) Ventilatory rate
          (2) Size of the tidal volume
          (3) Elastic resistance to ventilation
          (4) Nonelastic resistance to ventilation
          (5) Amount of positive end-expiratory pressure (PEEP), if any
      2. During positive pressure inspiration, intrathoracic pressure increases and thereby increases all pulmonary arterial and central venous pressures.
        a. This phenomenon is exaggerated by high ventilatory pressures and/or any PEEP.
      3. During positive pressure exhalation, intrathoracic pressure decreases and thereby decreases all pulmonary arterial and central venous pressures.
        a. This phenomenon is exaggerated by low ventilatory rates and lack of PEEP.
    C. Whether the patient is breathing spontaneously or receiving continuous positive airway pressure, intermittent mandatory ventilation, intermittent positive pressure ventilation, or continuous positive pressure ventilation, the forementioned effects on intrathoracic and subsequent hemodynamic pressures need to be considered. However, minimizing the artifact of positive-negative intrathoracic pressure swings is best accomplished by making the hemodynamic pressure recording at end exhalation regardless of the mode of ventilation.
  X. Representative Hemodynamic Profiles
    Note: The following examples represent numeric data consistent with the listed disorders; however, it should be fully appreciated that wide variations exist, and it is dangerous at best to come to any conclusions without viewing firsthand the patient's clinical presentation.

A. Pulmonary hypertension
    CVP = 7   BP* = 127/88
    PAP = 38/22   HR* = 105
    PWP = 10   CI = 3.5
B. Systemic hypertension
    CVP = 5   BP = 155/98
    PAP = 20/9   HR = 110
    PWP = 7   CI = 4.0
C. Right ventricular failure
    CVP = 28   BP = 120/100
    PAP = 30/8   HR = 130
    PWP = 4   CI = 2.3
D. Left ventricular failure
    CVP = 6   BP = 100/40
    PAP = 42/30   HR = 140
    PWP = 28   CI = 2.0
E. Hypervolemia
    CVP = 18   BP = 160/118
    PAP = 42/28   HR = 100
    PWP = 26   CI = 4.8
F. Hypovolemia
    CVP = 2   BP = 85/70
    PAP = 17/12   HR = 165
    PWP = 4   CI = 2.0

BIBLIOGRAPHY

Guyton AC: *Textbook of Medical Physiology*, ed 6. Philadelphia, WB Saunders Co, 1981.

Little RC: *Physiology of the Heart and Circulation*. Chicago, Year Book Medical Publishers, 1977.

McIntyre KM, Lewis AJ: *Textbook of Advanced Cardiac Life Support*. Dallas, American Heart Association, 1981.

McLaughlin AJ: *Essentials of Physiology for Advanced Respiratory Therapy*. St Louis, CV Mosby Co, 1977.

Mountcastle VB: *Medical Physiology*, ed 14. St. Louis, CV Mosby Co, 1980.

Ross G: *Essentials of Human Physiology*. Chicago, Year Book Medical Publishers, 1978.

Ruch TC, Patton HD: *Physiology and Biophysics*, ed 20. Philadelphia, WB Saunders Co, 1974.

Rushmer RF: *Cardiovascular Dynamics*, ed 3. Philadelphia, WB Saunders Co, 1970.

Schroeder JS, Daily EK: *Techniques in Bedside Hemodynamic Monitoring*, ed 2. St Louis, CV Mosby Co, 1981.

Shapiro BA, Harrison RA, Kacmarek RM, et al: *Clinical Applications of Respiratory Care*, ed 3. Chicago, Year Book Medical Publishers, 1985.

Spearman CB, Sheldon RL, Egan DF: *Egan's Fundamentals of Respiratory Therapy*, ed 4. St Louis, CV Mosby Co, 1982.

*BP = blood pressure; HR = heart rate.

Chapter 15

Fluid and Electrolyte Balance

I. Distribution of Body Fluids
   A. Percent of body weight made up by water:
      1. Adult men: 60%.
      2. Adult women: 55%.
      3. Newborn: 75%.
      4. Obese persons: 45% or less. Fat is much less vascular than muscle, thus the greater the fat content, the lower the water content.
   B. In the average adult, total body fluid volume is about 40 L.
      1. Intracellular (approximately two thirds of total body fluid): 25 L
         a. Red blood cell (RBC) volume: 2 L
         b. Other cellular compartments: 23 L
      2. Extracellular (approximately one third of total body fluid): 15 L
         a. Plasma volume: 3 L
         b. Other extracellular fluid: 12 L
II. Normal Intake and Output of Fluids
   A. In the healthy individual, intake and output should be in complete balance.
   B. Normal intake:
      1. Drink   1,200 ml/day
      2. Food   1,000 ml/day
      3. Metabolically produced   350 ml/day
      4. Total intake   2,550 ml/day
   C. Normal output
      1. Evaporation (lung and skin)   900 ml/day
      2. Sweat (on hot, humid days this
         can increase markedly)   50 ml/day
      3. Feces   100 ml/day
      4. Urine   1,500 ml/day
      5. Total output   2,550 ml/day
III. Composition of the Intravascular Space
   A. Normally, all compartments are in electrostatic balance; that is, cation and anion concentrations are equal.

1. Cation mean values (mEq/L):

Na^+	142
K^+	5
Ca^{+2}	5
Mg^{+2}	3
Total	155

2. Anion mean values (mEq/L):

HCO_3^-	27
Cl^-	103
Protein	16
Organic acids	6
PO_4^{-3}	2
SO_4^{-2}	1
Total	155

B. Plasma protein concentrations can be subdivided into:

	Mean values
Albumin	4.8 gm/100 ml
Globulin	2.5 gm/100 ml
Fibrinogen	300 mg/100 ml

C. In addition, the following substances are present in vascular fluid:

	Mean values
Glucose	90 mg/100 ml
Lipids	600 mg/100 ml

D. Anion gap: The difference between the commonly measured anions and cations, reflecting the quantity of unmeasured anions:

$$\text{Anion gap} = [[Na^+] + [K^+]] - [[Cl^-] + [HCO_3^-]] \qquad (1)$$
$$17 \text{ mEq/L} = [142 + 5] - [103 + 27]$$

Normally, the anion gap ranges from about 15 to 20 mEq/L.

IV. Composition of Extravascular (Interstitial) Fluid
   A. The extravascular concentrations of most substances are about the same as their intravascular concentrations.
   B. The major exception is protein. Since protein is not freely diffusible across the capillary membrane, extravascular protein concentrations are less than one third intravascular concentrations.
   C. As with all other compartments, electrostatic balance is maintained.
V. Composition of the Intracellular Compartment
   A. Electrostatic balance is maintained within the intracellular space.
   B. However, the composition of anions and cations differs considerably from intravascular levels.

C. 1. Cations, mean values (mEq/L):

$$
\begin{array}{ll}
Na^+ & 10 \\
K^+ & 140 \\
Ca^{+2} & 0 \\
Mg^{+2} & \underline{30} \\
Total & 180
\end{array}
$$

2. Anions, mean values (mEq/L):

$$
\begin{array}{ll}
HCO_3^- & 10 \\
Cl^- & 4 \\
Protein & 61 \\
PO_4^{-3} & 11 \\
SO_4^{-2} & 2 \\
Other\ anions & \underline{92} \\
Total & 180
\end{array}
$$

VI. Movement Across Membranes
   A. The following mechanisms are responsible for the movement of fluid and dissolved substances across membranes:
      1. Simple diffusion (see Chapter 2)
      2. Osmosis (see Chapter 2)
      3. Facilitated diffusion
      4. Active transport
   B. Facilitated diffusion (Fig 15–1) occurs from an area of high concentration of the diffusing substance to an area of low concentration. However, a carrier substance is necessary for movement to occur across the membrane.
      1. No energy is expended compared with active transport.
      2. Glucose moves across cell membranes by facilitated diffusion. Insulin allows a rapid attachment of glucose to the intramembrane carrier substance.
   C. Active transport is the movement of a substance from an area of low concentration to an area of high concentration.
      1. Movement is always uphill—low concentration to high concentration.
      2. Energy in the form of adenosine triphosphate (ATP) is necessary for transport to occur.

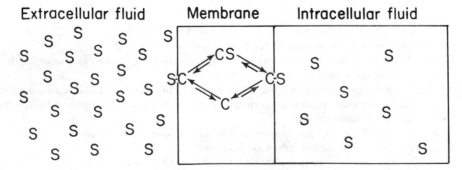

FIG 15–1.
Facilitated diffusion. *S*, substance diffusing; *C*, carrier substance. (From Sullivan LP: *Physiology of the Kidney.* Philadelphia, Lea & Febiger, 1975. Used by permission.)

3. The movement of many substances is controlled by active transport. Figure 15–2 depicts the most common active transport mechanism, the movement of Na^+ out of the cell and the movement of K^+ into the cell.

VII. Starling Law of Fluid Exchange
A. The Starling law of fluid exchange is the interrelationship among factors that determine the quantity and the direction of fluid movement across membranes.
B. The relationship is expressed as

$$J = k[(P_{cap} - P_{is}) - (\pi_{pl} - \pi_{is})] \qquad (2)$$

where J = net fluid movement
k = capillary membrane permeability
P_{cap} = capillary hydrostatic pressure
P_{is} = interstitial hydrostatic pressure
π_{pl} = plasma colloid osmotic pressure
π_{is} = interstitial colloid osmotic pressure

C. Theoretically, there are two pressures on each side of a capillary membrane.
1. Hydrostatic pressure: Blood pressure or interstitial fluid pressure.
2. Colloid osmotic pressure
a. Colloid osmotic pressure is the osmotic pressure caused by nondiffusible protein.
b. Since all dissolved substances except protein are readily diffusible, the effective osmotic pressure of either plasma or interstitial fluid is established by protein.
c. The quantity of protein is about three times greater in the plasma than in the interstitial fluid.
D. Capillary membrane permeability can be altered by many forms of physiologic stress, resulting in alterations in net fluid movement, given fixed hydrostatic and colloid osmotic pressures.
E. The pressures across the *pulmonary* capillary membrane are depicted in Figure 15–3.
1. Forces tending to move fluid *out* of the pulmonary capillary, mean values (mm Hg):

Capillary hydrostatic pressure	7
Interstitial hydrostatic pressure*	6
Interstitial colloid osmotic pressure	16
Total force moving fluid out of capillary	29

2. Forces tending to *maintain fluid in* the pulmonary capillary, mean values (mm Hg):

Plasma colloid osmotic pressure	28
Total force maintaining fluid inside the pulmonary capillaries	28

3. Net force causing fluid to leave pulmonary capillaries is 1 mm Hg (29–28 mm Hg).
4. The amount of fluid leaving the capillary as a result of the 1 mm Hg pressure gradient is dependent on the permeability of the pulmonary capillary membrane.
5. The negative interstitial hydrostatic pressure not only assists in moving fluid out of pulmonary capillaries but also maintains the alveoli "dry." This force, along with the interstitial colloid osmotic pressure, moves fluid from the lung into the interstitial space.

*This value is negative; however, with respect to direction of fluid movement, it is a force moving fluid out of the capillary; thus, a positive value is listed.

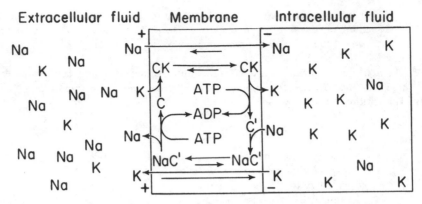

FIG 15–2.
Hypothetical scheme of active transport of sodium *(Na⁺)* and potassium *(K⁺)* across cellular membrane. *C,* carrier substance; *ATP,* adenosine triphosphate; *ADP,* adenosine diphosphate. (From Sullivan LP: *Physiology of the Kidney.* Philadelphia, Lea & Febiger, 1975. Used by permission.)

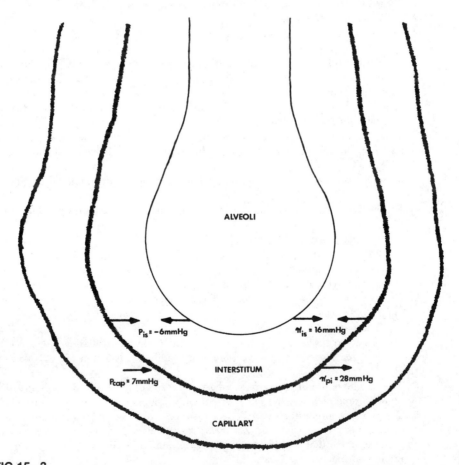

FIG 15–3.
Pressures affecting fluid exchange at the pulmonary capillaries. *Arrows* indicate direction individual pressures cause fluid movement. P_{is}, interstitial hydrostatic pressure; P_{cap}, interstitial hydrostatic pressure; π_{is}, interstitial colloid osmotic pressure; π_{pi}, plasma colloid osmotic pressure.

6. The pulmonary interstitial colloid osmotic pressure is much higher than the systemic interstitial colloid osmotic pressure because the pulmonary capillaries are much more permeable than the systemic capillaries.
7. Any alteration in the pressures listed can result in increased fluid movement into the interstitium or the alveoli.
8. The most common causes of increased fluid movement are:
   a. Increased capillary hydrostatic pressure
      (1) Left heart failure
      (2) Fluid overload
   b. Increased capillary permeability—any form of significant physiologic stress
      (1) Adult respiratory distress syndrome (ARDS)
      (2) Noxious gas inhalation
      (3) Pulmonary burns
      (4) Infection
   c. Decreased capillary colloid osmotic pressure
      (1) Hypermetabolic state
      (2) Starvation
      (3) Fluid overload

F. Forces affecting *systemic* capillary fluid movement, mean values (mm Hg)
   1. Forces moving fluid *out* of the capillary are:

Capillary hydrostatic pressure	16.0
Interstitial hydrostatic pressure	6.3
Interstitial colloid osmotic pressure	6.0
Total force moving fluid out of the capillary	28.3

   2. Forces moving fluid *into* the capillary are:

Capillary colloid osmotic pressure	28
Total force moving fluid into the capillary	28

   3. Net force causing fluid movement out of the capillary is 0.3 mm Hg (28.3–28 mm Hg).
   4. The amount of fluid leaving the capillary as a result of the 0.3 mm Hg pressure gradient is dependent on the permeability of the capillary membrane.
   5. Any alteration in the pressures listed can cause fluid to move into the interstitium.
   6. The most common causes of increased fluid movement are:
      a. Increased capillary hydrostatic pressure
         (1) Right ventricular failure
         (2) Fluid overload
      b. Increased capillary permeability—any significant physiologic stress
         (1) Bacteremia
         (2) Septicemia
         (3) Trauma
      c. Decreased capillary colloid osmotic pressure
         (1) Hypermetabolic state
         (2) Starvation
         (3) Fluid overload

VIII. Sodium
   A. Normal serum sodium levels range from about 135 to 144 mEq/L.
   B. Serum Na^+ concentration is normally a reflection of extracellular fluid volume.
   C. Approximately 70 to 100 mEq of Na^+ is excreted daily:
      1. In feces and skin: 5 to 10 mEq
      2. In sweat: 25 mEq
      3. In urine: about 40 mEq

D. Hyponatremia (decreased serum Na$^+$ concentration) is present if serum [Na$^+$] level is less than 130 mEq/L.
1. Hyponatremia may be reflective of:
   a. Decreased extracellular fluid volume
      (1) Excessive Na$^+$ loss
      (2) Decreased Na$^+$ intake
   b. Normal extracellular fluid volume
      (1) Excessive antidiuretic hormone (ADH) secretion
      (2) Glucocorticoid deficiency, Addison's disease
      (3) Severe hypothyroidism
      (4) Fluid overload with normal renal function
   c. Increased extracellular fluid volume
      (1) Cardiac failure
      (2) Renal failure
      (3) Nephrotic syndrome
      (4) Hepatic insufficiency
      (5) Trauma
2. The following clinical signs of hyponatremia are rare unless the [Na$^+$] level falls below 120 mEq/L:
   a. Headache
   b. Muscle cramps and weakness
   c. Thirst
   d. Nausea
   e. Agitation
   f. Anorexia
   g. Disorientation
   h. Apathy
   i. Lethargy
3. As the [Na$^+$] level falls below 110 mEq/L, drowsiness, progressing to coma, with convulsion occur.
4. Management
   a. In the presence of a decreased extracellular fluid volume, intravenous (IV) replacement is begun immediately to reestablish both Na$^+$ and fluid volume.
   b. In the presence of a normal extracellular fluid volume, management should focus on the underlying condition (i.e., diuretic therapy, excessive ADH production, glucocorticoid deficiency).
   c. In the presence of an expanded extracellular fluid volume, the treatment should focus on the cause of the fluid overload.
      (1) Congestive heart failure
      (2) Renal failure
      (3) Hepatic cirrhosis
E. Hypernatremia (increase in serum Na$^+$ concentration) always reflects a deficiency of water compared to total body solute volume ([Na$^+$] more than 145 mEq/L).
1. Etiology
   a. Water loss
      (1) Insensible loss
         (a) Increased sweating, fever, and exposure to high temperatures
         (b) Burns
         (c) Respiratory tract infections
      (2) Renal loss
         (a) Central diabetes insipidus
         (b) Nephrogenic diabetes insipidus
         (c) Osmotic diuresis

            (3) Hypothalamic disorders
                (a) Hypodipsia (diminished thirst)
                (b) Essential hypernatremia
        b. Sodium gain
            (1) Administration of hypertonic NaCl or $NaHCO_3$
            (2) Ingestion of Na^+
            (3) Primary hyperaldosteronism and Cushing's syndrome
  2. Clinical presentation
    a. Lethargy
    b. Muscle weakness
    c. Twitching
    d. Seizures
    e. Coma
    f. Death
  3. Since the brain adapts to the development of hypernatremia (hyperosmolal state) within 24 hours, the severity of symptoms is related to both the degree and rate of development of hypernatremia.
  4. Management
    a. Focus is on treating underlying problem and slowly returning Na^+ levels to normal by the administration of water.
    b. Rapid correction of hypernatremia with the administration of large quantities of water can result in cerebral edema, seizures, and death.

IX. Chloride
  A. Chloride balance is very similar to Na^+ balance.
  B. Normal serum levels range from about 95 to 105 mEq/L.
  C. Hypochloremia (decreased serum Cl^- concentration <95 mEq/L) may be caused by:
    1. Increased secretion and loss of gastric juices
    2. Increased renal excretion
    3. Aldosteronism
    4. Dilution
    5. Actual hyponatremia
    6. Bicarbonate ion retention
  D. Hyperchloremia (increased serum Cl^- concentration >105 mEq/L) may be caused by:
    1. Increased intake
    2. Decreased bicarbonate ion concentration
    3. Respiratory alkalosis
    4. Decreased renal excretion
    5. Dehydration
  E. Because of the exchange of Cl^- and HCO_3^- by the kidney, serum concentrations of these electrolytes are indirectly related. In addition, the pH of the urine and the plasma change in opposite direction as Cl^- levels change.
    1. Hypochloremia
      a. Increased serum HCO_3^-, alkalosis
      b. Decreased urine HCO_3^-, acidosis
    2. Hyperchloremia
      a. Decreased serum HCO_3^-, acidosis
      b. Increased urine HCO_3^-, alkalosis
  F. In chronic CO_2 retention with increased HCO_3^-, Cl^- is decreased.
  G. Since changes in $[Cl^-]$ closely mirror disturbances in $[Na^+]$ balance, symptoms of $[Cl^-]$ changes are similar to $[Na^+]$ changes.
  H. Treatment focuses on reversal of the underlying cause, along with the administration of either NaCl or water, depending on abnormality.

X. Potassium
  A. Normal serum K^+ concentrations are about 3.5 to 5.5 mEq/L.
  B. Normal K^+ loss
    1. Via skin and feces: 15–30 mEq/L
    2. Via urine: 10–30 mEq/L
  C. Normal K^+ ingestion: 50–100 mEq
  D. Minimum K^+ ingestion: 40 mEq
  E. Hypokalemia (decreased serum K^+ concentration <3.5 mEq/L)
    1. Causes
       a. Diuretic therapy
       b. Vomiting or nasogastric suction
       c. Malabsorption
       d. Laxative abuse
       e. Diarrhea
       f. Decreased intake
       g. Excessive output
       h. Hyperaldosteronism
       i. Steroid therapy
       j. Cirrhosis
       k. Liver failure
       l. Alkalosis
       m. Insulin-induced hypoglycemia
       n. Renal tubular acidosis
    2. Clinical signs and symptoms
       a. Metabolic alkalosis
       b. Acidic urine (because of exchange with H^+, as K^+ excretion decreases, H^+ excretion increases)
       c. Muscle weakness
       d. Fatigue
       e. Hypotension
       f. Confusion
       g. Cardiac arrhythmias (cardiac arrest)
       h. On ECG, flat or inverted T waves
       i. Loss of tendon reflexes
       j. Increased sensitivity to digitalis
    3. Treatment
       a. Treatment of underlying problem
       b. Administration of K^+
          (1) Essential if K^+ concentration is less than 3.0 mEq/L
          (2) May not be required if K^+ concentration is between 3.0 and 3.5 mEq/L
  F. Hyperkalemia (increased serum K^+ concentration >5.5 mEq/L)
    1. Causes
       a. Increased intake
          (1) Iatrogenic, rapid IV administration
          (2) Excess oral intake
       b. Reduced excretion
          (1) Acute renal failure
          (2) Severe chronic renal failure
          (3) Sodium depletion
          (4) Steroid deficiency
       c. Redistribution of K^+, release from cells
          (1) Acidosis
          (2) Muscle injury catabolism

(3) Leukemia chemotherapy
(4) Hemolysis
(5) Malignant hyperthermia
d. Others
   (1) Thrombocytosis
   (2) Massive leukocytosis
   (3) Muscle exercise during venous occlusion
2. Clinical signs and symptoms
  a. Metabolic acidosis
  b. Alkaline urine
  c. Muscle weakness
  d. Occasional paralysis
  e. Listlessness
  f. Nausea, vomiting
  g. Occasional ileus
  h. Confusion
  i. Paresthesia
  j. Cardiac arrhythmias (cardiac arrest)
  k. On ECG, spiked T wave
3. Treatment
  a. Increased urinary excretion of K^+ is essential (diuretic therapy).
  b. Intravenous calcium chloride or calcium gluconate is given to antagonize the cardiotoxic effects of hyperkalemia.
  c. Intravenous glucose and insulin are given to increase K^+ uptake by cells.

XI. Calcium
  A. Normal serum Ca^{+2} concentrations are about 5 to 10 mEq/L.
  B. About 50% of the calcium in the blood is bound to protein. The amount of Ca^{+2} bound to protein is affected by plasma pH.
    1. If plasma pH increases, more Ca^{+2} is bound to protein.
    2. If plasma pH decreases, less Ca^{+2} is bound to protein.
  C. Hypocalcemia (decreased serum calcium concentration)
    1. Causes
      a. Hyperthyroidism
      b. Vitamin D deficiency
      c. Magnesium deficiency
      d. Renal failure
    2. Clinical signs and symptoms
      a. Impaired neuromuscular function
        (1) Paresthesia
        (2) Muscle cramps
        (3) Tetany
      b. Tingling, numbness
      c. Cardiac arrhythmias
    3. Treatment of the underlying cause
      a. In acute hypocalcemia, calcium gluconate or calcium chloride can be administered intravenously.
      b. Adequate vitamin D ingestion must be assured.
  D. Hypercalcemia (increased serum Ca^{+2} concentration)
    1. Causes
      a. Malignancy
      b. Primary hyperparathyroidism
      c. Acute renal failure

        d. Vitamin D intoxication

        e. Hyperthyroidism

    2. Clinical signs and symptoms

        a. Tiredness, muscle weakness, neuromuscular paralysis

        b. Cardiac arrhythmias

        c. Anorexia, nausea and vomiting

        d. Weight loss

        e. Peptic ulcer, abdominal pain

    3. Management

        a. Correction of dehydration and electrolyte imbalance

        b. Diuretic therapy to increase Ca^{+2} excretion

        c. Administration of phosphate to increase Ca^{+2} movement into bone

        d. Steroid therapy to reduce intestinal absorption of Ca^{+2}

XII. Phosphate

  A. Normal serum PO_4^{-3} levels: are 1.5 to 2.5 mEq/L.

  B. Hypophosphatemia (decreased serum phosphate concentration <1.5 mEq/L)

    1. Causes

        a. Primary hyperparathyroidism

        b. Alkalosis

        c. Low intake

        d. Chronic alcoholism

        e. Beriberi

        f. Septicemia

        g. Vitamin D deficiency

        h. Hemodialysis

        i. Glucose and insulin administration

        j. Reduced intake

        k. Steroid therapy

    2. Clinical signs and symptoms

        a. Muscle weakness

        b. Paresthesia

        c. Rickets

        d. Impaired metabolism

        e. Seizures

        f. Reduced renal tubular bicarbonate reabsorption

        g. Impaired metabolism

        h. Coma

    3. Treatment

        a. Oral phosphate

        b. Intravenous K_2HPO_4

  C. Hyperphosphatemia (increased serum phosphate concentration >2.5 mEq/L):

    1. Causes

        a. Hypoparathyroidism

        b. Vitamin D toxicity

        c. Renal failure

        d. High intake

        e. Acidosis

        f. Severe catabolic state

        g. Acromegaly

    2. Clinical signs and symptoms

        a. Ectopic calcification

        b. Secondary hyperparathyroidism

        c. Renal osteodystrophy

3. Treatment
   a. Management of underlying cause
   b. Administration of aluminum hydroxide to decrease absorption
   c. Renal dialysis

XIII. Magnesium
   A. Normal serum Mg^{+2} concentration is 2.5 to 3.5 mEq/L.
   B. Hypomagnesemia (decreased serum Mg^{+2} concentration <2.5 mEq/L)
      1. Causes
         a. Decreased intake
         b. Gastrointestinal disturbances
         c. Endocrine disturbances
         d. Renal disease
         e. Alcoholism
      2. Clinical signs and symptoms
         a. Muscle weakness
         b. Nausea and vomiting, abdominal pain
         c. Neuromuscular excitability, tetany, cramp, paraesthesia
         d. Central nervous system depression, irritability
         e. Tachycardia
      3. Management
         a. Treatment of underlying cause
         b. Administration of magnesium sulfate
   C. Hypermagnesemia (increased serum Mg^{+2} concentration)
      1. Causes
         a. Acute or chronic renal failure
         b. Uncontrolled diabetes mellitus
         c. Adrenocortical insufficiency
         d. Metabolic acidosis
         e. Increased ingestion
      2. Clinical signs and symptoms
         a. Muscle weakness
         b. Loss of deep tendon reflexes
         c. Impaired autonomic nerve transmission
         d. Vasodilation
         e. Drowsiness
         f. Cardiac arrhythmias
      3. Management
         a. Renal dialysis (if renal failure is present)
         b. Diuretic therapy

XIV. Fluid Balance
   A. The venous system is referred to as the *capacitance system*, since it has the ability to store large quantities of blood.
   B. The storage capabilities of the venous system are depicted in Figure 15–4.
      1. Below minimum capacitance, large volume changes result in small pressure changes.
      2. Within the normal capacitance range, a volume change results in a small pressure change.
      3. Beyond the maximum capacitance level, a small volume change results in a large pressure change.
   C. Venous conductance is the ability of the venous system to conduct flow.
   D. Conductance is a reciprocal of resistance and is equal to flow divided by change in pressure.
   E. The greater the conductance, the greater the ability of the vessel to conduct flow.

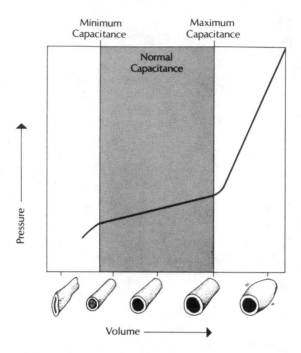

FIG 15-4.
Capacitance of the venous system (see text). (From Shapiro BA, Harrison RA, Kacmarek RM, et al: *Clinical Application of Respiratory Care,* ed 3. Chicago, Year Book Medical Publishers, 1985. Used by permission.)

   F. Venous return can be increased by either increasing driving pressure or increasing conductance.
     1. Physiologically the organism increases venotone to increase driving pressure, thus increasing venous return.
     2. Clinically, increasing conductance is the most common method of increasing venous return.
     3. Conductance can be increased by optimizing the vascular volume to vascular space relationship.
     4. This is achieved by maintaining a vascular volume that moves the venous system to a capacitance level that is near its maximum capacitance.
   G. Fluid administration (fluid challenge principle)
     1. This is an approach to fluid administration that results in optimization of the vascular volume to vascular space relationship.
     2. A general clinical and hemodynamic assessment of the patient is performed to establish baseline values. Specifically, the pulmonary wedge pressure (PWP) is determined.
     3. Approximately 50 to 200 ml of fluid is rapidly (over 10 minutes) administered. The volume used depends on the patient's clinical status.
     4. The patient is then assessed clinically for improvements in:
       a. Blood pressure
       b. Presence of crackles or wheezes
       c. Peripheral perfusion
       d. Urinary output
     5. The PWP is reassessed if:
       a. The PWP increases less than 3 mm Hg. This indicates that the capacitance is in the minimal range and the process should be repeated until:

        (1) Clinical improvement in circulation is noted

        (2) Abnormal breath sounds develop (crackles or wheezes)

    b. The PWP increase is between 3 and 7 mm Hg. Wait 10 minutes and reassess the PWP.

        (1) If the increase is now less than 3 mm Hg, repeat the entire process.

        (2) If the increase is still between 3 and 7 mm Hg, repeat with one half the original fluid volume used.

    c. If the increase is greater than 7 mm Hg, the capacitance is at or above the maximum level and additional fluid may be poorly tolerated.

6. The same guidelines may be applied to central venous pressure reading; however, a 2 to 5 cm H_2O pressure change is used as the guide.

BIBLIOGRAPHY

Deshpande VM, Pibeam SP, Dixon RJ: *A Comprehensive Review in Respiratory Care.* Norwalk, Mass, Appleton & Lange, 1988.

Ellerbe S: *Fluid and Blood Component Therapy in the Critically Ill and Injured.* New York, Churchill Livingstone, 1981.

Gabow PA: *Fluids and Electrolytes: Clinical Problems and Their Solution.* Boston, Little, Brown & Co, 1983.

Guyton AC: *Textbook of Medical Physiology,* ed 6. Philadelphia, Lea & Febiger, 1981.

Rose BD: *Clinical Physiology of Acid-Base and Electrolyte Disorders.* New York, McGraw-Hill Book Co, 1977.

Schrier RW (ed): *Renal and Electrolyte Disorders,* ed 2. Boston, Little, Brown & Co, 1980.

Smith K: *Fluids and Electrolytes: A Conceptual Approach.* New York, Churchill Livingstone, 1980.

Sullivan LP: *Physiology of the Kidney.* Philadelphia, Lea & Febiger, 1975.

Tepperman J: *Metabolic and Endocrine Physiology: An Introductory Text,* ed 3. Chicago, Year Book Medical Publishers, 1976.

Vanatta JC, Fogelman MJ: *Moyer's Fluid Balance: A Clinical Manual,* ed 2. Chicago, Year Book Medical Publishers, 1976.

Vander AJ: *Renal Physiology,* ed 2. New York, McGraw-Hill Book Co, 1980.

Weldy NJ: *Body Fluids and Electrolytes: A Programmed Presentation,* ed 3. St Louis, CV Mosby Co, 1980.

Chapter 16 _____

Cardiac Electrophysiology and ECG Interpretation

I. The electric conduction system of the heart functions in the:
   A. Provision of electric excitation of the myocardial fibers without extrinsic stimuli (automaticity).
   B. Conduction of electric impulses through the myocardium.
   C. Organized distribution of the electric impulses to the myocardium in a repetitive, sequential fashion.

II. Electroconduction System of the Heart (Fig 16–1)
   A. Sinoatrial (SA) node
      1. The SA node is located in the right atrium just inferior and posterior to the entrance of the superior vena cava.
      2. It is commonly referred to as the *pacemaker of the heart,* its *primary function.*
      3. The SA node has an intrinsic rate of depolarization of 60 to 100 per minute.
      4. The rate of depolarization ordinarily is under the control of the sympathetic and parasympathetic nervous systems.
         a. Sympathetic stimulation of the SA node increases the rate of depolarization-positive chronotropism.
         b. Parasympathetic stimulation of the SA node decreases the rate of depolarization-negative chronotropism.
      5. The wave of depolarization initiated from the SA node travels outwardly through the atrial musculature in concentric circles, thus depolarizing the atria and ultimately the atrioventricular node.
      6. For all practical purposes, the left and right atria depolarize simultaneously.
   B. Atrioventricular (AV) node
      1. The AV node is located in the right atrium between the opening of the coronary sinus and interatrial septum.
      2. Histologically it is comprised of cells identical to those of the SA node.
      3. The *function* of the AV node is threefold:
         a. Backup cardiac pacemaker because of its intrinsic depolarization rate of 40 to 60 per minute.
         b. The only electrical bridge between atria and ventricles.
         c. Responsible for delaying impulses from atria to ventricles.

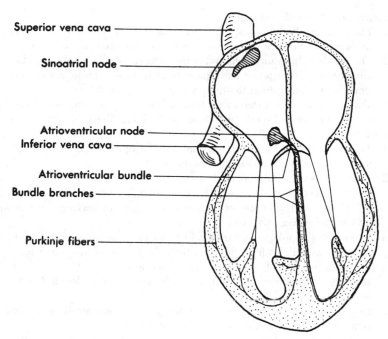

Superior vena cava

Sinoatrial node

Atrioventricular node

Inferior vena cava

Atrioventricular bundle

Bundle branches

Purkinje fibers

FIG 16–1.
The electrical conduction system of the heart (see text). (From Spearman CB, Sheldon RL, Egan DF: *Egan's Fundamentals of Respiratory Therapy,* ed 4. St Louis, CV Mosby Co, 1982. Used by permission.)

4. The AV node becomes continuous with the common bundle branch (bundle of His) and is the only normal pathway for electric conduction between atria and ventricles. The fibroskeleton of the heart electrically separates atrial from ventricular muscle. The AV node and common bundle penetrate the cardiac fibroskeleton.

5. That the tissue of the AV node slows the rate of electrical conduction accounts for the time delay between atrial and ventricular depolarization. This time delay also allows optimal ventricular filling prior to ventricular contraction (systole).

6. The rate of conduction of electrical impulses through the AV node is under the control of the sympathetic and parasympathetic nervous systems.
   a. Sympathetic stimulation decreases conduction time and allows overall increases in cardiac rate.
   b. Parasympathetic stimulation increases conduction time of the AV node. Strong parasympathetic stimulation may actually block all or a portion of the impulses originating from the atria.

C. Common bundle branch
   1. It is also known as the *AV bundle,* or *bundle of His.*
   2. It is located on the right side of the interventricular septum and penetrates the right fibrous trigone.
   3. Its *function* is twofold:
      a. To conduct impulses from the AV node to the left and right bundle branches.
      b. To penetrate the fibroskeleton of the heart, electrically bridging the atrial conduction system to the ventricular conduction system.
   4. The common bundle branch travels inferiorly in the interventricular septum for about 10 to 12 mm and then divides into one right and two left bundle branches.

D. Right and left bundle branches
  1. The right bundle branch appears simply as a continuation of the common bundle branch and follows an inferior course toward the apex of the heart.
  2. The left bundle branch penetrates the interventricular septum and divides into an anterior and posterior left bundle branch. Both bundle branches course inferiorly on the left side of the interventricular septum.
  3. The *function* of the three major bundle branches is to conduct electric impulses from the common bundle branch to the Purkinje fibers.
E. Purkinje fibers
  1. The Purkinje fibers are very fine ramifications of the bundle branches, which terminate on the endocardial layer of the heart.
  2. They are located throughout the entire endocardial layer of both ventricles and conduct the electrical impulses from the bundle branches to the ventricles. Depolarization of the ventricles begins when impulses leaving the Purkinje fibers invade the endocardial layer.
  3. The wave of depolarization travels from the endocardial layer outward toward the epicardium and also from the apex toward the base of the ventricles.
F. Summary of pathway of normal electrical conduction
  1. Impulses originate in the right atrium by spontaneous depolarization of the SA node.
  2. Impulses are conducted through atrial muscle, which results in depolarization of right and left atria and AV node.
  3. The impulse is delayed at AV node and then conducted through the cardiac fibroskeleton by the AV node and common bundle branch.
  4. The impulse is then conducted from the common bundle branch through right and left bundle branches to Purkinje fibers.
  5. The impulses exit the Purkinje fibers and cause depolarization of the ventricle from inside out and from apex to base.
  6. Design of the electrical conduction system of the heart allows simultaneous depolarization of right and left atria totally separate from simultaneous depolarization of the right and left ventricles. This fact has important implications for the mechanical function of the heart.

III. Electrocardiogram
  A. The ECG is a graphic display of current generated by the heart at the surface of the body. It depicts depolarization and repolarization of atria and ventricles.
  B. The ECG is used in assessing the electrical activity of the heart, which should be clearly delineated from the mechanical activity of the heart.
  C. Each portion of the cardiac cycle generates a specific type of electrical impulse. These impulses are repetitious and produce characteristic patterns on an ECG recording.
  D. The four major electrical cardiac events are atrial depolarization, atrial repolarization, ventricular depolarization, and ventricular repolarization.
    1. The polarized state is the normal resting state of cardiac muscle fiber. The extracellular charge is positive with respect to the intracellular charge (Fig 16–2, panel a).
    2. Depolarization is the process of reversing the normal state of polarity. Depolarization thus causes the extracellular charge to be negative with respect to the intracellular charge. This is largely because inflow of extracellular sodium ions is faster than outflow of intracellular potassium ions. Reversal of the cellular membrane charge is thus transmitted along cardiac muscle fiber, depolarizing subsequent fibers. If muscle fibers are normal, this electrochemical stimulation results in mechanical activity (shortening of muscle fibers and cardiac contraction) (Fig 16–2, panel b).

3. Repolarization is the process of reestablishing the normal state of polarity (i.e., reestablishing a positive extracellular charge with respect to the intracellular charge). The reestablishment of the resting cellular membrane charge is transmitted along the cardiac muscle fiber, repolarizing subsequent fibers. If muscle fibers are normal, this electrochemical stimulation results in lengthening of muscle fibers and cardiac relaxation (Fig 16–2, panel c). (*Note:* It is a mistake to assume that the mechanical activity of the heart is normal simply because the electric activity—ECG—is normal.)

E. The electric deflections of ECG in normal sequence are P wave, QRS complex, and T wave (Fig 16–3).

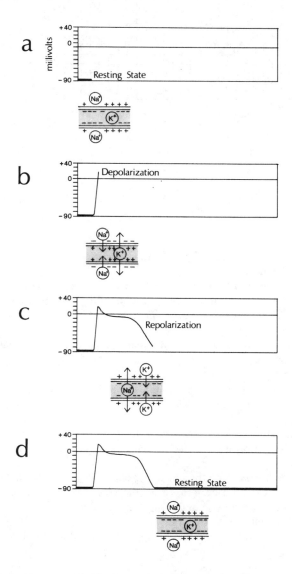

FIG 16–2.

Ion distribution and electric current (millivolt) generation in a myocardial cell: *a,* resting state; *b,* depolarization; *c,* repolarization; *d,* polarized (resting) state (see text). (From Shapiro BA, Harrison RA, Kacmarek RM, et al: *Clinical Application of Respiratory Care,* ed 3. Chicago, Year Book Medical Publishers, 1985. Used by permission.)

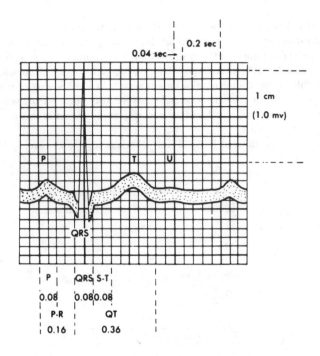

FIG 16–3.
Schematic representation of ECG tracing (see text). (From Spearman CB, Sheldon RL, Egan DF: *Egan's Fundamentals of Respiratory Therapy*, ed 4. St Louis, CV Mosby Co, 1982. Used by permission.)

1. The P wave is produced by atrial depolarization and usually is 0.06 to 0.11 second in duration.
2. The QRS complex is produced by ventricular depolarization and usually is 0.03 to 0.12 second in duration. Repolarization of the atria occurs simultaneously with ventricular depolarization and is masked by the overwhelming electric event of the QRS complex.
3. The T wave is produced by ventricular repolarization and usually is 0.14 to 0.26 second in duration.

F. PR, RR, and PP intervals
1. PR interval: Time from the beginning of atrial depolarization to the beginning of ventricular depolarization. The PR interval normally is 0.12 to 0.20 second in duration.
2. RR interval: Time from the peak of one QRS complex to the next QRS complex. It is used to measure the total cardiac cycle and normally is 0.6 to 1.0 second in duration.
3. PP interval: Time from the beginning of one P wave to the beginning of the next P wave. It can be used to measure the total cardiac cycle time and is normally equal to the RR interval (0.6–1.0 second in duration).

IV. Electrocardiogram Interpretation
A. The following system represents a simple organized approach to the evaluation of ECG tracings.
1. P waves
a. Should be present
b. Should have a configuration similar to that of other P waves.
c. Should be related on a one-to-one basis to the QRS complex.
2. PR intervals
a. Should have a normal duration of 0.12 to 0.20 second.

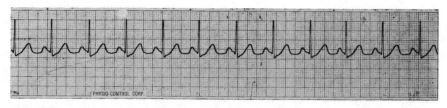

FIG 16–4.
Normal sinus rhythm.

      b. Should have consistent duration when compared with other PR intervals.
  3. QRS complexes
      a. Should have a duration of less than 0.12 second.
      b. Should have a similar configuration when compared with other QRS complexes.
  4. RR and PP intervals
      a. RR intervals should have a consistent duration when compared with other RR intervals.
      b. PP intervals should have a consistent duration when compared with other PP intervals.
      c. RR interval should be approximately equal to the PP interval in duration.
  5. Cardiac rate
      a. Should be 60 to 100/min.
        (1) Rates less than 60/min denote bradycardia.
        (2) Rates greater than 100/min denote tachycardia.
      b. Atrial rate should be equal to the ventricular rate.
  6. After careful evaluation of the previous five steps, the underlying aberration, if any, should be revealed and the rhythm easily identified.
  7. Treatment, if any, should then be guided by the mechanical consequences of the identified cardiac rhythm.
B. Normal sinus rhythm (Fig 16–4)
  1. P waves are present, have similar configurations, and are related to QRS complexes.
  2. PR interval is 0.12 to 0.20 second long and equal to other PR intervals.
  3. QRS complex is less than 0.12 second long and similar in configuration to other QRS complexes.
  4. RR intervals are regular and equal to PP intervals.
  5. Cardiac rate is 60 to 100/min.
  6. No treatment is warranted.
C. Sinus arrhythmia (Fig 16–5)
  1. P waves are present, have similar configuration, and are related to QRS complexes.
  2. PR interval is normal in duration and equal to other PR intervals.
  3. QRS complex is normal in duration and similar in configuration to other QRS complexes.

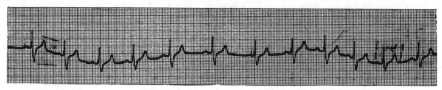

FIG 16–5.
Sinus arrhythmia.

4. PP and RR intervals both vary; however, they are equal to one another for a given cardiac cycle.
5. Cardiac rate varies; however, it generally averages 60 to 100/min.
6. Generally no treatment is warranted unless there are significant alterations in arterial blood pressure (i.e., symptomatic hypotension), in which case atropine may be employed to accelerate cardiac rate.

D. Sinus bradycardia (Fig 16–6)
1. P waves are present, have similar configuration, and are related to QRS complexes.
2. PR interval is normal in duration and equal to other PR intervals.
3. QRS complex is normal in duration and similar in configuration to other QRS complexes.
4. RR intervals are regular and equal to PP intervals.
5. Cardiac rate is less than 60/min.
6. Generally no treatment is warranted unless there are significant alterations in arterial blood pressure (i.e., symptomatic hypotension), in which case atropine is the drug of choice to accelerate cardiac rate.

E. Sinus tachycardia (Fig 16–7)
1. P waves are present, have similar configuration, and are related to QRS complexes.
2. PR interval is normal in duration (lower limits of normal) and equal to other PR intervals.
3. QRS complex is normal in duration and similar in configuration to other QRS complexes.
4. RR intervals are regular and equal to PP intervals.
5. Cardiac rate is greater than 100/min.
6. This rhythm is the normal physiologic response to stress; therefore, intervention should be aimed at treating the underlying cause.

F. Premature atrial contraction (PAC) (Fig 16–8)
1. P wave occurs earlier than expected and may have a normal or abnormal configuration.
2. PR interval is usually normal and equal in duration to other PR intervals.
3. QRS complex is usually normal in duration and similar in configuration to other QRS complexes; however, it may be absent if the P wave is not conducted through the AV node.
4. PP and RR intervals vary with the PAC; however, they are equal to one another for a given cardiac cycle.
5. Cardiac rate: Premature atrial contractions can occur at any rate.
6. No treatment is warranted if the PACs are infrequent. When they are frequent, discontinuation of stimulants such as tobacco, caffeine, and or sympathomimetics is generally indicated.

G. Atrial tachycardia (Fig 16–9)
1. P waves are present; however, they may be superimposed on a preceding T wave.
2. PR interval is usually normal in duration and equal to other PR intervals. However, with rapid rates it may be difficult to determine.
3. QRS complex is usually normal in duration and similar in configuration to other QRS complexes.
4. PP and RR intervals are regular and usually equal to each other.
5. Rate: atrial rate is usually 160 to 220/min, and ventricular rate is 160 to 220/min with 1:1 conduction; however, it may be 80 to 110/min with 2:1 conduction.
6. Conservative treatment such as vagal stimulation (i.e., carotid sinus massage, Valsalva's maneuver) should be employed in the symptomatic but hemodynami-

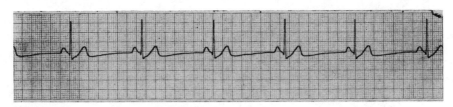

FIG 16–6.
Sinus bradycardia.

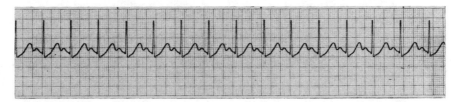

FIG 16–7.
Sinus tachycardia.

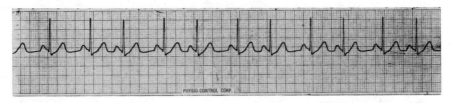

FIG 16–8.
Premature atrial contraction.

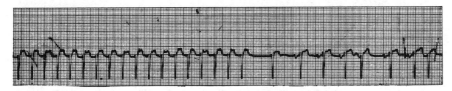

FIG 16–9.
Atrial tachycardia.

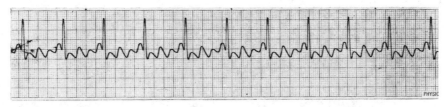

FIG 16–10.
Atrial flutter

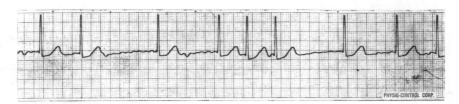

FIG 16–11.
Atrial fibrillation.

cally stable individual. In contrast, more aggressive intervention such as vera-
pamil administration or synchronized dc countershock is indicated in the hemo-
dynamically unstable individual.

H. Atrial flutter (Fig 16–10)
   1. P waves are present, have similar configuration, and resemble a sawtooth or
      picket fence pattern.
   2. PR interval is usually normal and equal in duration to other PR intervals; how-
      ever, it may be difficult to measure.
   3. QRS complex is usually normal in duration and similar in configuration to other
      QRS complexes.
   4. PP interval is regular and equal to other PP intervals; RR interval regular and
      equal to other RR intervals; PP interval is usually not equal to RR interval as a
      result of AV nodal block.
   5. Atrial rate is typically 220 to 350/min; ventricular rate is dependent on the de-
      gree of conduction through the AV node (i.e., 2:1, 3:1, 4:1 conduction).
   6. Synchronized dc countershock is the treatment of choice when a rapid ventricu-
      lar rate has resulted in hemodynamic instability.

I. Atrial fibrillation (Fig 16–11)
   1. P waves are not truly present; rather, fine or coarse irregular rapid baseline un-
      dulations called *fibrillatory waves* (f waves) occur.
   2. PR interval is not present.
   3. QRS complex is usually normal in duration and similar in configuration to other
      QRS complexes.
   4. PP interval is not measurable; RR interval is irregular and not equal to other RR
      intervals.
   5. Atrial rate is approximately 350 to 700/min; ventricular rate is 100 to 200/min.
   6. Initial treatment typically consists of increasing doses of digitalis in an attempt to
      block the number of impulses reaching the ventricles. However, as in atrial flut-
      ter, the treatment of choice is synchronized dc countershock when the individual
      is manifesting hemodynamic compromise.

J. First-degree heart block (Fig 16–12)
   1. P waves are present, are similar in configuration to other P waves, and are re-
      lated to the QRS complex.

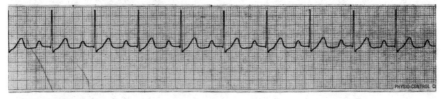

FIG 16–12.
First-degree heart block.

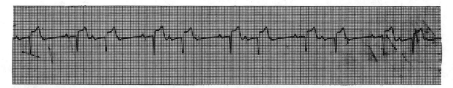

FIG 16–13.
Type I second-degree heart block.

2. PR interval is greater than 0.20 second and usually equal in duration to other PR intervals, but may vary.
3. QRS complex is normal in duration and similar in configuration to other QRS complexes.
4. RR intervals are regular and equal to PP intervals.
5. Rate: first-degree heart block can occur at any rate.
6. No treatment is warranted; however, monitoring for higher order forms of heart block (i.e. second or third degree) is generally advised.

K. Type I second-degree heart block (Fig 16–13)
   1. P waves are present, are similar in configuration to other P waves, and are related to QRS complexes, except for the nonconducted P waves.
   2. PR interval may begin with normal duration but lengthens progressively until one P wave is not conducted.
   3. QRS complex is normal in duration and similar in configuration to other QRS complexes.
   4. PP interval is regular and equal to other PP intervals. RR intervals vary, with absent QRS complexes.
   5. Atrial rate is typically 60 to 100/min; ventricular rate varies with degree of block (i.e., 2:1, 3:2, 4:3 conduction).
   6. Generally no treatment is warranted unless there are significant alterations in arterial blood pressure (i.e., symptomatic hypotension), in which case atropine should be employed to accelerate cardiac rate. A temporary pacemaker is indicated when atropine is either not effective or contraindicated. In any case, monitoring for complete heart block is advised.

L. Type II second-degree heart block (Fig 16–14)
   1. P waves are present, are similar in configuration to other P waves, and are related to QRS complexes, except for the nonconducted P waves.
   2. PR interval may be normal or prolonged; however, it is equal in duration to other PR intervals.
   3. QRS complex is usually normal in duration and similar in configuration to other QRS complexes.
   4. PP interval is regular and equal to other PP intervals. RR intervals vary, with absent QRS complexes; however, the PP and RR intervals are equal in cardiac cycles where the P wave is conducted.

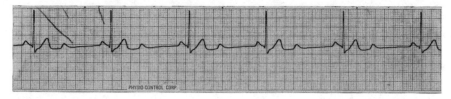

FIG 16–14.
Type II second-degree heart block.

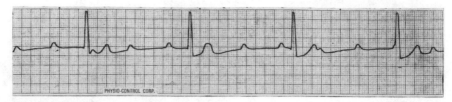

FIG 16–15.
Third-degree or complete heart block.

     5. Atrial rate is typically 60 to 100/min; ventricular rate varies with the degree of block.

     6. A permanent pacemaker is the treatment of choice to assure adequate ventricular rate. Use of intravenous atropine, isoproterenol, or both may be employed to assure an adequate ventricular rate in the interim.

  M. Third-degree or complete heart block (Fig 16–15)

     1. P waves are present, are similar in configuration to other P waves, but are unrelated to the QRS complexes.

     2. PR interval is completely variable and of no consequence.

     3. QRS complexes are normal in configuration and duration when block occurs at the AV node or bundle of His. QRS complexes are wide and aberrant when block occurs at the bundle branches.

     4. PP and RR intervals are regular but are not equal to each other.

     5. Atrial rate is typically 60 to 100/min; ventricular rate is typically 40 to 60/min with block at the AV node and less than 40/min with infranodal block.

     6. Treatment is the same as in type II second-degree heart block.

  N. Junctional or nodal rhythm (Fig 16–16)

     1. P waves are typically absent; however, they may be conducted retrogradely and appear anywhere in the cardiac cycle.

     2. PR interval is usually not measurable.

     3. QRS is usually normal in duration and is similar in configuration to other QRS complexes.

     4. PP interval usually not measurable. RR interval is regular.

     5. Ventricular rate is typically 40 to 60/min.

     6. Treatment is the same as in type II second-degree heart block.

  O. Supraventricular tachycardia (Fig 16–17)

     1. P waves are usually indiscernible. They may be absent, conducted retrogradely, or buried in the preceding T wave.

     2. PR interval cannot be measured.

     3. QRS complex is normal in duration and similar in configuration to other QRS complexes.

     4. PP interval is not measurable. RR interval is regular and equal to other RR intervals.

     5. Rate is typically greater than 150/min.

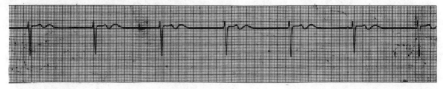

FIG 16–16.
Junctional or nodal rhythm.

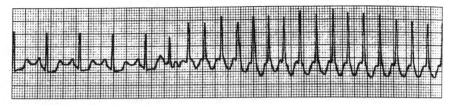

FIG 16–17.
Supraventricular tachycardia.

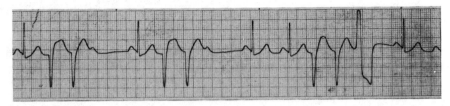

FIG 16–18.
Premature ventricular contraction.

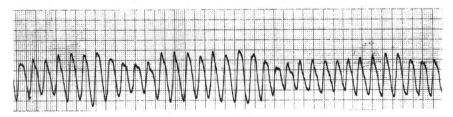

FIG 16–19.
Ventricular tachycardia.

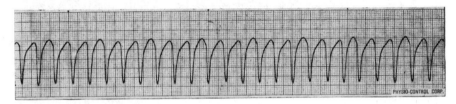

FIG 16–20.
Ventricular flutter.

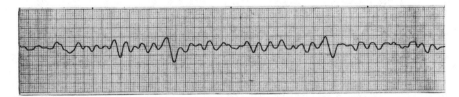

FIG 16–21.
Ventricular fibrillation.

    6. Intervention should be aimed at treating the underlying cause in the hemodynamically stable individual. However, in the instance of hemodynamic compromise, synchronized dc countershock is the treatment of choice.

P. Premature ventricular contraction (PVC) (Fig 16–18)
    1. P waves are typically absent.
    2. PR interval with PVC is not measurable.
    3. QRS complex is wide (greater than 0.12 second), bizarre, and unlike normal QRS complexes. It appears earlier in the cardiac cycle than expected and has a T wave on the opposite side of the baseline from the terminal portion of the QRS (PVC) complex.
    4. PP interval with PVC is not measurable. RR interval varies with the occurrence of PVC.
    5. PVCs can occur at any rate.
    6. Intravenous lidocaine is the treatment of choice; however, eventual identification and treatment of the underlying cause should be achieved.

Q. Ventricular tachycardia (Fig 16–19)
    1. P waves are generally indiscernible.
    2. PR interval is not measurable.
    3. QRS complex is wide, bizarre, and generally similar in configuration to other QRS complexes.
    4. PP interval is not measurable. RR interval is regular or slightly irregular.
    5. Ventricular rate is 100 to 250/min.
    6. Intravenous lidocaine is the treatment of choice in the hemodynamically stable individual. In contrast, synchronized dc countershock should be employed in the individual manifesting hemodynamic compromise.

R. Ventricular flutter (Fig 16–20)
    1. P waves are absent.
    2. PR interval is absent.
    3. QRS complex appears as a smooth sinusoidal wave with QRS complex and T waves merged and no clear separation of cardiac cycles.
    4. PP interval is absent. RR interval is regular.
    5. Ventricular rate is typically 200 to 300/min.
    6. Initially, support with CPR until defibrillation can be implemented and is successful.

S. Ventricular fibrillation (Fig 16–21)
    1. P waves are absent.
    2. PR interval is absent.
    3. QRS complexes are absent; however, there is low (fine) or high (coarse) amplitude undulation from the baseline that varies in shape and represents varying degrees of depolarization and repolarization.
    4. PP and RR intervals are absent.
    5. Rate is absent.
    6. Treatment is the same as in ventricular flutter.

BIBLIOGRAPHY

Conover MB: *Exercise in Diagnosing ECG Tracings,* ed 3. St Louis, CV Mosby Co, 1984.
Dubin D: *Rapid Interpretation of EKG's,* ed 3. Tampa, Fla, Cover Publishing Co, 1979.
Guyton AC: *Textbook of Medical Physiology,* ed 6. Philadelphia, WB Saunders Co, 1981.
Little RC: *Physiology of the Heart and Circulation.* Chicago, Year Book Medical Publishers, 1977.

Marriott HJL: *Practical Electrocardiography*, ed 6. Baltimore, Williams & Wilkins Co, 1980.

McIntyre KM, Lewis AJ: *Textbook of Advanced Cardiac Life Support*. Dallas, American Heart Association, 1981.

McLaughlin AJ: *Essentials of Physiology for Advanced Respiratory Therapy*. St Louis, CV Mosby Co, 1977.

Mountcastle VB: *Medical Physiology*, ed 14. St Louis, CV Mosby Co, 1980.

Phillips RE, Feeney MK: *The Cardiac Rhythms*. Philadelphia, WB Saunders Co, 1973.

Ross G: *Essentials of Human Physiology*. Chicago, Year Book Medical Publishers, 1978.

Ruch TC, Patton HD: *Physiology and Biophysics*, ed 20. Philadelphia, WB Saunders Co, 1974.

Rushmer RF: *Cardiovascular Dynamics*, ed 3. Philadelphia, WB Saunders Co, 1970.

Schroeder JS, Daily EK: *Techniques in Bedside Hemodynamic Monitoring*, ed 2. St Louis, CV Mosby Co, 1981.

Shapiro BA, Harrison RA, Kacmarek RM, et al: *Clinical Applications of Respiratory Care*, ed 3. Chicago, Year Book Medical Publishers, 1985.

Spearman CB, Sheldon RL, Egan DF: *Egan's Fundamentals of Respiratory Therapy*, ed 4. St Louis, CV Mosby Co, 1982.

Chapter 17 _____

Pulmonary Function Studies

- Pulmonary function studies include the study of all respiratory function: mechanics, lung volumes, exchange of gases across the alveolar-capillary membrane, and ventilatory drive during rest and exercise.
 I. Lung Volumes and Capacities
    A. The gas in the respiratory system is divided into four basic lung volumes and four lung capacities. All capacities are composed of two or more lung volumes.
        1. Lung volumes
            a. Residual volume (RV): Amount of gas left in the lung after a maximal exhalation.
            b. Expiratory reserve volume (ERV): Amount of gas that can be exhaled after a normal exhalation.
            c. Tidal volume (V_T or TV): Amount of gas inspired during a normal inspiration.
            d. Inspiratory reserve volume (IRV): Amount of gas that can be inspired above a normal inspiration.
        2. Lung capacities
            a. Total lung capacity (TLC): Volume of gas contained in the lung at maximum inspiration (RV + ERV + V_T + IRV).
            b. Inspiratory capacity (IC): Maximum volume of gas that can be inhaled after a normal exhalation (V_T + IRV).
            c. Vital capacity (VC): Maximum volume of gas that can be exhaled after a maximal inspiration (ERV + V_T + IRV).
            d. Functional residual capacity (FRC): Volume of gas that remains in the lung after a normal exhalation (RV + ERV).
    B. Normal lung volumes and capacities for a 165-lb, 6 ft tall, 25-year-old man are:
        1. TLC: 6,000 cc
        2. VC: 4,800 cc, about 80% of TLC
        3. IC: 3,600 cc, about 60% of TLC
        4. FRC: 2,400 cc, about 40% of TLC
        5. RV: 1,200 cc, about 20% of TLC
        6. ERV: 1,200 cc, about 20% of TLC
        7. V_T: 500 cc, about 3 cc per pound of ideal body weight (8%–10% of TLC)
        8. IRV: 3,100 cc, about 50% to 55% of TLC

C. All predicted lung volumes and capacities are based on statistical data from a group of individuals of the stated height, age, and sex.
   1. In addition, predicted normal values may vary for lung volumes due to:
      a. Race
      b. Ethnic background
      c. Socioeconomic factors
      d. Environmental exposures
      e. Occupation
      f. Place of residence (urban or rural)
   2. Values for a given subject may also vary from one measurement to another as a result of:
      a. Diurnal variation
      b. Seasonal variation
      c. Endocrine changes (menstrual cycle)
      d. Relationship of test to meals or exercise
      e. Quality of instruction and coaching
   3. The acceptable percent deviation from normal in all cases is ±20%. Thus, unless there is greater than 20% variance, the results will be reported as essentially normal.
   4. All lung volumes and capacities are expressed at body temperature and pressure saturated (BTPS). Thus, measured values at atmospheric temperature and pressure saturated (ATPS) must be converted to BTPS. Charles' Law (see Chapter 2) is used to make these conversions.
D. Normal values for vital capacities may be taken from various charts or derived from the following formulas:
   1. For males:

$$VC = 27.63 - (0.112 \times Age) \times (Height\ in\ cm) \tag{1}$$

   2. For females:

$$VC = 21.78 - (0.101 \times Age) \times (Height\ in\ cm) \tag{2}$$

E. All lung volumes and capacities depicted in Figure 17–1 can be measured by direct spirometry except:
   1. RV
   2. FRC
   3. TLC
F. Methods of measuring RV, FRC, and TLC are as follows:
   1. Determination of these volumes and capacities is accomplished by using indirect methods of measuring FRC; FRC is measured because it is the most stable of all lung volumes and capacities. Once the FRC is determined, it is used to calculate TLC and RV.
   2. Three basic methods of measuring FRC are nitrogen washout study (open circuit technique), helium dilution study (closed circuit technique), and body plethysmography (total thoracic gas volume determination). In addition, TLC or FRC may be determined radiographically.
      a. Nitrogen washout study
         (1) The test is always initiated and concluded at the patient's FRC level.
         (2) The patient is connected to a breathing circuit where he or she inspires 100% oxygen and the total volume of exhaled gas is collected.
         (3) Normally, the test is carried out for 7 minutes or until the percent of nitrogen expired is 1% to 2.5%.

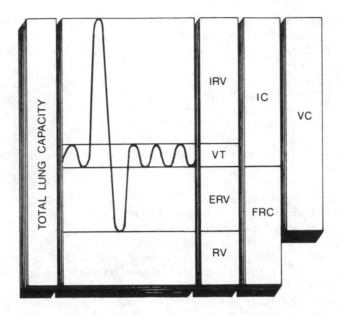

FIG 17–1.
Normal lung volumes and capacities and their relation to each other. Note that with normal spirometry the residual volume *(RV)* cannot be directly determined. Refer to text for further explanation. (From Shapiro BA: *Clinical Application of Blood Gases,* ed 3. Chicago, Year Book Medical Publishers, 1982. Used by permission.)

    (4) Since nitrogen makes up about 80% of FRC when the subject is breathing room air, the volume of nitrogen in the total exhaled gas will equal about 80% of the FRC.

    (5) Thus, the total gas exhaled is measured for volume and percent nitrogen present.
    Example:

Total volume collected	50 L
Measured nitrogen concentration	5%
Volume of nitrogen in FRC	2.5 L

    (6) The FRC is determined as follows:

$$\frac{2.5 \text{ L}}{0.80 \text{ FRC}} = \frac{x}{1 \text{ FRC}}$$
$$3.125 \text{ L} = x$$

    (7) Newer automated spirometers measure the percentage of N_2 and exhaled volume breath by breath so that FRC is calculated on an additive basis.

    (8) The RV is determined by subtracting ERV from FRC.

    (9) The TLC is determined by adding VC to RV.

    (10) Problems associated with the nitrogen washout study are as follows:

        (a) Atelectasis may result from washout of nitrogen from poorly ventilated, partially obstructed areas.

(b) Elimination of hypoxic drive in carbon dioxide retainers may result in apnea.

(c) Error in determinations if severe airway obstruction present. The error will be on the low side of actual FRC because of poor distribution of ventilation.

(d) A small system leak cannot be distinguished from severe uneven distribution of ventilation.

(11) It is generally considered reliable, reproducible, and simple for both patient and therapist.

b. Helium dilution study

(1) Since helium is metabolically inert (argon or neon are used in some systems), a given volume of helium may be distributed throughout the lung bellows system without absorption of a significant volume.

(2) The test is initiated and concluded at the patient's FRC level.

(3) The patient is connected to a rebreathing system, and a certain volume (%) of helium is placed into a bellows. The patient breathes through the system until a constant helium percentage is read in the lung bellows system.

(4) Normally the test takes up to 7 minutes to complete.

(5) A soda lime absorber is placed in the system to remove carbon dioxide. Oxygen is titrated into the system to meet the patient's oxygen demands.

(6) At the beginning of the test, the concentration of helium in the bellows and the volume of gas in the bellows are measured.

(7) At the completion of the test, the volume of gas in the bellows and the concentration of helium in the lung bellows system are measured.

(8) The FRC is calculated as follows:

(a) The amount of helium in the system is constant.

(b) The volume of helium at the beginning (B) of the test is equal to the volume of helium at the end (E) of the test. Thus:

$$\text{(Vol. lung}_B)(\text{Conc. lung}_B) + (\text{Vol. bellows}_B)(\text{Conc. bellows}_B) = \quad (3)$$
$$\text{(Vol. lung}_E)(\text{Conc. lung}_E) + (\text{Vol. bellows}_E)(\text{Conc. bellows}_E)$$

(c) If the volume of gas in the bellows at the beginning of the test is 2.0 L and the helium concentration is 10%, and at the end of the test the volume in the bellows is 2.0 L and the helium concentration is 3.5%, the patient's FRC can be calculated using equation 3, the unknown being equal to the FRC:

$$(x)(0.0\%) + (2.0\text{ L})(0.10) = (x)(0.035) + (2.0\text{ L})(0.035)$$
$$0.0 + 0.2\text{ L} = 0.035x + 0.07\text{ L}$$
$$\frac{0.13\text{ L}}{0.035} = \frac{0.035x}{0.035}$$
$$3.7\text{ L} = x$$

(d) A more commonly used modification of formula 3 is

$$\text{FRC} = \frac{(\%\text{ He}_{initial} - \%\text{ He}_{final})}{\%\text{ He}_{final}} \times \text{initial vol.} \quad (4)$$

where % $He_{initial}$ = initial helium concentration in the system and % He_{final} = final helium concentration at the conclusion of the test.

$$\text{Initial vol. of system} = \frac{\text{Vol. of He added}}{\text{Initial He conc.}} \tag{5}$$

(e) Using this same example:

% $He_{initial}$ = 10%
% He_{final} = 3.5%

$$\text{Initial vol.} = \frac{200 \text{ ml}}{10\%} = 2,000 \text{ ml, or } 2.0 \text{ L}$$

$$\text{FRC} = \frac{(10\% - 3.5\%)}{3.5\%} \times 2.0 \text{ L} = 3.7 \text{ L}$$

    (f) Some add 100 ml to the calculated FRC to account for absorbed He.

(9) A problem associated with the study is that gas distal to severely obstructed airways may not be measured because of poor distribution of ventilation.

    (a) System or patient leaks (punctured eardrum) will result in increased volume determination.

    (b) Uneven distribution and system leak are indistinguishable.

(10) Generally the He dilution study is considered reliable, reproducible, and simple for both patient and therapist.

c. Body plethysmography

  (1) The patient's total thoracic gas volume is determined. All of the gas contained in the thoracic cavity, even if it is distal to completely obstructed airways, or located in the abdomen or intestines, is measured.

  (2) The overall calculations are based on Boyle's law.

  (3) The total volume of the plethysmograph is known, and the volume displacement of the patient may be determined by body surface area charts. The volume of gas in the box surrounding the patient is determined by subtracting the volume the patient occupies from the volume of the box.

  (4) The patient is sealed in the box and ventilates through a mouthpiece with a pressure transducer attachment and a shutter valve allowing obstruction at the mouthpiece.

  (5) During the testing, the patient breathes gas from within the box.

  (6) At the FRC level, the shutter is closed, and the patient is instructed to pant at a low frequency of 20 to 40 breaths/min against an obstruction. As this occurs, proximal airway pressure and pressure in the plethysmograph are measured simultaneously. The low-frequency panting ensures that there is no difference between mouth and alveolar pressure. (Some use esophageal pressure measured with an esophageal balloon to reflect alveolar pressure changes instead of airway pressure.)

  (7) Boyle's law is used to determine the final volume in the plethysmography itself:

$$P_1V_1 = P_2V_2 \tag{6}$$

where P_1 = Original pressure in the plethysmograph is usually equal
to atmospheric, or 760 mm Hg

V_1 = Original volume in the plethysmograph minus the volume
occupied by patient (e.g., 1,000 L)

P_2 = Increased pressure in the plethysmograph as a result of
expansion of the thorax (e.g., 760.2 mm Hg)

V_2 = Final volume in the plethysmograph

$$(760 \text{ mm Hg})(1,000 \text{ L}) = (760.2 \text{ mm Hg})(x)$$

$$\frac{(760 \text{ mm Hg})(1,000 \text{ L})}{760.2 \text{ mm Hg}} = x$$

$$x = 999.737 \text{ L}$$

(8) The difference (V) between V_1 and V_2 is equal to the decreased volume in the plethysmograph after chest expansion. Since this is a sealed system, the change in volume in the plethysmograph is equal to the change in the volume in the patient's thorax.
Example:

$$V_1 - V_2 = V \qquad (7)$$
$$1,000 \text{ L} - 999.737 \text{ L} = 0.263 \text{ L}$$

(9) As the patient pants against an obstruction, the volume in the thorax increases, and the pressure in the thorax is decreased. Thus, again applying Boyle's law:

$$Pa_1 Va_1 = Pa_2 Va_2 \qquad (8)$$

where Pa_1 = Proximal airway pressure at resting FRC levels, which
would be equivalent to atmospheric (760 mm Hg)

Va_1 = Volume of FRC

Pa_2 = Pressure in airway after inspiring against an obstruction;
in this example: 700 mm Hg

Va_2 = Final volume in thorax is equal to the original volume
Va_1 plus results from equation 7 (V). Thus, Boyle's law
may be written as:

$$(Pa_1)(Va_1) = (Pa_2)(Va_1 + V) \qquad (9)$$
$$(760 \text{ mm Hg})(x) = 700 \text{ mm Hg } (x + 0.263 \text{ L})$$
$$760 \text{ mm Hg } x = 700 \text{ mm Hg } x + 184.1 \text{ mm Hg} \cdot \text{L}$$
$$\frac{60x}{60} = \frac{184.1 \text{ mm Hg} \cdot \text{L}}{60 \text{ mm Hg}}$$
$$x = 3.07 \text{ L}$$

(10) The thoracic gas volume is equal to 3.07 L.

(11) The measurement of extrapulmonary lung volume (abdominal gas, pneumothorax) is a major problem. Some patients become claustrophobic in the plethysmograph.

(12) Plethysmographic determinations correlate with radiographic studies.

3. The RV can be calculated from radiologic estimation of TLC and FRC.
   a. Estimations are made from standard posteroanterior (PA) and lateral chest x-ray films taken at a standard distance of 72 in. (183 cm).
   b. A transparency is placed over the x-ray film and the lung fields are traced.
   c. Two distinct methods are then available to estimate lung volumes: the ellipsoid method and the planimetry method.
      (1) The ellipsoid method considers the elliptical shape of the lungs and divides them into sections that may be geometrically assessed as cylinders, from which lung volume is determined.
      (2) The planimetry method makes use of regression equations for surface areas of radiologic lung fields that are based on plethysmography measurements.
   d. Patient cooperation and effort must be maximal for proper x-ray representation, regardless of the method employed.
   e. These methods compare well with plethysmographic methods.
      (1) Usually they are within 500 ml of the actual TLC.
      (2) They may be more accurate than inert gas methods if severe air trapping exists.
   f. Retrospective comparison with earlier chest x-ray films, if available, is possible.

G. Closing volume
   1. The closing volume is defined as the terminal portion of a slow exhaled VC that indicates the point at which the most gravity-dependent airways start to collapse.
   2. Normally during a maximal exhalation, there is a collapsing of peripheral bronchioles. In disease states, the volume of gas present in the lung when peripheral bronchioles begin to collapse increases.
   3. A single-breath nitrogen washout study is used to determine the closing volume (Fig 17–2).
   4. If an individual starts at RV level and inspires maximally, the first part of the inspired gas will move from the conducting airways into the apices. At this time, the apices fill only partially. Gas will then start to fill the bases. Toward the end of inspiration, both bases and apices fill. The lung fills in this manner due to transpulmonary pressure differences between apices and bases. An individual in the standing position has a higher transpulmonary pressure in the apices than in the bases. The lower transpulmonary pressure in the bases is essentially a result of lung position and gravity. Thus, the alveoli in the apices

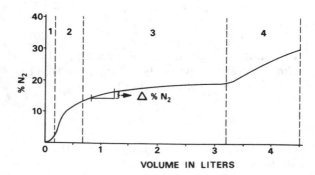

FIG 17–2.
Single-breath nitrogen washout curve shows the four phases associated with the study. Phase *4* is the volume referred to as the closing volume. $\Delta \% N_2$ is the percent change in nitrogen concentration between the first 750 ml and 1,250 ml of exhaled gas.

are considered slow alveoli: they fill first but empty last; the alveoli in the bases are considered fast alveoli: they fill last but empty first. (For further explanation, see Chapter 4.)

5. In the single-breath nitrogen washout study, the patient breathes 100% oxygen from RV level to TLC, then slowly exhales to RV level.
   a. The initial part of the inspiration will go to the apices. This gas will contain a high nitrogen concentration because the volume will be primarily from the conducting airways, which contains 80% nitrogen.
   b. The next volume of gas will move to the bases. This volume will contain nitrogen but to a lesser extent than the gas that originally moved to the apices.
   c. Finally, the bases and apices will fill to capacity with 100% oxygen.
   d. At maximal inspiration, the nitrogen concentration in the apices is much greater than in the bases.
   e. As the patient slowly exhales, gas leaves the area of the lung where compliance is least (i.e., the bases). The bases will empty until the peripheral bronchioles start to collapse. The volume of gas left in the airways at onset of collapsing is referred to as the *closing volume*.
   f. As the patient continues to exhale, gas starts to leave the apices where the nitrogen concentration is much higher.

6. When the nitrogen concentration is graphically plotted against the volume exhaled, a graph similar to that in Figure 17–2 results. This graph depicts the four phases of the single-breath nitrogen washout curve.
   a. Phase 1: The nitrogen concentration is zero, indicating that only gas from the conducting airways is being exhaled.
   b. Phase 2: The steep increase in nitrogen concentration indicates that the gas being exhaled is mixed bronchial and alveolar air.
   c. Phase 3: A very slow increase is evident, indicating that mostly alveolar air is being exhaled.
   d. Phase 4: At closing volume, gas is being exhaled primarily from the apices.

7. Normally the closing volume is expressed as a percentage of the VC.
   a. In young, healthy adults, closing volume is equal to about 10% of VC.
   b. This percentage increases normally with age. An individual aged 60 years or older may have a normal closing volume of 40%.
   c. Increases in closing volume appear to be one of the earliest indications of small airway obstruction.

8. Closing capacity is a term used to express the percentage of the TLC that the closing volume plus the RV represents. Normally in young, healthy adults this is equal to about 30%.

9. Delta percent nitrogen ($\Delta\%N_2$) is an expression used to indicate the change in nitrogen concentration between the first 750 ml and 1,250 ml exhaled.
   a. In normal, healthy adults it is equal to 1.5% or less.
   b. As the $\Delta\%N_2$ increases, it indicates uneven distribution of ventilation.

10. These tests were initially used to establish small airways disease. They do show abnormalities in most smokers and are normal in most nonsmokers, but they do not generally screen those who go on to develop clinically detectable airflow obstruction from those who do not.

11. Today, these tests are generally used for epidemiologic purposes; however, their clinical usefulness seems to go in and out of vogue.

II. Flow Rate Studies
  A. Forced vital capacity (FVC)
    1. The following flow rate determinations may be calculated from an FVC curve.
      a. The percentage of the vital capacity that is expired in 1 second ($FEV_1\%$) (Fig 17–3)

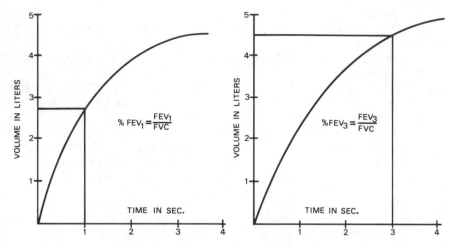

FIG 17–3.
Determination of *FEV₁%* and *FEV₃%* (see text).

    (1) The forced expired volume in 1 second (FEV₁) is divided by the FVC:

$$\text{FEV}_1\% = \frac{\text{FEV}_1}{\text{FVC}} \times 100 \tag{10}$$

    (2) Normally the FEV₁% is equal to at least 75% of the FVC.
    (3) Decreased values basically indicate obstruction of larger and moderate size airways.
    (4) The FEV₁%, along with the FEV₁ itself, are considered by many as the best indicators of clinically significant airways obstruction.
  b. The percentage of VC that is expired in 3 seconds (FEV₃%) (see Fig 17–3)
    (1) The forced expired volume in 3 seconds (FEV₃) is divided by the FVC:

$$\text{FEV}_3\% = \frac{\text{FEV}_3}{\text{FVC}} \times 100 \tag{11}$$

    (2) Normally the FEV₃% is equal to at least 97% of the FVC.
    (3) Decreased values basically indicate obstruction of smaller airways.
  c. Forced expiratory flow (FEF) determined between the first 200 ml and 1,200 ml of exhaled volume (FEF₂₀₀₋₁,₂₀₀) (Fig 17–4)
    (1) The slope of the line between the first 200 ml and 1,200 ml of exhaled volume is determined and reported as a flow:

$$\text{Slope in L/sec} = \frac{1\text{ L}}{\text{Time}} \tag{12}$$

    (2) The flow in L/sec is then converted to L/min:

$$(\text{L/sec})(60\text{ sec/min}) = \text{L/min} \tag{13}$$

    (3) Since the graph is determined at room temperature (ATPS), the flow must be corrected to body temperature (BTPS).

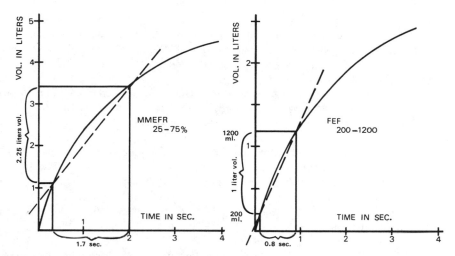

FIG 17–4.
Determination of $MMEFR_{25\%-75\%}$ and $FEF_{200-1,200}$ (see text).

        (4) Normally the $FEF_{200\ 1,200}$ for a young, healthy man is about 350 to 400 L/min; slightly lower values are noted in women.

        (5) Decreased values basically indicate obstruction of larger airways.

    d. Maximum midexpiratory flow rate ($MMEFR_{25\%-75\%}$) (see Fig 17–4)

        (1) The slope of a line between the first 25% and 75% of exhaled volume is determined and reported as a flow:

$$\text{Slope in L/sec} = \frac{\text{Volume}}{\text{Time}} \tag{14}$$

        (2) The flow in L/sec is then converted to L/min (see equation 13).

        (3) Since the graph is determined at ATPS, the flow must be converted to BTPS.

        (4) Normally the $MMEFR_{25\%-75\%}$ for a young, healthy man is 250 to 300 L/min; slightly lower values are noted in women.

        (5) Decreased values basically indicate obstruction of smaller airways.

B. Maximum voluntary ventilation (MVV) or maximum breathing capacity (MBC)

    1. This study is used to determine the maximum volume of gas that a patient can ventilate in 1 minute.

    2. The patient is directed to breathe as rapidly and as deeply as possible for 10 to 15 seconds.

    3. The total volume inspired or expired during the stated period is determined.

    4. This volume is converted to the volume per minute. For example, if the patient breathed 30 L in 10 seconds:

$$\frac{30\ \text{L}}{10\ \text{seconds}} = \frac{x}{60\ \text{seconds}} \tag{15}$$
$$x = 180\ \text{L}$$

    5. Normal MVV for young healthy men is 150 to 200 L/min; slightly lower values are noted in women.

    6. Decreased values basically indicate increased airway resistance or obstruction, decreased lung or thoracic compliance, or weakness of ventilatory muscles.

C. Peak expiratory flow rate
   1. Peak expiratory flow normally occurs during the early part of exhalation.
   2. Peak flows normally are equal to 400 to 600 L/min for young, healthy men and 300 to 500 L/min for young, healthy women.
   3. Decreased peak flows indicate larger airway obstruction.
D. *It is extremely important to remember that all volumes determined must be converted to body temperature and that flow studies are totally patient effort dependent. To ensure accuracy, results must be reproducible.*

III. Normal Values
   A. Normal values for all studies discussed are based on the averages of many healthy individuals of a particular sex, age, and height.
   B. Tables are available that give normal values for all tests for both sexes in all age and height categories.
   C. Determined values are considered normal unless they are 20% greater or less than predicted values.

IV. Flow-Volume Loops
   A. A flow-volume loop is the measurement of inspiratory and expiratory flows and volumes.
   B. The test is performed by having the patient maximally inspire, followed by a single forced exhaled vital capacity (FEVC) and forced inspired vital capacity (FIVC) loop).
   C. The following data can be determined from a flow-volume loop if a V$_T$ loop is superimposed on a VC loop (Fig 17–5):
      1. VC
      2. V$_T$
      3. IRV
      4. ERV
      5. IC
      6. Peak inspiratory and expiratory flows
      7. Inspiratory flows at 25%, 50%, and 75% of VC
      8. Expiratory flows at 25%, 50%, and 75% of VC
   D. The major advantage of flow-volume loops is that they give a quick visual impression of the general disease category (Fig 17–6).

V. Guidelines for the Performance of Standard Spirometry
   A. General equipment standards
      1. Volume of spirometer at least 7 L.
      2. Flow measuring capabilities 0 to 12 L/sec.
      3. Capable of accumulating volume for 30 seconds.
      4. Accuracy for all volume measurements is ±3% of reading or ±0.050 L, whichever is greater.
      5. Resistance and back pressure must be less than 1.5 cm H$_2$O/L/sec from 0 to 12/L/sec flow.
   B. Performance, reproducibility, and accuracy of spirometric studies
      1. Start of test (time zero)
         a. It ensures volume has not been exhaled before start of test.
         b. It ensures maximal effort was put forth during initial exhalation.
         c. Time zero is determined by back extrapolation of an FVC curve; that is, a straight line is drawn from the steepest part of the curve to zero volume.
         d. The volume before the intersect of the back extrapolation should be less than 5% of the FVC, or 0.100 L, whichever is greater, for the start to be acceptable (Fig 17–7).
      2. End of test is acceptable when one of the following occurs:
         a. A plateau of no volume change occurs for at least 2 seconds.

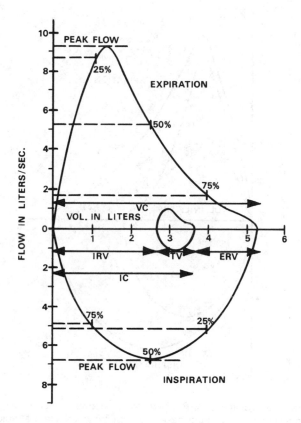

FIG 17–5.
Normal flow-volume loop with superimposed tidal volume *(TV)* loop. All normal spirometry values plus peak inspiratory and expiratory flows along with flow at 25%, 50%, and 75% of inspiration and expiration may be determined.

 b. A forced exhaled volume of reasonable duration has occurred (10–15 seconds) in patients with severe airways obstruction.
 c. If the patient cannot or should not (clinical stress) continue to exhale.
3. A minimum expiration of 6 seconds is required.
4. The maximum number of maneuvers performed to ensure reproducibility and accuracy is eight.
5. An acceptable FVC is one in which no. 1, 2, and 3 are met, and the following are absent:
 a. Cough
 b. Valsalva's maneuver
 c. Leak
 d. Obstructed mouthpiece with tongue
6. Reproducibility of the FVC maneuver requires that the largest and second largest FVC from acceptable curves not vary by more than 100 ml, or 5% of measurement, whichever is greater. The same criteria exist for FEV_1.
C. Reporting of spirometry results
 1. The largest FVC and FEV from acceptable curves are reported even if the two values are from different curves.
VI. Diffusion Studies
 A. Diffusion studies are used to determine how rapidly gases can move across the alveolar-capillary membrane.

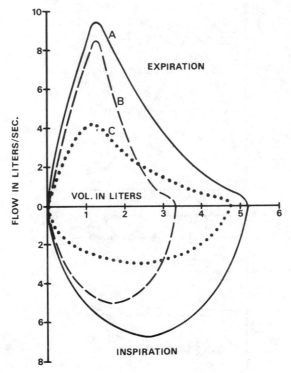

FIG 17–6.
A represents a normal flow-volume loop, *B* a flow-volume loop in restrictive lung disease, and *C* a flow-volume loop in an obstructive lung disease. Flow-volume loops afford a rapid visual evaluation of the overall disease state.

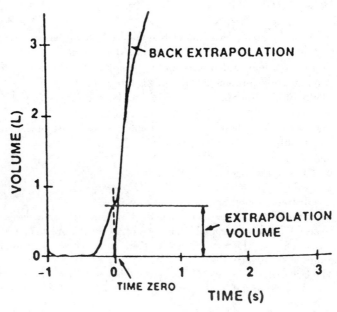

FIG 17–7.
Back extrapolation method to determine time zero on the FVC curve. (From ATS/ALA standardization of spirometry—1987 update. *Respir Care* 1987; 32:1039–1051. Used by permission.)

B. Oxygen and carbon monoxide (CO) are used because of their strong affinity for hemoglobin and poor solubility coefficients. Carbon monoxide is most commonly used in clinical practice.

C. There are two basic approaches to the measurement of CO uptake from the lung, or CO diffusing capacity (D_{LCO}): steady state and single breath.

D. During steady-state determinations, the subject breathes a fixed concentration of CO until a steady state is established (a constant value for exhaled CO).

   1. Then, D_{LCO} is calculated from the difference between inhaled and exhaled CO.

   2. This technique is rarely used clinically because of the prolonged time required for CO breathing.

   3. The single-breath method is more commonly used clinically.

E. Single-breath method: The patient maximally inhales a mixture of gases containing 0.1% to 0.3% CO with He, and air, followed by breath-holding for 10 seconds.

F. The pulmonary diffusing capacity for CO (D_{LCO}) is equal to

$$\frac{\text{ml CO transferred/min}}{\text{mean alveolar CO (mm Hg)} - \text{mean capillary CO (mm HG)}} \qquad (16)$$

G. Normal resting D_{LCO} for the average young man is 25 ml/min/mm Hg CO; for women this number is reduced (20 ml/min/mm Hg CO).

H. The D_{LO_2} may be computed by multiplying the D_{LCO} by 1.23:

$$D_{LO_2} = D_{LCO} (1.23) \qquad (17)$$

VII. Bronchial Provocation Tests

A. These tests are used to assess the responsiveness of bronchial airways and lung parenchyma to inhaled aerosols and fumes.

B. Methacholine or histamine inhalation tests

   1. Baseline FEV_1 measurements are made prior to the administration of the drug and following each dose administered.

   2. An aerosol of either drug is inhaled by the patient intermittently or on a continuous basis.

   3. Dosages begin at 0.03 mg/ml of aerosol and increase by doubling to a maximum dose of at least 20 mg/ml.

   4. Increasing dosages are administered and the response is evaluated by FEV_1 determinations until the FEV_1 falls by at least 20% of baseline.

   5. The provocation concentration of the drug producing the 20% or greater decrease in FEV_1 is referred to as the PC_{20}.

      a. A PC_{20} value of more than 20 mg/ml is considered asymptomatic for diagnosing asthma.

      b. A PC_{20} between 2 and 20 mg/ml generally corresponds to mild, episodic symptoms of asthma.

      c. Values less than 2 mg/ml are consistent with daily symptomatology and may require bronchodilator therapy.

   6. Uses of the test are:

      a. To substantiate the diagnosis of asthma in doubtful cases.

      b. To provide an indication of severity and determine treatment requirements.

      c. To document an inducing effect in occupational asthma and subsequent treatment.

C. Allergen inhalation tests
   1. Are used to determine specific allergic responses.
   2. Have a methodology similar to methacholine/histamine challenge.
   3. Normally require physician supervision during testing.
D. Occupational type exposure tests
   1. Are used to determine specific occupational sensitivities.
   2. Have a methodology similar to methacholine/histamine challenge.
   3. Require physician supervision.
VIII. Ventilatory Drive and Control of Breathing
   A. In healthy normals, CO_2 is the primary stimulus to breathe, and O_2 is a secondary stimulus.
   B. In disease, control of breathing is frequently altered, as is the drive to breathe.
   C. The following are used to evaluate a subje t's drive to breathe:
      1. Carbon dioxide
      2. Oxygen
      3. Inspiratory flow and inspiratory time
      4. Mouth occlusion pressure $(P_{0.1})$
   D. Ventilatory response to CO_2 (HCVR) is mediated by changes in extracellular $[H^+]$ via the central chemoreceptors (80% of response) and the peripheral chemoreceptors (20% of response).
      1. The HCVR is usually measured under hyperoxic conditions.
      2. Normally, a rebreathing technique is used, with 93% O_2 and 7% CO_2.
      3. As equilibrium is reached, minute ventilation demonstrates a linear change with CO_2, expressed as

$$\dot{V}_E = S(Pa_{CO_2} - B) \qquad (18)$$

   where S = the slope of the regression of $\dot{V}_E/Pa_{CO_2}$ and B = the x-axis intercept.
      4. The steeper the slope, the greater the ventilatory response.
      5. The slope of a normal response is 2.2 ± 0.2.
   E. The ventilatory response to O_2 or the hypoxic ventilatory response (HVR) is controlled primarily by the peripheral chemoreceptors.
      1. Normally, an inverse hyperbolic relationship exists between minute ventilation and Pa_{O_2} if begun at a hyperoxic state and continued to a Pa_{O_2} of 40 mm Hg.
      2. However, a linear inverse relationship between $HbO_2\%$ and minute ventilation exists as $HbO_2\%$ decreases below 90%.
      3. The HVR is genetically determined but may be altered by disease and environment.
      4. The relationship between $\dot{V}_E$ and $HbO_2\%$ is

$$HVR = \frac{\dot{V}_E}{HbO_2\%} \qquad (19)$$

      5. If the slope of the relationship between $\dot{V}_E$ and $HbO_2\%$ is expressed as a non-inversed relationship, the normal slope is 0.54 ± 0.07.
   F. Inspiratory flow and inspiratory time
      1. Ventilatory drive is directly related to peak inspiratory flow rate and the ratio of inspiratory time to total ventilatory cycle time. Ventilatory drive is inversely related to inspiratory time.
      2. Higher peak flow and shorter inspiratory time indicate greater ventilatory drive.

3. Normal peak inspiratory flows are 15 to 30 L/min but may increase to well over 100 L/min during increased cardiopulmonary stress.
4. Inspiratory times are normally 1 to 1.5 seconds in adults but may decrease to less than 0.5 second.
5. While the ratio of inspiratory time to total ventilatory cycle time is about 0.20 to 0.40 with stress, this ratio approaches 0.50.
6. Respiratory rate normally increases as ventilatory drive increases.

G. Mouth occlusion pressure
1. The $P_{0.1}$ is the amount of negative pressure generated in the first 100 msec of inspiration against an occluded airway. Occlusion must occur without the subject's awareness.
2. The $P_{0.1}$ correlates with minute ventilation.
3. The $P_{0.1}$ is an effective method of assessment of drive, even in the presence of severe respiratory muscle dysfunction.
4. For evaluation to be accurate, diaphragmatic innervation must be intact.
5. Normal $P_{0.1}$ is less than 4 cm H_2O.

H. Ventilatory drive is decreased in:
1. Patients with chronic obstructive pulmonary disease (blue bloaters)
2. Patients with obesity-hypoventilation syndrome (pickwickian syndrome)

X. Pulmonary Response to Exercise (see Chapter 22)
A. Pulmonary exercise testing is normally conducted to:
1. Evaluate work capacity and to provide rehabilitative, vocational, or recreational direction.
2. To describe the severity of the disease.
3. To differentiate pulmonary from cardiac limitation to exercise.
4. To aid in determining the effectiveness of treatment or surgery.

B. Method of exercise text
1. Twelve-minute walk (frequently used in hospitals or rehabilitation programs to determine estimated progress).
   a. The distance walked in 12 minutes is recorded.
   b. The number of stops in the period is recorded.
2. Stair climbing (used for the same purpose)
   a. The number of stairs climbed is logged.
   b. The time and number of rest periods are also recorded.
3. Numerous incremental protocols (using either a treadmill or cycle ergometer)
   a. The speed is variable, on a specific time reference.
   b. The incline of the treadmill or resistance to pedalling is increased over time.

C. Direct measurements made during exercise
1. Work output
2. Exercise time
3. Minute ventilation
4. Respiratory rate
5. Oxygen saturation
6. ECG
7. Oxygen consumption
8. Carbon dioxide production
9. Arterial blood gases

D. Derived values from basic data
1. Anaerobic threshold is that point during exercise when the oxygen demand exceeds oxygen delivery.
   a. Lactic acid increases.
   b. Carbon dioxide production markedly increases.

c. Minute ventilation markedly increases.
d. Oxygen consumption rate of increase is not altered.
2. Respiratory exchange ratio (R):

$$R = \frac{\dot{V}CO_2}{\dot{V}O_2} \tag{20}$$

3. Oxygen pulse is the $\dot{V}O_2$ divided by the heart rate.
E. Cardiac vs. pulmonary limitation to exercise
1. In cardiac diseases, the maximal voluntary ventilation is rarely reached, whereas with respiratory disease it is exceeded.
2. The anaerobic threshold is rarely reached in respiratory disease but is usually exceeded in cardiac disease.
3. Oxygen pulse and oxygen saturation decrease in both respiratory and cardiac disease but more so with cardiac disease.

BIBLIOGRAPHY

Altose MD: The physiological basis of pulmonary function testing. *Clin Symp* 1973; 3:3–10.
ATS/ALA standardization of spirometry—1987 update. *Respir Care* 1987; 32:1039–1051.
Ayers LN, Whipp BJ, Ziment I: *A Guide to the Interpretation of Pulmonary Function Tests.* New York, Roerig, Division of Pfizer Pharmaceuticals, New York Projects in Health, 1974.
Beauchamp RK: Pulmonary function testing procedures, in Barnes TA (ed): *Respiratory Care Practice.* Year Book Medical Publishers, Chicago, 1988.
Buist AS: Tests of small airways function. *Respir Care* 1989; 34:446–454.
Cherniack RN: *Pulmonary Function Testing.* Philadelphia, WB Saunders Co, 1977.
Chusid EL: The selective and comprehensive testing of adult pulmonary function. New York, Futura Publishing Co, 1983.
Clausen JL (ed): *Pulmonary Function Testing Guidelines and Controversies: Equipment, Methods, and Normal Values.* New York, Grune & Stratton, 1982.
Crapo RO: Reference values for lung function tests. *Respir Care* 1989; 34:626–637.
Ferris BG: Epidemiology standardization project: Recommended standardized procedure for pulmonary function testing. *Am Rev Respir Dis* 1978; 118:1.
Fluck RR: Flow and volume sensors. *Respir Care* 1989; 34:571–585.
Forster RE: Exchange of gases between alveolar air and pulmonary capillary blood: Pulmonary diffusing capacity. *Physiol Rev* 1957; 37:391.
Gardner RM: ATS statement: Snowbird workshop on standardization of spirometry. *Am Rev Respir Dis* 1979; 119:831–838.
Gardner RM: Pulmonary function laboratory standards. *Respir Care* 1989; 34:651–660.
Hepper GGN, Fowler WS, Helmholz HR Jr: Relationship of height to lung volume in healthy men. *Dis Chest* 1960; 37:314–320.
Irvin CG: Airways challenge. *Respir Care* 1989; 34:455–469.
Juniper RF, Frith PA, Hargreave FE: Airway responsiveness to histamine and metacholine: Relationship to minimum treatment to control symptoms of asthma. *Thorax* 1981; 36:575–579.
Kanner RE, Morris AH: *Clinical Pulmonary Function Testing.* Salt Lake City, Intermountain Thoracic Society, 1975.
Knudson RJ, Slatin RC, Lebowitz MD: The maximal expiratory flow-volume curve: Normal standards, variability, and effects of age. *Am Rev Respir Dis* 1976; 113:587–600.
Lough MD: Pulmonary response to exercise. *Respir Care* 1989; 34:517–523.
MacIntyre NR: Diffusing capacity of the lung for carbon monoxide. *Respir Care* 1989; 34:489–499.
Ruppel G: *Manual of Pulmonary Function Testing,* ed 3. St Louis, CV Mosby Co, 1982.

Ryan G, Dolovich MB, Roberts RS: Standardization of inhalation provocation tests: Two techniques of aerosol generation and inhalation compared. *Am Rev Respir Dis* 1981; 123:195–199.

Salome CM, Schoeffel RE, Waolcock AJ: Comparison of bronchial reactivity to histamine and metacholine in asthmatics. *Clin Allergy* 1980; 10:541–546.

Schoene RB: The control of ventilation in clinical medicine: To breathe or not to breathe. *Respir Care* 1989; 34:500–509.

Seltzer C, Siegelaub AB, Freidman GD: Differences in pulmonary function related to smoking habits and race. *Am Rev Respir Dis* 1974; 110:598–608.

Shapiro BA, Harrison RA, Cane R, et al: *Clinical Application of Blood Gases,* ed 4. Chicago, Year Book Medical Publishers, 1989.

Snow MG: Determination of functional residual capacity. *Respir Care* 1989; 34:586–596.

Spearman CB, Sheldon RL, Egan DF: *Egan's Fundamentals of Respiratory Therapy,* ed 4. St Louis, CV Mosby Co, 1982.

West JB: *Respiratory Physiology: The Essentials.* Baltimore, Williams & Wilkins Co, 1974.

West JB: *Pulmonary Pathophysiology: The Essentials.* Baltimore, Williams & Wilkins Co, 1977.

Wilson AF (ed): *Pulmonary Function Testing Indications and Interpretations.* New York, Grune & Stratton, 1985.

Chapter 18

Clinical Assessment of the Cardiopulmonary System

I. Initial Impression

    The overall condition of the patient is rapidly assessed by observation of the patient and by initial discussion.

  A. Level of consciousness or sensorium: Is the patient oriented to:

    1. Time

    2. Place

    3. Person

  B. Lack of orientation may indicate:

    1. Cerebral hypoxia

    2. Inadequate cerebral blood flow

  C. If the patient is falling asleep during discussions or is somnolent, Pa_{CO_2} levels may be elevated.

II. Vital Signs

  A. Temperature: An indicator of metabolic rate.

    1. Hyperthermia (fever): In the hospitalized patient it is normally indicative of infection, which is usually bacterial but may be viral.

      a. Fever increases overall metabolic rate:

        (1) For every 1°C increase in body temperature, O_2 consumption and CO_2 production increase by 10%.

        (2) Fever combined with hypoxemia may result in poor tissue oxygenation.

    2. Hypothermia is rare in hospitalized patients but may be a result of:

      a. Severe head injury affecting the hypothalamus

      b. Hypothyroidism

      c. Exposure to cold (emergency room)

    3. Hypothermia decreases O_2 consumption and CO_2 production.

      a. Shivering during hypothermia generates heat and consumes energy.

      b. Peripheral vasoconstriction minimizes heat loss secondary to convection.

  B. Pulse: A general reflection of pump capabilities of the heart.

    1. Heart rate in adults is normally 60 to 100/min.

      a. Heart rates greater than 100/min (tachycardia) may be a reflection of the following:

        (1) Fear

        (2) Anxiety

        (3) Low blood pressure

        (4) Anemia

        (5) Fever

        (6) Hypoxemia

        (7) Response to certain medications (e.g., sympathomimetics)

    b. Heart rates less than 60/min (bradycardia):

        (1) Are much less common than tachycardia.

        (2) May be a response of a diseased myocardium to severe stress.

        (3) May be a response to certain medications.

            (a) Parasympathomimetics (e.g., atropine)

            (b) β_1-Blockers (e.g., propranolol [Inderal])

            (c) Digitalis

  2. Rhythm: A regular rhythm should be noted. Irregular rhythm may indicate:

    a. Premature ventricular contractions

    b. Premature atrial contractions

    c. Heart blocks

  3. Strength: The force of the beat should be easily noted.

    a. A weak, thready pulse is normally associated with hypotension.

    b. A very strong bounding pulse may be associated with hypertension.

C. Blood pressure: The force exerted by the arterial pressure against the wall of the artery.

  1. Systolic pressure is normally 95 to 140 mm Hg in the adult.

  2. Diastolic pressure is normally 60 to 90 mm Hg in the adult.

  3. Pulse pressure is the difference between the systolic and diastolic pressure, normally 35 to 40 mm Hg. If it is less than 25 to 30 mm Hg, the peripheral pulse is difficult to palpate. This pressure provides the gradient for peripheral perfusion.

  4. Hypertension is a pressure greater than 140/90 mm Hg and may be reflective of:

    a. Hypoxemia

    b. Increased intracranial pressure

    c. Congestive heart failure (right sided)

    d. Fluid overload

    e. A response to medication (e.g., sympathomimetics)

  5. Hypotension is a pressure less than 95/60 mm Hg and may be reflective of:

    a. Fluid depletion

    b. Congestive heart failure (left sided)

    c. Peripheral vasodilation (sepsis)

    d. A response to medication (e.g., vasodilators)

    e. Positive pressure ventilation

    f. Positive end-expiratory pressure

D. Respiratory rate

  1. Normal adult respiratory rate is 12 to 20/min.

  2. Tachypnea rates greater than 20/min may be a result of:

    a. Hypoxemia

    b. Fever

    c. Metabolic acidosis

    d. Fear

    e. Anxiety

    f. Interstitial aveolar edema stimulating type J receptors

  3. Bradypnea rates less than 12/min may be a result of:

    a. Hypothermia

    b. Head trauma

    c. Narcotic overdose

    d. Sedative overdose

III. Physical Assessment of the Chest
    A. Chest assessment includes the following (sequentially performed as listed):
        1. Inspection
        2. Palpation
        3. Percussion
        4. Auscultation
    B. Inspection is the observation of the patient's chest configuration and pattern of breathing. During inspection, the following should be evaluated:
        1. Position
           a. Is the patient sitting comfortably, or does he or she require support to ventilate?
           b. The position assumed provides information about the patient's use of accessory muscles of ventilation or the presence of pain.
              (1) Use of accessory muscles results in positioning to support their use (i.e., sitting with elbows on bedside table, leaning forward)
              (2) If pain is present, the point of pain will be favored, and a position to minimize movement of affected area is assumed.
        2. Chest configuration
           a. Anteroposterior to lateral diameter is normally in a 1:2 ratio. If the patient is barrel chested, the ratio approaches 1:1, a common finding in patients with chronic obstructive pulmonary disease (COPD).
           b. Bony deformities of the thorax
              (1) Kyphosis: Posterior curvature of the thoracic vertebral column.
              (2) Scoliosis: Lateral curvature of the spinal column.
              (3) Kyphoscoliosis: Combination of kyphosis and scoliosis.
              (4) Pectus carinatum: Protrusion of the sternum anteriorly.
              (5) Pectus excavatum: Depression of the sternum.
              (6) Any thoracic deformity may result in restriction of ventilation.
        3. Ventilatory pattern
           a. Sequence of lung expansion
              1. Abdominal protrusion
              2. Lateral costal expansion
              3. Upper chest expansion
              4. Abnormal sequencing may be a result of underlying lung disease or an increase in cardiopulmonary stress.
                (a) Paradoxical breathing: Abdomen retracted during inspiration, usually indicative of fatigue of the diaphragm.
                (b) Respiratory alternans: The periodic change from a normal ventilatory pattern to a paradoxical pattern, indicative of impending or early fatigue of the diaphragm.
           b. Uniform bilateral chest expansion
              (1) The chest cage should move equally bilaterally.
              (2) Splinting of an area of the chest may be a result of:
                (a) Pain
                (b) Pneumonia
                (c) Atelectasis
                (d) Pleural effusion
                (e) Pneumothorax
           c. Use of accessory muscles of ventilation
              (1) Normal inspiration requires only contraction of the diaphragm and external intercostals.
              (2) Exhalation is passive.

   (3) Use of accessory muscles is an indication of increased work of breathing (see section III).
   d. Acute cardiopulmonary stress normally results in an increased ventilatory rate.
   e. Patients with chronic obstructive lung disease may have a decreased ventilatory rate, whereas patients with chronic restrictive lung disease may have an increased ventilatory rate.
   f. Pursed lipped breathing is indicative of chronic airway obstruction.
   g. Inspiratory/expiratory ratios should be about 1:2.
   h. The presence of audible wheezes, cackles, or rhonchi is indicative of secretions or bronchospasm.
   i. Cough
      (1) Present without request
      (2) Forceful or weak
      (3) Productive or nonproductive
      (4) A chronic cough may be an indication of chronic bronchitis, congestive heart failure, or tuberculosis.
      (5) A productive cough may indicate acute infection or chronic bronchitis.
      (6) The strength of the cough is reflective of overall ventilatory muscle strength and reserve.
C. Palpation is the touching of the chest to evaluate movement and underlying lung function.
   1. Symmetric movement of the thoracic cage
   2. Tone of ventilatory muscles
   3. Presence of consolidation, pneumothorax, atelectasis, or pleural effusion. These may cause a shift in the mediastinum. Palpation of the trachea at the suprasternal notch identifies shifting.
      a. Pneumothorax shifts the trachea and lungs away from the area of the pneumothorax.
      b. Consolidation and atelectasis shifts the trachea and lungs toward the affected area.
      c. Unilateral pleural effusion shifts the trachea and lungs away from the effusion. A bilateral effusion may not affect position.
   4. Fremitus: The vibration produced over the thoracic cage by the conduction of sound waves.
      a. Evaluation of fremitus is performed bilaterally to compare the tactile vibrations between sides of the chest.
      b. Normally, fremitus is equal throughout all lung fields; however, it may be increased over the apex of the right lung.
      c. Femitus is increased if lung density is increased (pneumonia, consolidation).
      d. Fremitus is decreased if atelectasis from obstruction is present or if fluid or air accumulates in the pleural space.
      e. A generalized or diffuse decrease in fremitus is noted in COPD and muscular or obese chest walls.
   5. Subcutaneous emphysema: If it is present, an air leak has allowed gas to enter the tissue.
D. Percussion is the production of audible and tactile vibrations over the chest by tapping the chest wall (Fig 18–1).
   1. If lung tissue is normal, percussion produces a moderately low-pitched sound.
   2. The presence of increased air in the thoracic cavity produces a lower-pitched, more muffled drumlike sound, frequently referred to as *hyperresonance*.

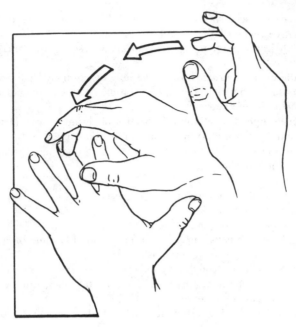

FIG 18–1.
Chest percussion technique. (From DesJardins T: *Clinical Manifestations of Respiratory Diseases.* Chicago, Year Book Medical Publishers, 1984. Used by permission.)

3. Decreased air in the thoracic cavity, consolidation, atelectasis, or a pleural effusion causes the percussion note to be higher pitched but dull or flat.

E. Auscultation is the evaluation of breath sounds with a stethoscope.
1. Normal breath sounds (Fig 18–2)
   a. Over the trachea, the sound is loud with a tubular quality, referred to as *bronchial* or *tracheal breath sounds.*
   b. Auscultation of the parenchyma reveals a soft muffled sound referred to as *vesicular breath sounds.* These are usually heard during inspiration but only minimally during exhalation.

Breath sound	Pitch	Intensity	Location	Diagram of sound
Vesicular or normal breath sounds	Low	Soft	Peripheral lung areas	
Bronchovesicular	Moderate	Moderate	Around upper part of sternum, between scapulae	
Bronchial	High	Loud	Over trachea	

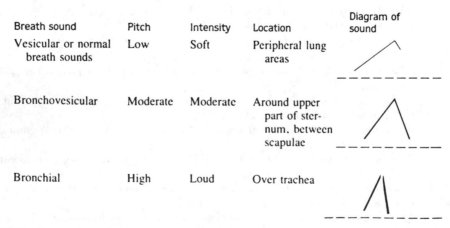

FIG 18–2.
Characteristics of normal breath sounds. (From Wilkens RL, Sheldon RL, Krider SJ: *Clinical Assessment in Respiratory Disease.* St Louis, CV Mosby Co, 1985. Used by permission.)

TABLE 18–1.

Recommended Terminology for Lung Sounds Versus Terminology in Other Publications*

Recommended Term	Classification	Terms Used in Other Publications
Crackles	Discontinuous	Rales Crepitations
Wheezes	High-pitched, continuous	Sibilant rales Musical rales Sibilant rhonchi
Rhonchi	Low-pitched, continuous	Low-pitched wheeze Sonorous rales

*From Wilkens RL, Sheldon RL, Krider SJ: *Clinical Assessment in Respiratory Disease*. St Louis, CV Mosby Co, 1985. Used by permission.

    c. The sound heard over the airways is termed *bronchovesicular*. It is softer than bronchial breath sounds and lower in pitch, being heard during both inspiration and expiration.

  2. Adventitious or abnormal breath sounds (Tables 18–1 and 18–2)

    a. *Crackles (rales):* A discontinuous sound (less than 20 msec) that is perceived as a wet, crackling, bubbling sound associated with gas moving through liquid. Normally they are heard during:

      (1) Pulmonary edema

      (2) Congestive heart failure (CHF)

      (3) The opening of collapsed airways during inspiration

      (4) In the presence of excessive secretions

    b. *Rhonchi:* A continuous sound (longer than 25 msec) that is low in pitch and normally indicative of secretions in large airways. In patients who can successfully mobilize their own secretions, rhonchi clear with coughing.

TABLE 18–2.

Application of Adventitious Lung Sounds*

Lung Sounds	Possible Mechanism	Characteristics	Causes
Wheezes	Rapid airflow through obstructed airways caused by bronchospasm, mucosal edema	High-pitched; most often occur during exhalation	Asthma, congestive heart failure
Rhonchi	Rapid airflow through obstructed airway caused by excess sputum, bronchospasm	Low-pitched; often occurs during exhalation	Bronchitis, asthma
Crackles			
Inspiratory and expiratory	Excess airway secretions moving with airflow	Coarse and often clear with cough	Bronchitis, respiratory infections
Early inspiratory	Sudden opening of proximal bronchi	Scanty, transmitted to mouth; not affected by cough	Bronchitis, emphysema, asthma
Late inspiratory	Sudden opening of peripheral airways	Diffuse, fine; occur initially in the dependent regions	Atelectasis, pneumonia, pulmonary edema, fibrosis

*From Wilkens RL, Sheldon RL, Krider SJ: *Clinical Assessment in Respiratory Disease*. St Louis, CV Mosby Co, 1985. Used by permission.

      c. *Wheezes:* A continuous sound (longer than 25 msec) that is high pitched and normally indicative of bronchospasm or mucosal edema in medium to larger airways. Wheezes do not clear with coughing.

      d. *Pleural friction rub:* A creaking or grating sound as a result of inflamed pleural surfaces rubbing together during breathing.

IV. Work of Breathing

  A. During normal breathing the muscles of ventilation consume 5% to 10% of the total oxygen consumed to perform the work of breathing.

  B. The effort required to perform the work of breathing is dependent on the following:

    1. Airway resistance (increased; increases work)

    2. Compliance (decreased; increases work)

    3. Respiratory rate (increased; increases work)

    4. Tidal volume (both increase and decrease may increase work)

    5. Use of accessory muscles (increases work)

    6. Ventilatory pattern (abnormal patterns increase work)

  C. Normally the ventilatory pattern a patient assumes is that which requires the least work.

    1. Figure 18–3,A relates the components of the work of breathing to the respiratory rate and tidal volume.

    2. Resistance work refers to the amount of work necessary to overcome nonelastic resistance to ventilation. If nonelastic resistance were the only force opposing ventilation, the ideal ventilatory pattern would be a slow rate and a large tidal volume.

    3. Elastic work refers to the amount of work necessary to overcome elastic resistance. If elastic resistance were the only force opposing ventilation, a rapid ventilatory rate with a small tidal volume would be ideal.

    4. Total work refers to actual work expended with varying ventilatory rates and tidal volumes. Note the ideal rate is about 12 to 16/min with an ideal tidal volume of about 350 to 550 ml.

    5. Figure 18–3,B illustrates the effect an increase in elastic work has on ventilatory pattern.

      a. Since elastic resistance to ventilation has increased, the least amount of work is accomplished at a high ventilatory rate and a small tidal volume.

      b. With most acute pulmonary diseases there is an increase in elastic work; therefore, ventilatory rates increase and tidal volumes decrease.

    6. If resistance work were increased, the total work curve (see Fig 18–3,A) would shift to the left.

      a. That is, the ideal respiratory pattern would produce a slow rate with large tidal volumes. This pattern minimizes the effect of the increased resistance.

      b. This would be the ideal ventilatory pattern for patients in asthmatic attacks. However, fear and anxiety frequently result in the opposite pattern (fast and shallow) being assumed.

    7. Refer to Chapter 4 for quantification of work of breathing.

V. Ventilatory Reserve

  A. Ventilatory reserve is the ability of the organism to respond to increased levels of cardiopulmonary stress.

  B. During normal breathing, the efficiency of the ventilatory muscles is poor. About 90% of the oxygen consumed to perform the work of breathing is lost as heat.

  C. The efficiency of the ventilatory muscles is further reduced with chronic pulmonary disease and with an increased minute ventilation.

  D. Figure 18–4, A depicts the relationship between minute volume and percentage of oxygen consumed for breathing in patients without chronic pulmonary disease (solid line) and patients with chronic pulmonary disease (dotted line).

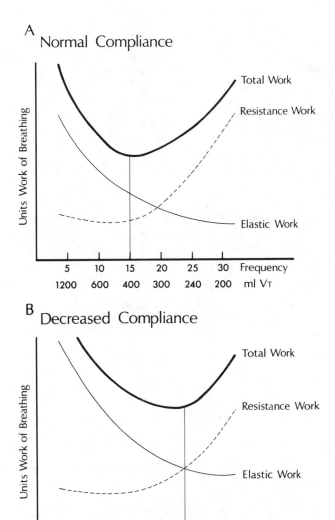

FIG 18–3.
A is a graphic representation of total work of breathing when minute ventilation is unchanged but ventilatory pattern (tidal volume and frequency) is varied. Note that for any minute ventilation there is a ventilatory pattern that requires minimal work. Of course, total work is the summation of resistance work (nonelastic resistance) and elastic work (elastic resistance). If elastic work is increased, as in **B,** the pattern of ventilation at which the minute volume can be achieved with minimal work is dramatically altered. This is a schematic representation of the principle that work of breathing is a major factor determining ventilatory pattern (see text). (From Shapiro BA, Harrison RA, Kacmarek RM, et al: *Clinical Application of Respiratory Care,* ed 3. Chicago, Year Book Medical Publishers, 1985. Used by permission.)

1. The percentage of oxygen consumed for breathing markedly increases as minute volume increases.
2. In patients with chronic pulmonary disease the percentage of oxygen consumed for breathing at basal level is already increased (20%). With increased minute volume there is a tremendous increase in oxygen consumption. These patients have lower reserves than patients without chronic pulmonary disease.

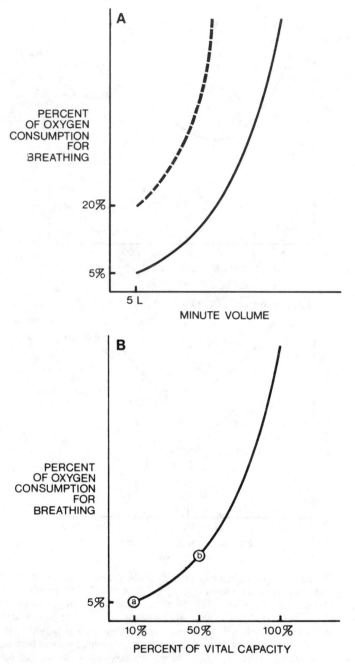

FIG 18–4.
A, the work of breathing in relation to vital capacity (see text). In **B,** point *a* represents a Vт of 500 ml with a VC of 5 L; point *b* represents a Vт of 500 ml with a VC of 1 L. (From Shapiro BA, Harrison RA, Walton JR: *Clinical Application of Blood Gases,* ed 3. Chicago, Year Book Medical Publishers, 1982. Used by permission.)

E. Figure 18–4,B illustrates the relationship between percentage of oxygen consumed for breathing and the percentage of the vital capacity that is the tidal volume.
   1. As the tidal volume becomes a greater percentage of the vital capacity, the amount of oxygen consumed for breathing increases.
   2. When the tidal volume is 50% of the vital capacity, limited ventilatory reserves exist, and the likelihood of sustained spontaneous ventilation is questionable.

VI. Vital Capacity/Maximum Inspiratory Pressure (VC/MIP)
   A. A normal VC is about 70 to 90 ml/kg of body weight.
   B. Vital capacities are frequently used as an estimate of the patient's ventilatory reserve.
   C. If the VC is more than 15 ml/kg of ideal body weight, it is assumed that the individual has the capability to respond to increased levels of cardiopulmonary stress.
   D. However, if the VC is less than 10 ml/kg, prolonged sustained spontaneous ventilation is questionable. This individual has virtually no reserves.
   E. At vital capacities between 10 and 15 ml/kg, reserves are marginal, and appropriate monitoring should be instituted.
   F. Maximum inspiratory pressure is also a parameter used to assess ventilatory reserves.
   G. If the MIP is more negative than -20 to -25 cm H_2O in a 20-second period and the patient has normal lungs and is recovering from anesthesia, neuromuscular or neurologic disease, or an overdose, sustained spontaneous ventilation is probable.
   H. In patients with chronic pulmonary disease or acute respiratory failure associated with multiorgan system failure, the use of a -20 to -25 cm H_2O range for MIP becomes less reliable.
      1. In this population, MIP or VC values provide a daily guide to ventilatory muscle capability but are unreliable as a specific indicator of spontaneous ventilatory capability.
      2. The measurement of MIP before and after weaning trials provides information on the development of fatigue. A lower value after a weaning trial compared with initial values indicates fatigue of ventilatory muscles.
   I. During the measurement of MIP, the diaphragm must be at its resting level for maximum performance. Thus, the greater the length of the diaphragmatic, muscle fibers (smaller lung volume), the greater their contractile force.
      1. In the intensive care unit, evaluation of MIP is difficult if a one-way valving system is not employed (Fig 18–5).
      2. The use of a one-way valve allows the patient to exhale after each attempted inspiration, resulting in a lower lung volume and greater force generation.
      3. Normally, inspiratory occlusion is maintained for 20 seconds, unless adverse reaction occurs.
         a. Cardiac arrhythmias
         b. Tachycardia, bradycardia
         c. Arterial desaturation
      4. In general, MIP should be measured only in patients with stable cardiopulmonary status who can withstand the stress.

VII. Assessment of Peripheral Perfusion
   A. Adequacy of peripheral perfusion can be estimated by:
      1. Sensorium
      2. Urinary output
      3. Capillary refill
      4. Skin turgor
      5. Cyanosis
      6. Peripheral pulses
      7. Skin temperature

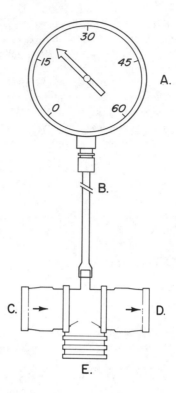

FIG 18–5.
Technical setup for performance of maximum inspiratory pressure measurement. *A,* pressure manometer; *B,* connecting tubing; *C,* one-way valve; *D,* one way-valve; *E,* patient connection of Briggs T piece. (From Kacmarek RM, Chapman C, Palazzo P, et al: Comparison of two techniques for the determertation of maximal inspiratory pressure [MIP] in mechanically ventilated patients. *Respir Care* [in press]. Used by permission.)

   B. Sensorium
      1. Confusion, agitation, and disorientation are all signs of cerebral hypoxia that can be caused by decreased oxygen carriage or decreased cerebral perfusion.
      2. Somnolence and drowsiness are signs of increased arterial Pco_2 levels.
   C. Urinary output
      1. Normal urinary output is about 40 to 60 ml/hour.
      2. Decreased urinary output is frequently a sign of decreased peripheral perfusion.
   D. Capillary refill decreases as peripheral perfusion decreases.
   E. Skin turgor also decreases as peripheral perfusion decreases.
   F. Cyanosis
      1. Cyanosis is a bluish discoloration of nail beds, lips, mucous membranes, and skin.
      2. Cyanosis is present if 5 gm% of hemoglobin is reduced.
      3. Decreased peripheral perfusion may cause sufficient pooling of blood, also allowing cyanosis to be noticed.
      4. However, cyanosis is normally noted when oxygen content is decreased in arterial blood.
      5. Anemic patients are least likely to demonstrate cyanosis, whereas polycythemic patients are most likely.
   G. Thready, faint, or distant peripheral pulses are noted as peripheral perfusion decreases.

VIII. Clubbing
- A. Clubbing is a painless enlargement of the terminal phalanges (fingers and toes) that develops over years.
- B. Its development is associated with significant cardiopulmonary disease and chronic decrease in oxygen supply to tissue.
- C. Clubbing is frequently noted in association with:
  1. Cystic fibrosis
  2. COPD
  3. Bronchogenic carcinoma
  4. Chronic cardiovascular disease

IX. Pedal Edema and Jugular Vein Distention
  1. Both are associated with increased vascular volumes and CHF.
  2. Pedal edema is seen with right-sided heart failure and may be a direct result of chronic hypoxemia resulting in pulmonary vasoconstriction, right ventricular hypertrophy, and eventually, right ventricular failure.
  3. Jugular vein distention is seen in right-sided failure.

X. Physical signs associated with common abnormal pulmonary pathology are listed in Table 18–3.

XI. Laboratory Assessment in Cardiopulmonary Disease
- A. Hematology
  1. Complete red blood cell count (CBC)
     - a. Red blood cell (RBC) count (normal levels)
       - (1) Men: 4.8 to 6.0 $\times$ 10^6/cu mm
       - (2) Women: 4.1 to 5.1 $\times$ 10^6/cu mm
     - b. Hemoglobin (normal levels)
       - (1) Men: 13 to 16 gm/dl or gm%
       - (2) Women: 12 to 14 gm/dl or gm%
     - c. Hematocrit (normal levels)
       - (1) Men: 40% to 54%
       - (2) Women: 37% to 47%
     - d. White blood cell (WBC) count: 5,000 to 10,000/cu mm
     - e. Differential of WBCs
       - (1) Neutrophils: 50% to 75%
         - (a) Segmented neutrophils: 90% to 100% of total neutrophils
         - (b) Bands: 0% to 10% of total neutrophils
       - (2) Eosinophils: 2% to 4%
       - (3) Basophils: Less than 0.5%
       - (4) Lymphocytes: 20% to 40%
       - (5) Monocytes: 3% to 8%
     - f. Platelet count: 200,000 to 350,000/cu mm
  2. Anemia: A below-normal quantity of hemoglobin, RBC count, or hematocrit and greatly decreases oxygen-carrying capacity. It may be a result of:
     - a. Hemorrhage (bleeding)
     - b. Deficiency in cell formation
     - c. Abnormal cell formation
  3. Polycythemia: An increase in hemoglobin, RBC count, or hematocrit. It may result from:
     - a. Chronic hypoxemia
     - b. Altered production by bone marrow
  4. Abnormalities in WBC count and their differential: A result of infection, allergic reaction, or leukemias.
     - a. An increase in overall WBC count (leukocytosis) is normally noted in bacterial infections.

TABLE 18–3.

Physical Signs of Abnormal Pulmonary Pathology*

Abnormality	Initial Impression	Inspection	Palpation	Percussion	Auscultation	Possible Causes
Acute airways obstruction	Appears acutely ill	Use of accessory muscles	Reduced expansion	Increased resonance	Expiratory wheezing	Asthma, bronchitis
Chronic airways obstruction	Appears chronically ill	Increased anteroposterior diameter, use of accessory muscles	Reduced expansion	Increased resonance	Diffuse reduction in breath sounds; early inspiratory crackles	Chronic bronchitis, emphysema
Consolidation	May appear acutely ill	Inspiratory lag	Increased fremitus	Dull note	Bronchial breath sounds; crackles	Pneumonia, tumor
Pneumothorax	May appear acutely ill	Unilateral expansion	Decreased fremitus	Increased resonance	Absent breath sounds	Rib fracture, open wound
Pleural effusion	May appear acutely ill	Unilateral expansion	Absent fremitus	Dull note	Absent breath sounds	CHF
Local bronchial obstruction	Appears acutely ill	Unilateral expansion	Absent fremitus	Dull note	Absent breath sounds	Mucous plug
Diffuse interstitial fibrosis	Often normal	Rapid shallow breathing	Often normal; increased fremitus	Slight decrease in resonance	Late inspiratory crackles	Chronic exposure to inorganic dust
Acute upper airway obstruction	Appears acutely ill	Labored breathing	Often normal	Often normal	Inspiratory and/or expiratory stridor	Epiglottitis, croup, foreign body aspiration

*From Wilkens RL, Sheldon RL, Krider SJ: *Clinical Assessment in Respiratory Disease.* St Louis, CV Mosby Co, 1985. Used by permission.

b. A decrease in overall WBC count (leukopenia) is normally noted in leukemias, radiation therapy, and chemotherapy.
c. Neutrophilia (increased neutrophils): A common response to stress and the body's first response to:
(1) Bacterial infection
(2) Inflammation
d. A *leftward shift* of the neutrophils: Increased levels of bands (immature neutrophils) as a result of stress. The greater the stress, the greater the percent bands.
e. Eosinophilia: An increase in the number of eosinophiles, usually a result of:
(1) Allergic reaction
(2) Parasitic infection
f. Lymphocytosis: An increase in the number of lymphocytes, usually a result of a viral infection.
g. Monocytosis: An increase in the number of monocytes, usually a result of:
(1) Chronic infections
(2) Malignancies
h. Basophilia: An increase in the number of basophiles usually seen in:
(1) Leukemias
(2) Other myeloproliferative disorders
(a) Polycythemia vera
(b) Essential thrombocysthemia
(c) Myelofibrosis
5. Platelet count
a. Platelets are necessary for normal coagulation of blood. If the platelet count is low, small skin hemorrhages are noted:
(1) Petechiae
(2) Ecchymoses
(3) Oozing from mucosal surfaces
b. Platelet counts are reduced by:
(1) Various drug therapies
(2) Bone marrow diseases
(3) Idiopathic thrombocytopenic purpura (ITP)
c. An increase in platelets may be a result of:
(1) Stress
(2) Bone marrow disease
d. Increased platelet levels increase the likelihood of thrombosis (blood clots).
B. Coagulation studies
1. In general, four distinct tests are used to evaluate the tendency of blood to clot.
a. Bleeding time
b. Platelet count (see earlier)
c. Activated partial thromboplastin time (APTT)
d. Prothrombin time (PT)
2. Bleeding time: Evaluates the ability of small skin vessels to constrict and evaluates the function of platelets. Normal time is up to 6 minutes.
3. APTT: Evaluates the amount of time it takes plasma to form a fibrin clot once the body's intrinsic clotting pathways are activated. Normal time is 32 to 51 seconds.
4. PT: Evaluates the amount of time it takes extrinsic blood factors to form a clot, once activated. Normal PT is 12 to 15 seconds.
5. All times are lengthened during hemophilia.
6. APTT: Monitored during heparin therapy.
7. PT: Monitored during warfarin sodium (Coumadin) therapy.

    C. Electrolytes (see Chapter 15)
    D. Blood urea nitrogen and creatinine levels urinalysis (see Chapter 9)

BIBLIOGRAPHY

Barnes T: *Respiratory Care Practice*. Year Book Medical Publishers, Chicago, 1988.

Cherniack RM, Cherniack L: *Respiration in Health and Disease*, ed 3. Philadelphia, WB Saunders Co, 1983.

Deshpande VM, Pibeam SP, Dixon RJ: *A Comprehensive Review in Respiratory Care*. Norwalk, Mass, Appleton & Lange, 1988.

Eubanks DH, Bone RC: *Comprehensive Respiratory Care*. St Louis, CV Mosby Co, 1985.

George RB, Light RW, Matthay RA: *Chest Medicine*. New York, Churchill Livingstone, 1983.

Kacmarek RM, Chapman M, Palazzo P, et al: Comparison of two techniques for the determination of maximal inspiratory pressure (MIP) in mechanically ventilated patients. *Respir Care* (in press).

Pare JAP, Fraser RG: *Synopsis of Diseases of the Chest*. Philadelphia, WB Saunders Co, 1983.

Parot S, Miara B, Milic-Emili J, et al: Hypoxemia, hypercarbia, and breathing pattern in patients with chronic obstructive pulmonary disease. *Am Rev Respir Dis* 1982; 126:882–886.

Petty TL: *Intensive and Rehabilitative Respiratory Care*, ed 3. Philadelphia, Lea & Febiger, 1982.

Rarey KP, Youtsey JW: *Respiratory Patient Care*. Englewood Cliffs, NJ, Prentice-Hall, 1981.

Shapiro BA, Harrison RA, Kacmarek RM, et al: *Clinical Application of Respiratory Care*, ed 3. Chicago, Year Book Medical Publishers, 1985.

Tisi GM: *Pulmonary Physiology in Clinical Medicine*, ed 2. Baltimore, Williams & Wilkins Co, 1983.

Wilkens RL, Sheldon RL, Krider SJ: *Clinical Assessment in Respiratory Care*. St Louis, CV Mosby Co, 1985.

Whitcomb ME: *The Lung: Normal and Diseased*. St Louis, CV Mosby Co, 1982.

Nutrition

I. Metabolic Pathways
   A. Carbohydrate metabolism
      1. Carbohydrate usually makes up 40% to 45% of the total food intake but may reach 60%.
      2. Amylases and disaccharidases hydrolyze complex starches and sugars to monosaccharides before they are absorbed in the small intestine.
         a. One half of the ingested carbohydrate is digested to glucose and the rest mainly to fructose and galactose.
         b. Most of the glucose circulates as blood sugar and is taken up by the body cells and metabolized for energy.
         c. Fructose, galactose, and some glucose are converted to glycogen—some in the liver and the rest in muscle.
            (1) There are about 500 gm of glycogen stored.
               (a) Of this total, 200 gm is in the liver and is available for systemic use.
            (2) The large glycogen stores in muscle are not available to provide glucose to the rest of the body.
      3. Glucose is also manufactured from amino acids and other products of intermediary metabolism by a process called gluconeogenesis, which protects the glycogen reserves.
         a. In the fasting state, liver glycogen is stimulated by catecholamine and glucagon to undergo glyconeonolyse and form blood glucose.
         b. Glucose then undergoes glycolysis to pyruvate.
            (1) Pyruvate may undergo one of three basic metabolic processes:
               (a) It can move into the mitochondria and be converted to acetylcoenzyme A (acetyl-CoA) for oxidation in the citric acid cycle.
                  1. Diversion of pyruvate for oxidation to CO_2 and H_2O in the citric acid cycle and the respiratory chain is known as *aerobic glycolysis*.
            (2) When O_2 is not present for aerobic glycolysis, pyruvate is reduced to lactate.
               (a) This process is known as *anaerobic glycolysis*.
                  1. Anaerobic glycolysis commonly occurs in periods of stress or severe exercise when demand for energy exceeds the supply of O_2.
                     a. When O_2 becomes available, lactate (which has built up in muscle and blood) can be reconverted to pyruvate for oxidation in the citric acid cycle.

        b. Anaerobic glycolysis is a rapid method for energy production.
          (1) It does not need large quantities of O_2.
          (2) However, only limited energy production occurs via this mechanism.
          (3) Pyruvate can also be carboxylated to oxaloacetate in the mitochondrea by pyruvate carboxylase.
            (a) Oxaloacetate can then form glucose in a process that is the reverse of glycolysis, known as *gluconeogenesis.*

B. Lipid (fat) metabolism
  1. Lipid is the main energy substrate in the body.
    a. Lipid provides about 90% of the total body caloric reserve.
      (1) In the average individual, 150,000 calories are in reserve.
      (2) In obese individuals, more than 150,000 calories are in reserve.
    b. Most body fat exists as fatty acids that are esterified with glycerol to form triglycerides.
      (1) Adipose tissue is about 90% triglycerides.
  2. Dietary lipid is hydrolyzed in the intestinal tract, absorbed, and then resynthesized to triglycerides.
    a. These are transported from the jejunal wall as lipid-protein complexes called *chylomicrons.*
      (1) Chylomicrons are a form of lipoproteins.
    b. Chylomicrons enter the blood via the intestinal lymphatics (lacteal) and thoracic duct.
    c. Short- and medium-chain free fatty acids enter directly into the portal blood without conversion into chylomicrons.
      (1) Medium-chain triglycerides are more easily hydrolyzed than long-chain triglycerides and can be easily absorbed.
  3. Lipoproteins may be modified in the liver before going to adipose tissue or may go there directly.
    a. In adipose tissue, lipoproteins are hydrolyzed, releasing fatty acids.
    b. The fatty acids are reesterified and stored as triglycerides.
  4. Triglycerides may also be formed from carbohydrate by lipogenesis.
    a. When carbohydrate intake is decreased, triglycerides are mobilized to glyceral and fatty acids.
    b. The glycerol is partly converted to glucose by gluconeogenesis.
      (1) The free fatty acids are oxidized to produce acetyl-CoA, which is converted to energy via the Krebs cycle.
        (a) When more acetyl-CoA is produced than the Krebs cycle can oxidize, it is converted to ketone bodies.
        (b) A ketone body: β-Hydroxybutyrol acetoacetate and acetone.
          1. Ketone production and gluconeogenesis both take place in the liver.
          2. In starvation, ketones are the main source of body fuel.
            a. Ketones minimize amino acid release from muscle and aid in protein conservation.

C. Protein metabolism
  1. Protein normally comprises about 20% of the lean body mass, or about 15% of the total body weight.
  2. An intake of about 0.8 to 1 gm/kg of body weight is needed each day in a normal individual.
  3. If energy demands are met by carbohydrate and lipids, protein is used entirely for:
    a. Protein replacement
    b. Growth and repair of tissues

c. Maintenance of circulating proteins

d. Manufacture of enzymes

4. Specific enzymes in the intestinal tract hydrolyze ingested protein to peptides and ultimately to amino acids.

5. The body cannot synthesize essential amino acids:
   a. Isoleucine
   b. Leucine
   c. Lysine
   d. Methionine
   e. Phenylalanine
   f. Threonine
   g. Tryptophan
   h. Valine

6. Amino acids not used anabolically for protein synthesis undergo catabolism (e.g., they may be transaminated or deaminated). After deamination, the residue may be converted by way of either:
   a. Acetyl-CoA to lipid (ketogenesis)
   b. Or oxaloacetate to glycogen

7. The nitrogen released is excreted in the urine as urea.
   a. One gram of urinary urea nitrogen (UUN) is derived from 6.25 gm of protein.

8. Branched chain amino acids (valine, leucine, and isoleucine) are used by muscle for metabolism.
   a. Valine is glycogenic.
   b. Leucine is ketogenic.
   c. Isoleucine is both.
   d. Branched chain amino acids given intravenously can be used as a source of energy for muscles and can preserve lean body mass.

9. Alanine is the major gluconeogenic amino acid.
   a. It is formed by transamination of pyruvate from branched chain amino acids.

10. Carbohydrates have a specific protein-sparing effect.
    a. Carbohydrates inhibit the catabolism of glycogenic amino acids.

11. Amino acids form the building blocks of proteins.
    a. One must ingest a ratio of between 100 and 150 nonprotein calories to 1 gm of nitrogen to ensure protein synthesis.
    b. This ratio is much higher in sepsis.

D. Summary of energy metabolism

1. Glucose is the principal energy source of anaerobic metabolism:
   a. During shock
   b. During tissue anoxia

2. The Krebs cycle is the main source of aerobic metabolism.
   a. It requires some glucose to prime it.
   b. Total energy needs cannot be supplied by fatty acid metabolism.

3. Glucose can be provided:
   a. From hydrolysis of carbohydrate
   b. By glycogenolysis
   c. By hydrolysis of lipids to glycerol and gluconeogenesis
   d. By conversion of some amino acids to carbohydrate

4. Triglycerides can be manufactured from excess carbohydrate, lipid, and protein intake.

5. All fuel sources can be used for energy.

II. Determination of Caloric and Protein Needs

A. Clinical energy measurement

     1. Energy is commonly measured in units of calories or joules.
       a. A calorie is the amount of energy (heat) needed to raise the temperature of 1 gm of water 1°C.
       b. One kilocalorie (1 Kcal) equals 1,000 calories.
     2. Selected caloric requirements of various substances:
       a. Protein and carbohydrate: 4 Kcal/gm
       b. Fat: 9 Kcal/gm
       c. Alcohol: 7 Kcal/gm
B. Energy used by the body can be measured by direct or indirect calorimetry.
     1. Direct calorimetry is based on the postulate that all energy expended in the body eventually becomes heat.
       a. In a resting person, the amount of energy expended over a given time or metabolic rate can be determined by measuring the heat liberated.
     2. Indirect calorimetry is based on the postulate that more than 95% of the energy expended by a person is derived from the reaction of oxygen with food (oxidation).
       a. For the average diet, 4,825 Kcal is produced for every liter of oxygen consumed.
       b. Various devices have been developed for indirect calorimetry.
         (1) Metabolic cart
         (2) Gas collection hood
C. Basal metabolic rate (BMR)
     1. The BMR is defined as the rate of energy expenditure under a given set of basal conditions.
       a. Absolute rest
       b. Awake
       c. After an overnight fast
       d. Rested
       e. Reclining for 30 min
       f. Relaxed
     2. The BMR gives an estimate of energy expended when no extra demands are placed on a patient and would include such functions as:
       a. Ion pump
       b. Synthesis and degradation of cell constinuents
       c. Substrate cycles
       d. Leakage of protons across the mitochondrial membrane
       e. Postural, respiratory, and heart muscle activity
     3. The BMR is related to body cell mass.
D. Resting energy expenditure (REE)
     1. If energy expenditure is measured after eating, energy expenditure is increased.
       a. This is known as the *specific dynamic action* (SDA) of food.
         1. It is due primarily to protein consumed.
         2. It amounts to an increase of about 10% of the BMR.
     2. The REE is defined as the BMR plus the component of SDA of food.
     3. The Harris-Benedict equation will give an estimation of REE:
       a. Male REE = 66.4230 + 13.7516W + 5.033H − 6.7750A   (1)
       b. Female REE = 655.0955 + 9.6534W + 1.8946H − 4.6756A   (2)
         where A = age in years, H = height in centimeters, and W = weight in kilograms.
E. Total energy expenditure
     1. The final factor that must be included to determine the total energy expenditure (TEE) is exercise or physical work performance and degree of stress.

2. The TEE = (REE × Activity factor) × Stress factor (Table 19–1)
3. The BMR has been found to increase under certain conditions (see Table 19–1).
   a. Trauma
   b. Infection
   c. Fever
   d. Stress
   e. Burns
F. Protein requirement
   1. The normal man engaging in an average amount of exercise requires 0.8 to 1.0 gm of protein/kg of body weight/day.
   2. In the moderately stressed individual (e.g., infection, major surgery), protein requirement is 1.5 to 2.0 gm/kg/day.
   3. In the severely stressed (e.g., burns, major trauma), protein requirement is 2.0 to 4.0 gm/kg/day.
   4. A calorie/nitrogen ratio of 150:1 is adequate for most catabolic patients. Higher ratios are used in severe stress.
   5. Daily protein requirements are:

$$\text{Protein gm} = 6.25 \times \frac{\text{Energy requirements}}{150} \tag{3}$$

III. Vitamin Requirements and Deficiency States
   A. General functions of vitamins
      1. Vitamins generally participate in metabolism in the interconversion and degradation of protein and amino acids.
      2. They also participate in the extraction of energy from carbohydrate and fat sources.
         a. Anabolic purposes
         b. Bone formation
   B. Fat-soluble vitamins
      1. Vitamin A (retinal)
         a. Natural occurrence
            (1) Liver, kidney
            (2) Butter, cream
            (3) Whole milk, cheese
            (4) Egg yolks
            (5) Fish liver oils
            (6) Dark green, leafy and yellow vegetables and fruit

TABLE 19–1.

Factors Indicating Increases in Basal Metabolic Rate Under Certain Physiologic Conditions

Condition	Factor
Confined to bed	1.2
Normal activity	1.3
Minor operation	1.2
Skeletal trauma	1.35
Major Sepsis	1.6
Severe thermal burn	2.1

    b. Function in biochemical system
      (1) Dim light vision
      (2) Cell membrane stability
    c. Requirement increases with increasing protein intake.
    d. Deficiency symptoms
      (1) Night blindness
      (2) Keratomalacia
  2. Vitamin D (calciferol)
    a. Natural occurrence
      (1) Synthesized by skin
      (2) Butter, cream
      (3) Egg yolk
      (4) Liver
      (5) Fish liver oil
      (6) Fortified milk
    b. Function in biochemical system
      (1) Necessary for endochondral bone formation
      (2) Intestinal Ca^{+2} absorption
    c. Bile necessary for absorption
    d. Deficiency symptoms
      (1) Childhood rickets
      (2) Adult osteomalacia
  3. Vitamin E
    a. Natural occurrence
      (1) Wheat germ
      (2) Nuts
      (3) Green plants
      (4) Egg yolks
      (5) Liver
      (6) Butter, fat
    b. Function in biochemical system
      (1) Primarily an antioxidant
    c. Requirement increases with increased ingestion of unsaturated oil.
    d. Deficiency symptoms
      (1) Muscular weakness
      (2) Hemolysis
  4. Vitamin K (phytonadione)
    a. Natural occurrence
      (1) Green leafy vegetables
      (2) Wheat bran
      (3) Soybeans
      (4) Cheese
      (5) Egg yolk
      (6) Liver
    b. Function in biochemical systems
      (1) Regulation of coagulation system
      (2) Synthesis of prothrombin
    c. Microbiologic production by intestinal flora account for 50% of requirement.
    d. Deficiency symptom
      (1) Hemorrhage
C. Water-soluble vitamins
  1. Vitamin B_1 (thiamine)

  a. Natural occurrence
     (1) Beef, pork, organ meats
     (2) Wheat grains
     (3) Fish
     (4) Dried beans and peas
     (5) Peanuts
  b. Function in biochemical systems
     (1) Ketoacid metabolism
  c. Deficiency symptoms
     (1) Beriberi
     (2) Anorexia
     (3) Ataxia
     (4) Weakness
     (5) Depression
     (6) Irritability
     (7) Lethargy
     (8) Heart failure
2. Niacin
  a. Natural occurrence
     (1) Beef
     (2) Milk
     (3) Wheat flour
  b. Function in biochemical systems
     (1) Cellular hydrogen transport
     (2) Component of coenzymes nicotinamide adenine dinucleotide (NAD) and nicotinamide adenine dinucleotide phosphate (NADP)
     (3) Glycolipis
     (4) Tissue respiration and synthesis
  c. Requirements vary directly with energy intake.
  d. Deficiency symptoms
     (1) Weakness
     (2) Anorexia
     (3) Dermatitis
     (4) Diarrhea
     (5) Dementia
3. Pantothenic acid
  a. Natural occurrence
     (1) Meat
     (2) Dairy products
     (3) Broccoli
  b. Function in biochemical systems
     (1) Component of CoA
  c. Deficiency symptom
     (1) Fatigue
4. Vitamin B_2 (riboflavin)
  a. Natural occurrence
     (1) Milk
     (2) Meat products
  b. Function in biochemical systems
     (1) Oxidative enzyme systems
     (2) Combines with phosphoric acid to become part of the flavin coenzymes flavin mononucleotide (FMN) and flavin adenine dinucleotide (FAD)

    c. Deficiency symptoms
      (1) Poor growth
      (2) Alopecia
  5. Pyridoxine (vitamin B_6)
    a. Natural occurrence
      (1) Yeast
      (2) Wheat germ, whole grain cereals
      (3) Pork, granular meats
      (4) Legumes
      (5) Potatoes
      (6) Bananas
      (7) Oatmeal
    b. Function in biochemical systems
      (1) Transamination in amino acid decarboxylation
      (2) A primary coenzyme in metabolism of protein, carbohydrate, fat, and nonoxidative degradation of amino acids
    c. Deficiency symptoms
      (1) Seborrheic dermatitis
      (2) Glossitis
      (3) Lymphopenia
  6. Folic acid
    a. Natural occurrence
      (1) Dark green leafy vegetables
      (2) Asparagus
    b. Function in biochemical systems
      (1) Synthesis of DNA and RNA
    c. Synthesis by intestinal flora may satisfy requirement.
    d. Deficiency symptom
      (1) Megaloblastic anemia
  7. Vitamin B_{12} (Cyanocobalamin)
    a. Natural occurrence
      (1) Animal meat
      (2) Dairy products
    b. Function in biomedical systems
      (1) Synthesis of DNA
      (2) Intimate link to folate metabolism
    c. Requires gastric intrinsic factor and distal ileum for absorption
    d. Deficiency symptoms
      (1) Decreased proprioception
      (2) Megaloblastic anemia
  8. Vitamin C (ascorbic acid)
    a. Natural occurrence
      (1) Citrus fruits
      (2) Tomatoes
      (3) Raw leafy vegetables
    b. Function in biochemical systems
      (1) Coenzyme or cofactor in hydroxylation of collagen
      (2) Essential to normal functioning of all cellular units, including ribosomes and mitochondria
      (3) Promotes healing of wounds
    c. Deficiency symptoms
      (1) Swollen, inflamed gums
      (2) Loosened teeth

(3) Capillary hemorrhages

(4) Subcutaneous and subperiosteal hemorrhages

IV. Interrelationship Between Pulmonary Disease and Nutritional Status

    A. Pulmonary function and nutritional status are closely interrelated.

        1. Malnutrition increases the risk of acute and chronic respiratory failure (CRF).

            a. A common complication of malnutrition is pulmonary infection.

        2. Inattention to nutritional requirements in patients with CRF results in increased morbidity and mortality.

            a. Inadequate or inappropriate nutrient intake exacerbates pulmonary dysfunction.

            b. Pulmonary distress limits nutritional intake.

    B. Pulmonary function can be enhanced by providing nutrients essential for respiratory function.

        1. Calories and protein should be provided in proportions to place the least stress on respiratory capacity.

        2. The amount of O_2 consumed and the amount of CO_2 produced are different for each major nutrient (Table 19–2).

            a. For each calorie of carbohydrate (CHO) metabolized, 0.20 L of O_2 is consumed and 0.20 L of CO_2 is produced.

            b. For each calorie of protein metabolized, 0.24 L of O_2 is consumed and 0.19 L of CO_2 is produced.

            c. For each calorie of fat metabolized, 0.22 L of O_2 is consumed and 0.15 L of CO_2 is produced.

        3. The ratio of CO_2 produced to O_2 consumed is called the *respiratory quotient* (RQ).

        4. A diet with a decreased amount of CHO and a proportionally increased amount of fat (50%) should be provided to the hypercapnic patient.

            a. When fat replaces CHO calories, CO_2 and minute ventilation are reduced.

            b. The RQ is reduced.

    C. Protein requirements and ventilatory drive

        1. Protein intake should match requirement.

            a. Inadequate protein intake can lead to:

                (1) Protein-calorie malnutrition

                (2) Wasting of lean body mass

        2. Low protein intake and high CHO intake will:

            a. Decrease elimination of theophylline.

            b. Require adjustment in dosage to avoid theophylline toxicity.

        3. Long-term use of steroids promotes:

            a. Protein catabolism and gluconeogenesis

            b. Generalized muscle wasting

            c. A negative nitrogen balance

        4. Excessive protein intake can be detrimental to a person who is unable to increase minute ventilation.

TABLE 19–2.

Respiratory Quotient, Oxygen Consumption, and Carbon Dioxide Production of Major Food Stuff

	O_2 Consumption (L)	CO_2 Production (L)	RQ
CHO	0.20	0.20	1.0
Protein	0.24	0.19	0.8
Fat	0.22	0.15	0.7

5. High protein diets stimulate ventilatory drive and minute ventilation.
   a. For patients without alveolar reserves, the stimulus can result in:
      (1) Increased work of breathing
      (2) Dyspnea
6. High-protein diets may increase the clearance of theophylline.
   a. Dosage requirements will be affected.
7. Adequate protein should be provided to allow for anabolism.
   a. Overfeeding of protein should be avoided.
   b. A calorie/nitrogen ratio of 150:1 should be provided.
8. Nitrogen balance is a useful means of determining the adequacy of protein intake (see section VII).

V. Weight Loss and Pulmonary Disease
   A. Decreased body weight is a complication of chronic obstructive pulmonary disease (COPD).
      1. The incidence varies between 25% and 65% of patients with COPD.
      2. Body weight correlates with the percent of predicted diffusion capacity and forced expiratory volume in 1 second.
      3. Sustained weight loss is associated with a poor prognosis.
         a. Weight loss of 10% or more is an antecedent of heart failure in hypercapnic patients with COPD.
         b. Mortality is significantly increased.
   B. Factors that result in decreased calorie intake
      1. Twenty percent to 25% of patients with COPD have peptic ulcers, and gastrointestinal discomfort may cause these patients to shun food.
      2. Bronchodilators, both sympathomimetic and theophylline derivatives, are gastric irritants.
         a. Nausea and vomiting may occur with toxic doses of theophylline.
      3. Chronic sputum production may alter the desire for and taste of food.
      4. A full stomach restricts descent of the diaphragm and makes breathing difficult after large meals.
      5. Shortness of breath may hamper the patient's ability to prepare meals or to eat with comfort.
      6. Depression is associated with decreased food intake.
   C. Factors that increase caloric expenditure
      1. Infections common in acute respiratory illness increase metabolic demand.
      2. The respiratory disease itself is capable of increasing energy expenditure.
      3. The elevated energy requirement may be related to the increased work of breathing in patients with respiratory disease.
         a. With diffuse bronchial obstruction, the mechanical work necessary to overcome nonelastic resistance increases.
         b. The respiratory muscles require oxygen to perform this mechanical work.
      4. The caloric cost of breathing increases in patients with pulmonary disease.
         a. Normal expenditure: 43 to 72 Kcal/day
         b. Pulmonary disease: 430 to 720 Kcal/day

VI. Muscle Mass and Strength
   A. Respiratory muscles are catabolized to meet the body's energy needs in malnutrition.
      1. Autopsy studies provide evidence of decreased weight of the diaphragm muscle in emphysema patients.
      2. Malnutrition decreases the degree to which the diaphragm can contract.
         a. Weakness of the diaphragm can contribute to respiratory failure.
   B. Respiratory muscle function is decreased in malnutrition.
      1. The loss in respiratory muscle strength occurs in both inspiratory and expiratory muscles.

TABLE 19–3.

Anthropometric Standards*

	Triceps Skinfold (mm)	Arm Muscle Circumstance (cm)
Male	12.5	25.3
Female	16.5	23.2

*% deficit in anthropometric measurements =

$$100 - \left[\frac{\text{Actual value}}{\text{Standard value}} \times 100 \right].$$

2. The loss in respiratory muscle strength is directly related to weight loss.
3. A major goal in the care of the patient with respiratory failure and nutritional depletion is restoration of lean body mass.

VII. Nutritional Assessment
    A. The systematic evaluation of a patient's current state of nutrition using both physical and biochemical means
        1. Nutritional assessment includes three major parameters:
           a. Nutrition history
           b. Anthropometrics
           c. Laboratory analysis
    B. Nutrition history parameters
        1. Diet history and interview
           a. Dietary patterns prior to illness and during any past treatments
           b. Usual weight prior to illness
           c. Recent weight changes
           d. Changes in sense of taste or smell related to food and to past treatments
           e. Changes in appetite and food likes and dislikes related to onset of disease and to previous treatments
           f. Twenty-four-hour dietary recall
    C. Anthropometric parameters (somatic compartment) (Table 19–3)
        1. Height and weight
           a. Determine premorbid and hospital admission weights.
           b. Determine ideal body weight.
        2. Triceps skinfold (TSF) (see Table 19–3)
           a. Measure of body's fat stores and nonprotein caloric reserves
           b. Measured using skinfold calipers
         3. Arm muscle circumference (AMC) (see Table 19–3)
           a. Indicator of lean body mass or muscle tissue
           b. AMC = midarm circumference = (TSF × 0.314)
    D. Laboratory parameters (visceral compartment)
        1. Serum albumin (Table 19–4)
           a. Normal serum albumin is 3.5 to 5.0 gm/dl.

TABLE 19–4.

Visceral Protein Levels

	Normal	Mild Deficit	Moderate Deficit	Severe Deficit
Albumin (gm/dl)	3.5–5.0	<3.5	<3.0	<2.5
Transferrin (mg%)	>200	<200	<180	<160
Total lymphocyte count (number/cu mm)	2,000–4,000	<1,800	<1,500	<900

(1) Normal serum albumin level is the equilibrium point between production, distribution, and degradation.

(2) Decreased albumin levels result from:

    (a) Inadequate synthesis

    (b) Increased catabolism

    (c) Extraordinary corporal losses of albumin

  b. Serum albumin levels are decreased in protein-depleted states.

  c. Count of 2.8 gm% is the cutoff point for albumin oncotic pressure; below 2.8 gm%, edema will usually be present.

2. Total iron-binding capacity or transferrin

  a. Values of 200 mg% or less correlate with malnutrition.

  b. Protein secreted by the liver

  c. Protein that transports iron

  d. Secretion declines in protein-depleted states.

  e. Protein manufactured by the endoplasmic reticulum in liver cells, which is dependent on adequacy of amino acid, whether from diet, muscle, gut, or cutaneous tissue

  f. First protein to increase as a result of nutritional repair

3. Total lymphocyte count (TLC) (see Table 19–4)

  a. Values of 1,800 or less correlate with malnutrition.

  b. Good indication of immune response

  c.

$$TLC = \% \; \frac{\text{Lymphocytes} \times \text{White blood cell count}}{100} \qquad (4)$$

4. Nitrogen balance

  a. The nitrogen balance is calculated to assess whether protein is being depleted and to assess the estimated degree of hypermetabolism.

  b. Twenty-four hour UUN is ordered.

  c. Nitrogen balance = N in − N out.

  d. In the healthy individual, nitrogen intake and nitrogen excretion are equal (about 11 gm/day) and in balance.

  e. Positive nitrogen balance more than +2 indicates net tissue growth.

  f. Negative nitrogen balance more than −2 indicates net tissue breakdown.

    (1) Negative nitrogen balance may be due to:

      (a) Trauma

      (b) Infection

      (c) Stress

      (d) Inadequate protein or CHO intake (or both):

$$\frac{\text{Protein intake}}{6.25} = (UUN + 4) \qquad (5)$$

5. Creatinine height index (CHI)

  a. Creatinine is given off by muscle at a constant rate.

  b. It is an accurate indicator of lean body mass.

    (1) Increased creatinine in urine equals increased muscle mass.

  c. It uses 24-hour urine test for creatinine.

  d. Creatinine excreted in 24 hours is compared with normal creatinine/height ratios.

6. Delayed cutaneous hypersensitivity (DCH) skin testing

  a. The DCH skin test is used to evaluate the cell-mediated immunity (CMI) response.

  b. The patient is tested by injecting antigen skin tests intradermally.

c. The CMI multitest is injected.

d. The area of induration is read at 48 hours.

   (1) Cellular immune function is severely compromised by protein calorie malnutrition.

   (2) Cell-mediated immunity correlates significantly with morbidity and mortality.

E. Types of malnutrition

   1. When nutrient intake is insufficient to meet requirements, malnutrition develops.

   2. Kwashiorkor (protein malnutrition)

      a. The patient who has developed kwashiorkor is one whose caloric intake was adequate or more than adequate in carbohydrate and fat but contained little, if any, protein.

      b. The patient will have adequate somatic stores.

      c. The patient will have defects in visceral compartment.

      d. The patient may appear well nourished, even obese.

   3. Marasmus (protein calorie malnutrition)

      a. Marasmus develops in patients who cannot maintain adequate oral intake.

      b. Such patients have adequate visceral protein stores.

      c. They have depleted somatic stores.

      d. Marasmus presents with weight loss and fat and muscle wasting due to overall calorie protein deprivation.

   4. Kwashiorkor-marasmus mix

      a. The patient has depleted somatic and visceral stores.

VIII. Dietary Intervention

A. Basic goals of dietary intervention for patients with chronic pulmonary disease:

   1. Prevent nutritional depletion.

   2. Assure that the mix of nutrients can be handled easily by the impaired respiratory system.

      a. Modify the level of fat and CHO.

      b. Keep RQ 1.0 or less.

      c. Prevent overfeeding of calories, especially CHO.

      d. There is a rise in CO_2 production concurrent with the increase in RQ.

      e. The response of overfeeding CHO above energy needs is to convert the excess glucose to fat.

         (1) Conversion of CHO to fat is associated with an RQ of approximately 8.

         (2) There is a large increase in CO_2 production.

B. General principles of tube feeding the patient with chronic respiratory disease and/or who is mechanically ventilated

   1. Provide a caloric intake to meet caloric needs of nutritional maintenance.

   2. Gradually increase the caloric intake beyond maintenance and monitor the respiratory effect when nutritional rehabilitation is the goal.

   3. Avoid overfeeding of protein.

      a. Provide enough protein so that nitrogen intake equals nitrogen output when maintenance is the goal.

      b. Provide enough protein to achieve a positive nitrogen balance if repletion is the goal.

   4. Restrict fluid and/or sodium as needed to lower pulmonary vascular pressure and decrease extravascular lung water.

      a. Use enteral formulas with high nutrient density if fluid is restricted.

   5. Monitor serum phosphate levels to avoid hypophosphatemia.

      a. Lean muscle contains approximately 100 mEq of phosphate/kg of wet tissue.

    b. Phosphate deficiency occurs when the patient's prior state of malnutrition is underestimated or if inadequate phosphate is provided.

    c. Deficiencies can develop in less than 48 hours.

    d. Hypophosphatemia can occur if increased requirements for phosphorus are not met.

  6. Hypercapnic and ventilator-dependent patients should have less CHO and more fat to minimize the demand on the respiratory system to eliminate CO_2.

    a. They should have 50% or more fat calories and 30% or less CHO calories.

    b. Enough CHO should be provided to prevent ketosis.

      (1) If calorie intake is adequate, 50 to 100 gm of digestible CHO will prevent ketosis.

    c. The caloric distribution of the feeding can be manipulated by adding fat (corn oil) to a commercial feeding.

    d. Pulmocare, a commercial enteral product, contains more than 50% calories of fat.

C. Monitoring of tube-fed patients

  1. The nutritional regimen should be continually adjusted to the patient's changing medical and nutritional condition.

    a. Hydration

      (1) Monitor fluid input and output.

      (2) Monitor the specific gravity of urine.

    b. Utilization of glucose

      (1) Serum and urine glucose

    c. Utilization of protein

      (1) Nitrogen balance

      (2) Blood urea nitrogen

    d. Serum electrolytes and phosphate

      (1) Sodium

      (2) Potassium

      (3) Chloride

      (4) Phosphate

    e. Respiratory function

      (1) Arterial blood gases

      (2) Minute ventilation

IX. Oral Diet Intervention

A. Nonhypercapnic patients: Dietary recommendations

  1. Make food preparation easier so fatigue does not result.

  2. Rest just before eating so respiratory demand is low.

  3. Eat in a quiet, relaxed atmosphere.

  4. Emphasize the meals early in the day if fatigue becomes worse as the day continues.

  5. Avoid foods that produce gas or bloating, which will cause distention and displacement of the diaphragm.

B. Hypercapnic patients: Dietary recommendations

  1. Eat small, frequent feedings.

    a. The demand for O_2 and the volume of CO_2 that has to be expired will be reduced.

    b. A full stomach interferes with the descent of the diaphragm and makes breathing difficult.

C. Nutritional maintenance

  1. Provide caloric intake equal to caloric needs.

D. Nutritional rehabilitation
1. Gradually increase caloric intake and monitor respiratory effect.
2. Substitute lower cholesterol fat for high CHO foods.
3. a. Calories as fat: 45% to 50%
    b. Calories as CHO: 30% to 35%
    c. Monitor total calories to avoid excessive intake.
4. Avoid overfeeding of protein.
    a. Provide enough for N balance if maintenance is the goal.
    b. Provide enough protein to achieve a + N balance if repletion is the goal.
5. Restrict intake of fluid, sodium, or both.
    a. Vascular pressure will be lowered.
    b. Extravascular lung water will decrease.

REFERENCES

Angelillio VA, Bedi S, Durfee D, et al: Effects of low and high carbohydrate feedings in ambulatory patients with chronic obstructive pulmonary disease and chronic hypercapnia. *Ann Intern Med* 1985; 103:883–885.

Arora NS, Rochester DF: Respiratory muscle strength and maximal voluntary ventilation in undernourished patients. *Ann Rev Respir Dis* 1982; 126:5–8.

Askanazi J, Nordenstrom J, Rosenbaum SH, et al: Nutrition for the patient with respiratory failure: Glucose vs. fat. *Anesthesiology* 1981; 54:373–377.

Askanazi J, Rosenbaum S, Hyman A, et al: Respiratory changes induced by the large glucose loads of total parenteral nutrition. *JAMA* 1984; 243:1444–1447.

Askanazi J, Weissman C, Rosenbaum SH, et al: Nutrition and the respiratory system. *Crit Care Med* 1982; 10:163–172.

Bassili HR, Deitel M: Effects of nutritional support on weaning patients off mechanical ventilators. *JPEN* 1981; 5:161–163.

Bone RC: Treatment of respiratory failure due to advanced chronic obstructive lung disease. *Arch Intern Med* 1980; 140:1018–1021.

Braun SR, Keim NL, Dixon RM, et al: The prevalence and determinants of nutritional changes in chronic obstructive pulmonary disease. *Chest* 1984; 86:558–563.

Brown SE, Light RW: What is now known about protein energy depletion: When COPD patients are malnourished. *J Respir Dis* 1983; 4:36–50.

Brown RO, Heezer WD: Nutrition and respiratory disease. *Clin Pharm* 1984; 3:152–161.

Calloway DH: Dietary components that yield energy. *Environ Biol Med* 1971; 175–186.

Carlsson M, Nordenstrom J, Hedenstierna G: Clinical implications of continuous measurement of energy expenditure in mechanically ventilated patients. *Clin Nutr* 1984; 3:103–110.

Cherniack RM: Ventilation, perfusion and gas exchange, in Frochlich ED (ed): *Pathophysiology: Altered Regulatory Mechanisms in Disease*. Philadelphia, JB Lippincott Co, 1976, pp 149–166.

Clark WR, Copeland RL, Bonaventura MM, et al: Ventricular tachycardia associated with hypophosphatemia. *Nutr Int* 1985; 102–106.

Dietary goals for the United States. *Nutr Today*, Sept-Oct 1977; 72:21–30.

Dietary guidelines Advisory Committee reports. *Nutr Today* May-June 1985; 252:8–15.

Dietel M, Williams VP, Rice TW: Nutrition and the patient requiring mechanical ventilatory support. *J Am Coll Nutr* 1983; 2:25–32.

Driver AG, McAleny MT, Smith JL: Nutritional assessment of patients with chronic obstructive pulmonary disease and acute respiratory failure. *Chest* 1982; 82:568–571.

Garfinkel F, Robinson S, Price C: Replacing carbohydrate calories with fat calories in enteral feedings for patients with impaired respiratory function [abstract]. *JPEN* 1985; 9:106.

Goldstein S, Askanazi J, Weissman C, et al: Ventilatory patterns, gas exchange and weight loss in patients with COPD [abstract]. *Fed Proc* 1985; 44:1384.

Goldstein SA, Askanazi J, Weissman C, et al: N balance during nutritional support in malnourished COPD patients [abstract]. JPEN 1986; 10:16S.

Goldstein SA, Thomashow B, Askanazi J: Functional changes during nutritional depletion in patients with lung disease. *Clin Chest Med* 1986; 7:141–151.

Heymsfield SB, Head CA, McManus CB III, et al: Respiratory, cardiovascular, and metabolic effects of enteral hyperalimentation: Influence of formula dose and composition. *Am J Clin Nutr* 1984; 40:116–130.

Hunter AMB, Carey MA, Larsh HW: The nutritional status of patients with chronic obstructive pulmonary disease. *Am Rev Respir Dis* 1981; 124:376–381.

Kelsen SG, Ference M, Kapoor S: The effect of inadequate caloric intake on diaphragm structure and function [abstract]. *Clin Res* 1982; 30:432A.

Kim WW, Kelsay JL, Judd JT, et al: Evaluation of long-term dietary intakes in adults consuming self-selected diets. *Am J Clin Nutr* 1984; 40:1327–1332.

Ingram RH: Chronic bronchitis, emphysema and airway obstruction, in Petersdorf RG, Adams RD, Braunwald E, et al (eds): *Harrison's Principles of Internal Medicine*, ed 10. New York, McGraw-Hill Book Co, 1983, pp 1550–1553.

Larca L, Greenbaum DM: Effectiveness of intensive nutritional regimens in patients who fail to wean from mechanical ventilation. *Crit Care Med* 1982; 10:297–300.

McCauley K, Weaver TE: Cardiac and pulmonary diseases: Nutritional Implications. *Nurs Clin North Am* 1983; 18:81–96.

McSweeney AJ, Grant I, Heaton RK, et al: Life quality of patients with chronic obstructive pulmonary disease. *Arch Intern Med* 1982; 142:473–478.

Newman JH, Neff TA, Ziporin P: Acute respiratory failure associated with hypophosphatemia. *N Engl J Med* 1977; 296:1101–1103.

Paaiw JD, McCamish MA, Dean RE, et al: Assessment of caloric needs in stressed patients. *J Am Coll Nutr* 1984; 3:51–57.

Rochester DF, Arora NS, Braun NMT: maximum contractile force of human diaphragm muscle, determined in vivo. *Trans Am Clin Climatol Assoc* 1981; 93:200–208.

Selwanov V, Sheldon GF, Fantini G: Nutrition's role in averting respiratory failure. *J Respir Dis* 1983; 4:29–32.

Thuurlbeck WM: Diaphragm and body weight in emphysema. *Thorax* 1978; 33:483–487.

Vandenbergh E, Van de Woestyne KP, Gyselen A: Weight changes in the terminal stages of chronic obstructive pulmonary disease: Relation to respiratory function and prognosis. *Am Rev Respir Dis* 1967; 95:556–566.

Winterbauer R, Durning RB Jr, Barron E, et al: Aspirated nasogastric feeding solution detected by glucose strips. *Ann Intern Med* 1981; 95:67–68.

Chapter 20

Obstructive Pulmonary Diseases

I. General Comments
   A. The acronym COPD is applied to patients with long-term chronic obstructive pulmonary disease, who show persistent airway obstruction, normally manifested by decreased expiratory flow rates.
   B. Prevalence
      1. From 1960 to 1970 the increase in deaths from emphysema was about 150% and is steadily increasing.
      2. In 1984, 70,000 deaths were attributed to emphysema.
      3. About 20 million Americans have been diagnosed with COPD. Of these, about:
         a. Forty-five percent have chronic bronchitis.
         b. Fifteen percent have emphysema.
         c. Forty percent have asthma.
      4. There seems to be a greater incidence of COPD in men than in women; however, the percentage of women with COPD is steadily increasing.
      5. On autopsy, some degree of emphysema appears in a large percentage of the population.
      6. Emphysema is the second leading cause of disability, arteriosclerotic heart disease being first.
   C. General causes of COPD
      1. Smoking. Of all risk factors, smoking shows the highest correlation with COPD; however, individual response to acute and chronic exposure varies considerably from individual to individual. The reasons for this variation in response is not well understood. Smoking:
         a. Inhibits ciliary function.
         b. Causes bronchospasm.
         c. Affects macrophage activity.
         d. Causes disruption of alveolar septal wall and capillary endothelium.
      2. Air pollutants, both particulate and gaseous.
      3. Passive smoking. Evidence indicates the passive inspiration of smoke from the environment increases risk. Passive smoking exposes the individual to the same toxic substance, although in lower concentration than the active smoker.
      4. Occupational exposure to dusts and fumes.
      5. Infection, which may cause decreased pulmonary clearance, resulting in an increased incidence of recurrent infection.

6. Heredity
   a. α_1-Antitrypsin deficiency, which results in emphysematous changes measurable in the third and fourth decades (see section II)
   b. Cystic fibrosis (see Chapter 26)
   c. Asthma (see section VI)
7. Allergies (e.g., chronic asthma), which can lead to permanent pulmonary changes.
8. Socioeconomic status. Higher incidence has been demonstrated in low socioeconomic groups.
9. Alcohol ingestion, although no direct link has been demonstrated. Alcohol ingestion:
   a. Decreases ciliary function.
   b. Decreases alveolar macrophage function.
   c. Decreases surfactant production.
   d. Alters antibacterial defenses of the lung.
10. Aging, which causes natural degenerative changes in the respiratory tract resembling emphysematous changes.

D. Physical appearance of patient
1. *Barrel-chested*, a result of increased air trapping (anteroposterior diameter increased)
   a. Increase in anteroposterior diameter
   b. Increase proportional to increase in functional residual capacity (FRC)
2. Frequently clubbing (pulmonary hypertrophic osteopathy), bulbous enlargement of terminal portion of the digits altering the angle of the nailbed
3. Cyanosis, a result of hypoxemia coupled with secondary polycythemia
4. Decreased and adventitious breath sounds
5. Often a hyperresonant chest
6. Ventilatory pattern
   a. Increased use of accessory muscles
   b. Paradoxical movement of the abdomen frequently observed
   c. Prolonged expiratory time
   d. Active exhalation
   e. Pursed-lip breathing
7. Malnourished, secondary to loss of appetite (anorexia)
8. Anxious
9. General muscle atrophy
10. May be edematous with jugular vein distention if congestive heart failure present

E. General pulmonary function changes (Table 20–1)
1. Frequently an increase in pulmonary compliance
2. Increased airway resistance as a result of mucosal edema and bronchiolar wall weakening
3. Prolonged expiratory times when no. 1 and 2 are present
4. Increased FRC
5. Increased RV
6. Increased RV/TLC ratio
7. Increased or normal TLC
8. Decreased or normal VC
9. Decreased or normal inspiratory capacity (IC) and inspiratory reserve volume (IRV)
10. Increased expiratory reserve volume (ERV)
11. Decreased expiratory flow studies: $FEV_1\%$, $FEV_3\%$, $MMEFR_{25\%-75\%}$, forced expiratory flow determined between the first 200 ml and 1,200 ml of exhaled volume ($FEF_{200-1,200}$), and maximum voluntary ventilation (MVV) all are reduced. The level of reduction is associated with severity of disease.

TABLE 20–1.

Comparison of Pulmonary Function Study Results
in Patients With Obstructive and Restrictive
Pulmonary Diseases

PFT Study*	Obstructive	Restrictive
TLC	↔ or ↑	↓
VC	↔ or ↓	↓
FRC	↑	↔ or ↓
RV	↑	↔ or ↓
RV/TLC ratio	↑	↔
$FEV_1\%$	↓	↔
$MMEFR_{25\%-75\%}$	↓	or ↓

*TLC = total lung capacity; VC = vital capacity; RV = residual volume; $FEV_1\%$ = percentage of forced vital capacity in 1 second; $MMEFR_{25\%-75\%}$ = maximum midexpiratory flow rate between 25% and 75%.

F. General x-ray findings
   1. Increased anteroposterior diameter
   2. Flattened hemidiaphragms
   3. Hyperinflation
   4. Pulmonary vascular engorgement with increased vascular markings
   5. Increased retrosternal airspace
   6. Normal or increased heart shadow
   7. Normal or thin elongated mediastinum
   8. Hypertranslucency
   9. Possible peripheral bullae or blebs
  10. In severe cases or end-stage disease, frequently right ventricular hypertrophy and congestive heart failure (CHF)

G. Dyspnea
   1. In all patients, dyspnea on exertion is one of the first noticeable symptoms.
   2. As the disease process progresses, dyspnea becomes apparent even at rest.
   3. Dyspnea normally increases as the work of breathing progressively increases.
   4. The percentage of the oxygen consumed to ventilate is increased, severely limiting the patient's level of physical exertion as the disease progresses.

H. Ventilatory drive and COPD
   1. The ventilatory drive of COPD patients may vary considerably.
   2. Some continue to increase their ventilatory efforts as the disease progresses, despite increases in work of breathing.
     a. These patients possess normal or increased ventilatory drives and are frequently referred to as "pink puffers."
     b. This group usually does not become carbon dioxide retainers, despite continual disease progression.
     c. As a result, administration of high F_{IO_2} does not depress ventilation. Normal carbon dioxide responsiveness continues until there is complete failure of ventilatory muscles.
     d. These patients present in acute distress, with normal or decreased P_{CO_2} levels.
     e. The level of P_{CO_2} rapidly increases when failure overwhelms ventilatory capabilities.
   3. Many COPD patients, on the other hand, have marked alterations in ventilatory drive.
     a. Frequently, their sensitivity to oxygen is increased and carbon dioxide is reduced.

    b. This group is commonly referred to as "blue bloaters."

    c. They experience progressive increases to baseline P_{CO_2} levels as their disease progresses.

    d. At presentation with an acute exacerbation of the disease, markedly elevated P_{CO_2} levels may be noted. Blood gas interpretation is usually acute ventilatory failure superimposed on chronic ventilatory failure with severe hypoxemia.

    e. These patients are classified as individuals who *will not* breathe during failure, whereas those with normal drives simply cannot breathe at the time of failure.

I. General pattern of arterial blood gas changes demonstrated by carbon dioxide retainers as their disease progresses from mild to severe

1. Because of the pathophysiology of COPD, ventilation/perfusion inequalities develop.

2. Mismatching of ventilation and blood flow results in hypoxemia. It should be noted that hypoxemia normally is the first measured blood gas abnormality (see Chapter 12).

3. Hypoxemia becomes increasingly worse as the disease process progresses, resulting in stimulation of peripheral chemoreceptors.

4. Stimulation of peripheral chemoreceptors may result in hyperventilation, the body's attempt to correct hypoxemia.

5. If hyperventilation persists, the kidneys compensate for the acid-base imbalance. Blood gas analysis reveals compensated respiratory alkalosis (chronic alveolar hyperventilation) with hypoxemia.

6. Hyperventilation continues until oxygen consumption by the patient's respiratory musculature exceeds the benefits received by hyperventilation.

7. The percentage of total oxygen consumption being used for ventilation becomes greatly increased because the efficiency of the respiratory system is greatly reduced by disease and increased accessory muscle use.

8. The body can no longer maintain the level of alveolar ventilation necessary to maintain adequate oxygen tensions without severely compromising oxygen delivery to other organs.

9. Because of the depressed ventilatory drive of the individual and the high cost of breathing, carbon dioxide is allowed to increase in an attempt to conserve energy.

10. This results in further progression of the hypoxemia.

11. The total oxygen reservoir may be decreased even further.

12. This is counterbalanced to a degree by a reduction in oxygen consumption by the respiratory muscles, a decrease in the patient's overall level of activity, and secondary polycythemia.

13. Alveolar ventilation continues to decrease. This is evidenced by increasing carbon dioxide levels and further development of hypoxemia.

14. With time, the patient begins to retain carbon dioxide. Blood gases at this time would reveal compensated respiratory acidosis (chronic ventilatory failure) with moderate to severe hypoxemia.

15. It is at the point where carbon dioxide starts to be retained that the patient's primary stimulus to breathe becomes oxygen. This abnormal primary stimulus to ventilation is known as the *hypoxic drive*.

16. If oxygen were administered in sufficient amounts, the hypoxic stimulus to breathe would be reduced, potentially to the point of apnea.

17. The disease continues to progress with increasing levels of carbon dioxide retention and more severe hypoxemia.

18. The disease process becomes end stage and terminal. The patient's level of physical activity is severely limited, and he or she is reduced to a pulmonary cripple.

J. Cor pulmonale
1. Cor pulmonale denotes right ventricular hypertrophy secondary to abnormalities of lung structure and function. Congestive heart failure may or may not be present.
2. It is a frequent sequel to chronic bronchitis and cystic fibrosis.
3. Pathogenesis
   a. Developing pulmonary disease results in increasing hypoxemia, which causes constriction of the pulmonary capillary system.
   b. Constriction causes pulmonary hypertension. The decreased capillary bed seen with advancing pulmonary disease also contributes to development of pulmonary hypertension.
   c. Pulmonary hypertension causes the right side of the heart to work harder. With time, right ventricular hypertrophy develops.
   d. Pulmonary hypertension, if not controlled, precipitates the development of right ventricular failure in addition to cor pulmonale.
   e. This results in peripheral edema due to increased resistance to venous return and decreased right ventricular function.
   f. Failure of the right side of the heart is more frequently seen in association with pulmonary disease than is left-sided heart failure.
II. Emphysema
A. Emphysema is characterized by enlargement of air spaces distal to terminal bronchioles, with loss of elastic fibers and destruction of alveolar septal wall.
B. Etiology
1. Smoking (high correlation with emphysema)
2. High correlation with environmental conditions (e.g., air pollution)
3. Occupational hazards, dust, fumes, and similar factors
4. Heredity
   a. Patient may have α_1-Antitrypsin deficiency, a lack of the enzyme that metabolizes trypsin, a digestive enzyme.
   b. If the trypsin is not metabolized, it will cause destruction of normal pulmonary tissue.
C. Types
1. Centrilobular
   a. Destructive changes occur primarily in the respiratory bronchioles.
   b. Incidence is much higher in men.
   c. Primary lesions appear in upper lobes.
   d. There is a very high correlation with centrilobular emphysema and smoking; frequently it is a sequel to chronic bronchitis.
   e. It rarely occurs in nonsmokers.
2. Panlobular
   a. Changes at alveolar level where destruction of septa predominates
   b. Effects seemingly generalized in distribution
   c. Seen with α_1-antitrypsin deficiency and the natural aging process
3. Bullous
   a. Destructive changes at the alveolar and respiratory bronchiolar level
   b. Prominent bleb and bullae formation
D. Clinical manifestations
1. Shortness of breath, developing very gradually
2. Nonproductive cough
3. Frequent respiratory infections
4. Cyanosis
5. Barrel-chested appearance
6. Hyperresonant chest

 7. Polycythemia
 8. Use of accessory muscles
 9. Clubbing
 10. Anorexia
 11. Muscle atrophy
 12. Suprasternal retractions
E. Chest x-ray findings
 1. Flattened hemidiaphragms
 2. Hypertranslucency
 3. Increased retrosternal air space
 4. Attenuated peripheral pulmonary vasculature
 5. Small heart
 6. Elongated cardiac silhouette
F. Pulmonary function studies: As outlined in section I.
G. Management: As outlined in section V.
III. Bronchitis
 A. Acute bronchitis
  1. Acute inflammation of tracheobronchial tree with production of excessive mucus
  2. Clinical manifestations
   a. Mucosal edema
   b. Increased sputum production
   c. Hacking paroxysms of cough
   d. Raw, burning substernal pain
  3. Causes
   a. Infectious: viral, bacterial, or fungal
   b. Allergic
   c. Chemical, smoke, irritant gases, and similar factors
  4. Treatment: Usually by administration of antibiotics, expectorants, aerosol therapy, and occasionally antitussives.
  5. Normally a self-limiting process without serious complications or residual effects
 B. Chronic bronchitis
  1. Chronic cough with excessive sputum production of unknown specific etiology for 3 months per year for 2 or more successive years
  2. Cause basically is frequent acute episodes of bronchitis, which may result from:
   a. Smoking (by far the leading cause)
   b. Air pollution
   c. Chronic infections
  3. Clinical manifestations
   a. Onset normally insidious, with patient rarely aware of its development
   b. Steps in development
    (1) Smoker's cough, followed by a
    (2) Morning cough, leading to
    (3) Continual cough, especially during cold weather and exacerbations
   c. Sputum
    (1) Normally sputum production increases slowly until there is continual abnormal production.
    (2) Sputum is usually thick, gray, and mucoid until chronic infections develop, then turning mucopurulent.
  4. Pathophysiology
   a. Mucosal glands
    (1) Size increases in relation to wall thickness; normally gland size is about one third of the height of the bronchial walls.

(2) In chronic bronchitis, gland size is about two thirds of the height of the bronchial walls.

(3) The number of mucus-secreting glands increases.

b. Submucosal gland hypertrophy

c. Increased population of goblet cells replacing ciliated columnar cells (epithelial metaplasia)

d. Submucosal infiltration

e. Mucosal edema

f. Smooth muscle hypertrophy

g. All the above collectively result in:

(1) Diminished airway lumen

(2) Secretion accumulation

(3) Submucosal infiltration

(4) General increase in sputum production

(5) Loss of ciliated cells

(6) Sputum production in nonciliated airways

(7) Impaired clearance mechanism

5. Chest x-ray findings

a. Early in the disease, x-ray changes are not significant, especially if the disease is associated only with larger airways.

b. If the disease has moved to the periphery, hyperinflation with a flattened hemidiaphragm may be noticed.

c. Peripheral pulmonary vasculature may be prominent.

d. Cardiac shadow is enlarged.

e. There is pulmonary vascular engorgement.

f. X-ray film usually is of little use in establishing diagnosis.

g. A positive patient history usually is the best diagnostic tool.

6. Pulmonary function studies

a. In early stages, all pulmonary function studies may be normal, except for slight decreases in expiratory flow rates.

b. As the disease process progresses, pulmonary function results are consistent with those presented in section I.

7. Treatment

a. Most important: Removal of patient from irritants

b. Aerosol and bronchodilator therapy

c. Antibiotics if indicated

d. Treatment regimen fairly consistent with that outlined in section V

IV. Bronchiectasis

A. Permanent abnormal dilation and distortion of bronchi and/or bronchioles

B. Classification

1. Cylindrical (tubular)

a. Bronchial walls are dilated, with regular outlines.

b. It is the least severe type, because bronchiectatic areas drain fairly well.

2. Fusiform (cystic)

a. Bronchial walls have large, irregularly shaped distortions with bulbous ends.

b. Evidence of bronchitis or bronchiolitis often is present.

3. Saccular

a. There is complete destruction of bronchial walls.

b. Normal bronchial tissue is replaced by fibrous tissue.

c. It is the most severe type and has worst prognosis.

C. Etiology

1. Despite controversy, probable contributing factors are as follows:

a. Recurrent infection, gram-negative infections being prominent

   b. Complete airway obstruction
   c. Atelectasis
   d. Congenital abnormalities
D. Pathophysiology
   1. Loss of cilia
   2. Inflammatory infiltration
   3. Sloughing of mucosa with ulceration and possible abscess formation
   4. Adjacent and distal lung tissue generally has reduced volume with patchy scarring and consolidation, all believed to be secondary to the obstruction of the bronchi.
E. Diagnosis
   1. The bronchogram is the only absolute diagnostic tool.
   2. Bronchoscopy may afford direct visualization of bronchiectatic lesions.
   3. Chest x-ray findings (see section IV–G)
   4. Sputum examination (see section IV–F)
F. Clinical manifestations
   1. Chronic loose cough, often exacerbated by change of position
   2. Clubbing of fingers
   3. Recurrent infections
   4. Increased sputum production of a characteristic three-layer nature upon standing
      a. Top layer: Thin, frothy
      b. Middle layer: Turbid, mucopurulent
      c. Bottom layer: Opaque, mucopurulent to purulent with mucous plugs (Dittrich's plugs), sometimes foul-smelling
   5. Hemoptysis (common)
   6. Severe ventilation/perfusion abnormalities
   7. Hallitosis
G. Chest x-ray findings
   1. Usually normal unless disease is advanced and associated with other types of COPD
   2. May show multiple cysts with associated fluid level
   3. May show cor pulmonale
H. Pulmonary function studies
   1. Cylindric type may show no changes or decreases in expiratory flow rates.
   2. The saccular or cystic type shows decreased flow rates, especially if associated with bronchitis, emphysema, or cystic fibrosis.
I. Management
   1. Aggressive bronchial hygiene with aerosol and chest physiotherapy
   2. Appropriate antibiotic therapy
   3. Possible lung resection if lesions are localized
V. General Management Principles in COPD
   A. Stable COPD
      1. Smoking cessation
         a. Regardless of level of disability, cessation of smoking is beneficial.
         b. Progress of disease is reduced if smoking stopped.
         c. However, no treatment can reverse or stop disease progression.
      2. Vaccination
         a. Influenza virus is recommended.
         b. Pneumococcal vaccination is controversial.
      3. Bronchodilators
         a. In general, response to bronchodilator therapy with pulmonary function studies should be demonstrated (15% or greater increase in baseline FEV_1 is considered positive).

    b. However, many believe bronchodilator therapy should be administered regardless of demonstrated response.

    c. Some patients respond to anticholinergics (atropine-like drugs) better than β-agonists because of altered autonomic receptor distribution with age (see Chapter 40).

      (1) Atropine

      (2) Ipratropium bromide (Atrovent)

      (3) Glycopyrrolate (Robinul)

  4. Corticosteroids

    a. Corticosteroids are used primarily to reduce mucosal edema.

    b. Aerosolized approaches are generally desired over systemic because of side effects of the systemic route.

    c. Aerosolized corticosteroids commonly used are:

      (1) Beclomethasone (Becotide, Vanceril)

      (2) Flunisolide (AeroBid)

      (3) Triamcinolone (Azmacort)

  5. Antibiotics

    a. Some recommend low-dose chronic antibiotic therapy in those with persistent and frequently reoccurring pulmonary infections.

    b. Agents frequently used are:

      (1) Ampicillin

      (2) Trimethoprim-sulfamethoxazole (Bactrium, Septra)

      (3) Tetracycline

      (4) Erythromycin

      (5) Chloramphenicol

  6. Oxygen therapy (see VB and Chapter 23)

  7. Mechanical ventilation (see VC and Chapters 23 and 36)

  8. Nocturnal nasal continuous positive airway pressure (CPAP) therapy (see Chapters 23 and 37)

  9. Improvement of patient's exercise tolerance by general graded body toning and stamina-developing exercises

  10. Maintenance of cardiovascular status by treatment of CHF

  11. Avoidance of exposure to all types of airway irritants

  12. Proper education and psychologic and sociologic support

B. Acute exacerbation of COPD

  1. Acute exacerbations may be associated with a number of specific concomitant problems (Table 20–2).

  2. Oxygen therapy: In general, $F_{I_{O_2}}$ is titrated to maintain P_{O_2} in the 60 mm Hg range. No need exists to increase P_{O_2} to the 90 mm Hg range.

  3. Antibiotic therapy: Acute exacerbations are commonly associated with pneumonia. Appropriate therapy should begin immediately.

  4. Bronchodilator therapy should be started immediately.

    a. Aminophylline

      (1) Loading dose: 5 to 6 mg/kg given intravenously

      (2) Maintenance dose: 0.5 to 0.6 mg/kg/hour given intravenously

    b. Aerosolized β$_2$-agonists

    c. Anticholinergics

    d. A combination of a through c is usually employed.

  5. Mucolytic therapy

    a. With some, mucolytic therapy represents appropriate systemic hydration, because some patients present dehydrated, increasing viscosity of pulmonary secretions.

    b. Acetylcysteine (Mucomyst) may also be administered by aerosol.

TABLE 20–2.

Comorbid Conditions That Present as Exacerbations of COPD*

Condition	Common Clinical Symptoms	Diagnostic Laboratory Tests	Treatment
Acute bronchitis	Productive cough, increased dyspnea, substernal discomfort, purulent sputum	Leukocytosis, sputum, Wright's stain, and Gram's stain	Antibiotics, systemic and airway hydration
Pneumonia	Fever, productive cough, pleuritic chest pain	As above, plus chest radiograph and blood cultures	As above; if toxic or in impending respiratory failure, hospitalization
Asthmatic bronchoconstriction	Increased cough, dyspnea, wheeze	Increased blood and sputum eosinophil count, elevated IgE in bronchial asthma	Corticosteroids, avoidance of causative agent if possible, desensitization when indicated, sodium cromolyn
Medication errors and noncompliance, tobacco smoke exposure; industrial smoke and fume exposure; failure to comply with exercise conditioning regime	Progressive dyspnea, "worsening"	Persistent eosinophilia, nontherapeutic serum theophylline levels, presence of carboxyhemoglobin, work history	Patient and family education, use of intelligent caregivers, job modification, closer work with pulmonary rehabilitation team
Malnutrition or weight gain	Weakness, weight loss or gain	Weight, characteristic blood chemistry and hematologic abnormalities	Nutrition counseling, dietary supplementation as indicated
Pneumothorax	Acute dyspnea, chest pain, syncope	Chest radiograph	Hospitalization, thoracotomy tube to suction
Acute myocardial infarction and/or CHF	Increasing dyspnea, may not have typical anginal chest	ECG, chest radiograph (may not be typical); cardiac enzymes	Hospitalization for cardiovascular monitoring
Pulmonary embolism and infarction	Acute dyspnea, hemoptysis (in infarction)	Chest radiograph, ventilation/ perfusion lung scan (may be difficult to interpret), pulmonary angiogram	Anticoagulation or thrombolysis
Bronchogenic carcinoma	Weight loss, recurrent pneumonia, hemoptysis, chest pain	Chest radiograph, computed tomography (CT) scan, sputum cytology, bronchoscopy	Thoracotomy and resection (if possible), radiation, chemotherapy

*From Burton GG: Exacerbations of chronic obstructive pulmonary disease: Pharmacologic management, in Kacmarek RM, Stoller JK (eds): *Current Respiratory Care.* Toronto, BC Decker, 1988. Used by permission.

6. Costicosteroid therapy
   a. Use of aerosolized steroids at home is common.
   b. During acute exacerbation, therapy consists of 75 to 125 mg of methylprednisone given intravenously every 6 hours for the first 24 hours, which is tapered to a maintenance dose of 25 to 50 mg/day.
7. Diuretic therapy
   a. Many COPD patients also have CHF.
   b. Appropriate diuretic therapy to normalize fluid balance is indicated.
8. Nutritional support
   a. Many COPD patients demonstrate chronic nutritional deficiencies.
   b. Preceding admission, nutritional maintenance decreases as respiratory symptoms progress.
   c. See Chapter 19 for details.
9. Bronchial hygiene techniques
   a. Chest physical therapy (see Chapter 31)
   b. Intermittent positive pressure breathing (see Chapter 32)
   c. Aerosol therapy (see Chapter 30)

C. Ventilatory management in acute exacerbations of COPD
   1. Indication for ventilatory support varies among experts but in general should be associated with reversibility of the event responsible for failure. Unless the state prior to the acute exacerbation can be reestablished, the likelihood of chronic ventilatory support is highly probable (Table 20–3; see also Chapter 23).
   2. General principles:
      a. During the first 48 to 72 hours, rest of ventilatory muscles should be assured.
         (1) Patients with COPD who are in acute exacerbation generally have acute and chronic respiratory muscle fatigue.
         (2) Recovery from fatigue requires rest and time.
         (3) Essentially, "controlled" ventilation should be provided by appropriate sedation. The control mode on the ventilator, however, should not be used. If sedation decreases, the control mode setting may result in the patient fighting the ventilator and thus in greater fatigue.
      b. Acid-base balance consistent with the patient's baseline level should be maintained.
         (1) To ensure depression of ventilatory drive and rest, mild hyperventilation (pH 7.40–7.45) during the first 48 to 72 hours, and subsequently during the night, may be necessary.
         (2) At other times, the Pco_2 should remain at the patient's normal level.
         (3) Chronic alteration of the Pco_2 from the patient's baseline will ensure failure during weaning trials.
         (4) If a Pco_2 of only 60 mm Hg is the level the mechanical properties of the lung are capable of maintaining, a Pco_2 of 40 mm Hg with a normalized pH will result in an acute respiratory acidosis when weaning is attempted as a result of suppressed ventilatory drive.
   3. Rate and tidal volume
      a. A mechanical ventilatory rate of between 6 and 12/min should be maintained.
         (1) Rates higher than this frequently result in air trapping and intrinsic positive end-expiratory pressure (auto-PEEP).
         (2) Generally, the lowest mechanical rate that prevents excessive spontaneous ventilation should be used (see Chapter 36).
      b. Tidal volume
         (1) Tidal volumes should be maintained at 12 to 15 ml/kg.

TABLE 20–3.

Indications for Mechanical Ventilation*

Physiologic Mechanism	Best Indicators (Normal Values)	Values Indicating Need for Mechanical Ventilation
Inadequate alveolar ventilation	Arterial P_{CO_2} (36–44 mm Hg)	Acute increase from normal or from patient's baseline
	Arterial pH (7.36–7.44)	<7.25–7.30
Hypoxemia	Alveolar-to-arterial P_{O_2} gradient breathing 100% O_2 (25–65 mm Hg)	>350 mm Hg
	$Pa_{O_2}/F_{I_{O_2}}$ ratio (350–400 mm Hg)	<200 mm Hg
Inadequate lung expansion	Tidal volume (V_T, 5–8 ml/kg)	<4–5 ml/kg
	Vital capacity (60–75 ml/kg)	<10 ml/kg
	Respiratory rate (12–20 breaths/min)	>35 breaths/min
Respiratory muscle weakness	Maximum inspiratory force (80–100 cm H_2O)	<25 cm H_2O
	Maximum voluntary ventilation (120–180 L/min)	<2 × resting ventilation requirement
	Vital capacity (60–75 ml/kg)	<10–15 ml/kg
Excessive work of breathing	Minute ventilation volume required to keep arterial P_{CO_2} normal (5–10 L/min)	>15–20 L/min
	Ratio of deadspace to tidal volume (25%–40%)	>60%
	Respiratory rate (12–20 breaths/min)	>35 breaths/min
Unstable ventilatory drive	Breathing pattern; clinical setting	No readily available measurement

*From Pierson DJ: Exacerbation of chronic bronchitis and emphysema: Ventilatory management, in Kacmarek RM, Stoller JK (eds): *Current Respiratory Care*. Toronto, BC Decker, 1988. Used by permission.

    (2) Since compliance is usually higher than normal, excessive airway pressure rarely develops.

    (3) The use of large V_Ts allows mechanical rate to be kept minimal and expiratory time lengthy.

  c. Generally, the more severe the COPD, the greater the concern about mechanical rate and V_T. In mild COPD, higher rates may not present problems.

4. Mode of ventilation

  a. To minimize the development of air trapping and auto-PEEP, intermittent mandatory ventilation/synchronized intermittent mandatory ventilation should be used to:

    (1) Ensure low mechanical rate.

    (2) Allow the patient to breathe spontaneously around the set rate, if needed.

  b. In mild COPD, assist/control may be used but is generally discouraged because of the potential for the development of air trapping and auto-PEEP.

5. Inspiratory time/peak flow rate

  a. Inspiratory time should match the patient's spontaneous inspiratory time.

  b. If inspiratory time is inappropriately long, the patient's work of breathing during mechanical ventilation can equal spontaneous work of breathing.

      c. Thus, inspiratory times are generally about 1.0 second.

      d. Peak inspiratory flow should be high enough to ensure gas delivery in the desired inspiratory time.

      e. Generally, peak flow should be set at 60 L/min or greater.

    6. The $F_{I_{O_2}}$ is set to provide adequate oxygenation (P_{O_2} between 60 and 80 mm Hg).

    7. Positive end-expiratory pressure

      a. In general, therapeutic PEEP levels should not be used in COPD patients because of concerns associated with:

        (1) Increasing FRCs

        (2) Cardiovascular embarrassment

        (3) Risk of barotrauma

      b. However, low levels of PEEP (3–7 cm H_2O) may be useful too.

        (1) The effect of auto-PEEP on work of breathing should be minimized (see Chapter 36).

        (2) Diseased airways should be stabilized.

        (3) The FRC loss associated with bypassing the glottic mechanism as a result of intubation should be reestablished.

VI. Asthma

  A. Asthma, according to the American Thoracic Society, is "characterized by an increased responsiveness of the trachea and bronchi to various stimuli and is manifested by widespread narrowing of the airways that changes in severity either spontaneously or as the result of treatment."

  B. Categories

    1. *Allergic or extrinsic:* Implies that asthma is a result of an antigen-antibody reaction on mast cells of the respiratory tract. This reaction causes release of histamine, bradykinins, eosinophilic chemotactic factor of anaphylaxis (ECF-A), and slow-reacting substance of anaphylaxis (SRS-A). These substances then elicit the clinical responses associated with an asthmatic attack and cause high serum IgE levels along with sputum and serum eosinophilia.

    2. *Idiopathic or intrinsic:* Implies that asthma is a result of imbalance of the autonomic nervous system, that is, the response of β- and α-adrenergic sites, as well as cholinergic sites of the autonomic nervous system are not properly coordinated.

    3. *Nonspecific:* Implies that the origin of asthmatic reactions is unknown. The asthmatic attack may follow viral infection, emotional changes, or exercise.

  C. Etiology

    1. In general, the complete causes are unknown, but heredity plays a significant role. Allergies and environmental factors also are frequently implicated.

    2. If the disease develops between ages 5 through 15 years, it usually has an allergic basis.

    3. If onset is after age 30 years, the disease normally is considered nonspecific.

    4. Incidence

      a. About 5% to 15% of the population under age 15 years is asthmatic.

      b. About 1% of the adult population is asthmatic.

      c. Normally at the onset of adolescence, the disease begins to disappear.

  D. Diagnosis

    1. Diagnosis depends on skin testing for antibodies and on the patient's and family history.

    2. In allergic asthma, antibody IgE serum levels are about six times that of normal.

    3. In idiopathic asthma, patients show an abnormal response to drug therapy: decreased beta sympathetic response and increased alpha sympathetic response.

4. In nonspecific asthma, frequent presenting symptoms are nasal polyps and aspirin intolerance.
5. Eosinophilia of sputum and blood are common.

E. Pathophysiology
  1. Thickening of subepithelial membranes
  2. Hypertrophy of mucous glands
  3. Eosinophilic infiltrates common in both sputum and serum
  4. Decrease in number of pulmonary mast cells
  5. Mucosal edema and bronchoconstriction
  6. Increased production of thick viscid secretions

F. Clinical manifestations
  1. Severe respiratory distress
  2. Rapid, shallow respiratory pattern
  3. Wheezing that is often audible without a stethoscope
  4. Weak cough
  5. Tachycardia and hypertension
  6. Sometimes diaphoresis
  7. Possibly cyanosis
  8. Barrel-chested appearance with hyperresonance
  9. Anxious
  10. Intercostal, substernal, subcostal retractions
  11. Paradoxical chest movement
  12. Accessory muscle usage
  13. Shortness of breath
  14. Prolonged expiratory time

G. Chest x-ray findings
  1. During an attack a classic hyperinflation pattern is seen.
  2. Between attacks the chest x-ray findings may be normal.

H. Pulmonary function studies
  1. During an attack expiratory flow rates and vital capacity are decreased. Bronchodilator therapy during pulmonary function testing often results in a significant improvement in test results.
  2. Between attacks pulmonary function studies may be normal or show decreased expiratory flow rates.

I. Status asthmaticus
  1. Status asthmaticus is a sustained asthmatic attack that does not respond to conventional therapy.
  2. Severe hypoxemia is normally present.
  3. Possible results
    a. Lactic acidosis
    b. Respiratory failure
    c. Mechanical ventilation
    d. Death

J. Management of stable asthma
  1. In general, treatment is primarily preventive and pharmacologic.
    a. Preventive
      (1) Avoid irritants and allergens.
      (2) Avoid occupational and environmental causes.
    b. Pharmacologic
      (1) β_2-Adrenergic agents
      (2) Methylxanthines (theophylline)
      (3) Cromolyn sodium

      (4) Anticholinergics

      (5) Corticosteroids

  2. Immunotherapy is used against identified antigens. Immunotherapy can be expected to:

    a. Increase serum and/or secretory IgG and IgA levels that block IgE capacity to bind to mast cells.

    b. Decrease IgE levels.

    c. Decrease mast cell sensitivity.

  3. Many approach treatment in a stepwise manner, adding additional approaches as severity increases and decreasing therapy as the patient improves (Table 20–4).

K. Management of acute exacerbation and status asthmaticus

  1. Pharmacologic management centers on relief of airway obstruction.

    a. Subcutaneous epinephrine

    b. Inhaled β_2-adrenergic agents

    c. Aminophylline

    d. Anticholinergic agents

    e. Corticosteroids (normally do not demonstrate efficacy until 6 to 8 hours after administration)

    f. In general, management is similar to stable asthma, except dosages and frequencies are increased, and more invasive routes of administration are chosen (Table 20–5).

TABLE 20–4.

Stepwise Management of Stable Asthma*

Step 1
    Avoid potential irritants and allergens.
    Treat concurrent sinusitis or esophageal reflux.
    Discontinue oral or ophthalmic β-blockers.
    Consider occupational causes of asthma.
    Consider aspirin or metabisulfite sensitivity.
Step 2
    Prescribe inhaled β-adrenergic agonist,
      metered dose inhaler.
      (If not effective, try spacer device, then
        nebulized or oral β-adrenergic agonist.)
Step 3
    Add oral theophylline.
Step 4
    Add trial of inhaled cromolyn.
Step 5
    Add corticosteroids:
      Begin inhaled steroids when patient is
       stable.
      Taper oral steroids off, and switch to
       alternate-day therapy or to the lowest daily
       dose, as tolerated.
As the patient improves, decre setherapy by a
    step.

*From Marcy TW, Matthay RA: Stable asthma, in Kacmarek RM, Stoller JK (eds): *Current Respiratory Care.* Toronto, BC Decker, 1988. Used by permission.

TABLE 20–5.

Treatment Guidelines in Acute Asthma*

Initial bronchodilator treatment
    Inhaled β-adrenergic agonists every 20–30
        min for three or four doses
                or
    Subcutaneous epinephrine every 20–30 min
        for three or four doses
Treatment for persistent airflow obstruction
    (status asthmaticus)
    Inhaled β-adrenergic agonists every 1–2 hr
    Intravenous aminophylline
    Intravenous corticosteroids
    Subcutaneous β-adrenergic agonists, in some
        patients
Ancillary measures
    Antibiotics for fever and sputum purulence
    Supplemental oxygen for:
        Documented hypoxemia
        FEV_1 or PEFR† ≤50% of predicted value in
            patients >45 yr old
Measures of uncertain benefit
    Hydration
    Inhaled saline mists
    Chest physiotherapy
    Expectorants
    Mucolytics

*From Fanta CH: Acute exacerbations of asthma and status asthmaticus: Pharmacologic management, in Kacmarek RM, Stoller JK (eds): *Current Respiratory Care.* Toronto, BC Decker, 1988. Used by permission.
†PEFR = peak expiratory flow rate.

    2. Systemic hydration demonstrates variable results depending on the length of time the asthmatic attack has been in progress before admission and on the level of dehydration.
    3. The use of chest physiotherapy, expectorants, and mucolytics during the acute phase is questionable. However, after resolution of the acute phase, chest physiotherapy is helpful in mobilizing retained secretions.
    4. Oxygen therapy should be administered liberally by cannula or simple mask if hypoxemia is present. A cannula is normally much better tolerated than a mask.
  L. Ventilatory management in status asthmaticus
    1. Indications for mechanical ventilation
      a. Acute ventilatory failure P_{CO_2} more than 50 mm Hg is always an indication for ventilation.
        (1) If P_{CO_2} level is more than 50 mm Hg, ventilatory muscle fatigue has occurred.
        (2) Airflow obstruction may be nearly complete.
      b. Many institute mechanical ventilation when patients present in impending acute ventilatory failure.
        (1) Normally, asthmatic individuals are relatively healthy prior to an acute attack; thus, they can be expected to hyperventilate in the presence of hypoxemia.

(2) If the severity of the attack persists or increases in spite of treatment; that is, if
  (a) Hypoxemia persists
  (b) Peak flow decreases
  (c) FEV_1 decreases
  (d) Abnormal breath sounds increase
  (e) Aeration decreases
  (f) Pco_2 will begin to rise because of fatigue.
(3) Once Pco_2 returns to normal (40–45 mm Hg), with persistent symptomatology failure is imminent in the presence of continued acute asthma.
(4) Intubation and mechanical ventilation should be immediately instituted to prevent further clinical deterioration.
2. Once the airway is established, pharmacologic control of ventilation is necessary.
  a. Paralyze with nondepolarizing agents.
  b. Sedate. Avoid the use of morphine and thiopental, because both may enhance bronchospasm.
3. During mechanical ventilation, major problems include air trapping and auto-PEEP.
4. To avoid air trapping and auto-PEEP, consider the following when ventilating:
  a. Long expiratory time to allow complete exhalation.
  b. However, long inspiratory time may be necessary to allow distribution of ventilation and the avoidance of high peak airway pressure.
  c. Slow ventilatory rates.
  d. Tidal volumes between 10 and 12 ml/kg.
5. In general, the following guidelines apply in most patients:
  a. Ventilatory rate: 6 to 10/min
  b. Tidal volume: 10 to 12 ml/kg
  c. Inspiratory time: 1.5 to 2.0 seconds
  d. Expiratory time: 4.0 to 8.0 seconds
  e. Peak flows set to achieve inspiratory time
  f. FI_{O_2} to maintain Po_2 at 60 to 70 mm Hg
  g. Positive end-expiratory pressure to modify the effects of auto-PEEP and to decrease air trapping
    (1) In general, PEEP is contraindicated in asthma, because it may increase air trapping.
    (2) However, in mechanically ventilated patients demonstrating auto-PEEP, low levels of PEEP (3–7 cm H_2O) may reduce air trapping and improve ventilation (see Chapters 36 and 37).
6. If bronchospasm persists, consider the use of anesthetic agents that are potent bronchodilators.
  a. Ether
  b. Halothane
  c. Enflurane
  d. Isoflurane
7. If persistent and progressive difficulty in maintaining a normal Pco_2 level (35–45 mm Hg) is noted, allow the Pco_2 level to increase to 50 to 60 mm Hg before increasing the ventilatory rate significantly.
  a. Increasing the rate will most likely:
    (1) Increase air trapping.
    (2) Increase deadspace.
    (3) Further increase Pco_2.
    (4) Increase peak airway pressure.
    (5) Increase the likelihood of barotrauma.

      b. Administer $NaHCO_3$ to maintain normal pH as the Pco_2 level is allowed to rise.

      c. Once the acute attack resolves, slowly adjust the ventilator to achieve a normal Pco_2 level as the kidney normalizes the HCO_3^- and pH levels.

8. Once the acute attack is resolved, ventilator discontinuance should progress rapidly.

9. Many asthmatics respond adversely (increase in bronchospasm) to an artificial airway when sedation has been reversed. Once it has been established that spontaneous ventilation is feasible, rapidly extubate.

BIBLIOGRAPHY

Abraham AS: The management of patient with chronic bronchitis and cor pulmonale. *Heart Lung* 1977; 6:104.

Bates DV, Macklem PT, Christie RV: *Respiratory Function in Disease.* Philadelphia, WB Saunders Co, 1971.

Bracchi G, Barbaccio P, Vezzoli F, et al: Peripheral pulmonary wedge sengiography in chronic obstructive pulmonary disease. *Chest* 1977; 71:718–724.

Burton GG: Exacerbations of chronic obstructive pulmonary disease: Pharmacologic management, in Kacmarek RM, Stoller JK (eds): *Current Respiratory Care.* Toronto, BC Decker, 1988.

Cherniack RM, Cherniack L: *Respiration in Health and Disease*, ed 3. Philadelphia, WB Saunders Co, 1983.

Committee of the Oregon Thoracic Society, Chronic Obstructive Pulmonary Disease: *C.O.P.D. Manual.* New York, American Lung Association, 1977.

Crofton J, Douglas A: *Respiratory Diseases*, ed 2. Boston, Blackwell Scientific Publications, 1975.

Fanta CH: Acute exacerbations of asthma and status asthmaticus: Pharmacologic management, in Kacmarek RM, Stoller JK (eds): *Current Respiratory Care.* Toronto, BC Decker, 1988.

Farzan S: *A Concise Handbook of Respiratory Diseases.* Reston, Va, Reston Publishing Co, 1978.

Gates AJ: Bronchiolitis or asthma: Differential diagnosis and treatment. *Respir Care* 1975; 20:1153.

George RB, Light RW, Matthay RA: *Chest medicine.* New York, Churchill Livingstone, 1983.

Goldsmith JR: *Health Effects of Air Pollution.* New York, American Thoracic Society. *Basics of Respiratory Diseases*, vol 4, 1975.

Hedley-Whyte J, Burgess GE, Feeley TW, et al: *Applied Physiology of Respiratory Care.* Boston, Little, Brown & Co, 1976.

Higgins MW, Keller JB, Metzner HL: Smoking, socioeconomic status and chronic respiratory disease. *Am Rev Respir Dis* 1977; 116:403–409.

Joint Committee of the Allergy Foundation of America and the American Thoracic Society: *Asthma: A Practical Guide for Physicians.* New York, National Tuberculosis and Respiratory Disease Association, 1973.

Marcy TW, Matthay RA: Stable asthma, in Kacmarek RM, Stoller JK (eds): *Current Respiratory Care.* Toronto, BC Decker, 1988.

Martin TR, Lewis SW, Albert RK: The prognosis of patients with chronic obstructive pulmonary disease after hospitalization for acute respiratory failure. *Chest* 1982; 82:310–314.

Pare JAP, Fraser RG: *Synopsis of Diseases of the Chest.* Philadelphia, WB Saunders Co, 1983.

Parot S, Miara B, Milic-Emili J, et al: Hypoxemia, hypercardia, and breathing pattern in patients with chronic obstructive pulmonary disease. *Am Rev Respir Dis* 1982; 126:882–886.

Petty TL: *Intensive and Rehabilitative Respiratory Care*, ed 3. Philadelphia, Lea & Febiger, 1982.

Pierson DJ: Exacerbation of chronic bronchitis and emphysema: Ventilatory management, in Kacmarek RM, Stoller JK (eds): *Current Respiratory Care*. Toronto, BC Decker, 1988.

Pontoppidan H, Geffin B, Lowenstein E: *Acute Respiratory Failure in the Adult*. Boston, Little, Brown & Co, 1973.

Rarey KP, Youtsey JW: *Respiratory Patient Care*. Englewood Cliffs, NJ, Prentice-Hall, 1981.

Shapiro BA, Harrison RA, Kacmarek RM, et al: *Clinical Application of Respiratory Care*, ed 3. Chicago, Year Book Medical Publishers, 1985.

Said SI: *The Lung in Relationship to Hormones*. New York, American Thoracic Society, *Basics of Respiratory Diseases*, vol 1, no 3, 1973.

Tisi GM: *Pulmonary Physiology in Clinical Medicine*, ed 2. Baltimore, Williams & Wilkins Co, 1983.

Thurlbeck WM: *Chronic Bronchitis and Emphysema*. New York, American Thoracic Society, *Basics of Respiratory Diseases*, vol 3, no 1, 1974.

Ward J: Cromolyn sodium: A new approach to treatment of asthma. *Heart Lung* 1975; 4:415.

West JB: *Pulmonary Pathophysiology: The Essentials*. Baltimore, Williams & Wilkins Co, 1977.

Whitcomb ME: *The Lung: Normal and Diseased*. St Louis, CV Mosby Co, 1982.

Wintrobe MM, Thorn GW, Adams RD, et al: *Harrison's Principles of Internal Medicine*, ed 7. New York, McGraw-Hill Book Co, 1974.

Witek TJ, Schachter EN: Air pollution and respiratory health. *Respir Care* 1983; 28:442–446.

Chapter 21

Restrictive Lung Diseases

I. General Comments
   A. A restrictive lung disease is any disease in which the ability to inhale is affected. Generally the characteristic feature is an inability to expand the lung fully.
   B. Restrictive diseases of pulmonary origin are frequently associated with an increase in pulmonary fibrous tissue. The result is an overall increase in pulmonary elastance and a decrease in pulmonary compliance.
   C. Characteristic pulmonary function findings (Table 21–1)
      1. Decreased or normal tidal volume (VT).
      2. Decreased or normal residual volume (RV).
      3. Decreased or normal expiratory reserve volume (ERV).
      4. Decreased or normal inspiratory reserve volume (IRV).
      5. Decreased total lung capacity (TLC).
      6. Decreased vital capacity (VC).
      7. Decreased inspiratory capacity (IC).
      8. Decreased or normal functional residual capacity (FRC).
      9. In pure restrictive lung diseases flow rate studies usually are normal; however, flow rates may be decreased when an obstructive component is also present.
      10. Pulmonary and/or thoracic and total compliance is usually severely decreased.
      11. There is a progressive increase in the work of breathing as the severity of the disease increases.
         a. Initially alveolar minute ventilation is normal or increased but, as the disease progresses, alveolar minute ventilation progressively decreases.
         b. Arterial blood gases may follow the same pattern as that seen in obstructive lung disease. The initial presenting symptom may be chronic respiratory alkalosis with hypoxemia but, as the disease progresses, chronic respiratory acidosis with hypoxemia may develop.
   D. Categories of restrictive diseases
      1. Pulmonary
      2. Thoracoskeletal
      3. Neurologic-neuromuscular
      4. Abdominal
II. Pulmonary Restrictive Lung Diseases
   A. Interstitial pulmonary fibrosis: A disease characterized by the excessive formation of connective tissue in the process of repairing chronic or acute tissue injury.
      1. Etiology: Any permanent injury to the lung, inflammation, allergy, and so forth.

TABLE 21–1.

Comparison of Pulmonary Function Study Results in Obstructive and Restrictive Pulmonary Diseases

PFT Study	Obstructive	Restrictive
TLC	↔ or ↑	↓
VC	↔ or ↓	↓
FRC	↑	↔ or ↓
RV	↑	↔ or ↓
RV/TLC	↑	↔
$FEV_1\%$	↓	↔
$MMEFR_{25-75}$	↓	↔ or ↓

2. Type: Localized or diffuse
  a. Causes of localized fibrosis
    (1) Tuberculosis
    (2) Unresolved pneumonias
    (3) Fungal infections
    (4) Abscess formation
  b. Causes of diffuse fibrosis
    (1) Chronic exposure to various inhalants. Specific pneumoconioses are listed in Table 21–2.
    (2) Acute exposure to toxic inhalants may also cause diffuse fibrosis (e.g., chlorine gas, ammonia, polyvinyl chloride, smoke inhalation, radiation therapy).
    (3) Diseases of unknown etiology that often show diffuse fibrosis:
      (a) Hamman-Rich syndrome
      (b) Eosinophilic granuloma
      (c) Sarcoidosis
      (d) Familial fibrocystic dysphagia
      (e) Chronic interstitial pneumonia
      (f) Collagen diseases
3. Pathophysiology
  a. Inflammatory reaction in response to organic or inorganic foreign agents.
  b. Inflammation is followed by cellular infiltration and acute vasculitis with local hemorrhage and thrombus formation, resulting in scar tissue.

TABLE 21–2.

Specific Pneumoconioses

Disease	Causative Agent
Silicosis	Silica dust
Farmer's lung	Moldy hay
Stannosis	Tin dust
Silo-fillers' disease	Nitrogen dioxide
Coal workers' pneumoconioses	Coal dust
Asbestosis	Asbestos
Berylliosis	Beryllium
Siderosis	Iron dust
Talcosis	Talc
Barritosis	Barium
Aluminosis	Aluminum

4. Clinical presentation
   a. Primary symptom: Progressive dyspnea on exertion and ultimately at rest.
   b. Nonproductive cough.
   c. As disease continues, progressive respiratory impairment and often cor pulmonale.
   d. Physical examination findings:
      (1) Clubbing
      (2) Cyanosis
      (3) Restricted chest wall and diaphragmatic movement
      (4) Diffuse, dry, crackling rales
      (5) Increased work of breathing
      (6) Use of accessory muscles of ventilation
      (7) Tachypnea with shallow tidal volumes
   e. Chest x-ray film
      (1) Small lung with large heart and elevated diaphragm
      (2) Fine reticular or nodular pattern involving entire lung but predominantly the lower lobes
   f. Arterial blood gases and pulmonary function studies as outlined in section I.
5. Treatment
   a. Removal of patient from environment causing the fibrotic changes if possible
   b. Therapy for underlying disease entity
   c. Corticosteroids
   d. Immunosuppressants
      (1) Azathioprine
      (2) Cyclophosphamide
   e. Oxygen therapy: As disease progresses, increased dyspnea is reported. Many are relatively refractory to oxygen therapy.
   f. Penicillamine therapy has improved subjective assessment of patients.
   g. Cyclosporine is used in late stages.
   h. Plasmapheresis is effective in a very small number of cases with high titers of immune complexes in later stages.
   i. Total heart-lung transplant has been successful in some cases.
   j. Mechanical ventilation: If these patients progress to mechanical ventilation, tidal volume delivery is limited because of decreased compliance.
      (1) V_T: 8 to 12 ml/kg.
      (2) Rate: 12 to 20/min.
      (3) Inspiratory time: About 1 second.
      (4) $F_{I_{O_2}}$ and positive end-expiratory pressure (PEEP) settings follow normal guidelines.
      (5) See Chapters 36 and 37 for details.
B. Pleural effusion: Accumulation of fluid in pleural space.
   1. Normally the fluid lining of the pleura is produced by the capillary network of the visceral pleural surface, and any excess is removed by the lymphatic system.
   2. Any disturbance in production of this fluid or in its removal can lead to development of pleural effusion.
   3. Primary causes: Inflammation and circulatory disorders.
      a. Malignancy
      b. Congestive heart failure
      c. Infection
      d. Pulmonary infarction
      e. Trauma
   4. The effusion compresses the lung on the affected side.

5. The effusion is gravity dependent and may shift with positional change.
6. Types of effusions
   a. Hydrothorax: A thin clear transudate caused by congestive heart failure, chronic nephritis, or pulmonary neoplasm.
   b. Empyema (pyrothorax): An effusion consisting entirely of pus caused by a bacterial infection.
   c. Hemothorax: Frank blood caused by a malignancy, pulmonary infarction, or ruptured blood vessel.
   d. Chylothorax: Accumulation of chyle resulting from the obstruction or trauma of the thoracic duct.
   e. Fibrothorax: An accumulation of fibrous tissue normally secondary to a prolonged effusion.
7. Treatment
   a. Primary: Removal of fluid from pleural space.
      (1) Thoracentesis or insertion of chest tubes.
      (2) Fluid allowed to reabsorb into pulmonary lymphatic system.
   b. Secondary: Treatment of underlying disease.
C. Pneumothorax: Accumulation of air within the pleural space.
   1. If air enters the pleural space, the pressure within the space changes from subatmospheric to atmospheric or supra-atmospheric pressure.
      a. The increased pressure compresses lung tissue and results in atelectasis.
      b. Ventilation of the lung on the affected side is decreased as a result of elimination of the subatmospheric intrapleural pressure.
   2. Types: Open and under tension.
      a. In an open pneumothorax, there is no buildup of pressure because the gas is allowed to move freely in and out of the pleural space.
      b. A tension pneumothorax results from the presence of a one-way valve, which allows gas only to enter the pleural space, not to leave it. This results in significant increases in pressure within the pleural space.
         (1) Clinical signs
             (a) Increased difficulty in ventilation: If patient is mechanically ventilated, airway pressure increases with each breath.
             (b) Patient's vital signs begin to deteriorate as mean intrathoracic pressure increases.
             (c) Breath sounds are absent on the affected side.
             (d) The affected side is hyperresonant to percussion.
             (e) Trachea and mediastinum may be shifted toward the unaffected side as the extent of tension pneumothorax increases.
             (f) Possible pleuritic pain.
             (g) Dry, hacking cough.
             (h) These clinical signs are more predominant if the patient is using a mechanical ventilator than if he or she is ventilating spontaneously. This is due to the greater pressure gradients developed, forcing more gas into the pleural space.
         (2) Treatment: Decompression of the thorax by chest tube insertion.
D. Cardiogenic pulmonary edema: Active movement of fluid across alveolar capillary membrane into alveoli as a result of increased capillary hydrostatic pressures.
   1. Normally a fine balance exists among capillary colloid osmotic (oncotic) pressure, capillary hydrostatic pressure, interstitial hydrostatic pressure, and interstitial colloid osmotic (oncotic) pressure across the pulmonary capillary bed (see Chapter 15).
   2. Usually a very small net pressure forces fluid into the interstitial space. This interstitial fluid is drained by the lymphatics.

3. If capillary hydrostatic pressure increases significantly, the net pressure forcing fluid into the interstitial space increases and eventually fluid moves directly into the alveoli.
4. Primary cause: Acute left ventricular failure (congestive heart failure).
   a. The hydrostatic pressure of the pulmonary vascular bed is increased because of the inability of the left side of the heart to accept the blood presented to it.
   b. This increased pressure offsets the normal pressure dynamics at the alveolar capillary membrane.
5. Secondary cause: Increased vascular volume causing an increase in pulmonary capillary hydrostatic pressure.
6. Acute right ventricular failure (congestive heart failure)
   a. Systemic edema develops as a result of right ventricular failure.
   b. The inability of the right side of the heart to accept the blood presented to it results in blood pooling in the periphery.
   c. Dependent edema (pedal edema), neck vein distention, and hepatomegaly are common clinical findings.
   d. It is not unlikely for patients with right-sided heart failure to eventually develop left-sided heart failure and those with left-sided heart failure to develop right-sided heart failure.
7. Treatment
   a. Primary: Pharmacologic
      (1) Furosemide (Lasix)
      (2) Morphine
      (3) Digitalis
   b. Interaortic balloon counterpulsation
   c. Oxygen therapy: Frequently high $F_{I_{O_2}}$ is required.
   d. Mask continuous positive airway pressure (CPAP) at 10 to 12 cm H_2O has been helpful in some patients and may avoid intubation if pulmonary edema can be stabilized quickly.
   e. Mechanical ventilation
      (1) Mechanical ventilation with PEEP can both improve and further worsen cardiac function.
      (2) The increased mean airway pressure (as with CPAP) decreases venous return in left-sided heart failure.
      (3) Marked increases in mean airway pressure can markedly reduce pulmonary perfusion and increase deadspace ventilation.
      (4) When mechanical ventilator settings are titrated, markedly increasing minute ventilation should be avoided, because P_{CO_2} raises with hemodynamic instability.
      (5) Stabilization of cardiac function improves the deadspace volume/tidal volume (V_D/V_T) ratio and thus returns P_{CO_2} to normal.
      (6) If increases in minute ventilation result in no change or an increase in P_{CO_2}, lack of pulmonary perfusion is most likely the cause of the P_{CO_2} increase.
      (7) In general, ventilator settings are similar to those of all patients without lung disease.
         (a) Rate: 8 to 12/min
         (b) V_T: 12 to 15 ml/kg
         (c) Inspiratory time: 1 to 1.2 sec
         (d) PEEP: 5 to 10 cm H_2O.
         (e) $F_{I_{O_2}}$: 1.0 until stabilization
      (8) In general, these patients require pharmacologic control during ventilation.

(9) Spontaneous breathing at this stage:
    (a) Diverts up to 40% of cardiac output to ventilatory muscles.
    (b) Enhances $\dot{V}/\dot{Q}$ mismatchings.
    (c) Because of marked ventilatory drive, peak airway pressure limits are frequently met or exceeded.
    (d) May contribute to cardiac instability.

E. Noncardiogenic pulmonary edema
1. The development of interstitial or true pulmonary edema from noncardiogenic origins.
2. Pathophysiologic etiologies
  a. Altered permeability of capillary endothelial cells, allowing an increased quantity of fluid into the interstitial space.
  b. Decreased capillary colloid osmotic pressure, which increases the pressure gradient, allowing more fluid to enter the interstitial space.
  c. Altered lymphatic function, preventing normal drainage of the pulmonary interstitium, thereby allowing fluid to accumulate.
  d. Alveolar epithelial damage, allowing fluid to enter the alveoli.
3. Clinical etiologies
  a. Neurogenic origin
    (1) Neurogenic origin is primarily a result of an acute insult to the central nervous system (CNS).
    (2) It causes an increased sympathetic discharge, leading to a sudden intravascular fluid shift into the pulmonary circulation.
    (3) The imbalance in hydrostatic and osmotic pressures created causes fluid to enter the interstitial space.
  b. Drug overdose
    (1) The exact mechanism poorly defined.
    (2) It is presumed that drugs, especially narcotics and sedatives, have a direct effect on increasing pulmonary capillary membrane permeability.
  c. High-altitude pulmonary edema
    (1) The mechanism is poorly understood.
    (2) It is thought to be the result of severe hypoxemia and vasoconstriction of the microcirculation.
    (3) As blood flows under high pressure through the patent portion of the microvasculature, edema develops.
  d. Reexpansion edema
    (1) It develops after the sudden reexpansion of a lung that had been collapsed for several hours.
    (2) The sudden reexpansion causes a negative pressure in the interstitium, creating a large pressure gradient across the capillary membrane and an increased transudation of fluid.
    (3) The rapid removal of pleural effusion fluid (greater than 1,000 ml) may produce edema.
  e. Pulmonary edema associated with renal disease
    (1) The mechanism is poorly defined.
    (2) It may occur in patients with acute glomerulonephritis or nephrotic syndrome.
    (3) It is also seen in chronically uremic patients and in patients on long-term hemodialysis.
  f. Other clinical conditions known to lead to noncardiogenic pulmonary edema:
    (1) Sepsis
    (2) Shock

(3) Pancreatitis

(4) Toxic gas or smoke inhalation

(5) Aspiration

(6) Pulmonary infections

4. Clinical presentation

   a. Responsive hypoxemia

   b. Decreased compliance

   c. Diffuse atelectasis

   d. Minimal decrease in FRC

5. Treatment (see section II–F)

   a. Oxygen therapy

   b. Fluid therapy

   c. Diuretics

   d. Low levels of PEEP therapy

6. Many consider noncardiogenic pulmonary edema to be the early form of adult respiratory distress syndrome.

F. Adult respiratory distress syndrome (ARDS)

1. Terms representing the same clinical syndrome

   a. Oxygen toxicity

   b. Oxygen pneumonitis

   c. Wet lung

   d. Congestive atelectasis

   e. Stiff lung syndrome

   f. Respiratory lung syndrome

   g. Postpump lung

   h. Posttraumatic pulmonary insufficiency

   i. Shock lung

2. Clinical features of the syndrome's pathophysiologic processes

   a. Refractory hypoxemia (hypoxemia that does not respond to an increasing $F_{I_{O_2}}$)

   b. Decrease in pulmonary compliance

   c. Decrease in FRC

   d. Chest x-ray film: Diffuse alveolar infiltrates throughout entire lung field (honeycomb effect)

   e. Complete reversal of disease process except for any residual fibrotic changes

3. Postmortem pulmonary findings

   a. Beefy lung, which does not collapse on removal from thoracic cavity

   b. Hyaline membrane formation on pulmonary parenchyma

   c. Interstitial edema and fibrosis

   d. Pneumocyte hyperplasia

4. Cause

   a. It is probably a reaction of the respiratory tract to high levels of physiologic stress for prolonged periods. This stress may be associated with any of the organ systems.

   b. Clinical problems associated with the development of ARDS are:

      (1) Oxygen toxicity

      (2) Chest trauma

      (3) Aspiration

      (4) Chemical irritation of respiratory tract

      (5) Blood transfusion

      (6) Emboli formation

      (7) Sepsis

      (8) Shock

      (9) Radiation injury

        (10) Near drowning

        (11) Pancreatitis

5. Pathophysiology of ARDS resulting from oxygen toxicity

   a. F_{IO_2} maintained above 0.50 to 0.60 for prolonged periods may cause acute pulmonary changes (see Chapter 24).

     (1) Interference with pulmonary enzyme systems, which disrupts pulmonary metabolism.

     (2) Type II alveolar cell dysfunction, which results in altered surfactant production.

     (3) Inhibition of mucociliary activity.

     (4) Increased permeability of capillary endothelium.

     (5) Nitrogen washout and atelectasis (absorption atelectasis).

   b. Primary symptoms noted by patient

     (1) Substernal distress

     (2) Cough

     (3) Nausea and vomiting

     (4) Paresthesia

     (5) Shortness of breath

     (6) Tachypnea

     (7) Tachycardia

   c. Functional changes

     (1) Decrease in compliance secondary to:

       (a) Altered surfactant levels

       (b) Dilution of surfactant by transudate

       (c) Atelectasis

     (2) Decrease in FRC secondary to:

       (a) Altered surfactant levels

       (b) Nitrogen washout atelectasis

     (3) Increased work of breathing

     (4) Refractory hypoxemia

   d. Pathophysiology of ARDS resulting from clinical problems presented in section II–F, 4 follows the general pattern seen with oxygen toxicity. The actual mechanism by which these changes develop is unclear.

6. Treatment

   a. Maintain adequate oxygenation state (see Chapter 37).

     (1) Administer PEEP therapy.

     (2) Titrate PEEP in an attempt to reduce F_{IO_2} below 0.50.

     (3) Maintain Po_2 at a minimum of approximately 60 mm Hg.

     (4) Maintain adequate tissue perfusion.

   b. Mechanical ventilation is indicated if the work of breathing becomes excessive and an adequate ventilatory state cannot be maintained.

     (1) In general, the initial setup is similar to the setting of the average patient requiring mechanical ventilation.

       (a) Rate: 8 to 12/min

       (b) V_T: 12 to 15 ml/kg

       (c) Inspiratory time: 1 to 1.2 sec

     (2) As the disease progresses, the lung becomes stiffer and the V_T/rate relationship requires alteration. In addition, physiologic deadspace increases because of destruction of pulmonary capillary blood vessels. As a result:

       (a) Rates more than 12 to 20 may be necessary.

       (b) Tidal volumes less than 10 ml/kg may be necessary.

       (c) Minute ventilation of greater than 15 to 20 L may be necessary.

(3) Alternate ventilatory methods are being used for the treatment of ARDS by some (see Chapter 36 for details).

(a) Airway pressure release ventilation.

(b) Inverse ratio ventilation.

(c) Apneic oxygenation with extracorporeal CO_2 removal.

(d) Hemofiltration (controversial treatment).

(e) Fluid therapy.

(f) Diuretic therapy.

(g) Steroid therapy: In early stages of management, steroids, especially methylprednisolone sodium succinate (Solu-Medrol), may help stabilize endothelial cells and type II pneumocytes if administered in large doses for short periods (controversial treatment).

G. Pneumonia: Pneumonitis caused by a microorganism.

1. Pneumonias are a leading cause of death in the United States and account for 10% of admissions to general medical floors.

2. Pathophysiology of pneumonia

a. Microorganisms cause inflammation of pulmonary mucosa, resulting in edema and phagocytic infiltration.

b. Exudation and consolidation result.

c. Consolidation is typically localized, as in lobar pneumonias.

3. Bacterial pneumonia (Table 21–3)

a. Common clinical signs and symptoms

(1) Abrupt onset (normally)

(2) Very high fevers, with chills, sometimes lasting longer than 20 min

(3) Large volumes of thick, purulent sputum

(4) Frequently tachypnea and tachycardia, sometimes a pleuritic type pain

(5) X-ray film: Consolidation

(6) White blood cell count: Frequently greater than 10,000/cu mm

(7) Hypoxemia secondary to shunting

4. Nonbacterial (viral or fungal) pneumonia (see Table 21–3)

a. Clinical signs and symptoms (occasionally mild and frequently undiagnosed)

(1) Onset normally is very gradual.

(2) Fevers normally are low grade; chills are uncommon.

(3) Sputum production is minimal, usually thin and mucoid.

(4) Tachypnea and tachycardia are rare; pleuritic pain is uncommon.

(5) X-ray film: Consolidation is uncommon.

(6) White blood cell count commonly is less than 10,000/cu mm.

TABLE 21–3.

Comparison of Clinical and Laboratory Manifestations of Bacterial and Viral Pneumonias

Symptom	Bacterial	Viral
Onset	Abrupt	Gradual
Fever	High	Low grade
Chills	Common	Uncommon
Sputum	Purulent, thick	Thin, mucoid
Tachycardia	Frequent	Rare
Hypoxemia	Common	Uncommon
Chest x-ray results	Consolidation	Consolidation uncommon
WBC count	>10,000/cu mm	<10,000/cu mm
Pleuritic pain	Occasional	Uncommon

5. Treatment
   a. Appropriate antibiotic therapy (bacterial and fungal)
   b. Oxygen therapy
   c. Fluid therapy
   d. Aerosol and chest physiotherapy, if indicated
H. Pulmonary embolism
   1. Pulmonary embolism is the occlusion of the pulmonary artery or one of its branches by a substance carried in the blood, normally a blood clot.
   2. A blood clot that is attached to its site of origin is referred to as a *thrombus*. Once detached, it is referred to as an *embolus*.
   3. The actual substance may be fat, blood, air, amniotic fluid, or a tissue fragment.
   4. Etiology and pathogenesis
      a. The most common sites of thrombus formation are the deep veins of the lower extremities and pelvis and within the right side of the heart.
      b. Thrombus development is most prevalent in patients who are immobilized due to pain or who are debilitated, paralyzed, or require prolonged bed rest.
      c. Factors facilitating thrombus formation
         (1) Abnormal vessel wall
         (2) Stagnation of blood
         (3) Increased coagulability
      d. Dependent lung regions are most commonly involved with pulmonary emboli.
      e. Pulmonary infarction occurs in about 10% of patients with pulmonary emboli, especially if there is a history of cardiac disease.
   5. Pathophysiology
      a. Deadspace ventilation is significantly increased.
      b. Total ventilation markedly increases in an effort to maintain normal P_{CO_2}.
      c. A minute volume–P_{CO_2} disparity develops (see Chapter 12).
      d. With large emboli, pulmonary artery pressures increase, especially if there is underlying cardiac disease.
   6. Clinical presentation
      a. Patient has dyspnea and chest pain.
      b. Hemoptysis may develop.
      c. Frequently cough, faintness, and anxiety accompany pulmonary embolus.
      d. Thrombophlebitis is often noted (frequently at the site of embolus formation).
      e. If a massive embolus is present, there may be:
         (1) Tachypnea
         (2) Tachycardia
         (3) Cyanosis
         (4) Decreased breath sounds
         (5) Wheezing and rales
         (6) Pleural friction rub
      f. Less common findings are:
         (1) Fever
         (2) Cardiac arrhythmias
         (3) Shock
   7. Chest x-ray films
      a. In some cases decreased lung volume, atelectasis, pleural effusion, and signs of pulmonary infarction may be present.
      b. In rare cases there is a local reduction in vascular markings and an enlarged pulmonary artery.

8. Laboratory findings
   a. Lung volumes and capacities are decreased.
   b. Flow studies are usually normal.
   c. Arterial blood gases usually reveal hypoxemia with a normal acid base balance or a respiratory alkalosis.
   d. Electrocardiogram may reveal arrhythmias.
9. Radioisotope lung scanning
   a. Ventilation/perfusion scans may help differentiate pulmonary embolism from other perfusion abnormalities.
   b. Findings must be correlated with patient's clinical findings and history.
10. Pulmonary angiography is considered definitive in the diagnosis of pulmonary embolism.
11. Treatment
    a. Intravenous streptokinase or urokinase.
    b. Anticoagulation therapy with heparin.
    c. Oxygen therapy.
    d. Intubation and ventilation in severe cases.
    e. Occasionally embolectomy is performed; however, this procedure is controversial.

I. Pulmonary alveolar proteinosis
   1. A disease characterized by alveoli filled with a liquid high in protein and lipid.
   2. Alveolar walls are normal but only scattered macrophages are noted.
   3. Pathogenesis
      a. The origin is unknown, but it is theorized that type II alveolar epithelial cells produce an excess of surfactant, lipid, and protein.
      b. This substance is poorly cleared by defective macrophages.
   4. Prevalence
      a. Most commonly develops in age groups 20 to 50 years, with 2:1 male/female ratio
      b. Some cases described in infants
   5. Clinical manifestations
      a. One third of all patients are asymptomatic.
      b. Common clinical findings:
         (1) Shortness of breath on exertion
         (2) Cough
         (3) Fatigue
         (4) Weight loss
         (5) Pleuritic pain
         (6) Possible low-grade fever
         (7) Clubbing of digits
   6. Chest x-ray film reveals infiltrates in perihilar regions and bases of the lung.
   7. Pulmonary function studies may be normal but diffusing capacity is decreased.
   8. Diagnosis is made primarily by open lung biopsy, bronchoalveolar lavage, or the measurement of lactic dehydrogenase levels.
   9. Prognosis
      a. Clinical course is variable.
      b. Disease may spontaneously resolve but reappear at a later date.
      c. One third of patients die, primarily due to predisposition to infection.
   10. Treatment
      a. No specific therapy is defined.
      b. Corticosteroids are used but are controversial.
      c. Lung lavage is helpful in some patients.

III. Thoracoskeletal Restrictive Lung Diseases
   A. Deformities of thoracic cage that result in limited movement of the chest demonstrate pulmonary function patterns consistent with restrictive lung disease.
   B. If the deformity is severe enough, a significant increase in the work of breathing results.
   C. Increased work of breathing eventually leads to hypoxemia, hypercapnia, and possible heart failure.
   D. Most commonly encountered thoracic abnormalities leading to restrictive lung disease are:
      1. Scoliosis: Gradual curvature of vertebral columnn in lateral plane of body.
         a. Is one of the most common thoracic deformities.
         b. May occur at various levels of the vertebral column.
         c. May develop with age as a result of poor posture.
      2. Kyphosis: Posterior curvature of thoracic vertebral column, resulting in a bony hump.
         a. Frequently develops in older individuals with degenerative osteoarthritis.
         b. May develop in individuals with chronic obstructive pulmonary disease.
      3. Kyphoscoliosis: Combination of thoracic scoliosis and kyphosis.
         a. In severe cases of kyphoscoliosis, one lung becomes severely compressed, the other overdistended.
         b. Cardiopulmonary disability may be very pronounced in severe kyphoscoliosis.
   E. Treatment
      1. No primary treatment is indicated in most cases.
      2. Scoliosis may be treated surgically.
      3. Most treatment centers on secondary pulmonary problems (e.g., pneumonia, asthma)
      4. Some patients with severe kyphoscoliosis develop progressive ventilatory muscle weakness and fatigue and may require nocturnal mechanical ventilatory assistance and oxygen therapy.
      5. During acute pulmonary problems that require mechanical ventilation, rates and tidal volume settings differ from normal because of decreased lung volumes.
         (a) Rate: More than 12 to 18/min
         (b) V_T: less than 10 to 12 ml/kg
         (c) Inspiratory time: 1.0 sec
IV. Neurologic-Neuromuscular Restrictive Lung Diseases
   A. Weakness or paralysis of the muscles of ventilation results in a pulmonary function pattern consistent with restrictive lung disease.
   B. Myasthenia gravis: A disease of the myoneural junction in which transmission of impulses across the motor end-plate is inhibited.
      1. Etiology: Unknown. Functionally it appears that acetylcholine is improperly released, synthesized, or prematurely hydrolyzed before crossing the neuromuscular junction (see Chapter 8).
      2. The disease is most common in women in their 20s to 40s, but it affects individuals of both sexes and of all ages, with about 10% of patients having a tumor of the thymus gland.
      3. The disease is manifested by generalized muscle weakness and most commonly demonstrates a descending paralysis.
      4. The primary symptoms normally are ocular, progressing to facial muscle weakness or paralysis followed by pharyngeal and laryngeal weakness and finally respiratory muscle weakness.
      5. Patients frequently present with a chief complaint of easy fatigability.

6. Diagnosis
    a. Diagnosis is based primarily on history and symptomatology.
    b. The administration of a parasympathomimetic of the cholinesterase inhibitor type confirms the diagnosis. Increased muscle strength is normally noted shortly after the administration of the drug.
7. Treatment
    a. Patients are maintained with cholinesterase inhibitors therapy.
        (1) Neostigmine (Prostigmine) is the drug of choice, but also:
        (2) Pyridostigmine (Mestinon)
        (3) Ambenonium (Mytelase)
    b. Treatment with atropine to reverse the side effects of the cholinesterase inhibitor.
    c. Thymectomy is performed in severe cases. In some patients complete remission has been reported.
    d. A 10-day course of adrenocorticotropic hormone (ACTH) is prescribed. Symptoms deteriorate during administration; however, remission is frequent after a 10-day course.
    e. In severe cases, intubation and mechanical ventilation are used as supportive measures until drug therapy is titrated.
8. Myasthenic vs. cholinergic crisis
    a. An acute exacerbation of the disease process producing weakness is termed a *myasthenic crisis*.
    b. An acute decrease in muscle strength as a result of the excessive use of cholinesterase inhibitors is termed a *cholinergic crisis*.
    c. The Tensilon (generic name edrophonium chloride) test is used to differentiate between a myasthenic and cholinergic crisis. Tensilon is a short-acting (5-min) cholinesterase inhibitor.
        (1) If the patient is suffering from a myasthenic crisis, the administration of Tensilon will improve muscle strength.
        (2) If a cholinergic crisis is present, Tensilon will increase muscle weakness and exacerbate symptomatology.
        (3) Muscle strength can be evaluated by serial vital capacity or maximum inspiratory pressure (MIP) measurements.
9. Monitoring of cardiopulmonary status
    a. Patients in acute exacerbation require very close cardiopulmonary monitoring.
    b. Evaluation of the patient's ventilatory reserve (see Chapter 18) is used to determine changes in ventilatory muscle strength.
    c. Vital capacity is monitored as frequently as every hour in acute situations.
    d. Deterioration of the vital capacity may signal the need for further medical intervention.
C. Guillain-Barré syndrome: Polyneuritis primarily affecting the peripheral motor and sensory neurons.
    1. The etiology is unclear. The disease may be viral or traumatic in nature. An increase in the number of cases has been reported following vaccination against poliomyelitis and swine flu.
    2. The syndrome affects all ages but is more prevalent in adults.
    3. The signs and symptoms show a symmetric ascending pattern of sensory abnormalities that may progress to actual paralysis.
    4. The disease is normally self-limiting and is reversible with time. The amount of residual effects is dependent on the extent of demyelination occurring during the active disease state.

5. Diagnosis is made by the presentation of the disease, a high protein content in the cerebral spinal fluid, and the reversible nature of the disease.

6. Treatment is purely symptomatic, the patient frequently requiring ventilatory support.

7. As with myasthenia gravis, careful monitoring of the patient's ventilatory reserves is indicated.

D. Other neuromuscular or neurologic diseases that may show a restrictive lung disease pattern
  1. Spinal cord diseases
     a. Paraplegia or quadriplegia
     b. Poliomyelitis
  2. Tetanus
  3. Muscular dystrophy
  4. Tick bite paralysis
  5. Congenital myotonia

E. Ventilatory management
  1. Some of these patients require mechanical ventilation for varying periods of time.
  2. Unless compounding pulmonary problems develop, the lungs of these patients are normal. As a result, mechanical ventilation is relatively uncomplicated.
  3. Many of these patients want to feel the ventilator expand their lungs; thus, tidal volume should be large, 12 to 15 ml/kg or more.
  4. As a result, the rate is frequently slow, 8 to 10 min.
  5. All other variables are titrated, based on the patient's response.

V. Abdominal Restrictive Lung Diseases
  A. Increased size of abdominal contents results in limited movement and elevation of the diaphragm.
  B. The limited diaphragmatic movement will demonstrate pulmonary function findings consistent with those of restrictive lung disease.
  C. Conditions that may show a restrictive pattern
     1. Abdominal tumors
     2. Obesity
     3. Third-trimester pregnancy
     4. Diaphragmatic hernias
     5. Ascites
  D. Pickwickian syndrome
     1. It is also referred to as obesity-hypoventilation syndrome.
     2. The syndrome is characterized by:
        a. Severe obesity
        b. Alveolar hypoventilation (more pronounced with sleep), with episodes of sleep apnea
        c. Somnolence
        d. Severe hypoxemia (more pronounced with sleep)
        e. Polycythemia
        f. Pulmonary hypertension (not related to hypoxemia)
        g. Cor pulmonale
     3. Etiology is unclear.
        a. Weight loss may reverse the syndrome.
        b. A high percentage of patients experience upper airway obstruction during sleep, especially in the supine position. The obstruction is believed to be soft tissue obstruction.

4. Frequently the hypoxemia and hypoventilation develop only during sleep.
   a. A significant decrease in total compliance is present at all times and is decreased further when the subject assumes the supine position.
   b. This results in an increased work of breathing, followed by decreased tidal volumes. This, coupled with possible soft tissue upper airway obstruction, leads to hypoventilation and hypoxemia.
   c. The sleep of these patients is commonly broken and restless, leading to generalized somnolence.
5. Treatment
   a. Primary treatment is weight loss.
   b. Respiratory stimulants have been used but with questionable success.
   c. Tracheostomy may be done when obstruction is identified by sleep studies.
   d. Continuous positive airway pressure by nasal mask helps to relieve airway obstruction and prevents arterial desaturation and hypercarbia at night.

VI. Smoke Inhalation and Carbon Monoxide Poisoning
   A. Smoke inhalation
      1. Etiology: The inhalation of byproducts of a fire (smoke and other noxious gases).
         a. Aldehydes
         b. Oxides of nitrogen and sulfur
         c. Ammonia
      2. Pathophysiology
         a. Edema, congestion, sloughing of mucosal membranes of the oral and nasal pharynx, larynx, trachea, and bronchi
         b. Obliterative bronchiolitis and alveolar edema
         c. Development of pulmonary edema
         d. Atelectasis caused by airway obstruction with fibrin, edema, fluid, carbon particles, white blood cells, and epithelial debris
      3. Clinical presentation (it may take 24 to 48 hours for symptoms to develop fully)
         a. Coughing and dyspnea
         b. Hypoxemia
         c. Tachypnea and tachycardia
         d. Facial burns, singed nasal hairs, stridor, and grunting (all indicative of upper airway burns)
         e. Results of x-ray studies are normal for the first 24 to 48 hours; however, signs of pulmonary edema, atelectasis, and infiltrates subsequently develop.
      4. Treatment
         a. Establishment of an artificial airway. This is imperative if upper airway burns accompany the smoke inhalation. If an airway is not established early, subsequent edema may prevent cannulation of the airway.
         b. Oxygen therapy (100% if CO poisoning is also present)
         c. Fluid and electrolyte therapy
         d. Bronchodilator therapy
         e. Steroid therapy
         f. Antibiotic therapy
         g. Mechanical ventilation if pulmonary burns present
            (1) Since pulmonary burns result in severe mucosal edema, air trapping and auto-PEEP frequently develops
            (2) As a result, mechanical rates should be low, 8 to 10/min, and expiratory times should be long.
            (3) In general, the approach used is similar to that in chronic obstructive pulmonary disease (see Chapter 20).

B. Carbon monoxide poisoning
   1. A result of inspiring byproducts of the incomplete combustion of carbon or carbon-containing material
   2. Pathophysiology
      a. Carbon monoxide combines strongly with hemoglobin to form carboxyhemoglobin (hemoglobin's affinity for CO is 210 times that of O_2).
      b. The total capability of the organism to carry oxygen to the tissues is reduced (anemic hypoxia).
      c. In addition, the oxyhemoglobin dissociation curve is shifted to the left, further limiting the amount of O_2 available at the tissue level.
      d. The likelihood of tissue hypoxia increases as COHb% sat increases.
   3. Clinical manifestations (symptomatology based on carboxyhemoglobin levels):
      a. Normally asymptomatic: less than 20%.
      b. Headache, exertional dyspnea, impaired judgment, nausea and vomiting: 20% to 60%.
      c. Loss of consciousness, convulsions, deep coma: 60% to 80%.
   4. X-ray findings: Chest x-ray film may show abnormalities consistent with pulmonary edema, usually interstitial in location.
   5. Diagnosis
      a. Analysis of arterial blood for carboxyhemoglobin levels.
      b. History.
      c. Frequently a metabolic acidosis caused by lactic acid accumulation is noted.
   6. Treatment
      a. Oxygen therapy: One-hundred percent O_2 is indicated until COHb% levels reach 10% or less. Increasing the arterial Po_2 decreases the half-life of COHb%. On inhalation of room air, the half-life of COHb is about 5 to 6 hours, whereas the inhalation of 100% O_2 decreases the half-life to about 90 min. Hyperbaric conditions (3 atm) can decrease the half-life of COHb to 23 min.
      b. With high COHb levels (> 40%–50%), intubation and mechanical ventilation may be necessary.
VII. Drug-induced Pulmonary Disease
   A. Many drugs used in the management of various problems have been linked to pulmonary side effects.
   B. Pulmonary response is usually one of three types:
      1. Chronic pneumonitis with fibrosis
      2. Allergic reactions
      3. Acute lung injury
   C. Response and magnitude of a response are dependent on many factors.
      1. Individual susceptibility
      2. Dose dependency
      3. Association with other therapies
         a. Oxygen
         b. Gamma irradiation
   D. The group of drugs most commonly inducing a pulmonary reaction are cytotoxic drugs used in chemotherapy for cancer. Specific agents commonly causing problems are:
      1. Antibiotics
         a. Bleomycin
         b. Mitomycin
         c. Zinostatin (neocarzinostatin)
      2. Alkylating agents
         a. Busulfan
         b. Cyclophosphamide

     c. Chlorambucil
     d. Melphalan
   3. Nitrosources
     a. Carmustine (BCNU)
     b. Semustine (methyl-CCNU)
     c. Lomustine (CCNU)
     d. Chlorozotocin
   4. Antimetabolites
     a. Methotrexate
     b. Azathioprine
     c. Mercaptopurine
     d. Cytarabine (cytosine arabinoside)
   5. Miscellaneous
     a. Procarbazine
     b. VM-26
     c. Vinblastine
     d. Vindesine
E. Other agents that have been reported to produce pulmonary side effects are:
   1. Antibacterial agents
     a. Nitrofurantoin
     b. Amphotericin
     c. Sulfasalazine
   2. Acetylsalicylic acid
   3. Opiates
     a. Heroin
     b. Methadone
   4. Sedatives
     a. Ethylorvynol
     b. Chlordiazepoxide
   5. Diuretics (hydrochorthiazide)
   6. Major tranquilizers
     a. Haloperidol
     b. Fluphenazine
   7. Antiarrhythmics
     a. Aminodarone
     b. Lidocaine
     c. Tocainide
   8. Miscellaneous
     a. Gold salts
     b. Penicillamine
     c. Colchicine

BIBLIOGRAPHY

Albert RK: Factors affecting transvascular fluid and protein movement in pulmonary edema and ARDS. *Semin Respir Med* 1981; 2:109–113.

Amandus HE, et al: The pneumoconioses: Methods of measuring progression. *Chest* 1973; 63:736.

Bates DV, Macklem PT, Christie RV: *Respiratory Function in Disease,* ed 2. Philadelphia, WB Saunders Co, 1971.

Bendixen HH, et al: *Respiratory Care.* St Louis, CV Mosby Co, 1965.

Brigham KL: Primary (high permeability) pulmonary edema. *Semin Respir Med* 1983; 4:285–288.

Brigham KL: Therapy of pulmonary edema. *Semin Respir Med* 1983; 4:313–316.

Cherniack RM, Cherniack L: *Respiration in Health and Disease*, ed 3. Philadelphia, WB Saunders Co, 1983.

Cooper JAD, White DA, Matthay RA: Drug-induced pulmonary disease, Part 1. *Am Rev Respir Dis* 1986; 133:321–340.

Cooper JAD, White DA, Matthay RA: Drug-induced pulmonary disease, Part 2. *Am Rev Respir Dis* 1986; 13:488–505.

Crofton J, Douglas A: *Respiratory Diseases*, ed 2. Boston, Blackwell Scientific Publications, 1975.

Cushing R: Pulmonary infections. *Heart Lung* 1976; 5:611.

Farzan S: *A Concise Handbook of Respiratory Diseases*. Reston, Va, Reston Publishing Co, 1978.

Fink JN, et al.: Clinical survey of pigeon breeders. *Chest* 1972; 62:277.

George RB, Light RW, Matthay RA: *Chest Medicine*. New York, Churchill Livingstone, 1983.

Gracey DR: Adult respiratory distress syndrome. *Heart Lung* 1975; 4:280.

Griswold K, Guanci MM, Ropper AH: An approach to the care of patients with Guillain-Barré syndrome. *Heart Lung* 1984; 13:66–72.

Hudson LD: Ventilatory management of patients with adult respiratory distress syndrome. *Semin Respir Med* 1981; 2:128–139.

Hycrs TM: Pathogenesis of adult respiratory distress syndrome: Current concepts. *Semin Respir Med* 1981; 2:104–108.

Kacmarek RM, Stoller J (eds): *Current Respiratory Care*. Toronto, BC Decker, 1988.

Kealy SL: Respiratory care in Guillaine-Barré syndrome. *Am J Nurs* 1977; 22:58.

Lakshminarayan S, Stanford RE, Petty TL: Prognosis after recovery from adult respiratory distress syndrome. *Am Rev Respir Dis* 1976; 113:7.

Mathewson HS: Oxygen: The specific antidote to carbon monoxide. *Respir Care* 1982; 27:986–987.

Murray JF, Nadel JA: *Textbook of Respiratory Medicine*. Philadelphia, WB Saunders Co, 1988, parts 1 and 2.

Pore JA, Fraser RG: *Synopsis of Diseases of the Chest*. Philadelphia, WB Saunders Co, 1983.

Petterson JE, Stewart RD: Absorption and elimination of carbon monoxide by inactive young men. *Arch Environ Health* 1970; 21:165–171.

Petty TL: Adult respiratory distress syndrome: Historical perspective and definition. *Semin Respir Med* 1981; 2:99–103.

Petty TL: *Intensive and Rehabilitative Care*, ed 3. Philadelphia, Lea & Febiger, 1982.

Safar P (ed): *Respiratory Therapy*. Philadelphia, FA Davis Co, 1965.

Selecky PA, Ziment I: Prolonged respirator support for the treatment of intractable myasthenia gravis. *Chest* 1974; 65:207.

Shapiro BA, et al: Case study: Myasthenia gravis. *Respir Care* 1974; 19:460.

Shapiro BA, Harrison RA, Kacmarek RM, et al: *Clinical Application of Respiratory Care*, ed 3. Chicago, Year Book Medical Publishers, 1985.

Shulman JA: Errors and hazards in the diagnosis and treatment of bacterial pneumonias. *Ann Intern Med* 1965; 62:41.

Snider GL: *Clinical Pulmonary Medicine*. Boston, Little, Brown & Co, 1981.

Solliday NH, Shapiro BA, Gracey DR: Adult respiratory distress syndrome. *Chest* 1976; 69:207.

Tisi GM: *Pulmonary Physiology in Clinical medicine*, ed 2. Baltimore, Williams & Wilkins Co, 1983.

Urbanitle JS: Carbon monoxide poisoning. *Prog Clin Biol Res* 1981; 51:355–385.

Whitcomb ME: *The Lung: Normal and Diseased*. St Louis, CV Mosby Co, 1982.

Wintrobe MM, Thorn GW, Adams RD, et al: *Harrison's Principles of Internal Medicine*, ed 7. New York, McGraw-Hill Book Co, 1974.

Ziskind MM: *The Acute Bacterial Pneumonia in the Adult*. New York, American Lung Association, 1974.

Chapter 22

Pulmonary Rehabilitation

I. Definition
- Pulmonary rehabilitation was defined in 1974 by the American College of Chest Physicians as:

an art of medical practice wherein an individually tailored, multidisciplinary program is formulated which through accurate diagnosis, therapy, emotional support, and education, stabilizes or reverses both the physio- and psychopathology of pulmonary diseases and attempts to return the patient to the highest possible functional capacity allowed by his pulmonary handicap and overall life situation.*

II. Pulmonary Rehabilitation Program
- A pulmonary rehabilitation program is structured according to the needs of the patient population being serviced as well as the resources available to the institution.
  A. Community assessment and planning before a program is started are crucial
  1. Assess the demographic profile of patients in the target community.
  2. Evaluate physician interest and awareness.
  3. Identify potential competition.
  4. Investigate transportation options for outpatients.
  5. Develop a marketing plan.
  B. Assessment of hospital resources
  1. Determine available vs. needed space and equipment.
  2. Identify clinical personnel desired vs. personnel available.
  3. Discuss financial expectations of the program.
  C. Alternatives in program structure
  1. Inpatient pulmonary rehabilitation
     a. Individual or group education and breathing retraining are scheduled for the patient in a general acute care unit, 5 to 7 days/week.
     b. Individual low-level bedside or ambulatory exercise is instituted.
     c. Patients may be prepared for follow-up in the outpatient phase.
     d. Few are structured as comprehensive multidisciplinary 1- to 2-week inpatient programs due to reimbursement limitations.
  2. Outpatient pulmonary rehabilitation
     a. Usually these programs involve two or three visits per week, but program lengths vary from 4 to 12 weeks.

*From the American Thoracic Society: *Am Rev Respir Dis* 1981; 124:663–666.

   b. Individual or small group (two to five patients) exercise and educational sessions are instituted.
   c. These programs are usually multidisciplinary.
3. Home-based pulmonary rehabilitation
   a. These programs may include education, breathing retraining, and a simple exercise routine.
   b. They may be included in the home care services of visiting nursing agencies or respiratory equipment providers.
   c. They are significantly less comprehensive in scope than hospital or clinic-based programs, with visits often less than once each week.
   d. They may be the only alternative for the homebound patient or when nearby hospitals are without a pulmonary rehabilitation program.
4. Office-based pulmonary rehabilitation
   a. These programs may include some components of outpatient programs, such as education, breathing retraining, and exercise testing and prescription.
   b. Usually they are implemented by a pulmonary physician or pulmonary nurse specialist.
D. Multidisciplinary team approach
   1. Clinicians from a variety of health care disciplines are necessary participants in a pulmonary rehabilitation program (see section II–E).
   2. If some or all of these disciplines are not represented, a simple team composed of the physician and respiratory therapist, nurse, or physical therapist can provide thorough pulmonary rehabilitation in any of the previously mentioned settings.
   3. Team members should have special interest or training in meeting the needs of chronic obstructive pulmonary disease (COPD) patients as well as skill in patient assessment and education in their respective clinical areas.
   4. Team conferences:
      a. Are attended by all team members at regular intervals (e.g., weekly or monthly).
      b. Provide a forum for initial goal setting and plan formation and for ongoing discussion of patients' progress and discharge goals.
      c. Facilitate dissemination of general program information to team members (quality assurance findings, policy and procedure changes, etc.).
E. Team members and their roles
   1. Pulmonary physician
      a. Serves as program medical director.
      b. Participates in the initial screening of patients.
         (1) Reviews the medical history, medications, and diagnostic test results.
         (2) Supervises and interprets the initial exercise test.
         (3) Performs or reviews the physical examination.
      c. Represents the program to hospital administration, medical staff colleagues, and the community.
      d. May initiate, review, participate in, and evaluate pulmonary rehabilitation research.
   2. Program coordinator (registered respiratory therapist, registered nurse, or registered physical therapist)
      a. May serve in combined role as program coordinator and primary patient care giver.
         (1) Develops and revises program policies and procedures.

(2) Implements daily program activities.
   (a) Assesses at each visit patient's weight, heart and lung sounds, respiratory and other symptoms, sleep, appetite, and adherence to home medication and exercise regime.
   (b) Carries out monitored exercise sessions.
(3) Maintains written and verbal communication with each patient's referring physician.
(4) Participates in the development and implementation of program marketing plan.
(5) Collects and reports program quality assurance data.
(6) Reviews current pulmonary rehabilitation literature and updates protocols and equipment as indicated.
(7) Represents the program to other hospital departments and to the community.

b. Provides patient education on select topics.
(1) Medications
(2) Respiratory anatomy and pathophysiology of chronic pulmonary disease
(3) Complications of chronic pulmonary disease
(4) Travel
(5) Sexuality
(6) Activities of daily living
(7) Breathing retraining and relaxation techniques
(8) Oxygen therapy and bronchial hygiene techniques

c. Performs assistance as needed with activities of daily living (inpatient program).
d. Assesses the need for home care (supplies and personnel).
e. May participate in exercise testing.

3. Dietitian
a. Evaluates nutritional status of patients.
(1) Weight
(2) Interview (diet history)
(3) Review of food record or calorie count
(4) Laboratory indices (total protein, albumin, cholesterol, phosphate, magnesium, transferrin, calcium values)
(5) Anthropometric measurements (e.g., skinfold thickness, arm muscle circumference)

b. Recommends individual dietary modifications, including calories, components, and supplements, if indicated.
c. Instructs patient and family on diet.
d. Develops individualized sample menus.

4. Social worker
a. Screens patients and families for evidence of psychosocial problems warranting referral or further treatment.
b. Assesses and discusses with patients and families the impact of COPD on self-esteem, lifestyle, and relationships.
c. Provides information on community resources to meet social, vocational, financial, transportation, and counseling needs.

5. Psychologist or psychiatrist
a. Most often serves the pulmonary rehabilitation program on a consultant basis for select patients and families.
b. Administers and interprets psychologic tests.
c. Conducts ongoing group or individual therapy.

d. Recommends or prescribes psychotropic medications (anxiolytic, antidepressants and sedative hypnotics).

6. Occupational therapist
   a. Evaluates the impact of chronic pulmonary disease on the patient's ability to perform activities of daily living as well as home maintenance, social, and vocational activities.
   b. Provides instruction and opportunities for practice in energy conservation and work simplification techniques.
   c. Includes instruction on coordinated breathing strategies.
   d. Recommends vocational alternatives or modifications for continued employment in the same setting.

7. Physical therapist
   a. Serves as program coordinator and primary patient care giver in some institutions.
   b. Teaches relaxation and biofeedback techniques.
   c. Provides consultation, treatment, and modified exercise recommendations for pulmonary rehabilitation patients with specific neuromusculoskeletal conditions.
   d. May design warm-up, strengthening, and toning exercise routines.

8. Pharmacist
   a. Provides consultation to program staff on medication selections, actions, and interactions.
   b. May provide group education to patients and families on medications.

9. Exercise physiologist
   a. Participates in exercise testing and prescription.
   b. May assist in conducting or monitoring group exercise sessions.

10. Clergyman
    a. May receive referrals as a consultant for patients and families with identified spiritual concerns.
    b. Provides spiritual counseling on issues such as death, dying, and quality of life.

III. Evaluation of the Pulmonary Rehabilitation Candidate
   A. Thorough screening of each patient is essential to the optimal planning and success of the individual treatment program.
   B. The ideal candidate meets the following criteria:
      1. Correctly diagnosed with symptomatic respiratory disease, usually COPD.
      2. Willing and motivated to participate in the program.
      3. Free from concurrent medical problems precluding safe, successful program participation.
         a. Recent myocardial infarction or ischemia
         b. Uncontrolled dysrhythmias
         c. Febrile or symptomatic infectious illness
         d. Recent gastrointestinal (GI) bleeding
         e. Severe disabling neuromusculoskeletal condition
         f. Psychiatric disorder or substance abuse, with significant impairment in concentration, motivation, judgment, or mood
   C. The program medical director and primary patient care giver (usually the program coordinator) should participate in the initial evaluation visit.
      1. The patient is given a physical examination (see Chapter 18).
      2. A patient and family medical history interview is conducted.
         a. Respiratory symptoms: Onset, duration, severity, and ameliorating or aggravating factors
         b. Family history of respiratory problems

      c. Childhood respiratory health and illness
      d. Environmental history
         (1) Travel
         (2) Occupations
         (3) Smoking
         (4) Allergies
      e. General medical and surgical history
    3. The goals and expectations of the patient and family are determined.
      a. Symptom control
      b. Functional improvement
    4. The program's overall goals, activities, and expected benefits (Table 22–1) as well as limitations and risks should be explained verbally and may be detailed on an informed written consent or program contract form.
  D. Preentry diagnostic tests should include:
    1. Complete pulmonary function test
      a. To establish correct diagnosis and severity of obstructive lung disease.
      b. To assess response to bronchodilators.
      c. To establish occupational disability.
    2. Chest roentgenogram
      a. To rule out acute cardiopulmonary congestion related to infection, heart failure, or interstitial lung disease.
      b. To assist in the diagnosis of cor pulmonale.
      c. To assist in assessment of the severity of hyperinflation and diaphragm flattening.
    3. Laboratory data
      a. Arterial blood gas analysis
      b. Laboratory and blood chemistry indices
         (1) Complete blood cell count
         (2) Electrolytes values
         (3) Nutritional-metabolic indices
         (4) Theophylline level (if applicable)
         (5) Sputum analysis (optional)
  E. A variety of reliable and valid tools can be used to assess psychologic status, motivation, and several aspects of quality of life in patients with chronic pulmonary disease.
    1. The Minnesota Multiphasic Personality Inventory (MMPI) assesses ten major dimensions of emotional distress and personality disturbance.

TABLE 22–1.

Benefits of Comprehensive
Pulmonary Rehabilitation

Increased physical energy and endurance
  Increased exercise capacity
  Improved ability to perform daily activities
Decreased anxiety and depression
  Improved understanding of the condition and
    its management
  Enhanced self-care and family support
  Acquisition of new coping skills
Improved quality of life
Decreased respiratory symptoms
Decreased hospital days
Decreased mortality

---

2. The Profile of Mood States (POMS) is a list of adjectives rated on a Likert-type scale to indicate recent mood.
3. The Katz Adjustment Scale (KAS) is composed of five subscales that focus on social adjustment, recreational activities, and general psychologic disturbance.
4. The Sickness Impact Profile (SIP) measures the effect of illness on behavioral function in 12 areas of daily living such as ambulation, home maintenance, social interaction, communication, alertness, and recreational pastime.
5. The Quality of Well-Being Scale (QWBS) is a subcomponent of the General Health Status index. The scaled score is derived based on symptom complexes and weighted functional level and indicates health-related life quality at one point in time.
6. The Eysenck Personality Inventory (EPI) is a simple instrument used to assess basic pertinent personality traits, such as extroversion and neuroticism.
7. The Additive Daily Activities Profile Test (ADAPT) is a self-administered test on which patients identify which of 105 activities (listed in order of descending estimated volume of oxygen utilization [VO_2] requirement) they currently perform and which they have stopped due to respiratory limitations.
8. Rotter's Locus of Control Scale evaluates the extent to which an individual perceives internal or external factors as responsible for outcomes and events in his or her life.

F. Exercise testing in pulmonary rehabilitation should include:
   1. Indications and purposes
      a. To diagnose the etiology of exercise limitation.
         (1) Rule out primary or concomitant cardiac disease (e.g., exercise-induced ischemia or dysrhythmias).
         (2) Assess ventilatory response to exercise.
         (3) Identify exertional hypoxemia (oxygen desaturation).
         (4) Rule out exercise-induced asthma.
      b. To determine the functional capacity and severity of exercise impairment.
         (1) Document baseline exercise capacity.
         (2) Obtain data for exercise prescription.
         (3) Establish occupational disability.
      c. To assess the effects of therapy.
         (1) Document postprogram exercise capacity (i.e., measure results of training).
         (2) Assess symptomatic or objective response to specific therapy (e.g., medication, oxygen therapy, and changes in exercise-induced bronchospasm).
   2. Contraindications
      a. Absolute
         (1) Heart failure
         (2) Unstable angina
         (3) Acute myocarditis
         (4) Uncontrolled hypertension (resting systolic pressure greater than 190 mm Hg, diastolic pressure greater than 120 mm Hg)
         (5) Myocardial ischemic changes on ECG not attributable to medications
         (6) Acute exacerbation of COPD
         (7) Other acute medical illnesses (e.g., febrile condition, recent pulmonary embolism or thrombophlebitis, GI bleeding).
      b. Relative
         (1) Aortic valve disease
         (2) Recent myocardial infarction (less than 6 weeks earlier)

(3) Medication effects (tachycardia greater than 120 beats/min, ST segment abnormalities)

(4) Seizure disorder

(5) Respiratory failure or insufficiency

(6) Cerebrovascular disease

3. Patient safety and monitoring during exercise testing

   a. Most exercise tests are conducted by two experienced clinicians, including a physician and respiratory therapist, exercise physiologist, or cardiopulmonary diagnostic technician.

   b. All persons should be certified in basic life support and, ideally, in advanced cardiac life support measures.

   c. Emergency resuscitation equipment should be available.

   d. Minimum requirements for noninvasive monitoring during exercise testing of the COPD patient include:

      (1) Blood pressure values, heart rate, and respiratory rate: baseline, every 2 to 3 min, at the end of exercise, and 3 to 5 min after exercise.

      (2) Continuous ECG: 12-lead rather than single-lead rhythm strip

      (3) Oxygen saturation: baseline, continuous during exercise, and for 3 to 5 min after exercise.

   e. Additional exercise diagnostic measurements and information derived (Table 22–2) include:

      (1) Expiratory flow measurements such as peak expiratory flow rate (PEFR), V_E, and V_T provide information regarding airflow limitation to exercise and the anaerobic threshold.

TABLE 22–2.

Selected Exercise Test Information: Results in Health and in COPD

Term	Explanation	Normal Values	Lung Disease
Maximal heart rate achieved	During exercise, heart rate normally rises linearly with increasing work rate up to an age-related maximum.	$\geq$ 85% of maximum	Decreased
$\dot{V}O_2$ maximum (L/min or ml/kg/min)	Maximal O_2 consumption indicates a subject's maximal exercise capacity or energy expenditure. It is expressed in volume per unit time. It may be roughly predicted based on exercise test work levels or directly calculated from exhaled gas measurements. $\dot{V}O_2$ maximum occurs when $\dot{V}O_2$ reaches a plateau despite continued increase in work rate.	Avg adult $\geq$ 24 ml/kg/min	Significantly below normal because ventilatory limitations end exercise at low levels of work; $\dot{V}O_2$ max recorded as symptom-limited $\dot{V}O_2$

Term	Explanation	Normal Values	Lung Disease
Anaerobic threshold	It is the level of work (exercise $\dot{V}O_2$) above which blood lactate levels show a sustained increase. It may occur at the exercise level (work rate) where respiratory minute volume ($\dot{V}_E$) and CO_2 output ($\dot{V}CO_2$) markedly increase but $\dot{V}O_2$ does not.	50%–60% of $\dot{V}O_2$ maximum	Threshold normal in COPD or may not be reached due to low maximal work capacity
V_D/V_T	This is the deadspace/tidal volume ratio. It normally decreases during exercise due to increased tidal volume and pulmonary blood flow and distribution.	Resting: 0.30–0.40 Exercise: 0.15–0.20	Above normal at rest and fails to decrease with exercise as V_T fails to increase significantly
$\dot{V}_E$ max/MVV	This is the ratio of maximum exercise minute ventilation to maximum voluntary ventilation.	Approximately 60%	Increased: may reach or exceed 100% of calculated MVV
MVV-$\dot{V}_E$ max	The difference between maximum voluntary ventilation and minute ventilation at maximum exercise reflects the breathing reserve.	20%–40% MVV	Significantly below normal (i.e., may be close to zero, indicating little or no ventilatory reserve)
$\dot{V}_E/\dot{V}O_2$	This is the ventilatory equivalent for oxygen (liters of ventilation for each liter of oxygen used). It reflects physiologic efficiency for ventilation.	30 $L_{\dot{V}E}/L_{\dot{V}O_2}$	Increased up to 60 due to ventilation/perfusion mismatch

(2) Measurements of exhaled gases (breath by breath, end-tidal carbon dioxide and oxygen) allow calculation of the maximal oxygen consumption (VO_2 max), respiratory quotient (R), and ventilatory equivalents for oxygen and carbon dioxide; these values indicate work efficiency and anaerobic threshold as well as the physiologic efficiency for oxygen transport and the adequacy of ventilation during exercise.

4. General exercise testing schemes
   a. *Constant time tests* require exercise at the highest possible work rate for a given period of time.
   b. *Single-stage tests* require exercise at a constant work rate for as long as possible; careful selection of the steady state, submaximum exercise level is important to allow test completion in approximately 8 to 12 min.
   c. In *discontinuous tests*, patients exercise at increasing work rates for constant time periods with rests of 15 min to 24 hours between exercise periods.

    d. *Continuous incremental tests* are used most commonly and employ stages that are 1 to 3 min long. The increase in workload between each stage may vary, and a 3-min stage is required for steady-state measurements.

5. Specific protocols
    a. The standard Bruce protocol consists of five 3-min stages beginning at 1.7 miles/hour (mph) and 10% grade but has been modified for use in pulmonary patients by lowering the starting grade and maximum speed. This protocol is used commonly in stress testing for cardiac disease.
    b. The lower-level Naughton protocol begins at 0% grade and 1 or 2 mph and after seven 2-min stages reaches the maximal level, 2.0 mph, 17.5% grade, or approximately a level of seven metabolic equivalents of the task, or 7 METs. The metabolic energy equivalent unit represents approximately 3.5 ml/kg of oxygen consumption at rest. Multiples of the MET unit are used to roughly indicate energy (oxygen consumption) required to perform various activities.
    c. A variety of continuous cycle ergometer protocols are each designed with workload increments of equal size (usually 8–25 W) imposed every 30 seconds to 4 min. (One watt [1 W] equals 1 joule.)
    d. The 12-min walking test requires that the patient cover as much distance as possible in a measured level corridor, resting only if necessary. At least two baseline measurements are recommended to account for a learning effect; through practice and pacing improvements, subjects may show a significant increase in distance, even before true training begins.
    e. The 2- or 6-min variation of the 12-min walking test is useful for patients unable to complete the latter.
    f. Many pulmonary rehabilitation teams design their own treadmill or cycle protocols; work rate intensity and increments should achieve the symptom-limiting end point in 10 to 15 min.

IV. Exercise Training
  A. Components of an exercise prescription: Type of exercise, frequency, intensity, and duration
    1. The type of exercise prescribed is determined by the patient's abilities and preferences as well as by the goals of training.
      a. Aerobic exercise aims to improve cardiopulmonary fitness through sustained activity of large muscle groups at an intensity raising the heart rate to a safe target range.
      b. Strengthening exercises aim to improve the tone and function of select muscle groups. Isolated muscle movements are repeated 10 to 30 times, often against resistance.
    2. Equipment and exercises commonly used in pulmonary rehabilitation include:
      a. Treadmill.
      b. Cycle ergometer.
      c. Level walking.
      d. Stair climbing.
      e. Rowing.
      f. Arm ergometer.
      g. Light weights.
      h. Swimming.
      i. Pulleys.
    3. The intensity of exercise is traditionally prescribed based on the heart rate or workload achieved on the baseline exercise test.
      a. The initial target heart rate is 60% to 70% of the maximum age-predicted heart rate (males: 205 minus one half their age; females: 220 minus their age) unless it exceeds the maximum heart rate achieved during exercise testing.

b. The Karvonen method is an alternative means for calculating exercise target heart rate.
   (1) Maximum heart rate achieved on the exercise test (MHR) minus the resting heart rate (RHR) equals the heart rate range (HRR):

$$MHR - RHR = HRR \qquad (1)$$
$$HRR \times 0.70 = Product \qquad (2)$$

   (2) In this equation, 0.60 or 0.80 may be substituted to derive the target heart rate at lower or higher levels.
   (3) Adding the *product* from equation 2 to the RHR will determine the target heart rate (THR):

$$Product + RHR = THR \qquad (3)$$

4. Intensity of exercise may also be selected based on the exercise test workload (treadmill speed and grade or cycle load) corresponding to the following measurements:
   a. 50% $\dot{V}O_2$ max
   b. 50% $\dot{V}_E$ max
5. In general, home or supervised exercise performed at any of these levels 30 min three to four times per week will produce training effects in 4 to 6 weeks (Table 22–3).
6. Some patients with chronic pulmonary disease may be unable to tolerate this traditional exercise conditioning scheme; some may fail to achieve target heart rates, whereas others achieve high heart rates at relatively low levels of exercise.
   a. Modify the exercise to each patient's tolerance.
   b. If necessary, begin with short exercise periods at a low intensity (e.g., 3–5 min walking or unloaded cycling) and aim to increase endurance before increasing the intensity of exercise.
7. Table 22–4 lists potential benefits from exercise reconditioning.
B. Implementation of pulmonary rehabilitation exercise sessions
   1. Patients are taught 10- or 15-second pulse taking.
   2. Each session begins and ends with stretching and warm-up or cool-down exercises.
      a. Rhythmic controlled breathing with head, neck, and shoulder exercises
      b. Arm lifts (small 1- to 5-lb weights optional)
      c. Side stretches for rib cage mobility
      d. Calf stretches
      e. Leg lifts (to forward, back, and sides)
   3. The following parameters are monitored:
      a. Heart rate, blood pressure, and respiratory rate at rest, at the end of exercise and 3 min after exercise
      b. Oxygen saturation (Sa_{O_2}) as needed
      c. The ECG rhythm as needed in patients with known (or at high risk for) cardiac arrhythmias
   4. The main exercise should be continuous and should involve large muscle groups.
      a. Level walking
      b. Treadmill, with or without incline
      c. Cycle ergometer

TABLE 22–3.

Exercise Testing Equipment: Advantages Versus Disadvantages

Type of Exercise Equipment	Advantages	Disadvantages
Level course, variable distance	Practical (utilizes walking, a familiar skill) Inexpensive No calibration after course distance measured Useful in repeated measurements in pulmonary rehabilitation programs Able to test more than one patient at a time	Difficult to perform certain physiologic assessments during testing (blood pressure, ECG, ventilation) Difficult to quantify workload
Steps	Simple, practical, applicable to daily living Inexpensive Relatively safe Transportable	Unable to vary work load Difficult to control patient's center of gravity to ensure full stepping excursion Some measurements difficult (blood pressure, ventilation)
Treadmill	Employs familiar exercise (walking) Easily calibrated Allows measurement of all important physiologic variables Use of incline allows stress to $\dot{V}O_2$ max in a relatively short period of time	Work rate dependent on body size Most expensive Noisy Motion may cause measurement artifact
Cycle ergometer	Safest Work rate independent of body size Less costly than treadmill Less artifact than treadmill Allows measurement of all important physiologic variables	Inability to pedal smoothly may affect determination of work rate Weak quadriceps muscles may stop test prematurely

       d. Stair climbing

       e. Swimming

    5. Supplemental oxygen is given during exercise.

       a. Flow rate or FI_{O_2} is titrated to achieve an Sa_{O_2} of at least 90% with exercise.

       b. The use of supplemental oxygen during exercise is mandatory for patients who receive oxygen at rest.

       c. It is indicated for patients not otherwise receiving oxygen if the Sa_{O_2} level falls below 88% to 90% with exercise.

       d. Traditionally it is provided via nasal cannula.

       e. Portable and oxygen-conserving systems (see Chapter 29) may be used.

  V. Respiratory Muscle Training

    A. Clinical assessment of respiratory muscles

      1. Maximal inspiratory pressure (MIP) and maximal expiratory pressure (MEP)

TABLE 22-4.

Potential Benefits From Exercise Reconditioning*

Accepted benefits for COPD patients
    Increased endurance
    Increased maximum O_2 consumption
    Increased skill in performance, with decreased
        ventilation, O_2 consumption, heart rate, and
        increased anaerobic threshold
Possible benefits (unusual in COPD patients)
    Increased sense of well-being
    Increased mucociliary clearance
    Increased hypoxic drive
    Increased left ventricular function
Unlikely, debated, or unknown benefits
    Improved survival
    Improved pulmonary function test results
    Lowered pulmonary artery pressure
    Improved blood gas values
    Improved blood lipid values
    Change in muscle O_2 extraction
    Change In step desaturation or apnea

*From Hughes RL, Davison R: *Chest* 1983; 83:241–249.
Used by permission.

    a. Measured during maximal static inspiratory or expiratory efforts into a mouthpiece connected to a pressure gauge.
    b. Indicate respiratory muscle strength.
    c. Measured from near residual volume and total lung capacity, respectively.
    d. Normal values for MIP in those aged 20 to 54 years:
       (1) Men: Approximately 100 to 150 cm H_2O
       (2) Women: Appproximately 75 to 125 cm H_2O
    e. Normal values for MEP in those aged 20 to 54 years:
       (1) Men: Approximately 200 to 250 cm H_2O
       (2) Women: Approximately 150 to 200 cm H_2O
    f. Decrease with age, chronic pulmonary disease, neuromuscular conditions, and nutritional depletion.
  2. Diaphragmatic excursion
    a. Measured as the distance between percussed levels of dullness on full inspiration and full expiration.
    b. Normally, approximately 3 to 5 cm.
    c. May be reduced in chronic pulmonary disease due to diaphragmatic weakness, severe hyperinflation, or both.
  3. Sustainable inspiratory pressure (SIP)
    a. Defined as the highest inspiratory presure (or % MIP) a patient can generate repeatedly over time (e.g., every breath for 10 min).
    b. Indicates inspiratory muscle endurance.
  4. Maximal sustained ventilatory capacity (MSVC)
    a. Defined as the highest level of ventilation (L/min or % MVV) a patient can sustain over time (usually 10–15 min).
    b. Indicates respiratory muscle endurance.
B. Types of training
  1. Isocapneic hyperpnea: Rapid deep breathing into a circuit maintaining end-tidal carbon dioxide level within normal limits.

      a. Respiratory muscle endurance training: Subject performs near-maximal breathing (rate and depth) for 15 to 30 min 3 to 5 days/week.

      b. Sophisticated equipment and supervision are required to regulate $F_{I_{O_2}}$ and prevent hyperventilation or respiratory alkalosis; *thus, it cannot be performed at home.*

   2. Inspiratory resistive breathing (IRB)

      a. The variable-orifice, flow-dependent device has multiple openings ranging from 1.8 to 5.3 mm in diameter.

      b. With the springload-type, flow-independent device, the patient must generate a prescribed threshold pressure to open a vent and allow inspiration.

      c. Optimal candidates and protocols for IRB are not firmly established.

         (1) One should begin with inspiratory resistive load corresponding to 25% to 30% of the MIP or the smallest orifice tolerated and monitor the Sa_{O_2} and respiratory rate.

         (2) Frequency and duration are 10 to 15 min once or twice daily for 4 to 8 weeks, then the resistance or threshold pressure is increased.

  C. Reported benefits of respiratory muscle training

   1. Increased inspiratory muscle strength (MIP)

   2. Increased inspiratory muscle endurance (SIP, MSVC)

   3. Increased exercise performance

   4. Improved ability to perform activities of daily living

VI. Patient and Family Education

  A. Major objectives of patient education in pulmonary rehabilitation

   1. Identifying and explaining the physical and psychosocial changes related to COPD in order to set realistic individual goals

   2. Identifying and developing skills in self-care techniques for optimal symptom management and overall health maintenance

  B. Factors that influence learning

   1. Acceptance of diagnosis

   2. Motivation and perceived need to learn

   3. Physical energy level

   4. Patient-professional relationship (learner-educator relationship)

   5. Cognitive functional level

   6. Health beliefs and values (e.g., locus of control)

   7. Level of emotional stability

  C. Teaching techniques used in pulmonary rehabilitation programs

   1. Lecture or panel presentation to group

   2. Individualized patient-family education sessions

   3. Demonstration of skills, practice, and return demonstration

   4. Group/family discussion

   5. Reading or written assignments

  D. Content or pulmonary rehabilitation education

   1. Respiratory anatomy and physiology and pathophysiology of COPD

      a. Upper and lower airway structures

      b. Respiratory muscles and the act of breathing

      c. Anatomic and functional changes in COPD

      d. Diagnostic tests and expected findings

      e. Origin of symptoms

      f. Complications of COPD (e.g., infection, cor pulmonale)

   2. Breathing retraining

      a. Techniques

         (1) Diaphragmatic breathing

      (2) Pursed lip breathing with prolonged controlled exhalation

      (3) Relaxation of accessory muscles

   b. Application of these techniques at rest, during exercise, and with daily activities

   c. Benefits

      (1) Decreased respiratory rate

      (2) Increased V_T

      (3) Decreased work of breathing

      (4) Improved subjective sense of control over breathing, especially during episodes of dyspnea or exertion

      (5) Decreased air trapping

      (6) Decreased airways closure

      (7) Improved Sa_{O_2} when used with exercise

3. Stress and relaxation

   a. Causes and effects of stress

   b. Techniques for stress reduction and relaxation

      (1) Jacobsen's progressive relaxation technique: Selected muscle groups are consciously relaxed in a systematic manner. The patient tenses, then relaxes muscles from head to toe, including face, neck, shoulders, arms, back, abdomen, legs, and feet.

      (2) Guided imagery: The coach (nurse, therapist, or family member) uses descriptive statements to aid the patient in visualizing relaxing scenes.

      (3) Biofeedback: Instrumentation is used to provide patients with signals regarding their control of select physiologic functions, such as respiratory rate and muscle tension.

      (4) Yoga

      (5) Physical exercise

      (6) Simple body positioning and controlled breathing

      (7) Self-relaxation using tapes, music, or self-talk

4. Medications

   a. Drug types

   b. Indications and actions

   c. Adverse effects

   d. Drug interactions

5. Energy conservation in activities of daily living

   a. Simplifying work tasks

   b. Planning daily schedules

   c. Using correct body mechanics

   d. Balancing work and recreation

   e. Getting adequate sleep and rest

6. Bronchial hygiene measures

7. Smoking cessation: Importance and methods available

   a. Behavior modification techniques (e.g., desensitization, gradual reduction, stimulus control)

   b. Individual counseling or psychotherapy

   c. Group smoking cessation clinics

   d. Hypnosis

   e. Cognitive approach (e.g., medical information, physician order)

   f. Acupuncture

   g. Relaxation

   h. Exercise

   i. Pharmacologic aids

8. Oxygen therapy (see Chapter 29)
   a. Purpose and expected benefit
   b. Use (dose, hours, adjustment with sleep and exercise)
   c. Care of equipment
   d. Safety information
9. Nutrition (see Chapter 19)
10. Fluid management
11. Sexuality and lung disease
    a. Sexuality and self-esteem
    b. Expected sexual changes with aging
    c. Effects of medications
    d. Techniques for sexual expression and energy conservation
12. Miscellaneous
    a. Environmental influences on breathing (e.g., temperature, humidity, indoor and outdoor pollutants, allergens)
    b. Handling medical emergencies (e.g., knowing when to call the physician)
    c. Travel tips
    d. Community resources

VII. Psychosocial Support
   • Psychosocial support in pulmonary rehabilitation aims to assist patients and families toward optimal understanding of and coping with COPD.
   A. Specific goals
      1. Help patients accept their condition and realistically assess strengths and limitations.
      2. Identify specific strategies for coping with stress, anxiety, and depression.
   B. Intervention methods
      1. Individual counseling
      2. Couple counseling
      3. Role playing
      4. Group discussion or therapy
      5. Better Breathers Clubs
      6. Spouse support group
   C. Activities and benefits in group support sessions
      1. Explore changes in individual image, family structure, and role functioning.
      2. Share problems and coping methods.
      3. Mobilize passive patients to participate.
      4. Enhance social interaction opportunity and skills.

VIII. Program Evaluation and Quality Assurance
   A. Program activities and goals should be monitored regularly in quality assurance audits (e.g., monthly or quarterly).
   B. Sample criteria include:
      1. Patient's achievement of goals (e.g., percent improvement in exercise capacity).
      2. Patient satisfaction assessments (postprogram interviews or questionnaires).
      3. Program attrition rates and reasons.
      4. Hospitalization days.
      5. Comparative scores on preprogram and postprogram tests of educational content presented.

IX. Post-program patient follow-up
   A. A summary letter is sent from the program coordinator to the primary or referring physician detailing the patient's goals and progress.
   B. The patient is encouraged to continue ongoing physician office visits for periodic medical assessment and regulation of medications.

C. Many outpatient pulmonary rehabilitation programs offer reevaluation visits at 3-, 6-, and 12-month intervals to assess and encourage compliance with home exercise and activity plans.

D. Ongoing education, support, and contact among patients is available through groups such as Better Breathers Clubs or other local lung association groups.

E. Home respiratory equipment vendors may also participate in patient follow-up through written or verbal reports to program coordinators and physicians.

BIBLIOGRAPHY

American Thoracic Society: Pulmonary rehabilitation. *Am Rev Respir Dis* 1981; 124:663–666.

Bell CW, Blodgett D, Goike CA, et al: *Home Care and Rehabilitation in Respiratory Medicine*. Philadelphia, JB Lippincott Co, 1984.

Belman M, Wasserman K: Exercise training and testing in patients with chronic obstructive disease. *Basics Respir Dis* 1981; 10:1–6.

Bergner M, Bobbitt, RA, Pollard WE, et al: The sickness impact profile: Validation of a health status measure. *Med Care* 1976; 14:57–67.

Better Breathing Today [audiotapes]. LaJolla, Calif, Health Communication Services, 1985.

Black LF, Hyatt RE: Maximum respiratory pressures: Normal values and relationship to age and sex. *Am Rev Respir Dis* 1969; 99:696–701.

Booker H: Exercise training and breathing control in patients with chronic airflow limitation. *Physiotherapy* 1984; 70:258–260.

Broussard R: Using relaxation for COPD. *Am J Nurs* 1979; 79:1962–1963.

Byrd RB, Hyatt RF: Maximal respiratory pressures in chronic obstructive lung disease. *Am Rev Respir Dis* 1968; 98:848–856.

Carrieri VK, Janson-Bjerklie S: The sensation of dyspnea: A review. *Heart Lung* 1984; 13:436–447.

Casciari RJ, Fairshter RD, Harrison A, et al: Effects of breathing retraining in patients with chronic obstructive pulmonary disease. *Chest* 1981; 79:393–398.

Daughton DM, Fix AJ, Kass I, et al: Maximum oxygen consumption and the ADAPT quality of life scale. *Arch Phys Med Rehabil* 1982; 63:620–622.

Davis JA, Convertino VA: A comparison of heart rate methods for predicting endurance training intensity. *Med Sci Sports* 1975; 7:295–298.

Dudley DL, Glasen EM, Jorgenson BN, et al: Psychosocial concomitants to rehabilitation in chronic obstructive pulmonary disease, part I. *Chest* 1980; 77:413–420.

Dudley DL, Glasen EM, Jorgenson BN, et al: Psychosocial concomitants to rehabilitation in chronic obstructive pulmonary disease, part II. *Chest* 1980; 77:544–551.

Dudley DL, Verhey JW, Masuda M, et al: Long-term adjustment, prognosis, and death in irreversible diffuse obstructive pulmonary syndromes. *Psychosom Med* 1969; 31:310–325.

Hansen JE: Exercise instruments, schemes, and protocols for evaluating the dyspneic patient. *Am Rev Respir Dis* 1984; 129(suppl):S25–S27.

Hanson EI: Effects of chronic lung disease on life in general and on sexuality: Perceptions of adult patients. *Heart Lung* 1982; 11:435–441.

Harris PL: A guide to prescribing pulmonary rehabilitation. *Primary Care* 1985; 12:253–266.

Hodgkin JE, Petty TL: *Chronic Obstructive Pulmonary Disease: Current Concepts*. Philadelphia, WB Saunders Co, 1987.

Hodgkin JE, Zorn EG, Connors GL (eds): *Pulmonary Rehabilitation: Guidelines to Success*. Stoneham, Mass, Butterworth, 1984.

Hughes RL, Davison R: Limitations of exercise reconditioning in COLD. *Chest* 1983; 83:241–249.

Jones NL, Campbell EJ: *Clinical Exercise Testing*, ed 2. Philadelphia, WB Saunders Co, 1982.

Kaplan RM, Atkins CJ, Timms R: Validity of a quality of well-being scale as an outcome measure in chronic obstructive pulmonary disease. *J Chronic Dis* 1984; 37:85–95.

Larson JL, Kim MJ, Sharp JT, et al: Inspiratory muscle training with a pressure threshold breathing device in patients with chronic obstructive pulmonary disease. *Am Rev Respir Dis* 1987; 138:689–696.

Leith DE, Bradley M: Ventilatory muscle strength and endurance training. *J Appl Physiol* 1976; 41:508–516.

McGavin CR, Gupta SP, McHardy GJR: Twelve-minute walking test for assessing disability in chronic bronchitis. *Br Med J (Clin Res)* 1976; 1:822–823.

McNair DM, Lorr M, Droppleman LF: *EDITS Manual for the Profile of Mood States.* San Diego, Calif, Educational Industrial Testing Service, 1971.

McSweeny, AJ, Grant I, Heaton RK, et al: Life quality of patients with chronic obstructive pulmonary disease. *Am J Med* 1982; 142:473–477.

Moser KM, Bokinsky GE, Savage RT, et al: Results of a comprehensive rehabilitation program. Physiologic and functional effects on patients with chronic obstructive pulmonary disease. *Arch Intern Med* 1980; 140:1596–1601.

Moser K: Shortness of breath, in *A Guide to Better Living and Breathing,* ed 3. St Louis, CV Mosby Co, 1983.

Mueller RE, Petty TL, Filley FG: Ventilation and arterial blood gas changes induced by pursed lips breathing. *J Appl Physiol* 1970; 28:784–789.

Neff TA, Petty TL: Outpatient care for patients with chronic airway obstruction. *Chest* 1971; 60(suppl): 115–175.

Nickerson BG, Keens TG: Measuring ventilatory muscle endurance in humans at sustainable inspiratory pressure. *J Appl Physiol* 1982; 52:768–772.

O'Ryan JA, Burns DG: *Pulmonary Rehabilitation: From Hospital to Home.* Chicago, Year Book Medical Publishers, 1984.

Paine R, Make BJ: Pulmonary rehabilitation for the elderly. *Clin Geriatr Med* 1986; 2:313–335.

Pattison EM, Rhodes RJ, Dudley DL: Responses to group treatment in patients with severe chronic lung disease. *Int J Group Psychother* 1971; 21:214–225.

Perry J: Effectiveness of teaching in the rehabilitation of chronic bronchitis and emphysema. *Nurs Res* 1980; 30:219–222.

Pulmonary Self-Care: A Program for Patients [videotapes]. Chicago, Encyclopedia Brittanica Educational Corp, 1980.

Ries AL, Moser KM: Comparison of isocapneic hyperventilation and walking exercise training at home in pulmonary rehabilitation. *Chest* 1986; 90:285–289.

Sahn SA, Nett LM, Petty TL: Ten year follow-up of a comprehensive rehabilitation program for severe COPD. *Chest* 1980; 77(suppl):311–314.

Shayewitz MB, Shayewitz BR: Athletic training in chronic obstructive pulmonary disease. *Clin Sports Med* 1986; 5:471–491.

Sinclair DJ, Ingram CG: Controlled trial of supervised exercise training in chronic bronchitis. *Br Med J (Clin Res)* 1980; 23:519–521.

Sonne LJ, Davis JA: Increased exercise performance in patients with severe COPD following inspiratory resistive training. *Chest* 1982; 81:436–439.

Tiep BL, Burns M, Kao D, et al: Pursed lips breathing using ear oximetry. *Chest* 1986; 90:218–221.

Tydeman DE, Chandler AR, Graveling BM, et al: An investigation into the effects of exercise tolerance training on patients with chronic airways obstruction. *Physiotherapy* 1984; 70:261–264.

Wasserman K, Whipp BJ: Exercise physiology in health and disease. *Am Rev Respir Dis* 1975; 112:219–249.

Weg JG: Therapeutic exercise in patients with chronic obstructive pulmonary disease. *Cardiovasc Clin* 1985; 15:261–275.

Wilson PK, Bell CW, Norton AC: *Rehabilitation of the Heart and Lungs.* Fullerton, Calif, Beckman Instruments, 1980.

Wright RW, Larsen DF, Monie RG, et al: Benefits of a community hospital pulmonary rehabilitation program. *Respir Care* 1983; 28:1474–1478.

Zack MB, Palonge AV: Oxygen supplemented exercise of ventilatory and nonventilatory muscles in pulmonary rehabilitation. *Chest* 1985; 88:669–675.

Chapter 23

Home Respiratory Care

I. Overall Goals of Home Respiratory Care
   A. Extend life
   B. Enhance the quality of life
   C. Reduce morbidity associated with disease
   D. Arrest the progress of chronic diseases
   E. Improve overall physiologic and psychologic function
   F. Provide an environment to enhance individual potential
   G. Provide cost-effective medical care
II. Primary Forms of Home Respiratory Care
   A. Oxygen therapy
   B. Aerosol therapy
   C. Mechanical ventilation
      1. Positive pressure
      2. Negative pressure
      3. CPAP
III. Oxygen Therapy
   A. Indication: Any cardiopulmonary disease resulting in chronic hypoxemia.
   B. Chronic hypoxemia: Defined in this situation by governmental reimbursement criteria.
   C. Reimbursement criteria include each of the following:
      1. Po_2 55 mm Hg or less
      2. Po_2 59 mm Hg or less with:
         a. Dependent edema or
         b. Cor pulmonale or
         c. Hematocrit 55% or more (polycythemia)
      3. Hemoglobin saturation 85% or less
      4. Hemoglobin saturation 86% to 89% or less and:
         a. Dependent edema or
         b. Cor pulmonale or
         c. Hematocrit 55% or more
   D. In general, because the relationship between Po_2 and hemoglobin saturation is variable and affected by a number of factors, criteria for home oxygen therapy should be based on Po_2, not on $HbO_2\%$ (Fig 23–1).
      1. Factors affecting Po_2 vs. $HbO_2\%$ (see Chapter 11)
         a. Temperature
         b. Pco_2

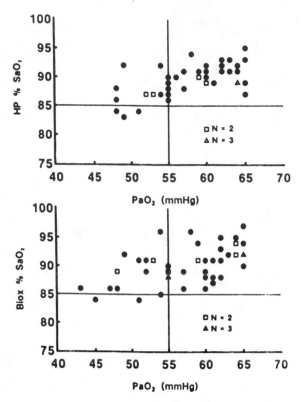

FIG 23–1.
The relationship between resting arterial oxygen tension (Pa$_{O_2}$) and arterial saturation (HbO$_2$%) measured by a Hewlett Packard HP47201A *(top)* or a Biox IIA *(bottom)* ear oximeter. *Solid lines* (Pa$_{O_2}$ 55 mm Hg; HbO$_2$% 85%) represent medicare criteria for long-term oxygen therapy prescription. (From Carlin BW, Clauser JL, Ries AL: *Chest* 1988; 94:239–241. Used by permission.)

    c. pH
    d. 2,3-Diphosphoglycerate levels
  E. Physiologic effects of long-term oxygen therapy
    1. Increased exercise capacity
    2. Decreased work of the myocardium
    3. Decreased work of breathing
    4. Decreased pulmonary hypertension
    5. Normalization of the hemoglobin level
  F. Oxygen containment systems used in the home (see Chapter 27 for details)
    1. System choice is based more on reimbursement than clinical efficiency.
    2. Oxygen concentrators are most commonly used.
    3. Liquid oxygen systems are especially useful for travel, work, and so forth.
    4. Tanks are the least commonly employed, are the most labor intensive, and are the most expensive.
  G. Oxygen therapy equipment (see Chapter 28)
    1. Simple oxygen cannula is the most common.
    2. Oxygen-conserving devices are used during high oxygen demand or travel.
      a. Oxygen reservoir systems
      b. Pulse dose or demand systems
    3. Transtracheal oxygen is useful during refractory hypoxemia or continued work away from home.
  H. Monitoring home oxygen therapy
    1. Patients who meet the criteria for oxygen therapy at discharge frequently do not require oxygen after a few months as a result of:
      a. Complete resolution of the acute precipitating problem
      b. Overall medical care

    c. Use of bronchodilator therapy

    d. Pulmonary rehabilitation programs

  2. Monthly monitoring of status should occur in the home.

    a. Pulse oximetry: After the need is established with Po_2 baseline, $HbO_2\%$ is determined with and without oxygen to establish $HbO_2\%$ to be used as baseline for home monitoring.

    b. Vital signs and ventilatory pattern

    c. Chest auscultation

  3. Office follow-up: Frequency is dependent on the severity of the overall disease process.

IV. Aerosol Therapy

  A. Patients with permanent artificial airways

    1. Some patients are capable of acclimating to artificial airways without the need for continuous aerosol therapy other than the use of artificial noses or heat and moisture exchangers.

    2. Many require nocturnal aerosol therapy. Whether heated or unheated, with or without oxygen, depends on the patient's medical status and tolerance.

    3. Few nonmechanically ventilated patients require continous aerosol therapy.

  B. Small-volume aerosolized drug therapy (see Chapters 30 and 40)

    1. Most non-tracheostomied nonmechanically ventilated patients are capable of co-ordinating the use of a metered dose inhaler with a spacer.

    2. Few require pneumatically operated small-volume nebulizers.

    3. Most common drugs delivered by aerosol in the home include:

      a. Bronchodilators.

      b. Corticosteroids.

      c. Parasympatholytes.

V. Mechanical Ventilation

  A. It is estimated that 7,000 individuals in the United States require long-term mechanical ventilatory assistance.

  B. It is likely that this number will increase over the next decade as a result of:

    1. Improved medical care.

    2. Cost effectiveness of elective nocturnal ventilatory support.

    3. Improved technology.

  C. Possible solutions to the increased need for long-term invasive ventilatory support in the home

    1. Meticulous consideration prior to initiation of mechanical ventilation in the acute care setting of the following:

      a. Reversability of the acute pulmonary disease process

      b. Chronicity of underlying disease

    2. Appropriate elective use of ventilatory assistance

      a. Negative pressure ventilation

      b. Noninvasive positive pressure ventilation

    3. Use of alternate care sites

      a. Alternate care sites include (listed in order of increasing independence and decreasing cost):

        (1) Chronic care hospitals

        (2) Skilled nursing facilities

        (3) Congregate living center

        (4) Home

  D. General indications for long-term ventilatory support

    1. Neuromusculoskeletal disorders: The best candidates have chronic, slowly progressive diseases.

2. Central hypoventilation: In general, those with sleep apnea are very good candidates.
3. Obstructive lung disease: Selective patients are good candidates. Many comply poorly, are difficult to manage, and suffer from many other organ system problems.
4. Restrictive lung disease: normally, such patients are never candidates; in general they have the highest respiratory needs.

E. The ideal patient for long-term ventilatory support:
1. Has a neuromuscular or neurologic disorder.
2. Is clinically stable.
3. Is well educated.
4. Is motivated or interested in self-care.
5. Has good support systems.
6. Has some ventilatory independence.

F. The keys to successful transition to the home are appropriate predischarge planning and a well-coordinated team effort. Key members of the discharge team include:
1. Physician
2. Respiratory therapist
3. Social worker
4. Home health agency
5. Durable medical equipment supplier

G. In general, patients requiring *nonelective* mechanical ventilatory assistance need about 4 weeks of in-hospital training and acclimation to equipment before movement into the home.

H. All respiratory care equipment used in the home should also be used in the hospital.

I. The need for skilled full-time care givers in the home is based on numerous factors.
1. Patient
   a. Adult, adolescent, infant; most infants require at least 8 hours/day of skilled care giver support.
   b. Condition: The number of hours requiring continuous support; the more the hours, the greater the need for skilled care givers.
   c. Ability to provide self-care.
   d. Rehabilitation potential.
2. Family
   a. The ability to provide care
   b. The ability to direct care
   c. The need for respite care
3. Third-party coverage
   a. Many insurers provide minimal home care support.
   b. Others reimburse only registered nurse care, even though the patient requires only a sitter.
   c. Most insurers have a maximum cap on monies available.
4. In general, infants require more care giver assistance than adults.

J. Invasive positive pressure ventilation
1. Discharge criteria
   a. Absence of sustained dyspnea or frequent episodes of severe dyspnea or frequent episodes of severe dyspnea and tachypnea
   b. Acceptable blood gases with $F_{I_{O_2}}$ level less than 0.40
   c. Psychologic stability
   d. Absence of life-threatening cardiac dysfunction or arrhythmias
   e. Manageable pulmonary secretions
   f. Protected airway

g. Absence of significant nutritional deficit

h. In general, overall medical stability

2. Evaluation of the home environment is essential before discharge.

   a. Location of ventilated patient in home. Room size related to equipment selection.

   b. Electrical capability of the home. Need for a backup electrical generator.

   c. Access for wheelchair into and out of the home.

   d. Availability of emergency help.

3. Home mechanical ventilators (general descriptions)

   a. Today, essentially five mechanical ventilators are designed and manufactured (see later discussion) for home use.

   b. In children and adults, ventilators designed primarily for hospital use should not be used in the home. With infants, exceptions are made (see later discussion).

4. Ideal characteristics of home care ventilators

   a. Designed exclusively with the home care patient in mind.

   b. User-friendly operation.

   c. Reliable operation.

   d. Absence of confusing digital readouts that change on a breath-by-breath basis.

   e. Available modes: control and assist/control.

   f. Respiratory rate: 6 to 40 breaths/min (bpm).

   g. Tidal volume: 100 to 2,000 ml.

   h. Peak flow capability: 30 to 100 L/min.

   i. Inspiratory time: 0.5 to 2.0 seconds.

   j. Internal battery capable of functioning for more than 2 hours.

   k. Appropriately alarmed.

      (1) High/low pressure

      (2) Ventilator failure to deliver gas as programmed

      (3) Ventilator inoperable

   l. Remote alarm capability.

   m. Remote "nurse" call capability.

   n. Compact (fits on wheelchair), light (less than 35 lb), access for titration of oxygen, and assisted breaths triggered by proximal patient airway pressure sensing.

5. None of the home care mechanical ventilators available today meets these criteria.

6. The internal gas flow pattern of modern home care ventilators is illustrated in Figure 23–2).

   a. Gas enters these units by way of an oxygen-accumulating device with a one-way valve.

   b. A one-way valve is also located just inside the unit's intake filter.

   c. From here, gas enters the piston chamber during the piston's back stroke.

   d. During the piston's forward stroke, gas exits the piston chamber via a one-way valve, which prevents gas from being drawn into the piston chamber during the piston's back stroke.

   e. A pop-off valve is located in the piston chamber (vent) to prevent excessive chamber pressurization.

   f. Once gas exits the piston chamber, it normally passes a pressure limit control adjustable by operator and a one-way inlet valve, allowing inspiration of gas from the unit's circuit during the piston's back stroke.

   g. Not all units include one-way inlet valve.

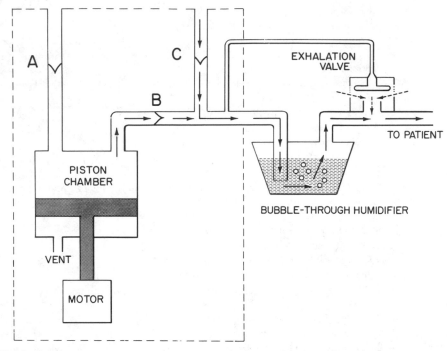

FIG 23–2.
Schematic of basic gas flow during spontaneous inspiration with a typical home care ventilator. **A,** one-way check valve allows gas entry into the piston chamber during piston back stroke. **B,** one-way check valve prevents negative ventilator circuit pressure from developing during back stroke of piston. One-way check valve allows patient to spontaneously inspire during closure of **(B)** when piston back stroke is in progress. Some gas may enter the system at the exhalation valve. *Arrows* depict gas flow during spontaneous inspiration. (From Kacmarek RM, Stanek KS, McMahon KM, et al: *Respir Care* [in press]. Used by permission.)

        h. *Note:* No demand or continuous gas flow system is included. During spontaneous breathing (synchronized intermittent mandatory ventilation, or SIMV) the patient must draw gas from:
           (1) The exhalation valve
           (2) The piston chamber
           (3) The one-way air inlet valve.
    7. Puritan-Bennett 2800
        a. Pressure: Positive.
        b. Powering mechanism: Electric.
        c. Driving mechanism: Piston system driven via rotary motion.
        d. Maintenance of gas flow pattern: Nonconstant flow generator.
        e. Circuit: Double.
        f. Gas flow and pressure pattern: Modified sine wave flow and modified sigmoidial pressure (see Chapter 35).
        g. Cycling parameter: Volume.
        h. Limits
           (1) Pressure
              (a) Relief/pop-off
              (b) Plateau inspiratory pressure limit
           (2) Time
        i. Modes

TABLE 23–1.

Alarm Systems of Positive Pressure Ventilators

Alarms	Puritan-Bennett 2800	Aequitron Medical LP-6	Life Care PLV-100	Life Care PLV-102	Intermed Bear 33	Medimex ARF 1500E
High inspiratory pressure	Yes*	Yes	Yes	Yes	Yes	Yes
Low inspiratory pressure	Yes	Yes	Yes†	Yes†	Yes	Yes
Apnea	Yes	Yes	Yes†	Yes†	Yes	No
Low battery	Yes	Yes	Yes‡	Yes‡	Yes	Yes
Inverse I:E ratio§	Yes	Yes‖	Yes	Yes	No	No
Ventilation malfunction	Yes	No	Yes	Yes	Yes	Yes
Low inspiratory flow	No	No	Yes	Yes	No	No
Revere external battery connections	No	No	Yes	Yes	No	No
Microprocessor failure	No	No	Yes	Yes	No	No
Switch to battery	No	No	Yes	Yes	Yes	No
Power failure	No	No	Yes	Yes	No	No
Oxygen	No	No	No	Yes	No	No

*High inspiratory pressure alarm is separate from high inspiratory pressure limit. No alarm is activated when limit is reached.
†The low inspiratory pressure and the apnea alarms are actually combined.
‡Has separate alarms for low internal and low external batteries.
§I:E ratio = inspiratory:expiratory ratio.
‖Actually referred to as setting error, controls set outside machine limits. An inverse I:E ratio will not be delivered.

        (1) Control
        (2) Assist/control
        (3) SIMV
        (4) Pressure limited plateau ventilation
    j. Inspiratory airway maneuvers: None.
    k. Expiratory airway maneuvers: None.
    l. Alarms (Table 23–1)
    m. Other features
        (1) Internal battery
        (2) Remote alarm
        (3) Patient call
    n. Size
        (1) Weight 31 lb
        (2) Dimensions 11⅜ by 10 by 12 in.
  8. Aequitron Medical Inc. LP-6
    a. Pressure: Positive.
    b. Powering mechanism: Electric.
    c. Driving mechanism: Piston system driven via rotary motor.
    d. Maintenance of gas flow pattern: Nonconstant flow generator.
    e. Circuit: Double.
    f. Gas flow and pressure pattern: Modified sine wave flow and modified sigmoidial pressure (see Chapter 35).
    g. Cycling parameter
        (1) Volume
        (2) Pressure
    h. Limits
        (1) Pressure (pop-off)
        (2) Time

      i. Modes
        (1) Control
        (2) Assist/control
        (3) SIMV
        (4) Pressure limited control or assist/control
      j. Inspiratory airway maneuvers: None.
      k. Expiratory airway maneuvers: None.
      l. Alarms (see Table 23–1)
      m. Other features
        (1) Internal battery
        (2) Remote alarm
        (3) Printer for tracking alarm conditions
      n. Size
        (1) Weight 32 lb
        (2) Dimensions 9¼ by 13½ by 12½ in.
  9. Life Care PLV-100
      a. Pressure: Positive.
      b. Powering mechanism: Electric.
      c. Driving mechanism: Piston system driven via rotary motor.
      d. Maintenance of gas flow pattern: Nonconstant flow generator.
      e. Circuit: Double.
      f. Gas flow and pressure pattern: Modified sine wave and modified sigmoidial pressure (see Chapter 35).
      g. Cycling parameter: Volume.
      h. Limits
        (1) Pressure (pop-off)
        (2) Time
      i. Modes
        (1) Control
        (2) Assist/control
        (3) SIMV
      j. Inspiratory airway maneuvers: None.
      k. Expiratory airway maneuvers: None.
      l. Alarms (see Table 23–1)
      m. Other features
        (1) Internal battery
      n. Size
        (1) Weight 28.2 lb
        (2) Dimensions 9 by 12½ by 12¼ in.
 10. Intermed Bear 33
      a. Pressure: Positive.
      b. Powering mechanism: Electric.
      c. Driving mechanism: Piston system driven via rotary motor.
      d. Maintenance of gas flow pattern: Nonconstant flow generator.
      e. Circuit: Double.
      f. Gas flow and pressure pattern: Modified sine wave and modified sigmoidial pressure (see Chapter 35).
      g. Cycling parameter: Volume.
      h. Limits
        (1) Pressure (pop-off)
        (2) Time

      i. Modes
        (1) Control
        (2) Assist/control
        (3) SIMV
      j. Inspiratory airway maneuvers: None.
      k. Expiratory airway maneuvers: None.
      l. Alarms (see Table 23–1)
     m. Other features
        (1) Internal battery
        (2) Touch pad control panel with locking feature
        (3) Remote alarm
     n. Size
        (1) Weight 32 lb
        (2) Dimensions 7½ by 14 by 12⅔ in.

11. Medimex ARF 1500E
    a. Pressure: Positive.
    b. Powering mechanism: Electric.
    c. Driving mechanism: Piston system driven via a rotary motor.
    d. Maintenance of gas flow pattern: Nonconstant flow generator.
    e. Circuit: Double.
    f. Gas flow and pressure pattern: Modified sine wave and modified sigmoidal pressure (see Chapter 35).
    g. Cycling parameter: Volume.
    h. Limits
      (1) Pressure (pop-off)
      (2) Time
    i. Modes
      (1) Control
      (2) Assist/control
      (3) Intermittent mandatory ventilation (IMV)
    j. Inspiratory airway maneuvers: None.
    k. Expiratory airway maneuvers: None.
    l. Alarms (see Table 23–1)
    m. Other features
      (1) Internal battery

12. Delivery of oxygen
    a. None of these units accepts a 50-psi oxygen or air source.
    b. All allow an oxygen-accumulating device to be attached to the gas entry port.
    c. The use of the accumulator produces the most precise and consistent $F_{I_{O_2}}$ (±3% to 4%).
    d. Oxygen may also be bled into the circuit by the use of a T attached between the ventilator and the humidifying device.

13. Positive end-expiratory pressure (PEEP)
    a. None of these units is designed for the application of PEEP.
    b. A PEEP valve may be placed at the exhalation valve.
    c. However, the patient's ability to trigger the machine would be grossly affected; the work of breathing (WOB) would increase (see Chapter 37).
    d. The use of PEEP devices with these ventilators is discouraged.

14. The SIMV/IMV mode
    a. None of these units actually provides SIMV/IMV as provided on intensive care unit ventilators.

b. No demand system or continous flow setup is included in the system's basic design.

c. When the unit is set on SIMV/IMV with the use of a bubble-through humidifier, the imposed WOB is excessive (Fig 23–3).

d. Even the use of passover humidifiers or heat and moisture exchangers does not sufficiently reduce the WOB.

e. If the SIMV/IMV mode is to be used, a one-way H-valve system placed before the system's passover humidifier should be used (Fig 23–4).

f. If an increased F_{IO_2} value is needed, oxygen can be titrated into the one-way H-valve system as shown in Figure 23–4.

g. The use of a one-way valve and a passover humidifier greatly reduces the imposed WOB of these systems in the SIMV/IMV mode.

15. Selection of ventilator parameters (adults)
   a. Criteria outlined in Chapters 20, 21, and 36 should be followed.
   b. The assist/control mode should be primarily used:
      (1) To decrease imposed WOB.
      (2) To improve ventilatory muscle rest.
      (3) Since adults normally do not wean from ventilatory support at home.
      (4) Muscular capabilities during periods independent of ventilator are enhanced if rest is maximized.

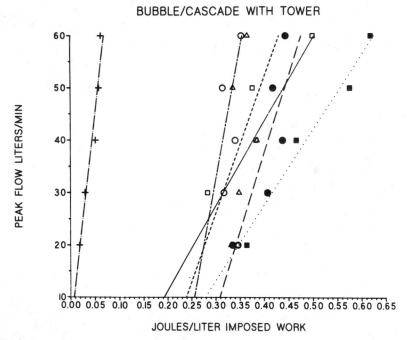

FIG 23–3.
Imposed WOB vs. peak inspiratory flow for five Home Care ventilators with a normally functioning Cascade humidifier (bubble-through) and the H-valve continuous flow system with a passover humidifier. The H-valve system produced the least imposed WOB. Positive sign and dashes and dots represent the H-valve continuous flow system with the passover humidifier. *Open circles* and *large* and *small dashes* represent the Intermed Bear 33. *Open triangles* and *small dashes* represent the Puritan Bennett 2800. *Open squares* and the *solid line* represent the Acquitron LP-6. The *closed circle* and *large dashes* represent the Medimax ARF 1500E. *Closed squares* and *small dots* represent the Life Care PLV-100. (From Kacmarek RM, Stanek KS, McMahon KM, et al: *Respir Care* 1990; 35:405–414. Used by permission.)

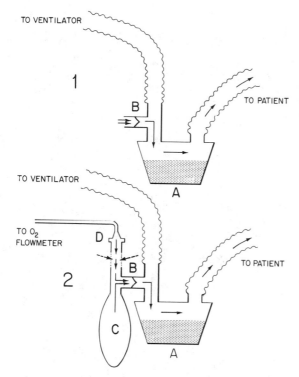

TO VENTILATOR

1

B

TO PATIENT

A

TO VENTILATOR

TO O₂
FLOWMETER

D

2

B

TO PATIENT

C

A

FIG 23–4.
Schematics of one-way H-valve
systems. **1,** valve open to atmosphere.
2, valve with 3-L reservoir bag attached
to 0.28 F_{IO_2} Venturi, powered by 4 L of
oxygen/min. **A** = passover humidifier;
B = one-way valve; **C** = reservoir; **D** =
0.28 F_{IO_2} Venturi. *Arrows* depict gas
flow during spontaneous inspiration.
(From Kacmarek RM, Stanek KS,
McMahon KM, et al: *Respir Care* [in
press]. Used by permission.)

16. Selection of ventilator parameters (infants)
    a. Many infants are weaned from mechanical ventilation in the home.
    b. Small, eventually weanable infants may require the use of pressure-limited
       continuous flow IMV.
    c. This can be accomplished by the addition of the one-way H-valve reservoir
       system depicted in Figure 23–4 and the use of a pop-off valve in the venti-
       lator circuit to maintain the pressure plateau.
    d. Criteria outlined in Chapters 25 and 26 should be followed during parame-
       ter selection.
K. Noninvasive approaches to mechanical ventilation
    1. Negative pressure ventilation
       a. Table 23–2 lists the capabilities of negative pressure generators currently
          available.
       b. Negative pressure can be provided with the use of:
          (1) Iron lung
          (2) Porta lung (full body chamber)
          (3) Poncho with chest shell
          (4) Pneumosuit with chest shell
          (5) Chest cuirass mass produced or customized
       c. Negative pressure ventilation functions best on individuals with neuromus-
          cular disease.
       d. It should not be used in patients with upper airway obstruction.
       e. For optimal use, respiratory rates and pressure must be high enough to cap-
          ture the diaphragm and inhibit spontaneous ventilation. Optimally the dia-
          phragm will work in synchrony with the ventilator.
       f. Most negative pressure units are controllers.
       g. The use of negative pressure ventilation is frequently successful when it is
          combined with other noninvasive approaches to ventilation.

TABLE 23–2.
Negative Pressure Generators

Ventilator	Mode	Rate	Maximum Negative Pressure (cm H_2O)	Maximum Positive Pressure (cm H_2O)	Power Failure Alarm	Low Pressure Alarm	I/E Ratio
33 CRE	Control	≤40	−50	No	No	No	Variable
33 CRX	Control	≤40	−60	No	No	No	Variable
33 CRA	Assistor	≤60	−50	No	No	No	Patient variable
Iron lung	Control	10–30	−60	—	—	—	1:1 (fixed)
Life Care 170C	Control	10–40	−60	+60	Yes	No	1:1.5 (fixed)
Puritan-Bennett Thompson Maxivent	Control	8–24	−70*	+70*	Yes	Yes	1:2 (fixed)

*The combined positive and absolute value of the negative pressure cannot exceed 70 cm H_2O.

2. Pneumobelt (Fig 23–5)
   a. This is a belt with an inflatable bladder designed to move the diaphragm up to assist exhalation.
   b. Inspiration occurs when the balloon deflates, allowing the diaphragm to move downward.
   c. It is effective only in the sitting position (at least 30 degrees).
   d. A pressure generator is used to inflate the bladder. Pressures of 50 to 70 cm H_2O are required, with the volume of gas entering the bladder approaching 2,000 ml to ensure appropriate movement.
   e. Tidal volumes of 300 to 500 ml can be achieved.
   f. All of these units function as controllers; they have no assist/control.
3. Rocking bed
   a. A rocking bed is a hospital-style bed designed to move the head and the foot of the bed in opposite directions rhythmically.
   b. Thus, head up, feet down tilt assists inspiration by moving the abdominal contents downward.
   c. Head down, feet up tilt assists exhalation by moving the abdominal contents upward.
   d. A maximum of a 60-degree arc is available.
   e. The rocking occurs at a rate between 8 and 34/min.
   f. It is most effective in neuromuscular disease patients.
   g. Normally it is ineffective in very thin patients.
   h. Frequently it is used with other noninvasive mechanical ventilation systems.
L. Elective noninvasive mechanical ventilatory assistance
   1. This is use of either positive pressure ventilation via mask (nasal or full face) or negative pressure ventilation at night or during the day for short periods (2–4 hours) to rest ventilatory muscles.
   2. Goals
      a. Rest ventilatory muscles.
      b. Increase muscle strength.
      c. Increase muscle endurance.
      d. Decrease resting P_{CO_2}.
      e. Increase exercise tolerance.
      f. Enhance activities of daily living.

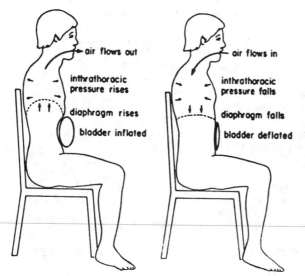

FIG 23–5.
Illustration of the function of the Pneumobelt. The Pneumobelt functions by exerting pressure on the abdominal contents by inflation of a rubber bladder. forcing the diaphragm upward and assisting exhalation *(left)*. When the bladder deflates, gravity pulls the diaphragm back down, assisting inhalation *(right)*. (From Hill NS: *Chest* 1986; 90:897–905. Used by permission.)

3. Indications
   a. Decreased FEV_1 (less than 25% predicted)
   b. Decreased forced vital capacity (less than 25% predicted)
   c. Decreased maximum voluntary ventilation (less than 25% predicted)
   d. Increased P_{CO_2}
   e. Decreased P_{O_2}
   f. Decreased maximum inspiratory pressure (less than 50 cm H_2O for chronic obstructive pulmonary disease; less than 25 cm H_2O for neuromuscular disease)
4. Although data on both negative and positive pressure ventilation appear promising, the use of nasal positive pressure ventilation seems to be most popular.
5. When nasal positive pressure ventilation is used:
   a. The assist/control mode should be used at a high enough backup rate to ensure control ventilation during sleep.
   b. Inspiratory time should be adjusted to equal the patient spontaneous inspiratory time (about 1.0 second).
   c. Peak flow should be 60 L/min or more.
   d. Tidal volume exhaled should be 8 to 12 ml/kg. Twice this level may need to be delivered because of leak.

BIBLIOGRAPHY

Bach JR, Alba AS, Bohatiak G, et al: Month intermittent positive pressure ventilation in the management of postpolio respiratory insufficiency. *Chest* 1987; 91:859–864.

Bach J, Alba A, Pilkington LA, et al: Long-term rehabilitation in advanced stage of childhood onset, rapidly progressive muscular dystrophy. *Arch Phys Med Rehabil* 1981; 62:328–331.

Banzett RB, Inbar GF, Brown R, et al: Diaphragm electrical activity during negative lower torso pressure in quadriplegic men. *J Appl Physiol* 1981; 51:654–659.

Banaszak EF, Travers H, Fazier M, et al: Home ventilator care. *Respir Care* 1981; 26:1262–1268.

Bolot JF, Robert D, Chemarin B, et al: Domiciliary-assisted ventilation by tracheostomy for chronic respiratory insufficiency. *Munch Med Wochenschr* 1977; 119:1641–1646.

Braun N: Respiratory muscle dysfunction. *Heart Lung* 1984; 13:327–332.

British Medical Research Council Working Party: Long-term domiciliary oxygen therapy in chronic hypoxic cor pulmonale complicating chronic bronchitis and emphysema. *Lancet* 1981; 1:681–686.

Carlin BW, Clausen JL, Ries AL: The use of cutaneous oximetry in the prescription of long-term oxygen therapy. *Chest* 1988; 94:239–241.

Dunkin LJ: Home ventilatory assistance. *Anaesthesia* 1983; 38:644–649.

Ellis ER, Grunstein RR, Chan S, et al: Noninvasive ventilatory support during sleep improves respiratory failure in kyphoscoliosis. *Chest* 1988; 94:811–815.

Feldman J, Tuteur PG: Mechanical ventilation: From hospital intensive care to home. *Heart Lung* 1982; 11:162–165.

Fischer DA, Prentice WS: Feasibility of home care for certain respiratory-dependent restrictive or obstructive lung disease patients. *Chest* 1982; 82:739–743.

Fraser IM, Berube CJ: Long-term positive-pressure ventilation. *Respir Technol* 1983; 19:13–18.

Gilmartin ME: Mechanical ventilation in the home: An overview, in Gilmartin ME, Make BJ (eds): *Mechanical Ventilation in the Home: Issues for Health Care Providers. Problems in Respiratory Care.* 1988, vol 1, pp 155–166.

Gilmartin M, Make B: Home care of ventilator-dependent persons. *Respir Care* 1983; 28:1490–1497.

Giovannoni R: Chronic ventilator care: From hospital to home. *Respir Ther* 1984; 14:29–33.

Goldberg AI: The regional approach to home care for life-supported persons. *Chest* 1984; 86:345–346.

Hughs RL: Home is the patient: A word of caution. *Chest* 1984; 86:344.

Kacmarek RM: Home care ventilators, in Bramson R, Hess D, Chatburn R (eds): *Respiratory Care Equipment.* Philadelphia, JB Lippincott Co (in press).

Kacmarek RM, Spearman CB: Equipment used for ventilatory support in the home. *Respir Care* 1986; 31:311–328.

Kacmarek RM, Stanek K, McMahon K, et al: Imposed work of breathing during synchronized intermittant mandatory ventilation using home care ventilations. *Respir Care* 1990; 35:405–414.

Kettrick RG, Donar ME: Ventilator-assisted infants and children, in Gilmartin ME, Make BJ (eds): *Mechanical Ventilation in the Home: Issues for Health Care Providers. Problems in Respiratory Care.* 1988, vol 1, pp 269–278.

Kopacz MA, Moriarty-Wright R: Multidisciplinary approach for the patient on a home ventilator. *Heart Lung* 1984; 13:255–262.

Maguire M, Vinz MT, Young P: Teaching patients' families to provide ventilator care at home. *Dimens Crit Care Nurs* 1982; 1:244–255.

Make B, Gilmartin M, Brody JS, et al: Rehabilitation of ventilator-dependent subjects with lung diseases: The concept and initial experiences. *Chest* 1984; 86:358–365.

Marino W, Braun N: Reversal of clinical sequelae of respiratory muscle fatigue by intermittent mechanical ventilation. *Am Rev Respir Dis* 1982; 125:830–836.

Leger P, Jennequin J, Gerard M, et al: Home positive pressure ventilation via nasal mask for patients with neuromuscular weakness or restrictive lung or chest-wall disease. *Respir Care* 1989; 39:73–80.

Nocturnal Oxygen Therapy Trial Group: Continuous or nocturnal oxygen therapy in hypoxemic chronic obstructive lung disease; a clinical trial. *Ann Intern Med* 1980; 93:391–398.

O'Donnel C, Gilmartin ME: Home mechanical ventilators and accessory equipment, in Gilmartin ME, Make BJ (eds): *Mechanical Ventilation in the Home: Issues for Health Care Providers. Problems in Respiratory Care.* 1988, vol 1, pp 217–240.

O'Donohue WJ: Patient selection and discharge criteria for home ventilator care, in Gilmartin ME, Make BJ (eds): *Mechanical Ventilation in the Home: Issues for Health Care Providers. Problems in Respiratory Care.* 1988, vol 1, pp 167–174.

O'Donohue WJ, Giovannoni RM, Goldberg AL, et al: Long-term mechanical ventilation. Guidelines of management in the home and at alternate community sites. *Chest* 1986; 90:1S–37S.

O'Leary J, King R, LeBlanc M, et al: Cuirass ventilation in childhood neuromuscular disease. *J Pediatr* 1979; 94:419–421.

O'Ryan JA, Burns DG: *Home ventilator care. Pulmonary rehabilitation: Hospital to home.* Chicago: Year Book Medical Publishers, 1984.

Rochester DF, Braun NMT, Laine S: Diaphragmatic energy expenditure in chronic respiratory failure. *Am J Med* 1977; 63:223–231.

Chapter 24

Assessment and Management of the Newborn

I. Clinical Evaluation of the Newborn
   A. Respiratory rate
      1. Normal rate: 30 to 60 breaths/min (bpm)
      2. Determined when newborn is not crying
      3. Tachypnea: Respiratory rates exceeding 60 bpm
   B. Apnea
      1. Apnea is often seen in premature newborns weighing less than 1,500 gm, with respiratory rates less than 30 bpm.
      2. It may be accompanied by bradycardia, cyanosis, or both.
      3. It may end with gently shaking or rubbing the newborn, or it may return spontaneously.
      4. Primary apnea may occur immediately after birth. The heart rate may fall during this time.
      5. Generally, newborns with primary apnea will resume breathing with stimulation.
      6. Secondary apnea is present when the newborn does not resume breathing on his or her own.
      7. The heart rate continues to fall, blood pressure falls, and the Pa_{O_2} level falls.
      8. Assisted ventilation is required.
   C. Retractions
      1. Retractions are present during increased inspiratory effort.
      2. They are visible around sternum, intercostal, and supraclavicular spaces.
      3. They result in a decrease in effective ventilation and an increase in deadspace ventilation.
      4. Increased respiratory rates may lead to seesaw breathing, which is dissynchrony between the abdomen and chest.
   D. Grunting
      1. Grunting is the sound heard on expiration created by the newborn exhaling through a partially closed glottis.
      2. In a newborn, grunting is created to maintain positive pressure in the lung to maintain alveolar stability.
      3. The more premature the newborn, the less the intensity of the grunt.

E. Cyanosis
   1. Acrocyanosis is present initially following birth. This is cyanosis of the hands and feet only.
   2. General or central cyanosis is found in the lips and mucosal lining of the mouth and is an indication of respiratory distress with hypoxemia.
F. Heart rate
   1. Normal rate is 120 to 160 beats/min.
   2. The heart rate is the most sensitive indicator of hypoxia. Since the stroke volume is relatively fixed, the cardiovascular system responds to all stress by increasing the heart rate.
   3. Outside stimuli (e.g., noise, cold, heat) affect the heart rate.
   4. The heart rate can be detected by palpation at the midclavicular line of the fifth intercostal space.
   5. Peripheral pulses are found by palpating the brachial, radial, and femoral arteries.
II. Apgar Score (Table 24–1)
   A. Following birth, the newborn is evaluated at 1- and 5-min intervals.
   B. The evaluation uses five factors:
      1. Heart rate
      2. Respiratory effort
      3. Muscle tone
      4. Reflex irritability
      5. Skin color
   C. The newborn is given a score of 0, 1, or 2 in all categories.
   D. The total score determines the newborn's condition at 1 and 5 min and assesses the resuscitative effort.
   E. Apgar scores of 7 to 10 (routine care)
      1. Put under radiant warmer.
      2. Dry.
      3. Suction mouth and nose.
   F. Apgar scores of 4 to 6
      1. Suction mouth and nose under radiant warmer.
      2. Stimulate by flicking soles of the feet and rubbing the back.
      3. If there is no improvement, provide supplemental oxygen with tubing over mouth and nose (flow rate 5 L/min).
      4. Reevaluate.
   G. Apgar scores of 0 to 3 (severe asphyxia)
      1. Suction mouth and nose.

TABLE 24–1.

Apgar Score

Sign	Score		
	0	1	2
Heart rate (beats/min)	Absent	<100	>100
Respiratory effort	Absent	Weak, irregular	Good, crying
Muscle tone	Flaccid	Some flexion of extremities	Well flexed
Reflex irritability	No response	Grimace	Cough or sneeze
Color	Blue, pale	Body pink, extremities blue	Completely pink

2. Bag and mask resuscitate with 100% oxygen.
3. If there is no improvement within 15 to 30 seconds, intubate.

III. Bag and Mask Resuscitation
    A. The appropriate-size mask and bag with an adjustable pressure popoff should be used.
    B. The jaw is moved upward and away from neck by placing a towel under the shoulders.
    C. Hyperextension should be avoided to prevent upper airway blockage because of the soft cartilage of the larynx.
    D. The patient is ventilated at a rate of 30 to 40 bpm.
    E. An orogastric tube may be required to aspirate air from the stomach.
    F. Effective ventilation is present when:
      1. Breath sounds are heard bilaterally.
      2. Heart rate increases (more than 100 beats/min).
      3. Chest is rising and falling.
      4. Color improves.
      5. Spontaneous movement and flexion of extremities occur.
    G. If no improvement occurs after 30 seconds:
      1. Reposition the head, neck, and mask.
      2. Reestablish ventilation.
    H. If after these maneuvers there is no improvement, intubate.

IV. Intubation
    A. Intubation should be done when:
      1. The heart rate is less than 100 beats/min.
      2. The Apgar score is less than 2.
      3. The birth weight is low.
      4. The infant is unresponsive to bag and mask ventilation.
      5. Transport of the unstable newborn is required.
    B. Estimations of tube sizes
      1. Weight
        a. Less than 1,000 gm = 2.5 mm inside diameter (I.D.)
        b. 1,000 to 2,000 gm = 3.0 mm I.D.
        c. 2,000 to 3,000 gm = 3.5 mm I.D.
        d. 3,000 to 4,000 gm = 4.0 mm I.D.
      2. Tubes smaller than 2.5 mm should not be used because of the high resistance to flow.
      3. Neonatal airways do not contain cuffs.
      4. Proper placement of the endotracheal tube can be assessed by:
        a. Increase in heart rate above 100 beats/min.
        b. Bilateral breath sounds
        c. Appropriate chest excursion
        d. Chest x-ray film
      5. Following intubation, the tube should be taped securely.
      6. Appropriate $F_{I_{O_2}}$ and humidification should be provided.

V. Complications of Intubation
    A. Hypoxia from incorrect tube placement or from the procedure taking too long
    B. Bradycardia from hypoxia
    C. Apnea from vagal response of laryngoscope, endotracheal tube stimulating posterior pharynx
    D. Trauma to airway, including mucosal damage, vocal cord damage, and perforation of the hypopharynx

VI. Procedure for Intubation
    A. Obtain proper equipment, which includes:
      1. Resuscitation bag and mask with pressure manometer.

2. Suction catheter (no. 5–6 French).
3. Bulb syringe.
4. Stylet with blunt end.
5. Proper size endotracheal tubes.
6. Laryngoscope and blade.
7. Tape.
8. Stethoscope.
9. Towel or diaper.
B. After obtaining equipment, suction the upper airway.
C. Oxygenate with resuscitation bag and mask and 100% oxygen.
D. Position the infant properly with a towel or diaper under the shoulders. This will help align the pharynx and trachea and put the infant in a "sniffing" position.
E. Insert appropriate-size blades and view vocal cords.
F. Insert appropriate size endotracheal tube through vocal cords into trachea.
G. After placement, ventilate at 30 to 40 bpm and pressures of 20 to 25 cm H_2O. Evaluate the position of the tube and the effectiveness of ventilation. Note the centimeter marking at the level of the upper lip.
H. If intubation is unsuccessful after 30 seconds and the heart rate drops to less than 100 beats/min, establish oxygenation with bag and mask resuscitation.
I. If no clinical improvement occurs following intubation:
1. Check for improper placement.
a. Esophagus: Remove tube and insert into trachea.
b. Right main stem: Withdraw 1 cm and reevaluate.
2. Increase ventilating rate.
3. Increase ventilating pressure.
4. Suction endotracheal tube to remove secretions.
VII. Maintenance of Artificial Airway
A. Respiratory water loss in newborns averages 41 ml/24 hours when they are breathing dry gas.
B. When a newborn is intubated, more than one fifth of the air conditioning surface is bypassed.
C. Humidification can reduce water loss down to 4 ml/24 hours.
D. Temperature of inspired gas should be between 35°C and 37°C with a relative humidity of 100%.
E. Reduction in the length of tubing and heating of tubes can help maintain the water content.
VIII. Suctioning
A. Perform suctioning as needed according to breath sounds and condition of the infant.
B. Use the appropriate-size catheter:

Endotracheal Tube Size	
mm I.D.	French Size
2.5	5
3.0	5–6
3.5	6–8
4.0	8

C. Saline can be instilled prior to suctioning to help thin secretions and keep the endotracheal tube patent.
D. Suction pressure should be less than 100 mm Hg.

    E. Remove thick secretions by repeated instillation of saline.

    F. Monitor the heart rate very closely during suctioning.

    G. After suctioning the endotracheal tube, remove secretions from the pharynx and nose as needed.

    H. Take care when suctioning deep into pharynx, because it may cause vomiting and aspiration around the endotracheal tube.

    I. The catheter should be marked following an initial suction attempt. Insert the catheter until it meets an obstruction. Pull back about 1 cm or until one of the markings on the catheter is in line with the universal adapter on the endotracheal tube.

    J. Turning the head from side to side may facilitate the introduction of the catheter into the opposite main stem bronchus.

    K. Apply suction only during withdrawal of the catheter and no longer than 10 seconds.

IX. Cardiopulmonary Resuscitation

    A. Initiate chest compressions when:

        1. The heart rate is less than 60 beats/min with 15 to 30 seconds of positive pressure ventilation with 100% oxygen.

        2. The heart rate is between 60 and 80 beats/min and not increasing.

        3. There is no heart rate.

    B. Two techniques may be used for cardiac compression on a normal-sized newborn.

        1. The first technique involves placing the thumbs of both hands on the middle third of the sternum just below the nipple line. The other fingers are wrapped around the neonate and are used to support the back.

        2. For a smaller newborn, the thumbs may be placed on top of one another.

        3. In a larger newborn, two-finger compression is done on the sternum with the ring and middle fingers. The compression on the sternum is done one finger below the nipple line. Support of the back is provided by the other hand.

        4. Compression should be done at a rate of 120 times/min and at a depth of ½ to ¾ in.

        5. With ventilation being delivered 40 times/min, this will give a 1:3 ratio of ventilation to compressions.

        6. Chest compressions are discontinued when the heart rate is 80 beats/min or greater.

    C. Various medications may be used during cardiopulmonary stress if there is no improvement of the heart rate and ventilation in the newborn.

        1. Best treatment for brief periods of bradycardia: Ventilation and 100% oxygen.

        2. Epinephrine:

            a. Has potent alpha and beta properties.

            b. Increases perfusion pressure, increases coronary blood flow, and increases oxygen delivery to the heart.

            c. Improves cardiac contractility and increases heart rate.

            d. Is given when the heart rate is less than 80 beats/min in spite of appropriate ventilation with 100% oxygen and chest compressions.

            e. Is given when the heart rate is 0 beats/min.

            f. Dosage is 0.1 to 0.3 ml/kg of a 1:10,000 solution.

            g. May be given every 5 min intravenously or by endotracheal tube instillation.

        3. Volume expanders are administered if:

            a. There is no return of color following oxygenation.

            b. The heart rate is good but the pulse is poor (shock).

            c. The response to resuscitation is poor in spite of good aeration.

            d. There is a decrease in blood pressure.

            e. Blood albumin, saline, normal saline, or Ringer's lactate may be administered intravenously (slowly over 5–10 min).

            f. Dosage is 10 ml/kg.

4. Sodium bicarbonate:
   a. Is administered for documented metabolic acidosis.
   b. Should not be used in brief episodes of cardiac arrest and when adequate ventilation is absent.
   c. For prolonged metabolic acidosis, a 0.5 mEq/L solution of sodium bicarbonate can be given (4 ml/kg) intravenously.
   d. If only 1.0 mEq/L is available, it should be mixed in a 1:1 solution with sterile water. This is administered intravenously and with a slow push.
   e. Dosage: 2 mEq/kg.
5. Naloxone hydrochloride (Narcan):
   a. Is a narcotic antagonist.
   b. Reverses respiratory depression induced by narcotics given to the mother up to 4 hours following birth.
   c. Dosage is 0.01 mg/kg.
   d. Administered via endotracheal tube, intravenously, or intramuscularly.
6. Dopamine:
   a. Increases blood pressure by increasing cardiac contractions, thereby increasing cardiac output.
   b. Administered intravenously when there is poor peripheral perfusion, thready pulse, and evidence of shock.
   c. Given after epinephrine, volume expander, and sodium bicarbonate.
   d. Dosage is begun at 5 μg/kg and may be increased up to 20 μg/kg.
   e. Heart rate and blood pressure should be monitored frequently.
7. Drugs that can be given via the endotracheal tube are atropine, lidocaine, isoproterenol (Isuprel), epinephrine, and naloxone (Narcan).

X. Other Newborn Assessment Scales
   A. Silverman score: Used to evaluate the level of respiratory distress of a neonate (Fig 24–1).
      1. Scores are based on a scale of 0 to 10.
         a. Scores of 0 to 3: No respiratory distress to mild respiratory distress
         b. Scores of 4 to 6: Moderate respiratory distress
         c. Scores of 7 to 10: Severe respiratory distress
      2. Scoring is performed in five areas and ranges from 0 to 2.
         a. Upper chest movement
            (1) Synchronized movement: 0
            (2) Lag of upper chest on inspiration: 1
            (3) Seesaw movement of upper chest: 2
         b. Lower chest movement
            (1) No retractions: 0
            (2) Retractions just visible: 1
            (3) Marked retractions: 2
         c. Xiphoid retractions
            (1) No retractions: 0
            (2) Retractions just visible: 1
            (3) Marked retractions: 2
         d. Dilation of nares
            (1) None: 0
            (2) Minimal dilation: 1
            (3) Marked dilation: 2
         e. Expiratory grunt
            (1) None: 0
            (2) Heard only with stethoscope: 1
            (3) Heard with naked ear: 2

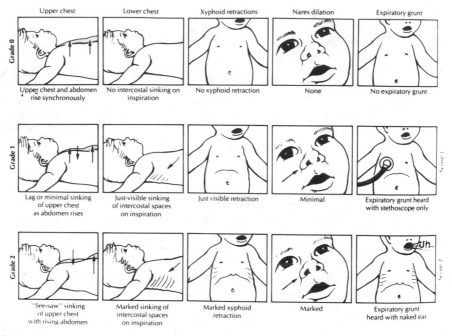

FIG 24–1.
Silverman scoring system for assessing and identifying breathing changes of the neonate. (From Eubanks D, Bone R: *Comprehensive Respiratory Care.* St Louis, CV Mosby Co, 1985. Used by permission.)

    B. Dubowitz scoring method
        1. The Dubowitz scoring method determines gestational age when used within the first 5 days of birth.
        2. It is accurate within 2 weeks of the newborn's gestational age.
        3. Each of the following categories is assessed on a grading scale. The higher the score assigned, the greater the gestational age of the newborn.
        4. Assessment is done bilaterally.
          a. External signs
            (1) Edema: Finger pressure on the dorsum of the foot is done for a few seconds. Assessment compares no edema to pitting edema (score 0–2).
            (2) Skin texture: Skin is assessed to determine skin texture. A transparent to leathery, cracked appearance is graded (score 0–4).
            (3) Skin color: Skin color is assessed during quiet time of the newborn. Scores are determined by a pale to dark red appearance over the ears, lips, palms, and soles of the feet (score 0–3).
            (4) Skin opacity: Skin of the abdominal trunk is assessed. More prominent skin veins are given a lower score and no skin veins seen given a higher score (Score 0–4).
            (5) Lanugo: The amount of fine hair over the back of the newborn. Premature infants have large amounts of hair, while term and post-term infants have no hair. Scores decrease with greater amounts of hair (score 0–4).
            (6) Plantar creases: Assessment is made on the soles of the feet. No creases are given a low score, and deep creases are given a high score (score 0–4).
            (7) Nipple formation: No nipple areola is given a low score, with areola raised and stippled given a higher score (score 0–3).

(8) Breast size: Assessment is done by palpating the nipple area and determining the approximate area of breast tissue. Measurements range from no breast tissue (low score) to more than 1 cm, which is given a high score (score 0–3).

(9) Ear form: Increase in scoring occurs as the form of the ear develops from the pinna being flat and shapeless to a well-defined, in-curving upper pinna (score 0–3).

(10) Ear firmness: Scores increase as the ear develops from a soft, easily folded ear to a firm ear with cartilage to the edge (score 0–3).

(11) Genitals:

   (a) Boys: Scores increase as the undescended testes develop into descended testes. Rugae, or wrinkles, in the scrotal sac are seen in the mature newborn.

   (b) Girls (with hips half abducted): Scores increase as the widely separated labia majora with protruded labia minora develops to where the labia majora is covered by the labia minora (score 0–2).

b. Neuromuscular/neurologic signs (Fig 24–2)

(1) Posture: Increased scores are assigned when greater flexion of the newborn is observed without touching.

(2) Square window: Scores are assessed by applying enough pressure to the hand to flex it to the forearm. Scores increase as that angle between the hypothenar eminence and forearm decreases from 90 to 0 degrees.

(3) Ankle dorsiflexion: The newborn's foot is flexed against the anterior aspect of the leg. Scores increase as this angle decreases from 90 to 0 degrees.

c. Arm recoil: The newborn's arms are flexed for a few seconds and then extended fully. Recoil is then observed by releasing the hands. Scores increase as the angle of the antecubital space reduces from 180 to less than 90 degrees.

d. Leg recoil: This assessment is done the same way as the arm recoil. The score increases as the angle between the knees and the hips decreases from 180 to less than 90 degrees.

e. Popliteal angle: The thigh is held in the high chest position. The leg is extended with the other hand. The scores increase as that angle behind the knee decreases from 180 to less than 90 degrees.

f. Heel to ear: The newborn's feet are drawn as close to the ears as possible. After releasing the feet, the score is then determined by assessing the popliteal angle and whether the feet can touch the ears.

g. Scarf sign: The newborn's hand is extended to the opposite shoulder. Scores increase if the elbow of the extended hand does not go past the middle of the chest.

h. Head lag: The newborn is pulled upward by both arms from a supine position. Scores increase if the newborn is able to hold the head forward. The newborn's head should be supported during this assessment.

i. Ventral suspension: The newborn, in a prone position, is suspended over one hand. The back, legs, arms, and neck are observed for extension. Scores increase as a curved back and neck with extended limp legs progress into a hyperextended back with good flexion of the arms and legs.

j. Scores indicate weeks of gestation (Table 24–2).

C. Ballard score (Fig 24–3)

1. The Ballard score includes six neuromuscular/neurologic and six physical signs.

a. Neuromuscular signs: Posture, square window, arm recoil, popliteal angle, scarf sign, and heal to ear.

b. Physical signs: Skin, lanugo, plantar creases, breast, ears, and genitals.

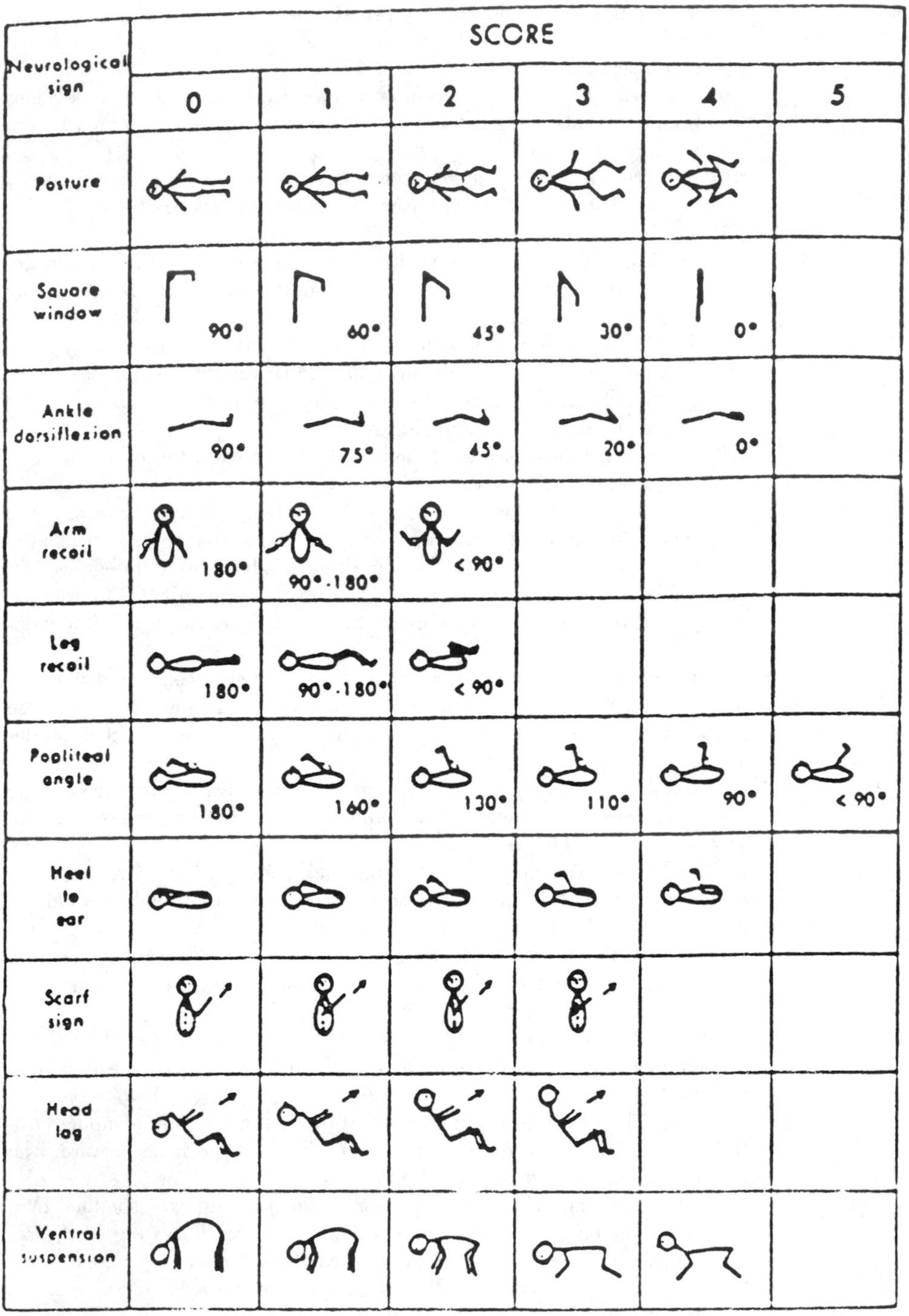

FIG 24–2.
Dubowitz scoring method. (From Dubowitz LMS, Dubowitz V, Goldberg C: Clinical assessment of gestational age in the newborn infant. *J Pediatr* 1970; 77:1–10. Used by permission.)

TABLE 24–2.
Dubowitz Scoring System

Score	Gestation (wk)
0–9	26
10–12	27
13–16	28
17–20	29
21–24	30
25–27	31
28–31	32
32–35	33
36–39	34
40–43	35
44–46	36
47–50	37
51–54	38
55–58	39
59–62	40
63–65	41
66–69	42

    2. It assesses the most useful items from the Dubowitz scoring system.

    3. Gestational age is assessable from 26 to 44 weeks.

XI. Oxygen Administration Equipment

  A. Isolette

    1. Ports in the back of the isolette allow oxygen to be connected by means of a connecting tube attached to a flowmeter.

    2. An internal blending device adjusts the F_{IO_2} that is delivered.

    3. An adjustable control provides alteration in the entrainment ports. When these ports are opened and oxygen is entering the unit, an F_{IO_2} of approximately 0.40 is achieved.

    4. The lever can be adjusted to occlude the ports, which increases the F_{IO_2} to 0.70 to 0.80.

    5. This system does not allow specific F_{IO_2} levels to be consistently delivered.

  B. Oxyhood

    1. If a specific F_{IO_2} level is desired, an oxyhood is preferred over an isolette.

    2. The device fits over the head of the newborn with an opening around the neck.

    3. The device is also used to provide warm humidity.

    4. The oxyhood has various small openings to allow temperature probes and oxygen-analyzing devices to be placed close to the newborn's head.

    5. This device, placed inside an isolette, allows a consistent and controllable F_{IO_2}, temperature, and humidity even when the integrity of the isolette has been altered.

    6. A minimum liter flow into the oxyhood of 4 to 6 L/min is needed to prevent rebreathing of exhaled carbon dioxide.

    7. An F_{IO_2} between 0.21 and 1.0 can be achieved.

  C. Other oxygen devices such as the Venturi mask, nasal cannula, simple, partial, and nonrebreather masks are not recommended for newborns.

  D. Nasal cannulas can be used for older newborns and infants who need continuous oxygen therapy because of bronchopulmonary dysplasia.

  E. Mist tent

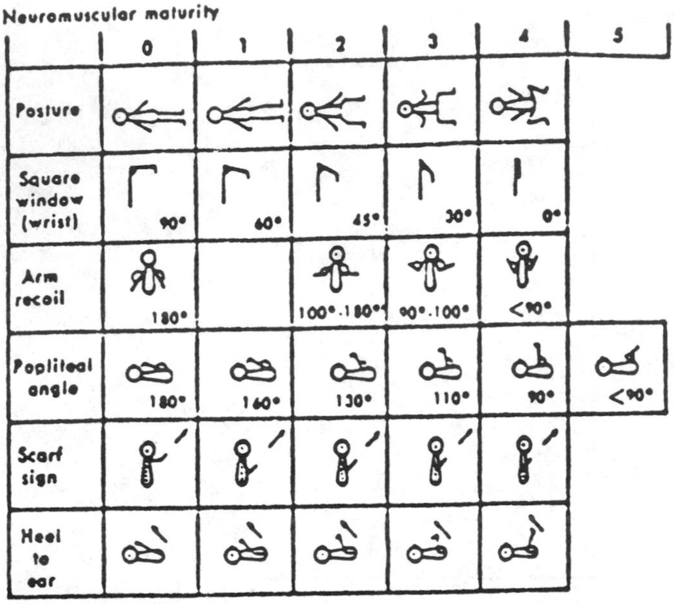

Neuromuscular maturity

	0	1	2	3	4	5
Posture						
Square window (wrist)	90°	60°	45°	30°	0°	
Arm recoil	180°		100°-180°	90°-100°	<90°	
Popliteal angle	180°	160°	130°	110°	90°	<90°
Scarf sign						
Heel to ear						

Physical maturity

Skin	Gelatinous red, transparent	Smooth pink, visible veins	Superficial peeling, &/or rash few veins	Cracking pale area rare veins	Parchment deep cracking no vessels	Leathery cracked wrinkled
Lanugo	None	Abundant	Thinning	Bald areas	Mostly bald	
Plantar creases	No crease	Faint red marks	Anterior transverse crease only	Creases ant. 2/3	Creases cover entire sole	
Breast	Barely percept.	Flat areola no bud	Stippled areola 1-2 mm bud	Raised areola 3-4 mm bud	Full areola 5-10 mm bud	
Ear	Pinna flat, stays folded	Sl. curved pinna; soft c̄ slow recoil	Well-curv. pinna; soft but ready recoil	Formed & firm c̄ instant recoil	Thick cartilage ear stiff	
Genitals ♂	Scrotum empty no rugae		Testes descending, few rugae	Testes down good rugae	Testes pendulous deep rugae	
Genitals ♀	Prominent clitoris & labia minora		Majora & minora equally prominent	Majora large minora small	Clitoris & minora completely covered	

Maturity rating

Score	Wks.
5	26
10	28
15	30
20	32
25	34
30	36
35	38
40	40
45	42
50	44

FIG 24-3.
Ballard scoring system. (From Ballard JL, Novak KK, Driver M: A simplified score for assessment of fetal maturation of newly born infants. *J Pediatr* 1979; 95:769–774. Used by permission.)

1. These devices are used for infants and children who require a cool environment and supplemental oxygen.
2. An FI_{O_2} of 0.30 to 0.50 can be achieved.
3. The temperature inside a well-functioning tent is about 7°C lower than room temperature.

4. Mist is provided by a baffle system that is powered by either air or oxygen at 12 to 15 L/min.
5. A fan or cooling unit inside the tent helps reduce the temperature.
6. The tent surrounds the bed and is tucked in under the mattress to maintain both temperature and F_{IO_2}.
7. If oxygen is being used, the child is not to have any toys that produce sparks within the tent.
8. Children with bronchiolitis, croup, and pneumonia commonly use mist tents with supplemental oxygen.

XII. Thermoregulation
  A. Skin temperature should be maintained between 35°C and 37°C.
  B. A newborn that is hypothermic will increase oxygen consumption and develop hypoxia, hypoglycemia, and periods of apnea.
  C. Heat loss can occur by:
    1. Evaporation: Loss of heat of evaporation.
    2. Conduction: Direct contact with cold surface.
    3. Radiation: Heat lost to cooler room.
    4. Convection: Heat lost to air currents (oxygen blown over face).
  D. Hyperthermia in the newborn may also cause hypoxemia and periods of apnea.
  E. Skin temperature should be monitored continuously to prevent wide fluctuations.

XIII. Equipment for Thermal Control
  A. Isolette or incubator
    1. It is used to administer oxygen, maintain proper temperature, and administer humidity.
    2. The temperature is monitored and maintained with a skin probe attached to the newborn.
    3. Newer isolettes are double walled. These monitor the inner surface of the isolette and the patient's skin. If either of these temperatures fall below a preset value, the incubator responds by increasing heat production.
    4. Access to the newborn is provided by hand holes on the side of the hood, or the hood can be lifted for complete exposure.
    5. The disadvantages of the isolette are that the device cannot maintain a consistent F_{IO_2} level, and humidification is provided by a system that blows air over standing water. A reduced relative humidity and infection are potential problems of these devices.
  B. Radiant warmers
    1. Radiant warmers use an open bed system that provides infrared heat from an overhead source.
    2. The device allows procedures to be performed on the newborn as well as greater accessibility during treatment.
    3. The wavelength of the infrared light does not harm the newborn's eyes.
    4. The amount of infrared heat is determined by a probe attached to the skin. The probe has a reflective patch to prevent inappropriate temperature adjustments.
    5. Heat loss can occur from evaporation and convection (personnel passing by create a breeze).
    6. The bed can be positioned to allow better access and therapeutic modalities to be provided to the newborn.
    7. Side shields can be placed around the bed to prevent convection and insensible water loss, or a plastic transparent sheet can be used to cover the newborn.

XIV. Blood Gas Monitoring (Invasive)
  A. Obtaining arterial blood gas (ABG) values
    1. Possible sites

  a. Radial artery stick
    (1) Use the radial artery on the thumb side.
    (2) Avoid the ulnar side because of the proximity of nerves.
    (3) Use a tuberculin syringe; a 25- to 26-gauge needle or butterfly may be used.
    (4) Transilluminate behind the wrist if you are unable to feel a pulse.
  b. Brachial, posterior tibial, temporal arteries
  c. Capillary heal stick
  d. Never use the femoral artery
  2. Normal ABG values (1–7 days after birth)
    a. pH: 7.37 to 7.40
    b. Pco_2: 33 to 35 mm Hg
    c. Po_2: 72 to 75 mm Hg
    d. HCO_3^-: 16 to 20 mEq/L
    e. Percentage of oxyhemoglobin ($HbO_2\%$): More than 90%
B. Complications of arterial blood gases
  1. Infection
  2. Hematoma
  3. Nerve damage
C. Obtaining capillary blood gas (CBG) values
  1. Possible sites: heel or finger
  2. Factors affecting CBG values
    a. Extrinsic factors
      (1) Improper technique
        (a) Application of pressure to puncture site
        (b) Inadequate warming of site (3–5 min for warming)
      (2) Excessive crying prior to puncture
    b. Intrinsic factors
      (1) Poor peripheral perfusion
      (2) Premature infant
      (3) Hypothermia
      (4) Hyperthermia
D. Comparison of CBG and ABG values
  1. Capillary blood gas Po_2 values are about 10 to 15 mm Hg less than actual ABG values. The difference between CBG and ABG Po_2 values become greater as the Po_2 values increase.
  2. The Pco_2 values are consistent in most circumstances but may differ up to 3 mm Hg (CBG values greater than ABG values).
  3. The CBG pH values tend to be consistent with the ABG pH values but may be 0.01 to 0.02 pH unit lower.
E. Umbilical artery line
  1. The umbilical artery line is inserted into either umbilical artery.
  2. The catheter is positioned at the level of lumbar vertebrae L3–4 on the chest x-ray film. (This may be referred to as *low position*.)
  3. The catheter placement is too high if it is in proximity of the diaphragm.
  4. Hazards include:
    a. Sepsis.
    b. Clot formation: If the clot occludes the line, the catheter should be removed. Never flush to remove the clot.
F. Blood gas abnormalities of the newborn
  1. Respiratory acidosis
    a. Ventilatory problem
    b. Chronic respiratory acidosis seen with bronchopulmonary dysplasia

2. Respiratory alkalosis
   a. Mechanical hyperventilation
      (1) Persistent fetal circulation
   b. Crying during blood gas puncture
3. Metabolic acidosis
   a. Metabolic acidosis normally is a result of hypoxemia (lactic acidosis).
   b. It is the most common acid-base problem of the newborn.
   c. Other causes include:
      (1) Dietary acid.
      (2) Keto acids.
      (3) Diarrhea.
      (4) Renal failure.
   d. These acids are excreted from the kidneys, not the lungs (nonvolatile acids).
   e. Premature newborns have immature phosphate and ammonia buffer systems and cannot handle the excessive buildup of metabolic acids.
   f. Newborns may develop persistent metabolic acidosis that:
      (1) Lasts longer than 3 days.
      (2) Has a base excess -7 to -15 mEq/L.
      (3) Is unrelated to asphyxia.
      (4) Is a dietary acid buildup.
   g. Signs include:
      (1) Poor weight gain.
      (2) Weight loss on adequate caloric intake.
      (3) Watery stools.
      (4) Lethargy in older infants.
      (5) Apnea in premature infants.
      (6) Gray pallor (not from anemia or hypoxia).
   h. Respiratory management includes oxygenation and ventilation if needed.
   i. Treatment of prolonged metabolic acidosis (not responsive to oxygenation) includes:
      (1) Giving sodium bicarbonate when the pH is less than 7.20 and the base deficit is more than -7 mEq/L.
      (2) Slowly infusing 4 ml of sodium bicarbonate/kg of a 0.5 mEq/L solution.
4. Metabolic alkalosis
   a. Metabolic alkalosis is commonly a result of:
      (1) Vomiting.
      (2) Nasogastric tube.
      (3) Hypokalemia.
      (4) Hypochloremia.
      (5) Diuretics.

BIBLIOGRAPHY

Aloan C: *Respiratory Care of the Newborn: A Clinical Manual.* Philadelphia, JB Lippincott Co, 1987.

American Heart Association: *Neonatal Resuscitation.* American Heart Association, 1988.

American Heart Association: *Pediatric Advanced Life Support.* American Heart Association, 1988.

Avery G: *Neonatalogy: Pathophysiology and Management of the Newborn,* ed 2. Philadelphia, JB Lippincott Co, 1981.

Bancalari E: Management of respiratory failure in the newborn, part I: Oxygen therapy and CPAP. *Curr Rev Respir Ther* 1980;(lesson 9):67–71.

Brill J: Resuscitation of the newborn. *Curr Rev Respir Ther* 1986; 9(lesson 6):43–51.

Curley M, Vaughn S: Assessment and resuscitation of the pediatric patient. *Crit Care Nurs* 1987; 7:26–42.

Hales R: New Directions in Pediatric Cardiopulmonary Resuscitation Section Connection. *Am Assoc Respir Care* 1989; 1(1):30–32.

Kaufman R, Van Fossan D, Aman Kwah K: A profile for testing fetal lung maturity. *Perinatal Neonatal* 1988; 5:35–38.

Koff P, Eitzman D, Neu J: *Neonatal and Pediatric Respiratory Care.* St Louis, CV Mosby Co, 1988.

Korones S: *High-risk Newborn Infants,* ed 4. St Louis, CV Mosby Co, 1986.

Lees M, King D: Recognition of cyanosis in the newborn. Pediatr Rev 1987; 9:36–42.

Malin S, Baumgart S: Optimal thermal management of low birth weight infants nursed under high-powered radiant warmers. *Pediatrics* 1987; 79:47–54.

Sendak M, Harris A: Oxygen saturation immediately after birth: An update on recent investigations. *Respir Manage* May/June 1988; 18:21–28.

Tucker S: Dopamine use in neonates. *Neonatal Network* October 1987; 5:21–24.

Wayman T: Factors affecting capillary blood-gas values. *Respir Ther* January/February 1980; 10:21–23.

Chapter 25

Respiratory Disorders of the Newborn

I. Transient Tachypnea in the Newborn (TTN)
  A. Transient tachypnea is seen in term or near-term newborns.
  B. It is considered type II respiratory distress syndrome (RDS).
  C. Symptoms begin 12 to 24 hours after birth and normally last only 24 hours.
  D. Respiratory rates may rise as high as 150 breaths/min (bpm).
  E. Predisposing factors
    1. Cesarean section
    2. Maternal analgesia
    3. Asphyxia in utero
    4. Maternal bleeding
    5. Prolapsed cord
    6. Maternal diabetes
  F. Clinical presentation and pathophysiology
    1. Newborn may be depressed at birth.
    2. Lung fluid is not absorbed, and clearing is delayed.
    3. Apgar scores are good at birth, but within 12 to 24 hours the newborn develops:
      a. Tachypnea.
      b. Nasal flaring.
      c. Grunting.
      d. Retractions.
      e. Cyanosis.
    4. Arterial blood gases show metabolic acidosis with mild hypoxemia.
  G. Radiologic findings
    1. There is pulmonary congestion after 12 hours.
    2. There are patchy infiltrates with a flattened diaphragm.
    3. X-ray findings may mimic cardiac problems, but the appearance resolves within 24 hours with TTN.
  H. Treatment
    1. Supplemental oxygen is given to maintain a Pa_{O_2} between 50 and 70 mm Hg and Sa_{O_2} at more than 90%.
    2. Continuous positive airway pressure may be used if there is no response from supplemental oxygen.

3. Mechanical ventilation is generally not required because resolution occurs within 12 to 24 hours, and the ability to ventilate is not normally impaired.

II. Meconium Aspiration Syndrome (MAS)
   A. Description
      1. Ten percent to 22% of newborns present with meconium aspiration.
      2. It is seen in full-term and postterm newborns.
      3. It is rarely seen in newborns less than 37 weeks of gestational age.
   B. Etiology
      1. Meconium is present in the colon late in gestation.
      2. Meconium is made up of undigested amniotic fluid and epithelial cells.
      3. Its consistency is highly viscous.
      4. If the newborn develops hypoxia in utero, several events occur:
         a. Redistribution of blood flow to vital organs
         b. Relaxation of anal sphincter and increased peristalsis
         c. Greater respiratory effort with gasping
         d. Passing of meconium into amniotic fluid
         e. Movement of meconium into the pharynx during increased respiratory effort
      5. Thick green "pea soup" appearance of the amniotic fluid normally indicates fetal distress and hypoxemia.
      6. Meconium is aspirated below the vocal cords during the newborn's first few breaths.
   C. Pathophysiology
      1. Aspiration of meconium causes a ball-valve obstruction.
      2. Hypoventilation and atelectasis normally follow.
      3. Alveolar edema and mucosal damage result from introduction of meconium into the lower airways.
      4. During the first few hours after aspiration, hypercarbia, hypoxemia, and metabolic acidosis develop.
      5. These may lead to persistent fetal circulation.
      6. As a result, a right-to-left shunt occurs, causing refractory hypoxemia.
      7. If mechanical ventilation is required, barotrauma and pneumothorax may complicate recovery.
   D. Radiologic findings
      1. Coarse irregular densities
      2. Diminished aeration
      3. Air bronchograms and consolidation in more severe cases
      4. Hyperexpansion with air trapping
   E. Clinical presentation
      1. Newborn presents with:
         a. Low Apgar score.
         b. Tachypnea.
         c. Grunting.
         d. Cyanosis.
         e. Nasal flaring.
         f. Hypoxia.
      2. Arterial blood gases (ABGs) show metabolic acidosis as a result of lactic acidosis.
      3. The chest is hyperexpanded from air trapping.
      4. Coarse rhonchi and rales occur.
      5. Expiration is prolonged.
      6. The newborn is stained with meconium fluid.

F. Treatment
   1. On presentation of the newborn's head and before the first breath is taken, the mouth, nose, nasopharynx, and oropharynx are suctioned.
   2. Heart rate is monitored.
   3. The vocal cords are viewed to determine if meconium is present at this level. If it is present, suctioning to the level of the vocal cords is performed.
   4. If meconium is aspirated, intubation and suctioning below the vocal cords are performed.
   5. Clearing of meconium by suction is always performed before assisted breaths are administered to facilitate removal of meconium and prevent further introduction into the lungs.
   6. Supplemental oxygen is provided to raise the P_{O_2} level above 50 mm Hg.
   7. Newborns that do not respond to increased $F_{I_{O_2}}$ (more than 0.60) normally require mechanical ventilation.
   8. Continuous positive airway pressure is seldom used because of the increased incidence of air leaks due to already overinflated alveoli.
   9. Mechanical ventilation is instituted when:
      a. The pH is less than 7.20.
      b. The Pa_{CO_2} is more than 70 mm Hg.
      c. The Pa_{O_2} is less than 50 mm Hg at an $F_{I_{O_2}}$ of 0.80 or greater.
   10. Goals of mechanical ventilation
      a. Maintain the Pa_{CO_2} at less than 50 mm Hg.
      b. Maintain the Pa_{O_2} at more than 50 mm Hg.
      c. Maintain the pH at more than 7.30.
   11. Ventilator settings
      a. High respiratory rates: More than 50 to 60 bpm
      b. Lowest peak inspiratory pressure necessary to keep blood gases in acceptable range
      c. Minimal positive end-expiratory pressure (PEEP): Less than 4 cm H_2O
      d. The $F_{I_{O_2}}$ to maintain the Pa_{O_2} at more than 50 mm Hg
   12. Recovery from MAS without mechanical ventilation takes place within 3 to 7 days.
   13. With mechanical ventilation assistance, 7 to 10 days may be required. More severe cases may take weeks.
   14. Extracorporeal membrane oxygenation is being used by some in very severe cases.
III. Pneumothorax
   A. Etiology
      1. Vigorous resuscitation
      2. Pulmonary disease requiring mechanical ventilation
         a. Meconium aspiration
         b. Respiratory distress syndrome
         c. Neonatal asphyxia
      3. High peak and mean airway pressures from mechanical ventilator, along with local hyperinflation
   B. Pathophysiology
      1. There may be air trapping and incomplete exhalation.
      2. More compliant alveoli adjacent to atelectatic alveoli may be overdistended from high intrapulmonary pressure.
      3. Ruptured alveolar blebs may be present.
      4. Improved lung compliance without a reduction in ventilator settings.
   C. Clinical presentation
      1. Irritability of newborn

    2. Sudden cardiopulmonary deterioration

    3. Tachypnea

    4. Tachycardia

    5. Cyanosis

    6. Pallor

    7. Increased respiratory efforts and appearance of cyanosis if the infant is on mechanical ventilation

    8. Change in cardiac impulse, shifting away from affected side

D. Diagnosis

    • Diagnosis can be determined with transillumination.

    1. Transillumination is the passage of light through body tissues for the purpose of examining a structure.

    2. The fiberoptic transilluminator is placed superior then inferior to the newborn's nipple bilaterally.

    3. A greater appearance of light under the chest suggests an abnormal amount of air in the thoracic cavity.

    4. If the lung is inflated, the tissue will absorb most of the light.

    5. If a pneumothorax is present, an outline of the collapsed lung will appear. The portion of the thorax containing air will appear brighter than the collapsed lung.

    6. A normal transillumination is confirmed by chest radiograph.

E. Treatment

    1. Decompression is performed promptly.

    2. A chest tube is placed at the second to third intercostal space lateral to the midclavicular line.

    3. The tube should be connected to an underwater seal drainage unit with −20 cm H_2O of suction

    4. Improvement of the newborn's condition is usually immediate.

IV. Persistent Fetal Circulation (PFC) or Persistent Pulmonary Hypertension in the Newborn (PPHN)

A. Description

    1. It is characterized by severe hypoxemia and cyanosis a few hours after birth.

    2. Right-to-left shunting, secondary to pulmonary hypertension, is present.

    3. It occurs as a result of the ductus arteriosus and foramen ovale failing to close or reopening after closure.

    4. No apparent lung disease is noted.

    5. Other causes include:

      a. Bacterial or viral pneumonia.

      b. Septecemia.

      c. Meconium aspiration.

      d. Transient tachypnea with hypoxemia.

      e. Intraventricular hemorrhage.

B. Pathophysiology

    1. Pulmonary hypertension occurs, causing increased pulmonary vascular resistance (PVR).

    2. Hypoxemia increases PVR, reducing pulmonary blood flow further.

    3. With the resultant hypoxemia, the ductus arteriosus opens, shunting blood from the pulmonary artery to the aorta and resulting in an increased right-to-left shunt.

    4. Because of the increased PVR and shunting, pulmonary venous return to the left side of the heart is reduced, reducing the left arterial filling pressure.

    5. Heart pressure on the right side exceeds heart pressure on the left side, reopening the foramen ovale and causing right-to-left shunting.

6. Blood gases show severe hypoxemia and acidosis with a normal CO_2 level.

C. Clinical presentation

1. Term and postterm newborn with severe respiratory distress and cyanosis
2. Hypoxemia
3. Tachypnea and cyanosis

D. Diagnosis

1. Need to differentiate between:
   a. Respiratory distress syndrome
   b. PFC or PPHN
   c. Congenital heart disease (cyanotic)

2. Tests to determine diagnosis:
   a. Hyperoxia test
      (1) Place infant in 100% oxygen for 5 to 10 min.
      (2) Determine the Pa_{O_2}. If the Pa_{O_2} is more than 100 mm Hg, lung disease is present. If the Pa_{O_2} is less than 50 mm Hg, a large right-to-left shunt is present.
      (3) If the Pa_{O_2} is less than 50 mm Hg, either PFC or cyanotic congenital heart disease is present.
      (4) To differentiate PFC from other anomalies, preductal and postductal ABG comparison is done.
   b. Preductal and postductal ABG comparison
      (1) Patient breathes 100% oxygen.
      (2) Blood gases are obtained from:
         (a) Preductal arteries: Right radial, brachial, and temporal.
         (b) Postductal arteries: Left radial, posterior tibial, and umbilical.
      (3) Also preductal and postductal $Tc_{P_{O_2}}$ measurements can be obtained by placing an electrode in a postductal position on the left lower quadrant of the chest and a preductal position on the right upper quadrant of the chest.
      (4) Results: A preductal and postductal Pa_{O_2} difference of more than 15 mm Hg indicates ductal shunting. A preductal and postductal Pa_{O_2} difference of less than 15 mm Hg indicates no significant ductal shunting.
   c. Hypoxemia-hyperventilation test
      (1) This is the most definitive test to determine PFC.
      (2) It may be performed on intubated and nonintubated patients.
      (3) The patient is hyperventilated with 100% oxygen using a resuscitator bag.
      (4) Respiratory rates of 100 to 150/bpm are delivered.
      (5) Watch the rise and fall of the chest; listen to breath sounds to determine ventilation.
      (6) If the patient is hyperventilated with 100% oxygen, the Pa_{CO_2} will decrease and the Pa_{O_2} will increase, thus reducing PVR and pulmonary hypertension.
      (7) Blood gases should show a reduced P_{CO_2} (20–25 mm Hg) and a significant increase in Pa_{O_2} (more than 100 mm Hg) if PFC is present.
      (8) Cyanosis diminishes or disappears.
      (9) No significant change in the Pa_{O_2} will occur with congenital heart disease.

E. Treatment

1. The goal is to reduce PVR and reverse right-to-left shunt.
2. The newborn can be put in an oxyhood with 100% oxygen.
3. If the infant is unresponsive, mechanical ventilation is instituted.
4. Settings are established from the hyperventilation test results.

5. Peak inspiratory pressures (PIPs) and rate are set to ensure hyperventilation. The ABGs are maintained as follows:
    a. P_{CO_2}: 20 to 25 mm Hg (critical P_{CO_2} level)
    b. pH: More than 7.45
    c. P_{O_2}: More than 120 mm Hg
6. Mechanical ventilator settings:
    a. PIP: 35 to 40 cm H_2O (determined from hyperventilation test)
    b. Inspiratory:expiratory ratio: Short inspiratory times (less than 0.5 seconds)
    c. $F_{I_{O_2}}$: 0.70 to 1.0.
    d. Respiratory rate: Adjust to maintain a "critical P_{CO_2} level" (rates may be as high as 150 bpm)
    e. Positive end-expiratory pressure: 4 cm H_2O or less (unless lung disease is present)
    f. Flow rate: Adequate to achieve short inspiratory time (less than 0.5 seconds)
7. Weaning
    a. Weaning may be initiated when the Pa_{O_2} is stable at more than 120 mm Hg.
    b. The $F_{I_{O_2}}$ is reduced by 0.01–0.02 and continued as long as the Pa_{O_2} is more than 120 mm Hg.
    c. Peak inspiratory pressures are reduced by 1 cm H_2O, again maintaining the Pa_{O_2} at more than 120 mm Hg and the P_{CO_2} at 20 to 25 mm Hg.
8. Pharmacology
    a. The α-adrenergic antagonist tolazoline can be used. It vasodilates pulmonary arteries to reduce pulmonary artery pressure (PAP). Side effects include pulmonary hemorrhage, gastrointestinal bleeding, and systemic hypotension.
    b. Volume expanders and dopamine may be given to correct hypotension.
9. Persistent fetal circulation is reversed when the PAP is less than the arterial pressure.
10. Other care
    a. Blood pressure (systolic) is maintained at 60 to 80 mm Hg.
    b. Muscle relaxants and sedatives may be used to prevent fighting the ventilator and fluctuation of Pa_{O_2}.
11. Extracorporal membrane oxygenation is being used by some in very severe cases.

V. Idiopathic Respiratory Distress Syndrome (IRDS), or Hyaline Membrane Disease (HMD)
  A. Incidence
    1. It occurs in 60% of premature infants weighing 1.0 to 1.5 kg at birth.
    2. It occurs in 5% of newborns of gestational age 35 weeks or less.
    3. Increased risk is associated with:
        a. Cesarean section delivery.
        b. Maternal hemorrhage.
        c. Maternal diabetes.
        d. Asphyxia at birth.
        e. Multiple births.
  B. Etiology
    1. Pulmonary hypoperfusion and ischemia
    2. Internal hemorrhage in the mother, causing reduced blood flow to the fetus
  C. Pathophysiology
    1. Reduction in lung volume from a lack of surfactant due to prematurity
    2. Reduced compliance
    3. Atelectasis

4. Hypoxemia and acidosis
5. Uneven ventilation/perfusion and hypoventilation
6. Increase in PVR
7. Pulmonary hypoperfusion
8. Increase in pulmonary capillary permeability
9. Plasma leakage
10. Protein and fibrin in fluid, which clots and forms a membrane lining alveoli and bronchioles (hyaline membranes)
11. Increased diffusion gradient
12. Increased intrathoracic pressures during mechanical ventilation
13. Right-to-left shunt with persistent fetal circulation
14. High $F_{I_{O_2}}$ levels and airway pressures during mechanical ventilation, causing further damage to tissues of the airways

D. Clinical presentation
   1. Onset of symptoms present at birth or 6 to 8 hours after birth
   2. Low Apgar score
   3. Expiratory grunting
   4. Nasal flaring
   5. Seesaw breathing
   6. Tachypnea
   7. Cyanosis when room air is breathed

E. Radiologic findings
   1. Classic appearance in the untreated newborn is reticulogranular infiltrates described as a "ground glass" appearance.
   2. Air bronchograms show collapsed alveoli surrounding air-filled bronchi.
   3. Lung volume is decreased.

F. Laboratory findings
   1. Elevated blood urea nitrogen level
   2. Arterial blood gas values
      a. Initially
         (1) pH: Less than 7.35 to 7.45
         (2) P_{CO_2}: Less than 35 to 45 mm Hg
         (3) P_{O_2}: Less than 50 to 70 mm Hg
      b. As IRDS progresses
         (1) pH: Less than 7.30
         (2) P_{CO_2}: Greater than 50 mm Hg
         (3) P_{O_2}: Less than 40 mm Hg
   3. Low urine output from lack of peripheral perfusion

G. Treatment
   1. Treat hypoxemia; keep the P_{O_2} at more than 50 mm Hg.
   2. Continuous positive airway pressure may be used initially when:
      a. The P_{CO_2} is normal, the P_{O_2} is less than 50 mm Hg at an $F_{I_{O_2}}$ of 0.60 or greater, and the pH is more than 7.30.
   3. Mechanical ventilation may be required when:
      a. The newborn is premature (less than 2,500 gm).
      b. The pH is 7.20.
      c. The Pa_{CO_2} is more than 60 mm Hg.
      d. The Pa_{O_2} is less than 40 mm Hg.
   4. Mechanical ventilation settings
      a. PIP: 25 to 35 cm H_2O
      b. Respiratory rates: 40 to 100/min
      c. $F_{I_{O_2}}$: More than 0.60
      d. PEEP: 4 to 8 cm H_2O

5. Maintain temperature at 35°C to 37°C.
6. Maintain fluid and electrolyte balance.
7. Maintain red blood cell count and glucose levels.
8. Reverse pulmonary hypertension with oxygen.
9. Watch for acute problems such as pneumothorax. When compliance starts to improve, the danger of pneumothorax from high ventilatory pressures is greatest.
10. Extracorporal membrane oxygenation is used by some in severe cases.

H. Prognosis
   1. The infant should recover in 10 to 14 days with minimal complications.
   2. If mechanical ventilation progresses longer than 2 weeks, the incidence of bronchopulmonary dysplasia increases.

VI. Bronchopulmonary dysplasia (BPD)
   A. It is a chronic disease in premature infants requiring supplemental oxygen to maintain a Pa_{O_2} level of more than 50 mm Hg.
   B. Etiology
      1. High levels of oxygen for a prolonged period
      2. Lengthy periods of positive pressure ventilation with high peak and mean airway pressures
   C. Infants weighing less than 1,500 gm have higher incidences.
   D. Pathophysiology
      1. Acute phase: 2 to 3 days after birth
         a. Classic RDS picture
         b. Ground glass (reticulogranular) appearance on chest x-ray film and air bronchograms
      2. Stage II: Up to 10 days
         a. Hyaline membrane formation
         b. Marked opacity of the lung
         c. Necrosis of alveolar epithelium
      3. Stage III: Up to 20 days
         a. Transition into chronic phase
         b. Alveolar emphysema and interstitial fibrosis
         c. Honeycomb pattern on chest x-ray film
         d. Development of cor pulmonale
      4. Stage IV: More than 1 month
         a. Formation of cysts throughout lung
         b. Marked respiratory distress, cyanosis, and diffuse rales
         c. Difficulty in weaning off ventilator
         d. Hyperinflation, flattened diaphragm, and atelectasis on chest x-ray film
         e. Cardiomegaly from cor pulmonale
         f. Thickened alveolar walls and increased diffusion gradient
   E. Clinical presentation
      1. Initially, typical appearance is that of an infant with respiratory distress who needs assisted ventilation.
      2. Multiple pneumothoracies are common.
      3. There is a lengthy ventilatory course associated with poor response to therapy.
         a. Increase in PIP: More than 25 cm H_2O
         b. Respiratory rates: More than 60 bpm
         c. $F_{I_{O_2}}$: 1.0
   F. Treatment
      1. Mechanical ventilation
      2. Maintain $F_{I_{O_2}}$ as low as possible by titrating PEEP to achieve PaO_2 above 50 mm Hg.

3. Bronchial hygiene: Suctioning, percussion and postural drainage, humidity
4. Bronchodilators
5. Digitalis and diuretics
6. Nutrition
G. Postmechanical ventilation
1. Use low flow oxygen.
2. Maintain the P_{O_2} 50 to 70 mm Hg.
3. Maintain the Pa_{CO_2} 40 to 60 mm Hg.
4. Pulmonary status normalizes by the age of 6 to 8 years.
VII. Pneumonia
A. Etiology
1. May be acquired during birth or after delivery.
2. May be viral, bacterial, or fungal in origin.
3. Most common neonatal infections: Herpes virus and cytomegalovirus.
B. Pathophysiology
1. Prenatal pneumonia may be acquired by transfer from the placenta or inhalation of amniotic fluid that is contaminated.
2. During birth the infant may aspirate contaminated materials (meconium).
3. Rupture of placental membranes greater than 12 hours prior to birth increases the incidence of infectious agents spreading to amniotic fluid and contaminating the fetus.
4. Postnatally, inhalation of contaminated aerosols or septicemia may lead to pneumonia.
5. Sepsis develops from gram-negative pulmonary infections more rapidly in premature infants than mature newborns because of greater lung involvement.
6. The most common pathogen is group B, β-hemolytic *Streptococcus* found in vaginal tissue.
7. Other pathogens include:
   a. *Escherichia coli*
   b. *Klebsiella*
   c. Enterococci
   d. *Pseudomonas* (after birth)
   e. *Staphylococcus* (after birth)
8. *Staphylococcus* is usually seen in newborns following birth and is spread by contact from health personnel.
C. Clinical presentation
1. Chest x-ray resembles RDS
2. Periods of apnea
3. Thermal instability
4. Dyspnea
5. Pallor or cyanosis
6. Poor weight gain (failure to thrive)
7. Respiratory distress
D. Laboratory findings
1. Hypoxemia with progressing metabolic acidosis
2. Increase in neutrophils and shift to the left of more than 15%
3. Sepsis (diagnosed by blood cultures)
E. Treatment
1. Oxygen therapy.
2. Aerosol therapy.
3. Broad-spectrum antibiotics (penicillin, ampicillin, kanamycin) are used initially.

4. Once the organism is identified, a specific agent is administered.

5. Hypotension is normally treated with dopamine and fluid.

6. Mechanical ventilation may be required in more severe cases.

VIII. Retinopathy of Prematurity (Retrolental Fibroplasia, or RLF)

    A. Etiology

        1. Lengthy exposure to oxygen in premature infants

            a. More than 1,000 gm: Eye damage occurs in 20% to 25%.

            b. 1,000 to 1,500 gm: Eye damage occurs in 2%.

        2. Pa_{O_2} of blood supplying retina more than 80–100 mm Hg

        3. Other risk factors

            a. Exchange transfusion

            b. Maternal hypertension

            c. Heavy cigarette smoking by mother

            d. Patent ductus arteriosus (PDA)

    B. Pathophysiology

        1. Immature blood vessels supplying the retina are constricted from one or more of the etiologies.

        2. Vascularization of the retina is reduced.

        3. Over the next few weeks, new capillary formation causes hemorrhage and peripheral retinal clouding and scarring.

        4. With minor scarring behind the retina, there may be normal vision if the causitive factor is removed. No permanent injury will result.

        5. After this time, further damage can occur with localized, peripheral, or total detachment of the retina.

        6. It can occur from extensive scarring behind the retina (cicatricial stacic).

    C. Treatment and prevention

        1. Maintaining Po_2 levels at 50 to 70 mm Hg.

        2. Reducing the time of exposure to high $F_{I_{O_2}}$ levels (more than 0.50).

        3. Using oxygen blenders to provide specific $F_{I_{O_2}}$ level during procedures (i.e., suctioning, apneic spell, endotracheal intubation).

        4. Performing frequent opthalmologic assessments.

        5. Using laser surgery to treat glaucoma.

IX. Cardiac Anomalies

    A. Patent ductus arteriosus (PDA) (Fig 25–1)

        1. It is an acyanotic anomaly (left-to-right shunt).

        2. It develops because of a failure of the ductus arteriosus to close at birth.

        3. Because of the difference between pulmonary artery and aortic pressures, left ventricular output flows into the pulmonary artery via the PDA.

        4. Right ventricular work greatly increases, resulting in congestive heart failure (CHF).

        5. This entity is most common among preterm infants with IRDS.

        6. Treatment

            a. Indomethacin (Indocin), a prostaglandin inhibitor that causes constriction of the ductus arteriosus, is prescribed.

            b. Surgical correction may be necessary.

    B. Atrial septal defects (ASDs) (Fig 25–2)

        1. It is an acyanotic anomaly (left-to-right shunt).

        2. It reflects failure of the foramen ovale to close or failure of the atrial septum to form correctly.

        3. Basic types of defects

            a. Ostium primum: Occurs low in the atrial wall and usually involves the mitral and tricuspid valves.

            b. Ostium secundum: Is an isolated defect occurring high in the atrial wall.

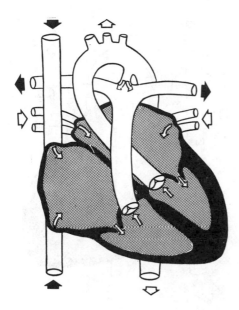

FIG 25–1.
Patient ductus arteriosus. (From Ross Laboratories
Clinical Education Aid no 7 [G163], Columbus, Ohio,
1978. Used by permission.)

4. Because of the pressure difference between the left and right atria, blood moves from the left atrium to the right atrium via the ASD.
5. Work of the right side of the heart frequently increases, resulting in CHF.
6. Treatment: Surgical correction by direct closure or by use of a plastic prosthesis via open heart surgery.

C. Ventricular septal defects (VSDs) (Fig 25–3)
   1. It is an acyanotic anomaly (left to right shunt).
   2. They vary considerably in size and may develop in either the membranous or muscular portion of the septal wall.
   3. Small defects may cause minor left-to-right shunting and normally close spontaneously.

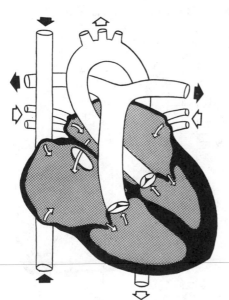

FIG 25–2.
Atrial septal defect. (From Ross Laboratories Clinical
Education Aid no 7 [G163], Columbus, Ohio, 1978.
Used by permission.)

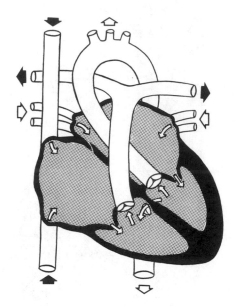

FIG 25–3.
Ventricular septal defect. (From Ross Laboratories
Clinical Education Aid no 7 [G163], Columbus, Ohio,
1978. Used by permission.)

    4. With large defects, significant left-to-right shunting occurs.
        a. Left and right ventricular pressures equilibrate.
        b. Since pulmonary vascular resistance is only about one fifth systemic vascular resistance, the majority of cardiac output is forced through the lung.
        c. As a result, CHF develops.
    5. Treatment
        a. Small defects: Spontaneous closure.
        b. Large defects: Surgical correction.
  D. Aortic stenosis (subaortic stenosis) (Fig 25–4)
    1. It is an acyanotic anomaly.
    2. It is an obstructive outflow lesion of the left ventricle.
    3. It develops as a result of a fibrous lesion at the aortic semilunar valve.

FIG 25–4.
Aortic stenosis. (From Ross Laboratories Clinical
Education Aid no 7 [G163], Columbus, Ohio, 1978.
Used by permission.)

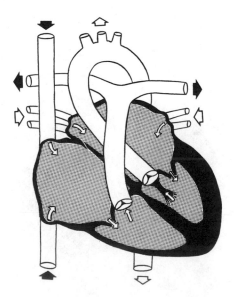

4. Left ventricular hypertrophy develops as a result of the increased resistance to cardiac output.
5. Treatment: Surgical correction may be necessary, which is achieved by performing an aortic valvulotomy or by dividing the fibrous obstruction below the aortic semilunar valve.

E. Coarctation of the aorta (Fig 25–5)
1. It is an acyanotic or cyanotic anomaly.
2. It is characterized by a narrowed aortic lumen.
3. The majority of cardiac output moves to the head and upper extremities.
4. Hypertension frequently develops in the upper extremities and hypotension in the lower extremities.
5. Types of coarctation
   a. Preductal coarctation: Stenosis of the aorta proximal to the entrance of the ductus arteriosus, which will cause cyanosis (right-to-left shunting).
   b. Postductal coarctation: Stenosis of the aorta distal to the ductus arteriosus, which will not cause cyanosis (left-to-right shunting).
6. Treatment
   a. Medical treatment with digitalis is given for heart failure.
   b. Surgical correction by resection of the coarctation is usually necessary.

F. Tricuspid Atresia (Fig 25–6)
1. It is a cyanotic anomaly (right-to-left shunting).
2. It is an obstructive lesion; the normal pathway of blood from the right atrium to the right ventricle through the tricuspid valve is partially blocked.
3. It is characterized by:
   a. Small right ventricle.
   b. Large left ventricle.
   c. Diminished pulmonary circulation.
4. Blood from the right atrium passes through an ASD into the left atrium, where it mixes with oxygenated blood from pulmonary veins.
5. Then blood flows into the left ventricle and can go into the aorta or through a VSD to the right ventricle and into the pulmonary circulation.
6. Treatment: Surgical correction is necessary and entails anastomosis of the aorta to the pulmonary artery and/or anastomosis of the superior vena cava to the right pulmonary artery to increase pulmonary blood flow.

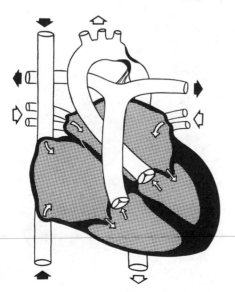

FIG 25–5.
Coarctation of the aorta. (From Ross Laboratories Clinical Education Aid no 7 [G163], Columbus, Ohio, 1978. Used by permission.)

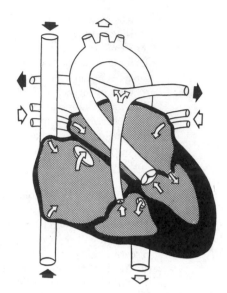

FIG 25–6.
Tricuspid atresia. (From Ross Laboratories Clinical
Education Aid no 7 [G163], Columbus, Ohio, 1978.
Used by permission.)

G. Tetralogy of Fallot (Fig 25–7)
1. It is a cyanotic anomaly (right-to-left shunt).
2. It is characterized by:
   a. Ventricular septal defect
   b. Stenosis of the pulmonic valve
   c. Dextroposition of the aorta
   d. Hypertrophy of the right ventricle
3. Obstruction to right ventricular outflow because of pulmonary stenosis causes
   right ventricular hypertrophy. Blood will then be shunted through the VSD
   into the dextropositional aorta. This will cause blood from the right side of the
   heart to pass directly into the systemic system unoxygenated. Right ventricular pressure will be equal to left ventricular pressure.
4. Treatment: It is managed medically, including adequate hydration. Surgery
   may be necessary to create an anastomosis between systemic and pulmonary
   circulations to increase pulmonary blood flow.

FIG 25–7.
Tetralogy of Fallot. (From Ross Laboratories Clinical
Education Aid no 7 [G163], Columbus, Ohio, 1978.
Used by permission.)

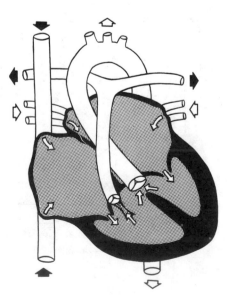

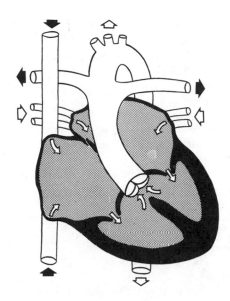

FIG 25–8.
Truncus arteriosus. (From Ross Laboratories Clinical Education Aid no 7 [G163], Columbus, Ohio, 1978. Used by permission.)

H. Truncus arteriosus (Fig 25–8)
  1. It is a cyanotic anomaly (right-to-left shunt)
  2. It is characterized by:
    a. Ventricular septal defect associated with a common blood vessel leaving both ventricles.
    b. Branching of pulmonary arteries from the common vessel (truncus), which continues as the aorta.
    c. Variable pulmonary blood flow, dependent on level of the stenosis distal to branching of the pulmonary arteries.
    d. Variable pulmonary symptoms, depending on amount of pulmonary circulation.
    e. Commonly both right and left ventricular hypertrophy.
  3. An admixture of venous and arterial blood from the right and left ventricles empties into a common vessel (bulbar trunk) at systemic pressure. Blood will

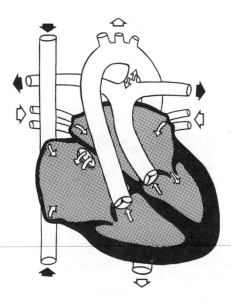

FIG 25–9.
Complete transposition of the great vessels. (From Ross Laboratories Clinical Education Aid no 7 [G163], Columbus, Ohio, 1978. Used by permission.)

either continue out the trunk to the systemic circulation or enter the pulmonary arteries. Pulmonary hypertension is often present.

4. Treatment: No surgical correction is available at this time. Medical management is used to reduce pulmonary hypertension and infections.

I. Complete transposition of the great vessels (Fig 25–9)
   1. It is a cyanotic anomaly (right-to-left shunt).
   2. It is characterized by:
      a. Reversed position of aorta and pulmonary arteries (i.e., the aorta comes off the right ventricle and the pulmonary artery comes off the left ventricle).
      b. Frequently the presence of a PDA and ASD.
   3. Two separate circulations occur, with the aorta emanating from the right ventricle and returning through systemic veins into the right atrium and the pulmonary artery emanating from the left ventricle and returning to the left atrium via the pulmonary veins. Venous and arterial blood may mix through an ASD, VSD, or PDA (Table 25–1).
   4. Treatment: Surgical correction may be necessary.

J. Anomalous venous return of the pulmonary veins (Fig 25–10)
   1. It is a cyanotic anomaly (right-to-left shunt).
   2. It is characterized by oxygenated blood returning from the lungs to the right atrium by one or more pulmonary veins.
   3. Types of anomalous return
      a. Complete: All pulmonary and systemic veins enter the right atrium. Interatrial communication is needed for oxygenated blood to reach the systemic circulation.
      b. Partial: Some pulmonary veins enter the left atrium.
   4. Treatment
      a. Complete anomalous return requires transplanting anomalous pulmonary veins from the right atrium to the left atrium and closing the ASD.
      b. With partial anomalous return, surgical correction may not be necessary.

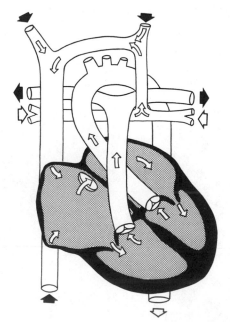

FIG 25–10.
Anomalous venous return of the pulmonary veins.
(From Ross Laboratories Clinical Education Aid no 7 [G163], Columbus, Ohio, 1978. Used by permission.)

TABLE 25–1.
Cardiac Anomalies

Defect	Characteristic Features	Direction of Shunt	Presence of Cyanosis	Treatment
PDA	Failure of ductus artericsus to close at birth	Left to right	Acyanotic	Indomethacin (Indocin); surgical correction
ASD	Failure of foramen ovale to close or septum to form correctly	Left to right	Acyanotic	Surgical correction
VSD	Failure of the septal wall to form properly	Left to right	Acyanotic	Surgical correction if large
Aortic stenosis	Fibrous lesion at the aortic semilunar valve causing ventricular hypertrophy	No shunt present	Acyanotic	Surgical correction if severe
Coarctation of aorta				
Preductal	Stenosis of aorta proximal to entrance of ductus arteriosus	Right to left	Cyanotic	Standard therapy for heart failure
Postductal	Stenosis of aorta distal to entrance of ductus arteriosus	Left to right	Acyanotic	Surgical resection
Tricuspid atresia	Blockage of the tricuspid valve: Small right ventricle Large left ventricle ASD	Right to left	Cyanotic	Surgical correction
Tetralogy of Fallot	VSD Stenosis of pulmonic valve Dextroposition of aorta Hypertrophic right ventricle	Right to left	Cyanotic	Surgical correction if necessary
Truncus arteriosus	VSD with common vessel leaving both ventricles; pulmonary arteries branch from common vessel, which continues as aorta Right and left ventricular hypertrophy	Right to left	Cyanotic	No surgical correction available Treat hypertension
Complete transposition of great vessels	Reversed position of aorta and pulmonary arteries Frequently PDA or ASD	Right to left	Cyanosis	Surgical correction usually necessary
Anomalous venous return	Pulmonary veins (one or more) returning to right atrium	Right to left	Cyanosis	Surgical correction usually necessary

X. Pulmonary Anomalies
  A. Choanal atresia: Blockage of the opening into the nasopharynx by a membranous tissue, usually with bony implants.
     1. If it is bilateral, the condition is a respiratory emergency because it inhibits nasal ventilation.
     2. If a nasal suction catheter cannot be passed, choanal atresia should be suspected in a neonate with severe respiratory distress.
     3. Treatment: Surgical correction is necessary.
  B. Esophageal atresia: Malformation of esophagus, with tracheoesophageal fistulas a common complication.
     1. Types
        a. Atresia of the upper esophagus, with the lower esophagus connected to the trachea or mainstem bronchi.
        b. An intact trachea, but unattached stomach and esophagus.
        c. H-type fistula: A normal trachea and esophagus connected by a small tube-like fistula.
     2. Clinical signs
        a. Accumulation of oral secretions
        b. Continuous or sporadic respiratory distress
        c. Abdominal distention as a result of air entry
     3. Treatment: Surgical correction is necessary.
  C. Diaphragmatic hernia: Result of incomplete development of diaphragm, allowing abdominal organs to enter the thoracic cavity.
     1. Respiratory and cardiovascular stress is pronounced.
     2. Most hernias occur on the left side, frequently causing a shift of the mediastinum and atelectasis.
     3. Treatment: Immediate surgical correction is necessary.
  D. Congenital laryngeal stridor or partial airway obstruction: Result of incomplete development of larynx
     1. May cause mild respiratory distress.
     2. Usually improves with maturing of laryngeal and tracheal cartilage.
  E. Lung hypoplasia and aplasia
     1. It is a partial (hypoplasia) or complete (aplasia) lack of development of the parenchyma of a lung.
     2. It results from in utero failure to develop an adequate circulation to the affected lung, lobe, or segment, causing a reduction in lung parenchyma.
     3. If only a small portion of the lung is involved, physiologic effects are minimal.
     4. If lungs are aplastic, the reduction in lung parenchyma means a reduction in pulmonary vasculature. This causes pulmonary hypertension and right-sided heart failure.
     5. Lung aplasia or hypoplasia can be seen with other anomalies.
     6. Treatment: Symptomatic; no specific intervention is specified.

BIBLIOGRAPHY

Achanti B, Pyati S, Yeh T: Indomethacin therapy in premature infants of advanced postnatal age. *J Perinatol* 1987; 7:235–237.

Aloan C: *Respiratory Care of the Newborn: A Clinical Manual.* Philadelphia, JB Lippincott Co, 1987.

Anton W: Bronchopulmonary dysplasia: Respiratory care components of successful transition to the home. *Respir Pract* 1987: 1(2):15–19.

Avery G: *Neonatalogy, Pathophysiology and Management of the Newborn*, ed 2. Philadelphia JB Lippincott Co, 1981.

Bancalari E: Respiratory failure in the newborn. *Curr Rev Respir Ther* 1979; 2(lesson 2):11–15.

Bancalari E: Respiratory failure in the newborn. *Curr Rev Respir Ther* 1979; 2(lesson 3):19–23.

Crouse D, Phillips J: Persistent pulmonary hypertension of the newborn. *Perinatol Neonatol* September–October 1987; 11:12–38.

Emmanouilides G, Baylen B: *Neonatal Cardiopulmonary Distress.* Chicago, Year Book Medical Publishers, 1988.

Fox W, Duara S: Persistent pulmonary hypertension in the neonate: Diagnosis and management. *J Pediatr* 1983; 103:505–514.

Goldberg R, Bancalari E: Bronchopulmonary dysplasia: Clinical presentation and the role of mechanical ventilation. *Respir Care* 1986; 31(7):591–598.

Hageman J, Adams S, Gardner T: Pulmonary complications of hyperventilation therapy for persistent pulmonary hypertension. *Crit Care Med* 1985; 13(12):1013–1014.

International Committee for the Classification of the Late Stages of Retonopathy of Prematurity. *Pediatrics* 1988; 82:37–43.

Koff P, Eitzman D, Neu J: *Neonatal and Pediatric Respiratory Care.* St Louis, CV Mosby Co, 1988.

Korones S: *High-Risk Newborn Infants,* ed 4. St Louis, CV Mosby Co, 1986.

Ling E: Persistent fetal circulation, direction and treatment. *Perinatol Neonatol* November–December 1985; 9:21–31.

Nickerson B: Bronchopulmonary dysplasia chronic pulmonary disease following neonatal respiratory failure. *Chest* April 1985; 87:528–534.

Pearlman S, Maisels J: Preductal and postductal transcutaneous oxygen tension measurements in premature newborns with hyaline membrane disease. *Pediatrics* 1989; 83:98–100.

Reidel F: Long-term effects of artificial ventilation in neonates. *Acta Paediatr Scand* 1987; 76:24–29.

Shapiro C: Retrolental fibroplasia: What we know and what we don't know. *Neonat Network* June 1986; 6:33–44.

Southwell S: Update on the treatment of persistent pulmonary hypertension of the newborn. *Neonat Network* April 1986; 4:19–25.

Spear M, Spitzer A, Fox W: Hyperventilation therapy persistent pulmonary hypertension of the newborn. *Perinatol Neonatol* September–October 1985; 9:27–34.

Stern L: *Diagnosis and Management of Respiratory Disorders in the Newborn.* Reading, Mass, Addison-Wesley Publishing Co, 1983.

Thibeault D, Gregory G: *Neonatal Pulmonary Care,* ed 2. New York, Appleton-Century-Crofts, 1988.

_____

Chapter 26

Respiratory Disorders of the Pediatric Patient

I. Pediatric patients are classified by age as follows:
   A. Newborn: Up to 30 days old
   B. Infant: 30 days to 12 months
   C. Child: 1 year to 8 to 12 years
II. Evaluation of the pediatric patient for respiratory distress
   A. Chief complaint
      1. Is the problem acute, recurrent, or chronic?
      2. Is the problem from ingestion, inhalation, trauma, or accident?
   B. History
      1. Current medications
      2. Past medical history
   C. Physical examination
      1. Airway
      2. Breathing
      3. Cardiovascular status
      4. Activity level
      5. Conscious or unconscious
   D. Common pediatric disorders
      1. One to 24 months
         a. Cystic fibrosis
         b. Bronchiolitis
         c. Croup
         d. Epiglottitis
         e. Ingestion of poison
         f. Foreign body obstruction
      2. Two to 5 years
         a. Croup
         b. Asthma
         c. Burns
         d. Cystic fibrosis (CF)
         e. Ingestion of poison
         f. Foreign body obstruction
   E. The majority of pediatric admissions are for respiratory problems.

F. Causes of respiratory problems
    1. Nasal
        a. Enlarged adenoids
        b. Deviated nasal septum
        c. Nasal polyps
    2. Oropharyngeal
        a. Enlargement of tonsils
        b. Tumors or cysts
    3. Larynx
        a. Epiglottitis
        b. Postendotracheal intubation (vocal cord problems)
        c. Croup
    4. Tracheal
        a. Stenosis
        b. Trauma
        c. Tumors
    5. Bronchi
        a. Excessive secretions (CF)
        b. Spasm of smooth muscle (asthma)
        c. Inflammation (bronchiolitis)
    6. Obstruction of airway
        a. Tongue
        b. Food
        c. Teeth, pins, coins, and so forth
        d. Vomitus
        e. Infection (croup, epiglottitis)
G. Clinical identification of respiratory distress
    1. Restless or irritable
    2. Nasal flaring
    3. Tracheal tug (sucking in of tissue lying over sternal notch)
    4. Retractions
    5. Seesaw (paradoxical) breathing
    6. Flaring of lower rib cage
    7. Diminished or absent breath sounds
    8. Tachypnea
        a. Newborn: More than 60 breaths/min (bpm)
        b. Up to 1 year: More than 35 bpm
        c. More than 1 year: More than 25 bpm
    9. Cyanosis on oxygen therapy ($F_{I_{O_2}}$ more than 0.30)
H. Other signs of significance
    1. Temperature
        a. Normal temperature: 36.1°C to 37°C
        b. Low-grade fever: Temperature of 37.1°C to 38.4°C (normally viral infection)
        c. High-grade fever: Temperature of 38.4°C or more (normally bacterial infection)
    2. Respiratory status
        a. Dyspnea
        b. Apnea
        c. Chest pain
        d. Hemoptysis
    3. Cardiovascular status
        a. Pulse: Normal
            (1) Up to 2 years: 130 to 140 beats/min

(2) Two to 10 years: 80 beats/min

(3) More than 10 years: 70 to 80 beats/min

b. Pulse: Tachycardia

(1) Up to 2 years: More than 140 beats/min

(2) Two to 10 years: More than 130 beats/min

(3) More than 10 years: More than 100 beats/min

c. Pulse: Bradycardia

(1) Up to 2 years: Less than 100 beats/min

(2) Two to 10 years: Less than 60 beats/min

(3) More than 10 years: Less than 50 beats/min

d. Blood pressure

(1) One to 24 months: 100/70 mm Hg

(2) More than 2 years of age

(a) Upper limits for systolic pressure: $90 + (2 \times \text{years in age})$ mm Hg

(b) Lower limits for systolic pressure: $70 + (2 \times \text{years in age})$ mm Hg

III. Croup (Laryngotracheobronchitis or LTB)(Table 26–1)

A. Description

1. Viral infection involving the larynx and subglottic area

2. Infectious agent: parainfluenza virus (most common) or *Mycoplasma pneumoniae*

3. Infants and children 6 months to 3 years of age (rarely occurs after this age)

4. Seasons: Fall and winter

B. Clinical presentation

1. Gradual onset from 2 to 3 days

2. Runny nose

3. Hoarseness

4. Barking cough

5. Retractions

6. Accessory muscle usage

7. Low-grade fever

8. Stridor

C. Radiologic presentation

1. Lateral neck x-ray film shows subglottic narrowing.

2. Haziness of this area indicates swelling.

D. Management

1. Use cool mist with an $F_{I_{O_2}}$ of 0.30 to 0.40.

2. Rest.

3. Use racemic epinephrine with a hand-held nebulizer every 1 to 2 hours as needed.

4. Let child sleep; do not awaken for treatment.

5. Helium-oxygen mixture may be used to reduce air flow resistance.

6. Glucocorticoids and dexamethasone may be used in severe cases.

TABLE 26–1.

Comparison of Croup and Epiglottitis

Factor	Croup	Epiglottitis
Etiology	Virus: Parainfluenza	Bacteria: *Haemophilus influenzae*
White blood cell count	Normal	Elevated
Onset	Gradual	Sudden
Cough	Dry, barking	Muffled
Lateral neck x-ray film	Subglottic inflammation	Supraglottic inflammation
Treatment	Symptomatic	Artificial airway

    7. Monitor pulse oximetry, and arterial blood gases (ABGs) after the patient is stabilized.

    8. If respiratory failure is impending, look for:

        a. Increasing pulse.

        b. Restlessness and lethargy.

        c. Increased retractions.

        d. Cyanosis on increased $F_{I_{O_2}}$.

        e. Decreased breath sounds.

    9. Intubate when:

        a. Signs of respiratory failure are present.

           (1) Pa_{O_2}: Less than 70 mm Hg at an $F_{I_{O_2}}$ of more than 0.40

           (2) Pa_{CO_2}: More than 55 mm Hg

   10. Care following intubation includes:

        a. Providing supplemental warm humidified oxygen to raise the Pa_{O_2} to more than 60 mm Hg and the Sa_{O_2} at more than 90%.

        b. Suctioning the airway.

        c. Maintain spontaneous ventilation if the patient is able to maintain a Pa_{CO_2} of less than 50 mm Hg.

IV. Epiglottitis

  A. Description

    1. It is a bacterial infection affecting the supraglottic area. The most common organism is *Hemophilus influenzae* type B.

    2. It produces an enlarged cherry-red epiglottis, which partially obstructs the airway.

    3. It commonly infects children 3 to 7 years of age.

  B. Clinical presentation

    1. Abrupt onset: 7 to 8 hours

    2. High fever

    3. Hoarseness

    4. Cough

    5. Hyperextension of neck and chest thrust forward (characteristic sitting position)

    6. Sore throat

    7. Drooling (unable to swallow from sore throat)

    8. Stridor

  C. Radiologic findings

    1. For typical clinical presentation, x-ray film may not be needed.

    2. A lateral neck x-ray film may differentiate croup from epiglottitis.

    3. The enlarged epiglottis looks like an enlarged thumb instead of a little finger.

    4. Valleculae are obliterated.

  D. Management

    1. Give 30% to 40% oxygen by mask.

    2. Disturb the child as little as possible.

    3. Prepare intubation and resuscitation equipment in case of obstruction.

    4. Take the patient to the surgical suite for nasotracheal intubation.

    5. Use an endotracheal tube 0.5 mm smaller than predicted to prevent trauma.

    6. Following intubation, provide humidification and supplemental oxygen (30%–40%).

    7. Suction the endotracheal tube frequently.

    8. Administer intravenous (IV) antibiotics such as chloramphenicol and ampicillin.

    9. Obtain blood cultures.

      10. Continuous positive airway pressure (CPAP) may be needed if the Pa_{O_2} is not responsive to oxygen therapy ($F_{I_{O_2}}$ more than 0.60). Initially the CPAP should be 4 to 6 cm H_2O.

      11. Mechanical ventilation may be needed if the Pa_{CO_2} is more than 55 mm Hg. Positive end-expiratory pressure (PEEP) may also be necessary.

      12. Most patients respond very well without the need of CPAP or mechanical ventilation with PEEP.

      13. If endotracheal intubation is needed, it is usually required for 24 to 72 hours.

  E. Extubation

    1. Extubation can occur when swelling diminishes and air can be heard around the endotracheal tube during quiet breathing.

    2. Provide cool humidity and aerosol therapy with supplemental oxygen.

    3. Monitor for airway obstruction.

    4. Reintubate if respiratory distress occurs.

    5. Racemic epinephrine may be given for tracheal swelling from the endotracheal tube immediately after extubation.

V. Bronchiolitis

  A. Description

    1. It is an inflammatory disease of the bronchioles.

    2. For those less than 2 years of age, the most common infectious agent is respiratory syncytial virus (RSV). Those who are 6 weeks to 6 months of age become the sickest.

    3. Other infections include parainfluenza types 1 and 3, adenovirus, and *M. pneumoniae*.

    4. Chemical factors may also contribute (most commonly cigarette smoke).

    5. Usually occurs in spring and winter.

  B. Clinical presentation

    1. An upper respiratory tract infection follows 2 to 3 days of:

      a. Cough.

      b. Tachypnea of more than 50 bpm.

      c. Low-grade fever.

      d. Intercostal retractions.

      e. Wheezing.

      f. Fine rales.

      g. Poor appetite.

      h. Cyanosis.

    2. It may be difficult to differentiate bronchiolitis from asthma in younger patients.

  C. Radiologic findings

    1. Hyperinflation

    2. Consolidation in lower lobes

  D. Diagnosis

    1. Use nasopharyngeal secretions.

    2. Use immunofluorescent antibody staining.

    3. Rule out cystic fibrosis. Perform sweat test.

  E. Management and treatment of mild symptoms

    1. Symptoms

      a. Respiratory rate: 30 to 45 bpm

      b. Wheezing

      c. Blood gases

        (1) P_{CO_2}: 35 to 50 mm Hg

        (2) P_{O_2}: More than 70 mm Hg when receiving 30% to 40% oxygen

      d. Mild retractions

    2. Isolation

3. Mist tent
4. Frequent suctioning
5. Bronchodilators
F. Management and treatment of severe symptoms
   1. Symptoms
      a. Respiratory rate: More than 45 bpm
      b. Distant or inaudible breath sounds
      c. Cyanosis
      d. Blood gases
         (1) Pco_2: More than 50 mm Hg
         (2) Po_2: Less than 70 mm Hg at an FI_{O_2} of 0.40
      e. Severe retractions
   2. Ribavirin (Virazole) aerosol may be used.
      a. Ribavirin is used if the RSV is associated with severe cyanotic congenital heart disease.
      b. It is used if the RSV patient has severe bronchopulmonary dysplasia.
      c. It is used to avoid intubation.
      d. It disrupts the RNA within the virus and prevents any further transmission or shedding.
      e. It comes in 100-ml vials containing 6 gm of lyphodized powder.
      f. It is reconstituted with 300 ml of sterile water, which gives 20 mg/ml (2% solution).
      g. It is administered by the SPAG-2 system (small particle aerosol generator) into a tent or head hood.
      h. The device puts out 95% of aerosol particles in therapeutic range with a median particle diameter of 1.2 to 1.3 μ.
      i. Therapy is commonly administered for 12 to 18 hours/day.
      j. Hazards and risks include:
         (1) Conjunctivitis in children.
         (2) Suppression of immunity.
         (3) Possible risks to health care personnel (use mask, gloves, and gown when in contact with aerosol).
      k. The manufacturer states that ribavirin should not be used with a mechanical ventilator due to rain-out in patient circuit and endotracheal tubing, potentially causing inadvertent PEEP or airway obstruction. However, many centers do aerosolize the drug via ventilator systems.
      l. If aerosol is used with mechanical ventilation, tandem particle filters are used in line on the expiratory side of the patient circuit.
      m. The filters require frequent change (1–2 hours), as do the ventilator circuits (every shift).
   3. Monitor the Pa_{O_2} and Pco_2 for impending respiratory failure.
   4. Monitor hydration and weight gain.
   5. Severe cases may require mechanical ventilation.
   6. Intubate when:
      a. The Pco_2 is more than 60 mm Hg.
      b. The pH is less than 7.25.
      c. The Pa_{O_2} is less than 70 mm Hg at an FI_{O_2} of more than 0.60.
      d. Breath sounds are absent.
      e. The patient is lethargic.
      f. The patient is exhausted.
      g. Apneic episodes occur.
VI. Cystic Fibrosis (Mucoviscidosis)
   A. Description
      1. It is inherited as a recessive disorder that involves the exocrine glands.

2. Both parents must have the recessive gene.
3. There is a 25% chance that asymptomatic parents with recessive genes will have a child with CF, a 50% chance the child will be a carrier and not have CF, and a 25% chance that the child will not have CF or be a carrier.
4. Cystic fibrosis causes exocrine glands to produce abnormally viscid secretions, there is pancreatic deficiency, and there is a high sweat electrolyte concentration.
5. Sixty percent of patients are diagnosed in the first year of life, with 90% being diagnosed by the age of 5 years. The median age of survival is slightly more than 20 years.

B. The etiology is a non-sex-linked autosomal recessive gene.
C. Clinical manifestations result from abnormal secretions from the sweat glands, bronchial glands, mucosal glands, small intestine, the pancreas, and bile ducts of the liver.
1. Sweat glands: There is abnormal absorption of sodium and chloride (two to five times normal), but water reabsorption is normal.
2. Pancreas: Eighty percent of patients with CF suffer from pancreatic deficiency. A low-volume, highly viscid fluid that has few enzymes to break down ingested fat is secreted. Insulin secretion is impaired as a result of fibrosis. Diabetes is often present in the older child.
3. Intestine: Mucous glands of the intestine are involved, causing tarry, viscous feces in the newborn. A distended abdomen results from failure to pass feces.
4. Liver: Lesions found in the liver are similar to those of the pancreas. Blockage of bile ducts and fibrosis results.
5. Bronchial glands: Excessive thick, tenacious mucus is produced, which obstructs small airways and produces respiratory insufficiency and pulmonary hypertension.

D. Pulmonary pathophysiology
1. At birth, the size of the bronchial gland is normal, but hypertrophy and hypersecretion quickly develop.
2. Obstruction of small bronchi and bronchioles from thick, tenacious secretions occur.
3. Overdistention of the lung and dilation of airways follow.
4. Infection from stagnant mucus, *Pseudomonas aeruginosa,* and *Staphylococcus aureus* is common.
5. Progression of the disease results in:
   a. Consolidation and atelectasis.
   b. Destruction of respiratory epithelium and simple squamous epithelium.
   c. Pneumonitis.
   d. Fibrosis.
   e. Abcesses.
6. Progressive respiratory failure occurs with marked hypercapnia, hypoxia, and pulmonary hypertension.
7. Congestive heart failure follows.
8. Ninety-eight percent of the patients die from cardiorespiratory involvement.

E. Diagnosis
1. Diagnosis is based on clinical symptoms and family history.
2. In the newborn, failure to pass meconium (the first feces) within 12 hours of birth is common.
3. The most reliable diagnostic test is the sweat chloride level. This test is performed by pilocarpine iontophoresis, which locally stimulates sweat glands. Collection and measurement of the NaCl in the sweat follow.

4. A minimum of 100 mg of sweat is collected from either the forearm, trunk, or thigh.
5. A concentration of NaCl greater than 60 mEq/L is consistent with the diagnosis of CF. The normal NaCl concentration is 28 mEq/L. Also potassium is measured. The normal K^+ content is 10 mEq/L; 22 mEq/L or greater is present with CF.
6. Two consecutive tests should be performed if the first results are positive. The results should be within 10% to 15% of each other.
7. Neonatal screening is currently used to detect CF. The present test used is the radioimmunoassay for immunoreactive trysinogen. The accuracy of this test has been questioned.

F. Physical presentation
  1. Earliest pulmonary symptoms
    a. Dry, hacking cough
    b. Progression of cough to more frequent coughing spells with production of large quantities of secretions (cough is paroxysmal)
    c. Failure to thrive
    d. Flattened diaphragms (older child)
    e. Recurrent wheezing
    f. Dyspnea on exertion
  2. The older child has muscular weakness and growth failure, short stature, reproductive tract underdevelopment, and clubbing of the digits.
  3. Pneumothorax frequently occurs in patients with advanced lung disease. Seventy percent to 100% of these patients will have recurring pneumothoracies, with 80% dying within 3 years of the first pneumothorax.
  4. Hemoptysis occurs as a result of changes in bronchial circulation. Massive hemoptysis of 300 ml within 24 hours frequently develops.

G. Pulmonary function studies
  1. Primary alteration is a decrease in compliance and increase in respiratory rate.
  2. Ventilation/perfusion mismatch develops.
  3. Expiratory flow rates are reduced.
  4. The Pa_{CO_2} level is reduced or near normal in the early stage of the disease, progressing to hypercapnea.
  5. The functional residual capacity (FRC) is increased.
  6. The residual volume (RV) is increased and the expiratory reserve volume decreased.
  7. The ratio of RV to total lung capacity (TLC) is increased in severe obstruction.
  8. The vital capacity is reduced.

H. Radiologic findings
  1. Atelectasis in the right upper lobe is common.
  2. Progression of the disease leads to hyperinflation and flattening of the diaphragm and increased anteroposterior diameter.
  3. There is thickening of the bronchi with areas of consolidation and atelectasis.
  4. The heart shadow is narrowed.

I. Treatment
  1. Good pulmonary hygiene
    a. Percussion and postural drainage
  2. Bronchodilator and mucolytic therapy
    a. β_2-Agonist for reversable airway obstruction
    b. Acetylcysteine (Mucomyst) to help reduce viscosity of secretions

3. Nebulization
   a. Mist tents to humidify air and administer oxygen in younger patients and older patients at night
   b. Ultrasonic nebulizers to add water to secretions to help in expectoration
4. Antibiotics
   a. Oral antibiotics (neostigmine) are given to prevent colonization of *S. aureus* and *H. influenzae.*
   b. Intravenous antibiotics include cephalosporins (gentamyacin, kanamyacin, and tobramycin).
5. Bronchial lavage
   a. Acetylcysteine and saline are used to remove mucous plugs.
6. Oxygen, low flow (maintain Sa_{O_2} at more than 90%)
7. Other supportive measures
   a. Supply good nutrition and increase calories 150%.
   b. Prescribe supplemental pancreatic enzymes (streptodornase, streptokinase) to metabolize fat.
   c. Increase carbohydrates and protein intake while reducing fat intake.
   d. Increase water intake.
   e. Physical therapy: Increase activity as tolerated (swimming, running, bicycling).
   f. Vitamins (fat-soluble A, D, E, and K).
   g. Supply supportive home therapy.

VII. Foreign Body Aspiration
   A. Description and etiology
      1. The greatest incidence is in children 6 months to 3 years of age.
      2. The majority of materials aspirated are radiolucent and cannot be seen on x-ray film.
      3. It is the major cause of death in children less than 6 years of age.
      4. Pins, coins, aspirin, nuts, and raisins are common materials aspirated.
   B. Manifestations
      1. Aspirated material obstructing the trachea is a medical emergency. Symptoms include:
         a. Choking.
         b. Retractions.
         c. Struggling and fighting for air.
         d. Gagging.
         e. Breath sounds that may vary from absent to rhonchi.
      2. Aspirated material lodged in bronchus usually stimulates a violent cough, sneezing, and possibly bloody sputum if the material is sharp.
   C. For treatment of upper airway obstruction in the child, refer to the American Heart Association Basic Life Support Guidelines.
   D. Aspiration of foreign body in lower airway
      1. Aspiration of a foreign body into the lower airway usually stimulates a violent cough that draws the material more distal.
      2. Coughing may cease if the foreign body becomes firmly lodged. The patient may become asymptomatic for several days.
      3. Eventually a chronic cough and fever develops. However, a chronic cough without fever is frequently present.
   E. Treatment
      1. Postural drainage and percussion therapy
      2. Bronchodilator therapy
      3. If there is no change in patient status and symptoms, bronchoscopy should be performed.

VIII. Asthma
    A. Etiology
        1. The most common mechanism for asthma is allergy.
        2. Other mechanisms include cold exposure, stress, exercise, infection, and other nonspecific inhaled irritants.
    B. Clinical manifestations
        1. Bronchoconstriction
        2. Increased production of secretions
        3. Increased airway resistance
        4. Air trapping
        5. Hyperinflation
    C. Pathophysiology
        1. Stimulation occurs.
        2. Stimulation is then transmitted by the vagus nerve to the brain stem and out parasympathetic pathways.
        3. Bronchoconstriction occurs.
        4. Histamine and other mast cell mediators are released to prolong reaction.
        5. Bronchial lumen is reduced, epithelium thickens, and there is hypertrophy of smooth muscle and mucous glands.
        6. Excessive secretions are produced.
        7. Air trapping and hyperinflation occur.
        8. Changes in pulmonary mechanics occur, including:
           a. Reduced compliance.
           b. Increased airway resistance.
           c. Increased FRC.
        9. Lack of airflow stagnates mucus, and plugging occurs.
      10. Sputum takes on a characteristic appearance of stringy casts from bronchiolar origin (Curschmann's spirals).
      11. Also contained in mucus are eosinophils and polymorphonuclear cells.
    D. Clinical presentation
        1. In the early stages, the child presents with:
           a. Dyspnea.
           b. Cough.
           c. Increased respiratory rate.
           d. Inspiratory wheezing.
           e. Barrel-chested appearance.
        2. Blood gases show:
           a. Hypoxemia and hypocarbia (mild asthma).
           b. Hypoxemia and hypercarbia (severe asthma).
        3. Pulmonary function
           a. Increased TLC.
           b. Greatly increased RV.
           c. Reduced ventilatory capacity.
           d. Reduced forced expiratory volume in 1 second and forced vital capacity.
           e. Reduced peak flow rate.
    E. Radiologic findings
        1. Hyperinflation
        2. Flattened diaphragms
        3. Infiltrates may be noted in children less than 6 years old.
    F. Treatment
        1. Initial treatment of mild asthma
           a. Oxygen therapy to keep the Pa_{O_2} at 60 to 70 mm Hg and Sa_{O_2} at more than 90%

      b. Theophylline to raise serum concentration to 10 to 20 mg/ml, 5 to 7 mg/kg intravenously every 6 hours

      c. Bronchodilator therapy (see Chapter 41)

  2. Management of severe asthma (status asthmaticus)

      a. Administer 0.01 ml of subcutaneous epinephrine 1:1,000. It can be administered every 15 to 20 min. Desired effects include:

        (1) Clearing of wheezing.

        (2) Reduced respiratory rate.

        (3) Reduced respiratory effort.

      b. Administer IV aminophylline.

      c. Provide IV hydration.

      d. Corticosteroid therapy may be instituted when the usual bronchodilators have not worked within 4 to 6 hours. Steroids such as Solu-Cortef, Solu-Medrol, dexamethasone, or betamethasone may be given intravenously.

      e. Clinical status should be monitored for signs of respiratory failure. These include:

        (1) Decreased breath sounds.

        (2) Cyanosis at an $F_{I_{O_2}}$ of 0.40 or more.

        (3) Depressed level of consciousness.

      f. Arterial blood gases should be monitored closely to identify CO_2 retention and severe hypoxemia.

      g. Intravenous isoproterenol may be started with worsening conditions. This is continued and titrated until the P_{CO_2} drops by 10% or if the pulse exceeds 170 beats/min.

BIBLIOGRAPHY

Allen W, Olsen G: Management of status asthmaticus. *Curr Rev Respir Ther* 1983; 3(lesson 21):91–94.

Burton G, Hodgkin J: *Respiratory Care, A Guide to Clinical Practice*, ed 2. Philadelphia, JB Lippincott Co, 1987.

Chameides L, et al: *Textbook of Pediatric Advanced Life Support*. Dallas, American Heart Association, 1988.

Curley M, et al: Assessment and resuscitation of the pediatric patient. *Crit Care Nurse* 1987; 7:26–42.

Daily E, Schroeder J: *Techniques in Bedside Hemodynamic Monitoring*, ed 4. St Louis, CV Mosby Co, 1989.

Downes J, et al: Acute respiratory failure in infants and children. *Pediatr Clin North Am* 1972; 19:423–445.

Frank M, et al: Theophylline: A closer look. *Neonat Network* 1987; 9:7–12.

Gioia R, Rogers M: The hospital management of asthma. *Curr Rev Respir Ther* 1979; 1(lesson 9):67–71.

Graef J, Cone T: *Manual of Pediatric Therapeutics*, ed 2. Boston, Little, Brown & Co, 1980.

Gregory G: *Respiratory Failure in the Child*. New York, Churchill-Livingstone, 1981.

Hughes J: *Synopsis of Pediatrics*, ed 5. St Louis, CV Mosby Co, 1980.

Koff P, et al: *Neonatal and Pediatric Respiratory Care*. St Louis, CV Mosby Co, 1980.

Kimmons H, Peterson B: Management of acute epiglottitis in pediatric patients. *Crit Care Med* 1986; 14:278–279.

Lough M, et al: *Pediatric Respiratory Care*, ed 3. Chicago, Year Book Medical Publishers, 1985.

Loughlin G: Cystic fibrosis. *Curr Rev Respir Ther* 1986; 4(lesson 15):115–118.

McIntosh K: Respiratory syncytial virus infections in infants and children: Diagnosis and treatment. *Pediatr Rev* 1987; 9:191–196.

Pascoe D, Grossman M: *Quick References to Pediatric Emergencies,* ed 3. Philadelphia, JB Lippincott Co, 1984.

Rau J: *Respiratory Care Pharmacology,* ed 3. Chicago, Year Book Medical Publishers, 1989.

Rothstein P, Johnson P: Pediatric intensive care factors that influence outcome, *Crit Care Med* 1982; 10:34–37.

Stern L: *Diagnosis and Management of Respiratory Disorders in the Newborn.* Reading, Mass, Addison-Wesley Publishing Co, 1983.

Steward DJ: Epiglottitis. *Curr Rev Respir Care* 1988; 10(lesson 19):147–151.

Taber L, et al: Ribavirin aerosol treatment of bronchiolitis associated with respiratory syncytial virus infection in infants. *Pediatrics* 1983; 72:613–618.

Tepper R, et al: Infants with cystic fibrosis, pulmonary function at diagnosis. *Pediatr Pulmonol* 1988; 5:15–18.

Wheeler W, Colten H: Cystic fibrosis, current approach to diagnosis and management. *Pediatr Rev* 1988; 9:241–248.

Wood D, et al: A clinical scoring system for the diagnosis of respiratory failure preliminary report on childhood status asthmaticus. *Am J Dis Child* 1972; 123:227–228.

Chapter 27

Gas Therapy

I. Medical, Laboratory, and Therapeutic Gases and Mixtures
   A. Ethylene (C_2H_4)
   B. Nitrous oxide (N_2O)
   C. Cyclopropane [$(CH_2)_3$]
   D. Oxygen (O_2)
   E. Nitrogen (N_2)
   F. Carbon dioxide (CO_2)
   G. Helium (He)
   H. Oxygen/nitrogen (21% O_2/79% N_2)
   I. Oxygen/carbon dioxide (90%–98% O_2/2%–10% CO_2)
   J. Helium/oxygen (40%–80% He/20%–60% O_2)
II. Flammable Gases
   A. Ethylene
   B. Cyclopropane
III. Nonflammable Gases
   A. Nitrogen
   B. Carbon dioxide
   C. Helium
IV. Gases That Support Combustion
   A. Oxygen
   B. Helium/oxygen
   C. Oxygen/carbon dioxide
   D. Oxygen/nitrogen
   E. Nitrous oxide
V. Gas Cylinders
   A. Cylinder types and composition
     1. Type 3AA: Seamless, high-quality, heat-treated steel, spun chrome molybdenum
     2. Type 3A: Seamless, low carbon, heat-treated steel (no longer produced)
   B. Cylinder markings: Markings are located at the neck of the cylinder in two groupings (Fig 27–1).
     1. Front
       a. Line 1: ICC or DOT, 3A or 3AA, 2015
         (1) ICC or DOT: The organization governing the transport of cylinder
           (a) ICC: Interstate Commerce Commission. The agency that regulated construction, transport, and testing of compressed gas cylinders from 1948 to 1970.

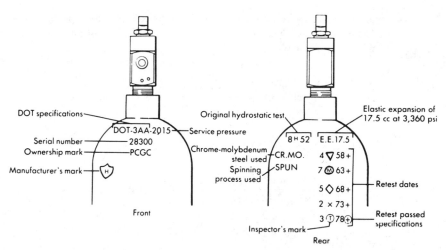

FIG 27–1.
Typical markings for cylinders containing medical gases, front and back views. (From Spearman CB, Sheldon RL, Egan DF: *Egan's Fundamentals of Respiratory Therapy,* ed 4. St Louis, CV Mosby Co, 1982. Used by permission.)

 (b) DOT: Department of Transportation. The federal agency responsible for construction, transport, and testing of compressed gas cylinders since 1970.
 (2) 3A or 3AA: Cylinder type
 (3) 2,015: Maximum working pressure in pounds per square inch (psi), which normally can be exceeded by 10% (2,200 psi).
 b. Line 2: 28300, Serial number
 c. Line 3: PCGC
  (1) PCGC: Initial of owner
 d. Line 4: Manufacturer's mark
 2. Rear: Refer to Figure 27–1.
C. Cylinder size
 1. Large cylinders using hexagonal nut connections
  a. H or K: 9-in. diameter, 55-in. height
  b. G: 8½-in. diameter, 55-in. height
  c. M: 7⅛-in. diameter, 46-in. height
  d. F: 5½-in. diameter, 55-in. height
 2. Small cylinders using yoke connections
  a. E: 4¼-in. diameter, 30-in. height
  b. D: 4¼-in. diameter, 20-in. height
  c. B: 3½-in. diameter, 16-in. height
  d. A: 3-in. diameter, 10-in. height
D. Cylinder capacities for oxygen
 1. D: 12.7 cu ft
 2. E: 22 cu ft
 3. G: 187 cu ft
 4. H or K: 244 cu ft
E. Maximum filling pressure of 3AA oxygen cylinders: 2,015 psi plus 10% (2,200 psi).
F. Calculation of duration of flow from oxygen and compressed air cylinders.
 1. One cubic foot of gas = 28.3 L.
 2. The volume of gas in liters in a full cylinder = cubic foot volume × 28.3 L/cu ft.

3. Dividing the above determined value by the maximum filling pressure of 2,200 psi results in the calculation of a factor indicating the number of liters per pound per square inch:

$$\text{Factor for duration of flow} = \frac{(\text{cu ft vol})(28.3 \text{ L/cu ft})}{2.200 \text{ psi}} \quad (1)$$

4. For a D size cylinder:

$$\frac{(12.7 \text{ cu ft})(28.3 \text{ L/cu ft})}{2,200 \text{ psi}} = 0.16 \text{ L/psi}$$

5. Liters per psi factors for oxygen cylinders
   a. D: 0.16 L/psi
   b. E: 0.28 L/psi
   c. G: 2.41 L/psi
   d. H or K: 3.14 L/psi
6. Calculation of duration of flow in minutes
   a. Gauge pressure multiplied by duration of flow factor (L/psi) equals the number of liters in the cylinder.
   b. Dividing the result of no. 6a by the flow in liters per minute results in the time in minutes that the cylinder will last:

$$\text{Time in minutes cylinder will last} = \frac{(\text{Gauge pressure})(\text{Duration of flow factor})}{(\text{Flow in L/min})} \quad (2)$$

   c. Example for E cylinder:

Gauge pressure	1,500 psi
Duration of flow factor	0.28 L/psi
Flow in L/min	10 L/min

$$42 \text{ min} = \frac{(1,500 \text{ psi})(0.28 \text{ L/psi})}{10 \text{ L/min}}$$

The cylinder will deliver 10 L/min for 42 min before it is completely empty.
   d. Clinically, it is advisable to subtract 500 psi from the gauge pressure to provide a safety margin before the duration of flow is calculated.
G. Color code for E cylinders (Color coding is mandatory for E size cylinders only; other size cylinders are not required to follow any coding system.)
   1. Oxygen: Green (universal code: white)
   2. Helium: Brown
   3. Ethylene: Red
   4. Cyclopropane: Orange
   5. Nitrous oxide: Light blue

　　　　6. Carbon dioxide: Gray
　　　　7. Oxygen and carbon dioxide: Green and gray
　　　　8. Oxygen and helium: Green and brown
　　H. Hydrostatic testing of cylinders
　　　　1. Perform periodic high-pressure testing of gas cylinder integrity.
　　　　2. Cylinder expansion is determined by measuring water displacement of an empty cylinder compared to that cylinder when filled to $\frac{5}{3}$ of its maximum pressure.
　　　　3. All cylinders must be retested every 5 to 10 years, depending on elastic expansion of the original testing.
　　I. Cylinder stem pop-off valves
　　　　1. Large cylinders use a frangible disk designed to rupture at a pressure within 5% of cylinder-bursting pressure.
　　　　2. Small cylinders use a fusable plug designed to melt at a temperature of 65.6°C to 76.7°C, (150°–170°F).
VI. Regulation of Gas Flow
　　A. High-pressure gas regulators
　　　　1. Regulators limit flow in a system by reducing maximum working pressure.

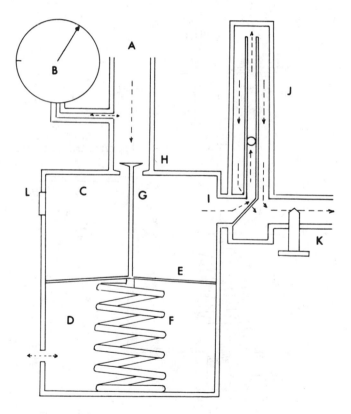

FIG 27–2.
Diagram of preset, high-pressure gas regulator. **A,** attachment to cylinder; **B,** pressure gauge; **C,** pressure chamber; **D,** ambient pressure chamber; **E,** flexible diaphragm; **F,** spring; **G,** valve stem; **H,** gas entry valve; **I,** outflow port; **J,** Thorpe tube flowmeter; **K,** needle valve; **L,** pop-off valve. (From Spearman CB, Sheldon RL, Egan DF: *Egan's Fundamentals of Respiratory Therapy,* ed 4. St Louis, CV Mosby Co, 1982. Used by permission.)

2. Regulators reduce cylinder pressures to a usable working pressure of 50 psi or less.
3. Single-stage regulators
    a. Cylinder pressure is reduced to a working pressure of up to 50 psi in one step or stage.
    b. One high-pressure pop-off valve is incorporated in the regulator and set at about 200 psi.
4. Multistage regulators
    a. Cylinder pressure is reduced to a working pressure of up to 50 psi in a series of steps or stages.
    b. A high-pressure pop-off valve is incorporated into each stage of the regulator, with the final stage pop-off set at about 200 psi.
5. Preset regulators (Fig 27–2)
    a. Pressure is reduced in one or more stages to a fixed working pressure of 50 psi.

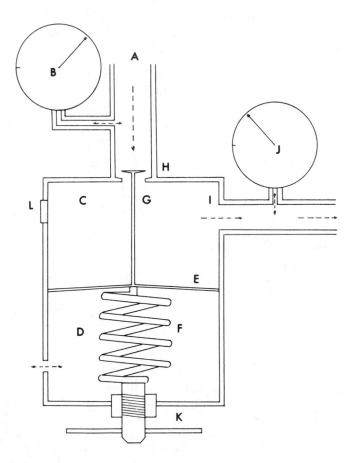

FIG 27–3.
Diagram of an adjustable, high-pressure gas regulator. **A,** attachment to cylinder; **B,** pressure gauge; **C,** pressure chamber; **D,** ambient pressure chamber; **E,** flexible diaphragm; **F,** spring; **G,** valve stem; **H,** gas entry valve; **I,** outflow port; **J,** Bourdon flow gauge; **K,** threaded gas flow control; **L,** pop-off valve. (From Spearman CB, Sheldon RL, Egan DF: *Egan's Fundamentals of Respiratory Therapy,* ed 4. St Louis, CV Mosby Co, 1982. Used by permission.)

    b. Normally a low-pressure gas-regulating device (e.g., Thorpe tube) is incorporated to reduce flows to working levels.

    c. Preset regulators are used without a Thorpe tube when connected to a system utilizing a 50-psi pressure source (e.g., ventilators).

  6. Adjustable regulators (Fig 27–3)

    a. Pressure is reduced in one or more stages to a final working pressure adjustable to between 0 and 50 psi.

    b. Normally a Bourdon pressure gauge calibrated in liters per minute indicates flow leaving the final stage of the adjustable regulator.

B. Low-pressure gas regulators (flowmeters)

  1. Bourdon gauge (Fig 27–4)

    a. The Bourdon gauge is a pressure-sensitive gauge that uses an expandable copper coil to indicate pressure readings.

    b. Bourdon gauges can be calibrated to indicate flow and are used as flow-measuring devices.

    c. If back pressure is applied distal to the gauge, it will indicate a flow higher than actual flow.

  2. Thorpe tube flowmeters (Fig 27–5): Gas flow is measured by the vertical displacement of a float in an increasing diameter tube. Flow is regulated by a needle valve placed proximal or distal to the float.

    a. Compensated Thorpe tubes are designed to function accurately at a working pressure of 50 psi at 21.1°C (70°F).

      (1) The needle valve is always located distal to the float.

      (2) If backpressure is applied distal to the needle valve, the float will indicate the actual flow delivered.

    b. Uncompensated Thorpe tubes are designed to function at variable working pressures.

      (1) The needle valve is always located proximal to the float.

      (2) If backpressure is applied distal to the float, the float will always indicate a flow lower than the actual flow delivered.

VII. Safety Systems Incorporated in Gas Flow Systems and Cylinders

A. Pin-Index Safety System (PISS) (Fig 27–6)

  1. This system is used only on *E size cylinders or smaller*.

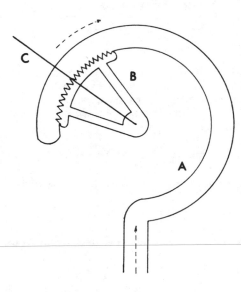

FIG 27–4.
Internal function of a Bourdon gauge. **A,** curved, flexible, closed tube; **B,** gear mechanism; **C,** indicator needle, reflecting flow or pressure on face of valve. (From Spearman CB, Sheldon RL, Egan DF: *Egan's Fundamentals of Respiratory Therapy,* ed 4. St Louis, CV Mosby Co, 1982. Used by permission.)

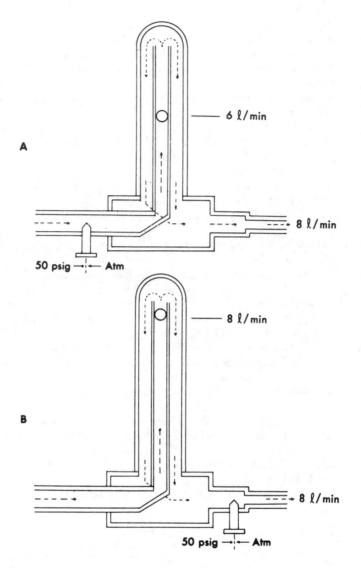

FIG 27–5.
Comparison of pressure-uncompensated **(A)** and pressure-compensated **(B)** flowmeters. In the former, the flow-control valve is proximal to the meter, and the gauge records less than the actual output. In the latter, location of the valve distal to the meter correlates the gauge reading with the output. (From Spearman CB, Sheldon RL, Egan DF: *Egan's Fundamentals of Respiratory Therapy*, ed 4. St Louis, CV Mosby Co, 1982. Used by permission.)

      2. It is used on connections where the maximum working pressure is greater than 200 psig (pounds per square inch gauge).
      3. It incorporates a yoke type of connection where two pins on the regulator connection (yoke) are matched to holes on the cylinder stem.
      4. Ten possible combinations are available, nine currently in use.
      5. Pin positions 2 and 5 are used for oxygen.
    B. American Standard Compressed Gas Cylinder Valve Outlet and Inlet Connections Safety System (Fig 27–7)
      1. This system is only used on cylinders *larger than E size.*

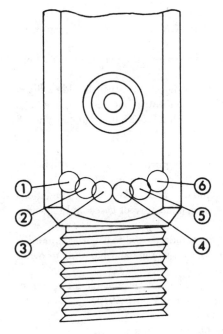

FIG 27–6.
Location of the Pin-Index Safety System holes in the cylinder valve face, various pairs of which constitute indices for different gases. See text for complete pairings. (From Spearman CB, Sheldon RL, Egan DF: *Egan's Fundamentals of Respiratory Therapy*, ed 4. St Louis. CV Mosby Co, 1982. Used by permission.)

2. It is used on connections where the maximum working pressure is greater than 200 psig.
3. It incorporates a hexagonal nut and specific nipple on the regulator fitted to an externally threaded cylinder connection.
4. For oxygen the connection is CGA-540, 0.903-14 NGO, RH-Ext. A Compressed Gas Association connection no. 540 is used with a 0.903-in. threaded outlet diameter and 14 threads/in. of the National Gas Outlet type. The threads are external and right handed.

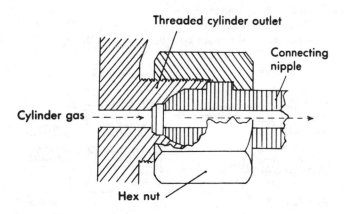

FIG 27–7.
Structure of a typical American Standard connection, such as might be used to attach a reducing valve to a large high-pressure cylinder. The hexagonal nut is held onto the nipple of the reducing valve by a circular collar, seen as a cross-sectional projection on the nipple. As the hexagonal nut is tightened on the threaded cylinder outlet, the end of the nipple is snugly seated into the conical outlet. (From Spearman CB, Sheldon RL, Egan DF: *Egan's Fundamentals of Respiratory Therapy*, ed 4. St Louis, CV Mosby Co, 1982. Used by permission.)

  C. Diameter-Index Safety System (DISS) (Fig 27–8)
   1. Used on all connections distal to the regulator where maximum working pressures are less than 200 psig.
   2. Used for connections of flowmeters to regulators or other connections where frequent equipment changes are made.
   3. It incorporates a hexagonal nut and a nipple designed with two shoulders fitted into a body and externally threaded with two concentric borings.
   4. The DISS connection for oxygen is no. 1240 with a 0.5625-in. diameter and 18 threads/in.
VIII. Agencies Regulating Medical Gases
  A. Food and Drug Administration (FDA): Determines purity standards and labeling for all medical gases listed in the United States Pharmacopeia (USP).
  B. Compressed Gas Association (CGA): Sets standards and makes recommendations to manufacturers and municipal authorities on manufacture of gases and on safety standards for cylinders.
  C. National Fire Prevention Agency (NFPA): Sets standards and makes recommendations to manufacturers and municipal authorities on storage and handling of cylinders.
  D. Department of Transportation (DOT): The federal agency responsible for construction, transport, and testing of compressed gas cylinders since 1970.
 IX. Fractional Distillation of Air
  A. The gas is filtered to remove all dust and impurities.
  B. The gas is dried to remove all water vapor.
  C. The gas is compressed to 200 atm pressure.
  D. The heat of compression is removed by heat exchangers until the temperature returns to ambient.
  E. The gas is then rapidly and repeatedly decompressed by dropping the pressure 5 atm. The reduction in pressure allows tremendous cooling by expansion to occur, bringing the temperature below the boiling point and liquifying all gases in the air.
  F. The temperature of the liquid is then increased and the various gases evaporated and collected at their respective boiling points.
  X. Portable Liquid Oxygen Systems
  A. These systems are used primarily for home oxygen therapy.

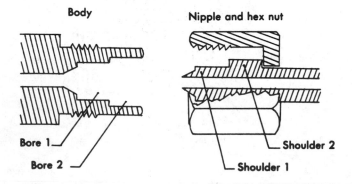

Body   **Nipple and hex nut**

Bore 1   Shoulder 2

Bore 2   Shoulder 1

FIG 27–8.
Components of a representative Diameter-Index Safety System connection. The two shoulders of the nipple allow the nipple to unite only with a body having corresponding borings. If the match is incorrect, the hexagonal nut willl not engage the body threads. (From Spearman CB, Sheldon RL, Egan DF: *Egan's Fundamentals of Respiratory Therapy,* ed 4. St Louis, CV Mosby Co, 1982. Used by permission.)

B. Since a larger volume of oxygen (860.6 L of gas/L of liquid) can be stored more easily as a liquid than as a gas, these systems are most useful for home care.

C. During storage there is evaporative loss of oxygen because of the continual conversion of the liquid to a gas.

D. Available oxygen flow rates are up to 8 L/min.

E. These units do not provide the 50-psi power source needed to drive other respiratory care equipment.

F. These units are generally stationary and can provide oxygen therapy for 4 to 12 days at 2 L/min.

G. Many companies also manufacture portable liquid oxygen systems.

    1. These systems contain approximately 0.5 to 1.5 L of liquid oxygen.

    2. They are generally lightweight (5–13.5 lb).

    3. Provision of oxygen at 1 L/min can be maintained for up to 24 hours with some units.

XI. Oxygen Concentrations

A. These systems incorporate molecular sieves to purify entrained ambient air.

B. Concentrations of 80% to 95% oxygen are generally available. The higher the delivered flow, the lower the F_{IO_2} level.

C. Maximum delivered flow is about 5 L/min.

D. These units are stationary and are designed for home use.

BIBLIOGRAPHY

Burton GG, Gee GN, Hodgkin JE: *Respiratory Care: A Guide to Clinical Practice*, ed 2. Philadelphia, JB Lippincott Co, 1985.

Christopher KL: At home administration of oxygen, in Kacmarek RM, Stoller JK (eds): *Current Respiratory Care*, Toronto, BC Decker, 1988.

Compressed Gas Association: *Handbook of Compressed Gases*. New York, Compressed Gas Association.

Compressed Gas Association: *Pamphlet V-1: American Standard Compressed Gas Cylinder Valve Outlet and Inlet Connections*. New York, Compressed Gas Association.

Compressed Gas Association: *Pamphlet V-5: Diameter Index Safety System*. New York, Compressed Gas Association.

Deshpande VM, Pilbeam SP, Dixon RJ: *A Comprehensive Review in Respiratory Care*. East Warwick, Conn, Appleton & Lange, 1988.

McPherson SP: *Respiratory Therapy Equipment*, ed 3. St Louis, CV Mosby Co, 1988.

Rarey KP, Youtsey JW: *Respiratory Patient Care*. Englewood Cliffs, NJ, Prentice-Hall, 1981.

Rau JL, Rau MY: *Fundamental Respiratory Therapy Equipment: Principles and Use of Operation*. Sarasota, Fla, Glenn Educational Medical Services, 1977.

Spearman CB, Sheldon RL, Egan DF: *Egan's Fundamentals of Respiratory Therapy*, ed 4. St Louis, CV Mosby Co, 1982.

Young JA, Croker D: *Principles and Practice of Respiratory Therapy*, ed 2. Chicago Year Book Medical Publishers, 1976.

Chapter 28 _____

Oxygen Therapy

I. General Characteristics of Oxygen
   A. Colorless
   B. Odorless
   C. Tasteless
   D. Molecular weight: 32 gm
   E. Density at STP: 1.43 gm/L
   F. Boiling point at 1 atm: $-183°C$ $(-297.4°F)$
   G. Melting point at 1 atm: $-216.6°C$ $(-361.1°F)$
   H. Critical temperature: $-118.4°C$ $(-181.1°F)$
   I. Critical pressure: 736.9 psia (pounds per square inch absolute)
   J. Triple point: $-218.7°C$ $(-361.89°F)$ at 0.2321 psia
   K. Forms oxides with all elements except inert gases
   L. Constitutes about 20.95% of atmosphere
   M. Used at cellular level as the final electron acceptor in electron transport chain located in mitochondria of cell
II. Hypoxia: Inadequate Quantities of Oxygen at the Tissue Level
   A. Anemic hypoxia: Decreased carrying capacity of blood for oxygen
      1. Anemia
      2. Carbon monoxide poisoning
      3. Methemoglobinemia
      4. Shift of the oxyhemoglobin dissociation curve to the right
      5. Hypoxemia may or may not be present
   B. Stagnant hypoxia: Decreased cardiac output, resulting in increased systemic transit time
      1. Shock
      2. Cardiovascular instability
      3. Regional vasoconstriction
   C. Histotoxic hypoxia: Inability of tissue to utilize available oxygen
      1. Cyanide poisoning
      2. Rarely accompanied by hypoxemia
   D. Hypoxemic hypoxia: Decrease in diffusion of oxygen across alveolar capillary membrane
      1. Low inspired $F_{I_{O_2}}$
      2. Ventilation/perfusion inequalities

3. Increased true shunt
4. Cardiac anomalies
5. Diffusion defects

III. Hypoxemia: Inadequate Quantities of Oxygen in the Blood
   A. Evaluation of hypoxemia
      1. Normal: Pa_{O_2} 80 to 100 mm Hg
      2. Mild hypoxemia: Pa_{O_2} 60 to 70 mm Hg
      3. Moderate hypoxemia: Pa_{O_2} 40 to 59 mm Hg
      4. Severe hypoxemia: Pa_{O_2} less than 40 mm Hg
      5. For individuals more than 60 years of age, the lower level of acceptable Pa_{O_2} decreases because the normal aging process of the lung effects oxygenation capabilities.
         a. The lower limit of normal Pa_{O_2} is decreased 1 mm Hg for each year over 60.
            Example: For a 70 year old patient, a Pa_{O_2} down to 70 mm Hg is acceptable.
            (1) Pa_{O_2} less than 60 to 65 mm Hg is always considered hypoxemia.
         b. More precisely, acceptable lower limits for Pa_{O_2} can be determined by the following (at sea level):
            (1) For patients in the supine position:
               $Pa_{O_2} = 103.5 - (0.42 \times age) \pm 4$ mm Hg
            (2) For patients in the sitting position:
               $Pa_{O_2} = 104.2 - (0.27 \times age)$ mm Hg
   B. Causes of hypoxemia (see Chapters 12 and 13)
      1. True shunting
      2. Ventilation/perfusion inequalities
      3. A decreased mixed venous Po_2 may intensify the hypoxemic effect of no. 1 and 2.
   C. Responsive vs. refractory hypoxemia
      1. Refractory hypoxemia is hypoxemia demonstrating a negligible increase in the Pa_{O_2} with the application of oxygen.
         a. If the Fi_{O_2} is greater than or equal to 0.50 while the Pa_{O_2} is less than 60 mm Hg, the hypoxemia is refractory.
         b. If a 0.20 increase in the Fi_{O_2} results in less than a 10 mm Hg increase in the Pa_{O_2}, the hypoxemia is refractory.
         c. Refractory hypoxemia is a result of true shunting.
      2. Responsive hypoxemia is hypoxemia that demonstrates a significant response to an increase in the Fi_{O_2}.
         a. A 0.20 increase in the Fi_{O_2} results in a greater than 10 mm Hg increase in the Pa_{O_2}.
         b. Responsive hypoxemia is a result of ventilation/perfusion inequalities.
   D. Clinical manifestations of hypoxemia
      1. Tachycardia and hypertension
         a. If cardiovascular status is poor, bradycardia and hypotension may result.
      2. Tachypnea and hyperpnea
      3. Pulmonary hypertension (constriction of pulmonary vascular bed)
      4. Vasoconstriction of vascular beds supplying skin, muscles, and abdominal viscera (with moderate to severe hypoxemia)
      5. Vasodilatation of vascular beds supplying heart and brain, resulting in increased blood flow
      6. Development of cyanosis (if hypoxemia is severe and hemoglobin content is increased or normal)
      7. Lactic acidosis if coupled with poor perfusion
      8. Confusion, disorientation, or both
      9. Secondary polycythemia (with chronic hypoxemia)

IV. Indications for Oxygen Therapy
    A. Hypoxemia
        1. Oxygen therapy increases alveolar P_{O_2}, thus increasing the pressure gradient for oxygen diffusion into the bloodstream.
        2. Increasing the pressure gradient may cause an increase in Pa_{O_2}.
    B. Excessive work of breathing
        1. Hypoxemia stimulates peripheral chemoreceptors, causing an increase in the rate and depth of ventilation and increasing the work of breathing.
        2. Oxygen therapy, by increasing alveolar P_{O_2}, may increase arterial P_{O_2}. This will reduce stimulation of peripheral chemoreceptors and reduce the work of breathing.
    C. Excessive myocardial work
        1. The primary compensatory response to hypoxemia is an increase in force and rate of contraction of the heart.
        2. Oxygen therapy may correct hypoxcmia and decrease the stimulus to increase cardiac output.

V. Hazards of Oxygen Therapy
    A. Retinopathy of prematurity (retrolental fibroplasia, RLF)
        1. The presence of opaque fibrotic tissue behind the lens of the eye, resulting in retinal detachment and blindness.
        2. A Pa_{O_2} greater than 80–100 mm Hg may result in RLF in the premature infant.
        3. Pathophysiology of RLF
            a. Phase 1: Hyperoxia causes vasoconstriction of the retinal blood vessels. This is followed by vascular obliteration if the hyperoxia persists (3 or more days).
            b. Phase 2: Vasoproliferation with elimination of the hyperoxic state; additional capillaries develop in the immature retina to the point that light penetration is impaired and blindness results.
        4. Normally seen only in neonates.
        5. Maintaining Pa_{O_2} values less than 80 mm Hg greatly reduces the risk of RLF.
    B. Oxygen toxicity
        1. A series of reversible pathophysiologic inflammatory changes of lung tissue
        2. Free radical theory of oxygen toxicity
            a. The following free radicals of oxygen can be produced at the cellular level:
                (1) Hydrogen peroxide: H_2O_2
                (2) Superoxide radical: O_2^-
                (3) Hydroxyl radical: $OH\cdot$
                (4) Singlet excited oxygen: $^1O_2$
            b. The following enzymes are important cellular defenses against oxygen free radicals:
                (1) Superoxide dismutase (SOD), which converts O_2^- to O_2.
                (2) Catalase (CAT), which converts H_2O_2 to H_2O and O_2.
                (3) Additional intracellular defenses against oxygen free radicals include:
                    (a) Glutathione peroxide
                    (b) Glutathione
                    (c) Cysteine
                    (d) Cysteamine
                    (e) Vitamin E in lipid membrane
                    (f) Vitamin C (intracellular)
            c. The quantity of oxygen free radicals is dependent on Pa_{O_2}. The greater the Pa_{O_2}, the greater the quantity of free radicals.
            d. Effects of oxygen free radicals
                (1) Inhibition of glycolysis
                (2) Interference with surfactant transport and production

          (3) Nucleic acid (DNA) damage
          (4) Cross-linkage of DNA molecules
          (5) Cell and organelle membrane disruption
          (6) Enzyme inhibition

    3. Pathophysiology of oxygen toxicity

      a. Cellular susceptibility to hyperoxia (100% O_2)
          (1) Pulmonary capillary endothelium (most susceptible)
          (2) Alveolar type I epithelial cells
          (3) Alveolar type II epithelial cells
          (4) Alveolar type III epithelial cells (least susceptible)
      b. With continued exposure to 100% O_2, type I alveolar cells are destroyed and replaced by type II cells.
      c. Early or acute exudative phase is characterized by perivascular, interstitial, and intra-alveolar edema with destruction and necrosis of endothelial cells. Alveolar congestion and fibrinous exudation (hyaline membrane) develop.
      d. Late or chronic proliferative phase is characterized by a progressive reabsorption of the exudate and a thickening of the alveolar septa.
      e. Clinical manifestations
          (1) Tracheobronchitis
          (2) Cough
          (3) Substernal pain
          (4) Nausea and vomiting
          (5) Anorexia
          (6) Paresthesia
          (7) Refractory hypoxemia
          (8) Diffuse patchy bilateral infiltrates
          (9) Alveolar atelectasis
          (10) Decreased compliance

    4. Susceptibility and risk factors associated with the development of oxygen toxicity:
      a. Exposure to $F_{I_{O_2}}$ levels greater than 0.40 for lengthy periods of time.
      b. Previous development of severe acute pulmonary disease, which decreases the risk of toxicity. The acute disease is believed to induce the production of SOD and glutathione, thus reducing the oxygen free radical levels.

    5. Prevention: Judicious use of oxygen therapy.

    6. Treatment: Appropriate use of positive end-expiratory pressure therapy, diuretics, and fluids while reducing the $F_{I_{O_2}}$ to "safe" levels (0.50 or less).

C. Oxygen-induced hypoventilation

    1. This is observed in patients with chronic CO_2 retention or central nervous system depression (see Chapter 20).

    2. The increased Pa_{O_2} decreases or eliminates the hypoxic drive, inducing greater levels of hypoventilation.

    3. Intermittent use of oxygen therapy may cause arterial P_{O_2} to fall below pretreatment levels.

D. Absorption atelectasis (Fig 28–1)

    1. Nitrogen is metabolically inactive and constitutes 80% of alveolar gas. Nitrogen is essential in maintaining alveolar stability.

    2. Administration of high $F_{I_{O_2}}$ (more than 0.70) washes out nitrogen.

    3. In poorly ventilated alveoli, more oxygen is removed per unit time by the perfused blood than can be replaced by normal ventilation.

    4. This results in a decrease in alveolar size.

    5. As alveoli reach their critical volume, collapse and atelectasis occur.

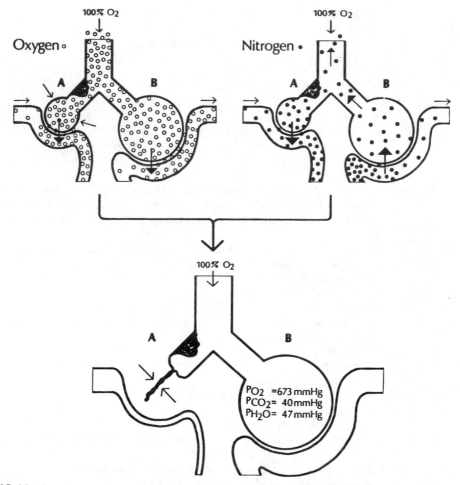

FIG 28–1.
Schematic representation of primary mechanisms causing denitrogenation absorption atelectasis. *Top drawings* represent the alveolar-capillary units shortly after administration of 100% inspired oxygen. *White circles* represent oxygen molecules that have increased in concentration in both units. **A** and **B.** The ablation of alveolar hypoxia in unit **A** results in loss of vasoconstriction with considerably increased blood flow. The increased blood flow to this still poorly ventilated alveolus results in significantly increased oxygen extraction, which results in diminished gas volume. *Black circles* represent nitrogen, which is rapidly depleted from all units secondary to the fact that inspired nitrogen concentration is now zero. Initially, more nitrogen leaves the blood and the body via unit **B** because it is better ventilated. However, as the blood P_{N_2} level progressively decreases, nitrogen will start to leave alveolus **A** via the blood. This results in further loss of gas volume from alveolus **A** since it remains poorly ventilated but well perfused. Thus, nitrogen is depleted from all units within 5 to 15 min. The *bottom drawing* represents the final steady state in which increased oxygen and nitrogen extraction has caused the alveolus to collapse. Thus, a poorly ventilated, poorly perfused unit **A** becomes a nonventilated, poorly perfused unit after administration of 100% inspired oxygen. (From Shapiro BA, Harrison RA, Walton JR: *Clinical Application of Blood Gas,* ed 3. Chicago, Year Book Medical Publishers, 1982. Used by permission.)

      6. This commonly occurs in patients with small tidal volumes or poor distribution of ventilation due to partial airway obstruction.

  VI. Oxygen Delivery Systems

    A. In general, delivery systems are divided into two categories: high-flow and low-flow.

TABLE 28–1.

Entrainment Ratios and Outputs of Specific Air Entrainment Systems*

System	$F_{I_{O_2}}$	Entrainment Ratio	Flow at Which Operated	Total Flow (L/min)
Ventimasks	0.24	1–25	4	104
	0.28	1–10	4	44
	0.31	1–7	6	48
	0.35	1–5	8	48
	0.40	1–3	8	32
	0.50	1–1.7	12	32
Mechanical	0.60	1–1	12	24
Aerosol	0.70	1–0.6	12	19

*Clinical trials indicate some variation in $F_{I_{O_2}}$ levels provided by air entrainment masks.

B. High-flow systems
   1. The patient's entire inspired atmosphere is consistently and predictably delivered by the system.
   2. To maintain a consistent $F_{I_{O_2}}$ the apparatus flow must exceed the peak inspiratory flow of the patient.
   3. Peak inspiratory flows are difficult to measure but may be approximated by delivering a total flow at least *four times* the patient's measured minute volume.
      a. Normal peak inspiratory flows are about four times the patient's measured minute volume.
      b. This flow usually will provide adequate volume in the face by a changing ventilatory pattern.
   4. Typical high-flow systems
      a. Air entrainment masks: Deliver a specific $F_{I_{O_2}}$ level up to 0.50 (Table 28–1 and Fig 28–2).

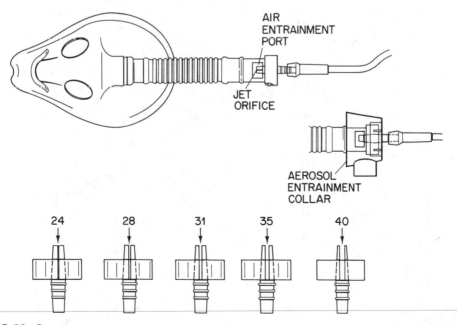

FIG 28–2.
Air entrainment mask with various jet orifices. Each orifice provides a specific delivered $F_{I_{O_2}}$. (From Kacmarek RM: Oxygen therapy techniques, in Kacmarek RM, Stoller J [eds]: *Current Respiratory Care*. Toronto, BC Decker, 1988. Used by permission.)

(1) Care should be taken to ensure the air entrainment mask provides sufficient flow to meet a patient's need. This is especially true with masks delivering higher $F_{I_{O_2}}$ levels.

b. Mechanical aerosol systems: Set up singly or in tandem to deliver high humidity along with a specific $F_{I_{O_2}}$ level (see Table 28–1 and Fig 28–3).

   (1) Again, care should be taken to ensure sufficient flow.

c. Cascade-type humidifier systems

   (1) Volume and concentration of gas are determined by titration of compressed air and oxygen or the use of an oxygen blender (Fig 28–4).

   (2) Virtually any $F_{I_{O_2}}$ level is available.

   (3) Virtually any flow is available.

   (4) Systems are extremely versatile and may be applied to a patient via an aerosol mask or standard artificial airway attachment.

d. Determinations of $F_{I_{O_2}}$ with any system combining gas flows:

$$F_{I_{O_2}} = \frac{(F_{I_{O_2}} \text{ of A})(\text{Flow of A}) + (F_{I_{O_2}} \text{ of B})(\text{Flow of B}) + \text{ etc.}}{\text{Total flow of combined systems}} \qquad (1)$$

e. High-flow systems can be attached to patients by a variety of devices in addition to the typical air entrainment mask (Fig 28–5).

   (1) Aerosol mask

   (2) Face hood

   (3) Tracheostomy collar

   (4) Briggs T piece

C. Low-flow systems

1. The total minute volume is not delivered by the apparatus.

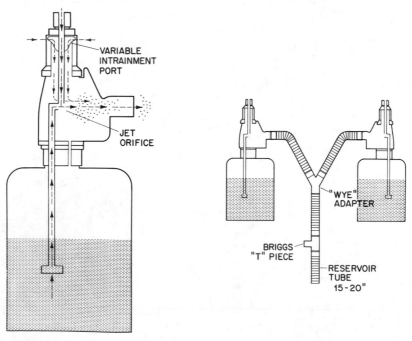

FIG 28–3.
Mechanical aerosol delivery system: Single unit and tandem arrangement. (From Kacmarek RM: Oxygen therapy techniques, in Kacmarek RM, Stoller J [eds]: *Current Respiratory Care.* Toronto, BC Decker, 1988. Used by permission.)

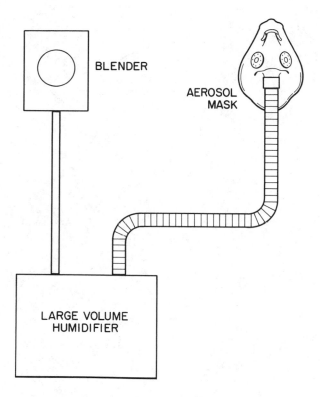

FIG 28–4.
High-flow large-volume (Cascade) humidifier setup. (From Kacmarek RM: Oxygen therapy techniques, in Kacmarek RM, Stoller J [eds]: *Currrent Respiratory Care.* Toronto, BC Decker, 1988. Used by permission.)

2. The $F_{I_{O_2}}$ delivered to the patient depends on:
   a. Flow of gas from equipment.
   b. Patient anatomic reservoir (oral and nasal cavity).
      (1) Normal anatomic reservoir in adults is about 50 ml.
      (2) Normal end-expiratory pause may allow for filling of anatomic reservoir with 100% oxygen.
   c. Reservoir of equipment.
   d. Paient respiratory rate, tidal volume, and minute volume.
3. *The $F_{I_{O_2}}$ delivered with any low-flow system is extremely variable and unpredictable.*
4. If the patient's minute volume were to increase on a particular low-flow system, the $F_{I_{O_2}}$ would *decrease.* The patient would entrain a larger percentage of room air in the minute volume.
5. If the patient's minute volume were to decrease on a particular low-flow system, the $F_{I_{O_2}}$ would *increase.* The patient would entrain a smaller percentage of room air in the minute volume.
6. The following is an example of the calculations used to *estimate* the $F_{I_{O_2}}$ delivered by low-flow oxygen therapy systems. This calculation is for a cannula at 6 L/min.
   a. Ventilatory variables
      (1) Respiratory rate: 20 breaths/min (bpm)
      (2) Tidal volume: 500 ml
      (3) Inspiratory: expiratory ratio: 1:2
      (4) Inspiratory time: 1 second

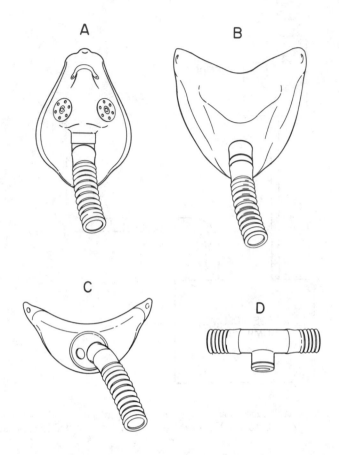

FIG 28–5.
Various appliances used to apply high-flow system. **A,** aerosol mask; **B,** face hood; **C,** tracheostomy collar; **D,** Briggs T piece. (From Kacmarek RM: In-hospital administration of oxygen, in Kacmarek RM, Stoller J [eds]: *Current Respiratory Care.* Toronto, BC Decker, 1988. Used by permission.)

   (5) Volume of patient's anatomic reservoir (volume of oral and nasal cavity): 50 cc
  b. Volume delivered by cannula per second
   (1) Flow is 6 L/min, which equals 6,000 ml/min.
   (2) Thus, 100 ml/sec is delivered to patient.
  c. Volume of 100% oxygen inspired per breath
   (1) In the 1-second inspiratory time, 100 ml is delivered by cannula.
   (2) A 50-ml volume of oxygen is accumulated in anatomic reservoir prior to inspiration (accumulates during expiratory pause).
   (3) If 150 ml is inspired from no. (1) and (2), 350 ml of room air would need to be entrained. Since about 20% of room air is oxygen. 70 ml of oxygen is entrained:

$$100 \text{ ml} + 50 \text{ ml} + 70 \text{ ml} = 220 \text{ ml} \qquad (2)$$

  d. Therefore, the inspired oxygen concentration is equal to:

$$\frac{220 \ (O_2)}{500 \ (V_T)} = F_{I_{O_2}} \text{ of } 0.44 \qquad (3)$$

  where V_T is tidal volume.

e. *It must be kept in mind that the $F_{I_{O_2}}$ listed for each low-flow system is purely speculative and that the $F_{I_{O_2}}$ is totally dependent on the patient's ventilatory pattern. The values provided should be used only as gross guidelines rather than as the exact $F_{I_{O_2}}$ delivered.*

7. Calculations similar to those in section VI–C, 6c have been used to determine the approximate $F_{I_{O_2}}$ levels for various low-flow systems:

a. *Oxygen cannula* (Fig 28–6)
   (1) 1 L/min $F_{I_{O_2}}$: 0.24
   (2) 2 L/min $F_{I_{O_2}}$: 0.28
   (3) 3 L/min $F_{I_{O_2}}$: 0.32
   (4) 4 L/min $F_{I_{O_2}}$: 0.36
   (5) 5 L/min $F_{I_{O_2}}$: 0.40
   (6) 6 L/min $F_{I_{O_2}}$: 0.44

b. *Simple O_2 mask:* Should be run between 5 and 8 L/min to ensure flushing and to prevent CO_2 accumulation in the face mask. This flow will result in an $F_{I_{O_2}}$ between 0.40 and 0.60, *depending on the patient's ventilatory pattern* (see Fig 28–6).

c. *Oxygen mask with bag* (partial rebreathing mask): Should be run between 7 and 10 L/min. The flow must be adequate to ensure that the bag deflates only about one third during inspiration to prevent CO_2 buildup in the system. This flow will result in an $F_{I_{O_2}}$ between 0.70 and 0.80 or more, *depending on the patient's ventilatory pattern* (Fig 28–7).

d. *Nonrebreathing mask:* Must be run with sufficient flow to prevent the bag from collapsing during inspiration. Nonrebreathing masks are difficult to use

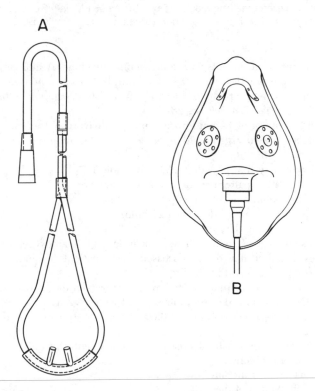

FIG 28–6.
A, nasal cannula; **B,** simple oxygen mask. (From Kacmarek RM: In-hospital administration of oxygen, in Kacmarek RM, Stoller J [eds]: *Current Respiratory Care.* Toronto, BC Decker, 1988. Used by permission.)

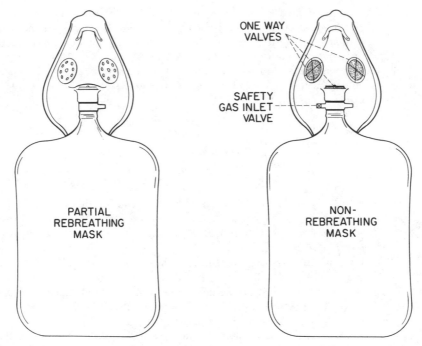

FIG 28–7.
Partial rebreathing and nonrebreathing masks. (From Kacmarek RM: In-hospital administration of oxygen, in Kacmarek RM, Stoller J [eds]: *Current Respiratory Care.* Toronto, BC Decker, 1988. Used by permission.)

properly on patients with a high minute volume. A high-flow cascade setup is more practical for 1.0 F_{IO_2} administration. If a nonrebreathing mask is functioning properly, the F_{IO_2} is 0.90 to 1.0, *depending on the patient's ventilatory pattern* (see Fig 28–7).

    D. Criteria for use of high- and low-flow oxygen delivery systems
        1. *Whenever a consistent and predictable F_{IO_2} is required, a high-flow system should be utilized.*
        2. A low-flow system provides relatively stable F_{IO_2} levels if the patient's:
           a. Ventilatory pattern is consistent and regular.
           b. Tidal volume is between 300 and 700 ml.
           c. Respiratory rate is less than 25 bpm.
    E. Oxygen-conserving devices
        1. These devices use either a reservoir designed into an oxygen cannula system or provide pulsed flow of oxygen based on the patient demand.
        2. Reservoir cannula (Fig 28–8)
           a. This device incorporates two reservoir bags in the body of the cannula.
           b. On exhalation, the reservoir bags fill with oxygen.
           c. Thus, a larger volume of 100% oxygen is available on the next inspiration.
           d. Oxygen use may be decreased up to 50% with this unit.
           e. Major problems
               (1) Size of the unit
               (2) Weight of the unit
               (3) Aesthetics of the unit
           f. It is designed for home oxygen delivery.

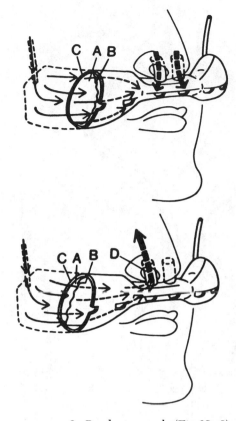

FIG 28–8.
Reservoir cannula. While the patient is exhaling *(top)*, oxygen is accumulating in the reservoir **(A)** formed by the inflated diaphragm **(B)** and the back wall of the conserver **(C)**. While the patient inhales *(bottom)*, the diaphragm **(B)** collapses, and the oxygen-enriched gas from the reservoir **(a)** is released to the patient **(D).** (From Tiep BC, Nicotra B, Carter R, et al: Evaluation of a low-flow oxygen conserving nasal cannula. *Am Rev Respir Dis* 1984; 130:500–502. Used by permission.)

3. Pendant cannula (Fig 28–9)
   a. It functions on the same principle as the reservoir cannula.
   b. Its reservoir is located in the pendant setting on the patient's chest.
   c. It may reduce oxygen use from 50% to 75%.
   d. Major problems are size, weight, and aesthetics.
   e. It is designed for home oxygen delivery.
4. Pulse dose oxygen or demand oxygen delivery system
   a. These systems provide delivery of oxygen only during inspiration.
   b. Negative pressure generated by the patient triggers gas delivery.
   c. Two general types exist: Variable pulsed volume and variable ratio of pulsed breaths to no oxygen delivery breaths.
      (1) Variable pulsed volume devices alter the volume of oxygen from about 10 to 40 ml/breath.
      (2) Variable ratio devices vary delivery of a fixed volume every breath to a fixed volume every fourth breath.
   d. Adequate oxygenation is maintained, since only that gas at the lung parenchymal level participates in gas exchange.
   e. Only the first one third of inspiration reaches the lung parenchyma.
   f. These devices may conserve 50% to 75% of the oxygen used.
   g. They are designed primarily for home use.
   h. A major concern regarding reliability of triggering still remains.
   i. Their function with every patient should be carefully evaluated.
F. Transtracheal oxygen catheter (Fig 28–10)
   1. With this system a no. 8 French catheter is inserted between the second and third tracheal rings and extended to about 2 cm above the carina.

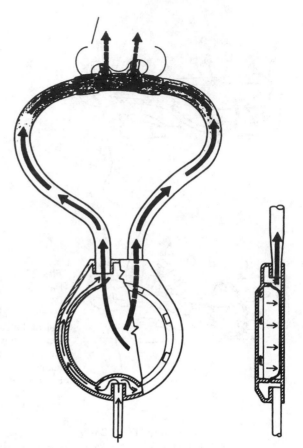

FIG 28–9.
Pendant cannula. Frontal view and cross-sectional view *(right)* of the pendant during inspiration. Negative pressure in the tubing causes the membrane to rapidly move posteriorly, thus providing a burst of oxygen-rich gas. During exhalation, the first part of exhalation enters the pendant (100% oxygen). Once it is filled (40 ml), exhaled gas enters the room. (From Gonzales SC, Huntington D, Romo R, et al: Efficiency of the Oxymizer Pendant in reducing oxygen requirements of hyporemic patients. *Respir Care* 1986; 31:681–688. Used by permission.)

2. Continuous delivery of oxygen is provided via the cannula.
3. Since oxygen is directly delivered into the trachea, oxygen use can be decreased by 50%.
4. In some patients refractory to oxygen therapy because of severe pulmonary fibrosis, transtracheal oxygen therapy has improved arterial oxygenation.
5. General indications
   a. Need for improved mobility.
   b. Compliance with nasal cannula (poor).
   c. Complications with nasal cannula (high).
   d. Hypoxemia refractory to nasal oxygen.
   e. Patient preference due to comfort or cosmesis.
6. Generally it is used for long-term oxygen therapy in the home.
7. Complications
   a. Bronchospasm
   b. Subcutaneous emphysema
   c. Keloids at site of insertion
   d. Penumothorax
   e. Infection
   f. Bleeding
   g. Obstruction from mucous balls on the catheter
VII. Selection of Oxygen System for Adults
   • Refer to Chapters 24, 25, and 26 for guidance regarding infants and children.

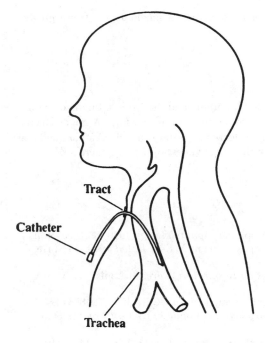

Tract

Catheter

Trachea

FIG 28–10.
Schematic of transtracheal oxygen catheter in place. It is inserted between the second and third tracheal rings and extended to about 2 cm above the carina. (From Spofford B, Christopher K, McCarty D, et al: Transtracheal oxygen therapy: A guide for the respiratory therapist. *Respir Care* 1987; 32:345–352. Used by permission.)

A. Patients with artificial airways
   1. Only high-flow systems are adaptable to artificial airways.
   2. With an endotracheal tube, a Briggs T piece is used.
   3. With a tracheostomy tube:
      a. A Briggs T piece is used if a consistent $F_{I_{O_2}}$ level is essential.
      b. If humidity is the primary concern, a tracheostomy mask or tracheostomy collar is more comfortable and produces less torque on the trachea.
      c. At lower $F_{I_{O_2}}$ levels (0.40 or less), aerosol generators provide sufficient flow.
      d. If the $F_{I_{O_2}}$ level needed is greater than 0.40 to maintain high flow, a Cascade large-volume nebulizer system may be necessary.
B. Patients without artificial airways
   1. Any system discussed may be used.
   2. The low-flow system, especially the O_2 cannula, is normally the best tolerated of all systems and the most complied with. If it can provide adequate oxygenation, it should be used before other systems.
   3. In the emergency room, a simple oxygen mask or partial rebreathing mask should be used if the cannula does not provide sufficient $F_{I_{O_2}}$.
   4. In the recovery room, an aerosol generator, normally unheated, with a face mask is usually sufficient.
VIII. Use of 100% Oxygen
   A. The use of 100% oxygen may result in:
      1. Oxygen toxicity.
      2. Absorption atelectasis.
      3. Oxygen-induced hypoventilation.
   B. In spite of these possibilities, 100% oxygen should always be used short term during:
      1. Cardiac arrest.
      2. Transport.
      3. Acute cardiopulmonary instability.

4. Carbon monoxide poisoning, whenever carboxyhemoglobin levels are greater than 10%.

IX. Monitoring of Oxygen Therapy
   A. Arterial blood gas analysis
   B. Tidal volume and respiratory rate
   C. Pulse and blood pressure
   D. It is important to evaluate the work of breathing and the work of the myocardium to determine the overall effectiveness of an increase in the F_{IO_2}. A minor change in the P_{O_2} may be accompanied by a decrease in the work of breathing and the work of the myocardium, indicating the effectiveness of the F_{IO_2} increase.

BIBLIOGRAPHY

Ashton N: The pathogenesis of retrolental fibroplasia. *Ophthalmology* 1979; 86:1695–1699.

Barber RE, Lee J, Hamilton WK: Oxygen toxicity in man. *N Engl J Med* 1970; 283:1478–1488.

Bendixen HH, Egert ID, Hedley-Whyte J, et al: *Respiratory Care*. St Louis, CV Mosby Co, 1965.

Block AJ: Neuropsychological aspects of oxygen therapy. *Respir Care* 1983; 28:885–888.

Burton GG, Gee GN, Hodgkin JE: *Respiratory Care: A Guide to Clinical Practice*. Philadelphia, JB Lippincott Co, 1984.

Christopher KL, Spoffort BT, Brannin PK, et al: Transtracheal oxygen therapy for refractory hypoxemia. *JAMA* 1986; 256:494–497.

Christopher KL: At home administration of oxygen, in Kacmarek RM, Stoller J (eds): *Current Respiratory Care*, Toronto, BC Decker, 1988.

Consensus Conference: National Conference on Oxygen Therapy Report. *Chest* 1984; 86:234–247.

Deneke SM, Fanburg BL: Normobaric oxygen toxicity of the lung. *N Engl J Med* 1980; 303:76–86.

Deshpande VM, Pilbeam SP, Dixon RJ: *A Comprehensive Review in Respiratory Care*. Norwalk, Conn, Appleton & Lange, 1988.

Eubanks DH, Bone BC: *Comprehensive Respiratory Care: Learning System*. St Louis, CV Mosby Co, 1985.

Fenley DC: Long-term home oxygen therapy. *Chest* 1985; 87:99–103.

Frank L, Massaro D: The lung and oxygen toxicity. *Arch Intern Med* 1979; 139:347–350.

Frank L, Massaro D: Oxygen toxicity. *Am J Med* 1980; 69:117–126.

Gibson RL, Comer PB, Beckham RW, et al: Actual tracheal oxygen concentration with commonly used oxygen equipment. *Anesthesiology* 1976; 44:71–73.

Gonzales SC, Huntington D, Romo R, et al: Efficiency of the Oxymizer Pendant in reducing oxygen requirements of hypoxemic patients. *Respir Care* 1986; 31:681–688.

Harkema JR, Mauderly JL, Hahn FF: The effects of emphysema on oxygen toxicity in rats. *Am Rev Respir Dis* 1982; 126:1058–1065.

Hedley-White J, Burgess GE III, Feeley TW, et al: *Applied Physiology of Respiratory Care*. Boston, Little, Brown & Co, 1976.

Kacmarek RM: In-hospital administration of oxygen, in Kacmarek RM, Stoller J (eds): *Current Respiratory Care*. Toronto, BC Decker, 1988.

McPherson SP: *Respiratory Therapy Equipment*, ed 3. St Louis, CV Mosby Co, 1986.

Mellemgaard K: The alveolar-arterial oxygen difference: Its size and components in normal man. *Acta Physiol Scand* 1966; 67:10–14.

O'Donohue WJ: Oxygen conserving devices. *Respir Care* 1987; 32:37–42.

Patz A: Studies on retinal neovascularization. *Invest Ophthalmol Vis Sci* 1980; 19:1133–1138.

Redding JS, McAfee DD, Parham AM: Oxygen concentrations received from commonly used delivery systems. *South Med J* 1978; 71:169–172.

Safar P (ed): *Respiratory Therapy*. Philadelphia, FA Davis Co, 1965.

Schacter EW, Littner MR, Luddy P, et al: Monitoring of oxygen delivery systems in clinical practice. *Crit Care Med* 1980; 8:405–409.

Shapiro BA, Harrison RA, Kacmarek RM, et al: *Clinical Application of Respiratory Care,* ed 3. Chicago, Year Book Medical Publishers, 1985.

Singer MM, Wright F, Stanley LK, et al: Oxygen toxicity in man. *N Engl J Med* 1970; 283:1473–1478.

Sobini CA, Grassi V, Solinas E: Arterial oxygen tension in relation to age in healthy subjects. *Respiration* 1968; 25:3–14.

Spearman CB, Sheldon RL, Egan DF: *Egan's Fundamentals of Respiratory Therapy,* ed 4. St Louis, CV Mosby Co, 1982.

Spofford B, Christopher K, McCarty D, et al: Transtracheal oxygen therapy: A guide for the respiratory therapist. *Respir Care* 1987; 232:345–352.

Tiep BL, Nicotra B, Carter R, et al: Evaluation of a low-flow oxygen conserving nasal cannula. *Am Rev Respir Dis* 1984; 130:500–502.

Woolner DF, Larkin J: An analysis of the performance of a variable venturi-type oxygen mask. *Anesth Intensive Care* 1980; 8:44–51.

Young JA, Crocker D: *Principles and Practice of Respiratory Therapy,* ed 2. Chicago, Year Book Medical Publishers, 1976.

Youtsey JW: Oxygen and mixed gas therapy, in Barnes TA (ed): *Respiratory Care Practice.* Year Book Medical Publishers, Chicago, 1988.

Ward JJ: Equipment for mixed gas and oxygen therapy, in Barnes TA (ed): *Respiratory Care Practice.* Year Book Medical Publishers, Chicago, 1988.

_____

Chapter 29

Airway Care

I. General Indications for Use of Artificial Airways
   A. To prevent or relieve upper airway obstruction.
   B. To protect the airway from aspiration.
   C. To facilitate tracheal suction.
   D. To provide a sealed, closed system for mechanical ventilation or continuous positive airway pressure (CPAP).
II. General Classification of Artificial Airways
   A. Oropharyngeal airway
      1. Used to relieve upper airway obstruction by maintaining the base of the tongue off the posterior wall of the oral pharynx.
      2. Used to prevent inadvertent laceration of the tongue in the incoherent or seizuring patient.
      3. Used as a bite block with oral endotracheal tubes.
      4. Poorly tolerated in alert patient due to stimulation of gag reflex.
   B. Nasopharyngeal airway
      1. It is used to relieve upper airway obstruction caused by tongue or soft palate falling against posterior wall of the pharynx.
      2. Suctioning via this airway is less traumatic than nasal suctioning.
      3. It is better tolerated than oropharyngeal airway.
      4. It should be alternated every 24 hours between right and left nares to minimize complications.
      5. Sinusitis, otitis media, and nasal necrosis are possible complications of its use.
   C. Oroendotracheal tube
      1. Advantages when compared with nasotracheal tubes
         a. It is easy to insert and is the airway of choice in an emergency.
         b. Ideally, it is used for short-term intubation of 24 hours or less.
         c. Tube size inserted can be larger than if a nasotracheal tube were inserted.
         d. Sinusitis and otitis media are not problems.
         e. The angle of curvature is less acute than with nasal tubes; it is easier to suction.
         f. Generally there is less resistance to gas flow, and less work of breathing is imposed.

g. A larger-diameter tube can be inserted via the nasal route.
  (1) Men: 8 to 9 mm inside diameter (I.D.)
  (2) Women: 7 to 8 mm I.D.
2. Problems associated with orotracheal tubes
  a. They are poorly tolerated in conscious and semiconscious patients.
  b. They are difficult to stabilize.
  c. Inadvertent extubation is common.
  d. A bite block is necessary to prevent biting of tube.
  e. Vagal stimulation is common.
  f. Oral hygiene is difficult.
  g. They require laryngoscopy during insertion.
  h. They are easily dislodged.
  i. Patients are unable to mouth words.
  j. Lips may be lacerated.
  k. There is a potential for laryngeal pathology.
  l. The tip of the tube moves when the patient's head position changes.
    (1) Extension of the head moves the tip toward the oropharynx (possible extubation).
    (2) Flexion of the head moves the tip toward the carina (possible right endobronchial intubation).
  m. Oral feeding is difficult.
D. Nasoendotracheal tube
  1. Advantages over oroendotracheal tube for long-term intubation
    a. Easier to stabilize.
    b. It is better tolerated.
    c. It may be inserted blindly (laryngoscopy is unnecessary in most cases).
    d. Oral hygiene is easily accomplished.
    e. The patient is able to swallow.
    f. The patient to able to mouth words.
    g. Attachment of equipment is easier and safer; there is less torque on the trachea.
  2. Problems associated with nasotracheal tubes
    a. The tip of the tube moves when the patient's head position changes.
    b. Pressure necrosis in area of the alae nasi may occur.
    c. Sinus drainage may be obstructed, and acute sinusitis may result.
    d. Eustachian tube drainage may be obstructed, and otitis media may result.
    e. The incidence of vocal cord damage after 3 to 7 days (also seen with oroendotracheal tubes) increases.
    f. Vagal stimulation is possible, but it occurs less frequently than with the oroendotracheal tube.
    g. Skilled personnel are necessary for placement.
    h. The nasal passage limits the tube size; a tube at least 0.5 mm I.D. smaller than the oral route is required.
      (1) Men: 7.5 to 8.5 mm I.D.
      (2) Women: 6.5 to 7.5 mm I.D.
    i. The angle of curvature is very acute, the resistance to gas flow is increased, there is difficulty in suctioning, and the work of breathing is increased when compared with an oral tube in the same patient.
    j. It is a potential for laryngeal pathology.
E. Tracheostomy tube
  1. Advantages over endotracheal tubes
    a. There are no complications with the upper airway or glottis.
    b. It is easier to suction.

    c. It is easier to stabilize.

    d. The tracheostomy tube is the best tolerated of all airways.

    e. The patient is able to mouth words, and talking or fenestrated tubes are available.

    f. The patient has the ability to swallow.

    g. With mature stoma, reinsertion is easy.

2. Problems associated with tracheostomy tube

    a. It requires surgery.

    b. There may be immediate complications.

        (1) Bleeding

        (2) Pneumothorax

        (3) Air embolism

        (4) Subcutaneous and mediastinal emphysema

    c. There may be late complications.

        (1) Infection of surgical wound

        (2) Innominate artery erosion

        (3) False passage into subcutaneous tissue

        (4) Hemorrhage may occur

        (5) Tracheal stenosis may occur

3. Frequent and routine changing of tracheostomy tubes is unnecessary if the airway is functioning properly, is properly humidified, and no infectious process is present in the tracheostomy wound.

4. If stomal infection exists, weekly changing of the tracheostomy tubes is recommended.

F. Fenestrated tracheostomy tube (Figs 29–1 and 29–2)

1. Fenestration is located in the outer cannula only.

2. The inner cannula is similar in design to the inner cannula of a normal tracheostomy tube.

3. Requisites for proper use include:

    a. Removal of inner cannula.

    b. Deflation of cuff.

    c. Corking of outer cannula.

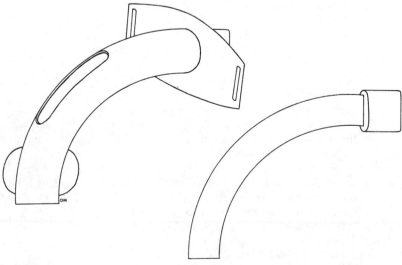

FIG 29–1.
Fenestrated tracheostomy tube. Inner and outer cannulas are depicted.

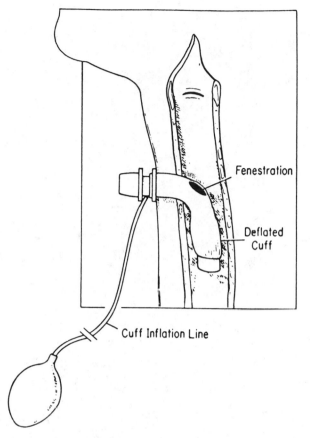

Fenestration

Deflated
Cuff

Cuff Inflation Line

FIG 29–2.
Fenestrated tracheostomy tube with
cuff deflated and inner cannula
removed as it sits in the airway.
(From Wilson D: Airway appliances
and management, in Kacmarek RM,
Stoller JK [eds]: *Current Respiratory
Care.* Toronto, BC Decker, 1988.
Used by permission.)

4. The patient is forced to ventilate via the upper airway through fenestration in the outer cannula of the tracheostomy tube and around the tube.
5. Problems associated with the fenestrated tube include:
   a. Possible formation of granular tissue at site of fenestration.
   b. Increased resistance to gas flow and work of breathing.
6. Commercial fenestrated tubes are available from many manufacturers; however, often these do not fit properly.
7. Many patients require the fitting of a customized tube.
G. Talking tracheostomy tube (Fig 29–3)
   1. It is designed to allow the patient to verbalize when the cuff is inflated.
   2. It functions by directing secondary gas flow through ports in the tube above the patient's cuff, allowing gas to move past the vocal cords while maintaining ventilation via the airway.
   3. The internal diameter of the airway is smaller than the standard tube of the same size.
H. Tracheal button (Figs 29–4 and 29–5)
   1. It is used to maintain patency of the tracheal stoma.
   2. The inner lip of the button lies on the internal anterior tracheal wall and the outer lip on the tissue of the neck.
   3. The tracheal button allows the patient to ventilate completely from the upper airway without tracheal obstruction.
   4. In an emergency, the patient may be suctioned or ventilated via the tracheal button.

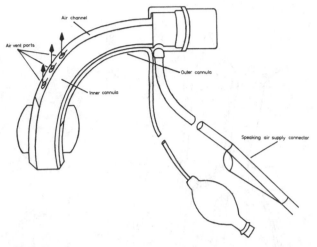

FIG 29–3.
Talking tracheostomy tube.

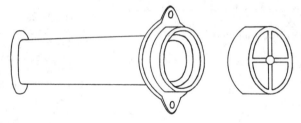

FIG 29–4.
Tracheal button with one-way valve, allowing inspiration but not expiration.

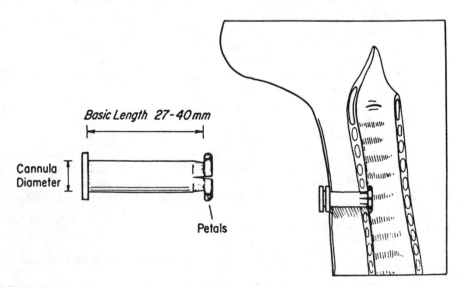

FIG 29–5.
Dimensions and actual positioning of an Olympic tracheostomy button. (From Wilson D: Airway appliances and management, in Kacmarek RM, Stoller JK [eds]: *Current Respiratory Care*. Toronto, BC Decker, 1988. Used by permission.)

   I. Esophageal obturator (Fig 29–6)
      1. The obturator is used only as an emergency airway.
      2. The obturator is a mask attached to a blind endotracheal tube, which has perforations along its length and a cuff at tip of tube.
      3. The obturator is inserted into the esophagus, and the cuff is inflated.
      4. It should be removed only after intubation of the trachea has been performed and cuff inflated.
      5. The patient is ventilated by forcing gas into the obturator. Gas moves out of perforations in the tube and is forced into the trachea.
      6. Problems associated with the esophageal obturator include:
         a. Intubation of the trachea during insertion.
         b. Regurgitation on removal of the airway.
         c. Rupture of the esophagus.
  J. Cricothyroidotomy
      1. Incision through the cricothyroid membrane located between the cricoid and thyroid cartilages
      2. Used as an emergency airway if upper airway obstruction prevents oroendotracheal intubation and ventilation
      3. Advantages
         a. Rapid establishment of airway
         b. Easily accomplished during cardiopulmonary resuscitation
      4. Disadvantages
         a. Perforation of thyroid gland
         b. Perforation of esophagus
         c. Mediastinal or subcutaneous emphysema
         d. Pneumothorax
         e. Hemorrhage
         f. Vocal cord damage if performed too high
         g. Increased airway resistance because of the small internal diameter of the tube
III. Laryngotracheal Complications of Endotracheal Intubation
  A. Sore throat and hoarse voice
  B. Glottic edema

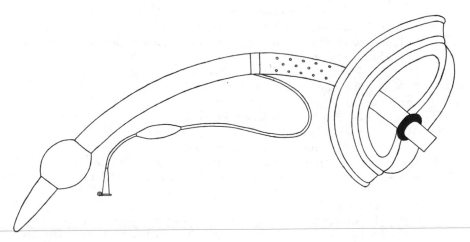

FIG 29–6.
Esophageal obturator airway.

    C. Subglottic edema

    D. Ulceration of tracheal mucosa

    E. Vocal cord ulceration, granuloma, and polyp formation

    F. Vocal cord paralysis

    G. Laryngotracheal web

IV. Postextubation Therapy

    A. Administration of 0.5 ml of 2.25% weight/volume racemic epinephrine, 1 mg of dexamethasone with 4 ml of normal saline solution may reverse or prevent glottic or subglottic edema.

    B. If symptoms of glottic or subglottic edema persist, reintubation may be necessary.

V. Airway Cuffs

    A. Uses

        1. Mechanically ventilate patient

        2. Protect airway from aspiration

    B. Tracheal wall pressures

        1. Intra-arterial pressure approximately 30 mm Hg (42 cm H_2O)

        2. Venous pressures approximately 18 mm Hg (24 cm H_2O)

    C. Lateral tracheal wall pressures:

        1. Greater than 30 mm Hg cause cessation of arterial blood flow.

        2. Greater than 18 mm Hg obstruct venous flow.

        3. Greater than 5 mm Hg inhibit lymphatic flow.

    D. Cuff pressures ideally should be maintained at less than 20 mm Hg to maintain tracheal capillary blood flow.

    E. Effects of high lateral tracheal wall pressures; sequence of tracheal changes:

        1. Mucosal ischemia

        2. Mucosal inflammation, hemorrhage, and/or ulceration

           a. Tracheal granuloma formation

        3. Exposure of cartilage

        4. Tracheal ring destruction

           a. Tracheomalacia

           b. Tracheal stenosis

               (1) At cuff site

               (2) At tip of airway

               (3) At stoma in tracheostomies

    F. Additional factors predisposing to tracheal damage

        1. High peak airway pressure or positive end-expiratory pressure (PEEP) requiring higher cuff pressures

        2. Too small or too large a cuff in relation to tracheal size

        3. Noncircular cross-sectional tracheal shape

        4. Cuff material

           a. Silicon: Requires least inflation pressure

           b. Polyvinyl chloride

           c. Latex: Requires greatest inflation pressure

    G. High-volume, low-pressure vs. low-volume, high-pressure cuffs

        1. High-volume, low-pressure cuffs are the cuffs of choice for long-term airway maintenance.

           a. Advantages

               (1) Intracuff pressures are lower than with high-pressure cuffs.

               (2) Lateral tracheal wall pressure is dissipated over a large surfaced area.

           b. Disadvantage: May form folds when inflated, allowing aspiration of liquids or entrapment of secretions that cause infection.

H. Special cuffs
    1. Kamen-Wilkinson cuff (Bivona cuff)
        a. It is made of polyurethane foam.
        b. It is inflated by atmospheric pressure.
        c. No positive pressure is added to cuff.
        d. Minimum pressures normally are applied to the tracheal wall.
        e. Deflation of the cuff with a syringe before insertion allows reexpansion by atmospheric pressure.
    2. Lanz cuff
        a. Dynamic cuff theoretically allows only 20 cm H_2O pressure to be developed in the cuff.
        b. Valve assembly on the pilot tube maintains constancy of intracuff pressure by allowing gas movement from the pilot balloon to the cuff.
I. Cuff inflation techniques
    1. Minimal leak technique: Cuff volume maintains the seal except at maximum inspiratory pressure.
        a. Insertion of enough air into the cuff prevents any leaks.
        b. While positive pressure is applied to the airway, gas should be withdrawn from the cuff until a slight leak develops. The leak should not be so great as to overcome the purpose of the cuff.
    2. Minimal occluding volume: A minimal volume of gas is required to maintain the airway seal at peak positive pressure during inspiration.
        a. Insert enough air to prevent any leak.
        b. Withdraw gas during inspiration until a leak occurs.
        c. Carefully inflate until the gas leak is stopped at peak inspiratory pressure.
    3. Monitoring of cuff pressures and volumes
        a. A pressure monitor is used to evaluate actual intracuff pressure.
        b. It is important to monitor intracuff pressures if high peak airway pressures are necessary or if high levels of PEEP are employed.
        c. If the minimal occluding volume technique is used, cuff pressures should be monitored. A 1- to 2-ml increase in cuff volume can cause a precipitous increase in intracuff pressure.
        d. Actual cuff pressures should be monitored and recorded routinely with ventilator checks or oxygen therapy equipment checks.
        e. Cuff volumes should be monitored less frequently. Frequent deflation and inflation of a cuff increase the likelihood of improper maintenance.
        f. Steadily increasing cuff volume necessary to maintain a specific cuff pressure may be indicative of:
           (1) An overdistended cuff.
           (2) Tracheomalacia.
    Note: Outside the operating room, only high-volume, low-pressure cuffs should be utilized.
VI. Cuff Deflation Technique
  A. Complete suctioning of lower airway
  B. Complete suctioning above cuff
  C. Deflation of cuff while positive pressure is applied to direct any pooled secretions above the cuff up and out of the airway
VII. Artificial Airway Emergencies
  A. Inadvertent extubation
  B. Airway obstruction
    1. Mucous plug
    2. Granuloma tissue
    3. Herniation of the cuff over the end of the tube

      C. Endobronchial intubation

      D. Kinking of the airway

VIII. Management of Acute Obstruction of Artificial Airway

      A. Manipulate tube (check for kinks).

      B. Attempt to suction airway.

      C. Deflate cuff.

      D. If all of these fail and tension pneumothorax is ruled out, remove the tube and ventilate with bag and mask.

  IX. Airway Suctioning

      A. Complications of airway suctioning

        1. Hypoxemia

        2. Arrhythmias

        3. Hypotension

        4. Lung collapse

        5. Cardiac arrest

      B. Requisites of suction catheters

        1. They should be constructed of a material that will cause minimal irritation and trauma to tracheal mucosa.

        2. Minimal frictional resistance when passing through the artificial airway is essential.

        3. They should be sufficiently long to easily pass the tip of the artificial airway.

        4. They should have smooth, molded ends and side holes to prevent mucosal trauma.

        5. The catheter diameter should be less than one half the internal diameter of the artificial airway.

          a. To convert French (Fr) size to size in millimeters (approximation):

$$mm = \frac{Fr - 2}{4} \tag{1}$$

          b. To convert the size in millimeters to French size (approximation):

$$Fr = (4)\,(mm) + 2 \tag{2}$$

      C. Suctioning technique

        1. Use completely sterile technique.

        2. Preoxygenate the patient.

        3. Insert the catheter without vacuum until an obstruction is met, and then slightly retract the catheter.

        4. Apply suction only during removal of the catheter.

        5. The suction catheter should remain in the airway no longer than 10 to 15 seconds.

        6. Reoxygenate and ventilate.

        7. In the event of catheter adherence to the wall of the airway, release suction, withdraw the catheter, and reapply suction.

        8. To minimize airway trauma, use the following suction pressures:

          a. Infants: 60 to 80 mm Hg

          b. Children: 80 to 120 mm Hg

          c. Adults: 120 to 150 mm Hg

      D. Closed suctioning system (Fig 29–7)

        1. This system is permanently affixed to the airway-ventilator tubing system.

        2. During suctioning, mechanical ventilation is still maintained.

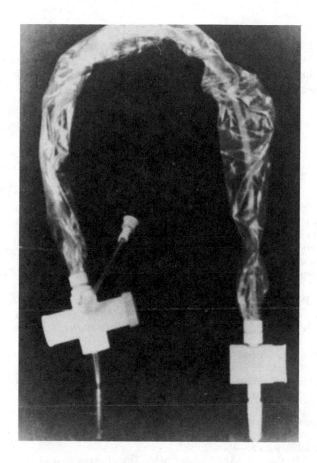

FIG 29–7.
Tracheostomy care suction catheter system. (From Wilkins RL: Suctioning and airway care, in Kacmarek RM, Stoller JK [eds]: *Current Respiratory Care*. Toronto, BC Decker, 1988. Used by permission.)

    3. The suction catheter is located in the plastic sleeve and is advanced into the airway at the time of suctioning.

    4. This system is useful:

        a. If disconnection from the ventilator, even for short periods of time, results in desaturation, bradycardia, and hypotension.

        b. In isolation patients with highly communicable diseases.

    5. Generally, this system reduces the risk of contamination of practitioners during suctioning.

    6. These systems should not be used if the mechanical ventilatory rate is less than 8 breaths/min. If rates are low the patient does not receive sufficient ventilatory support to prevent hypoxemia.

    7. In general, the $F_{I_{O_2}}$ with these systems does not require adjustment during suctioning; however, each patient's tolerance of the system should be evaluated with a pulse oximeter before the decision to maintain the $F_{I_{O_2}}$ level during suctioning is made.

  E. Instillation of normal saline

    1. The instillation of normal saline into the airway at the time of suctioning is normally unnecessary if:

        a. Proper systemic hydration is maintained.

    b. Proper bronchial hygiene is provided.

    c. Proper humidification of inspired gases is ensured.

2. However, if these criteria are not maintained, the instillation of 3 to 5 ml of normal saline solution prior to suctioning may help to mobilize thick, retained, difficult-to-suction secretions.

BIBLIOGRAPHY

Applebaum EL, Bruce DL: *Tracheal Intubation.* Philadelphia, WB Saunders Co, 1976.

Bendixen HH, et al: *Respiratory Care,* St Louis, CV Mosby Co, 1965.

Burton GG, Hodgkin JE: *Respiratory Care: A Guide to Clinical Practice* ed 2. Philadelphia, JB Lippincott Co, 1985.

Chapman GA, Kim CS, Frankel J, et al: Evaluation of the safety and efficiency of a new suction catheter design. *Respir Care* 1986; 31:889–895.

Conrardy PA, Goodman LR, Lainge F, et al: Alteration of endotracheal tube position, flexion and extension of the neck. *Crit Care Med* 1976; 4:8–12.

Demers RR: Complications of endotracheal suctioning procedures. *Respir Care* 1982; 27:453–457.

Deshpande VM, Pilbeam SP, Dixon RJ: *A Comprehensive Review in Respiratory Care.* Norwalk, Conn, Appleton & Lange, 1988.

Dobrin P, Canfield T: Cuffed endotracheal tubes: Mucosal pressure and tracheal wall blood flow. *Am J Surg* 1977; 133:562–568.

Glover DW, McCarthy-Glover M: *Respiratory Therapy—Basics for Nursing and the Allied Health Professions.* St Louis, CV Mosby Co, 1978.

Greisz H, Quarnstrom O, Willen R: Elective cricothyroidotomy: A clinical and histopathological study. *Crit Care Med* 1982; 10:387–389.

Heffner IE, Miller KS, Sahn SA: Tracheostomy in the intensive care unit: part 1. Indications, techniques, management. *Chest* 1986; 90:269–274.

Heffner IF, Miller KS, Sahn SA: Tracheostomy in the intensive care unit: part 2. Complications. *Chest* 1986; 90:430–436.

Holladay-Skelley FB, Deeren SM, Powaser MM: The effectiveness of two preoxygenation methods to prevent endotracheal suction-induced hypoxemia. *Heart Lung* 1980; 9:316–323.

Kastanos N, Miro RE, Perez AM, et al: Laryngotracheal injury due to endotracheal intubation: Incidence, evolution, and predisposing factors. A prospective long-term study. *Crit Care Med* 1983; 11:362–366.

Kress TD: Cricothyroidotomy. *Ann Emerg Med* 1982; 11:197–201.

Langrehe EA, Washburn SC, Guthrie MP: Oxygen insufflation during endotracheal suctioning. *Heart Lung* 1981; 10:1028–1036.

Lewis FR, Schlobohm RM, Thomas AN: Prevention of complications from prolonged tracheal intubation. *Am J Surg* 1978; 135:452–457.

MacKenzie CF: Compromises in the choice of orotracheal or nasotracheal intubation and tracheostomy. *Heart Lung* 1983; 12:485–492.

McDowell DE: Cricothyroidostomy for airway access. *South Med J* 1982; 75:282–284.

Nelson EJ, Morton EA, Hunter PM: *Critical Care Respiratory Therapy—A Laboratory and Clinical Manual.* Boston, Little, Brown & Co, 1983.

Off D, Braun SR, Tompkins B, et al: Efficacy of the minimal leak technique of cuff inflation in maintaining proper intracuff pressures for patients with cuffed artificial airways. *Respir Care* 1983; 28:1115–1120.

Palvin EG, Van Nimgegan D, Hornbein TF: Failure of a high compliance-low pressure cuff to prevent aspiration. New York, American Standards Association, 1975, vol 43, p 216.

Rarey KP, Youtsey JW: *Respiratory Patient Care.* Englewood Cliffs, NJ, Prentice-Hall, 1981.

Rindfleisch SH, Tyler ML: Duration of suctioning: An important variable [editorial]. *Respir Care* 1983; 28:457–458.

Safer P (ed): *Respiratory Therapy.* Philadelphia, FA Davis Co, 1965.

Shapiro BA, Harrison RA, Kacmarek RM, et al: *Clinical Application of Respiratory Care*, ed 3. Chicago, Year Book Medical Publishers, 1985.

Spearman CB, Sheldon RL, Egan DF: *Egan's Fundamentals of Respiratory Care*, ed 4. St Louis, CV Mosby Co, 1982.

Sinsheimer F: *Basics of Respiratory Therapy—a Laboratory Manual.* Boston, Little, Brown & Co, 1983.

Stauffer JL, Olson DE, Petty TL: Complications and consequences of endotracheal intubation and tracheotomy: A prospective study of 150 critically ill adult patients. *Am J Surg* 1981; 70:65–76.

Stauffer JL, Silvestri RC: Complications of endotracheal intubation, tracheostomy, and artificial airways. *Respir Care* 1982; 27:417–434.

Wilson DJ: Airway applicances and management, in Kacmarek RM, Stoller JK (eds): *Current Respiratory Care.* Toronto, BC Decker, 1988.

Wilkins RL: Suctioning and airway care, in Kacmarek RM, Stoller JK (eds): *Current Respiratory Care.* Toronto, BC Decker, 1988.

Young JA, Crocker D: *Principles and Practice of Respiratory Therapy*, ed 2. Chicago, Year Book Medical Publishers, 1976.

Chapter 30

Aerosol and Humidity Therapy

- An aerosol is a suspension of liquid or solid particles in a gas such as smoke or fog.
- Humidity refers to the addition of water vapor to a gas, that is, water in molecular form only.
 I. Stability
- Stability is the tendency of aerosol particles to remain in suspension. The following factors affect the stability of an aerosol:
    A. Size: The smaller the aerosol particle, the greater the tendency toward stability. The larger the particle, the greater the tendency to rain out of suspension.
    B. Concentration: The greater the concentration of particles, the greater the tendency for individual particles to coalesce into larger particles and rain out of suspension.
    C. Humidity: The greater the relative humidity of the gas carrying the aerosol, the greater the stability of the aerosol.
 II. Penetration and Deposition of an Aerosol in the Respiratory Tract
    A. Penetration refers to the depth within the respiratory tract that an aerosol reaches. Deposition is the rain-out of aerosol particles within the respiratory tract.
    B. Depth of penetration and volume of deposition depend on:
       1. Gravity: Gravity decreases penetration and increases premature deposition but has minimal effect on particles in the therapeutic range of 1 to 5 μ (Table 30–1).
       2. Kinetic energy: The greater the kinetic energy of the gas carrying the particles, the greater the tendency for premature deposition. This is because coalescence and impaction are increased.
       3. Inertial impaction: Deposition of particles is increased at any point of directional change or increased airway resistance. Thus, the smaller the airway diameter, the greater the tendency for deposition.
 III. Ventilatory Pattern for Optimal Penetration and Deposition
    A. The patient's ventilatory pattern is the most important variable that can be controlled to ensure maximum penetration and deposition of aerosol particles.
    B. Ideal ventilatory pattern
       1. Large, slowly inspired tidal volume (VT) over 3–4 seconds.
       2. During inspiration, the patient's mouth should be opened widely to decrease deposition of the aerosol in the mouth and oropharynx.
       3. After inhalation, a 3- to 4-second breath-holding period is advisable to ensure maximum deposition.

TABLE 30–1.

Penetration and Deposition Versus Particle Size

Particle Size (μ)	Deposition in Respiratory Tract
>100	Do not enter respiratory tract
100–10	Trapped in mouth
100–5	Trapped in nose
5–2	Deposited proximal to alveoli
2–1	Can enter alveoli, 95%–100% of particles 1 μ in size settling
1–0.25	Stable, with minimal settling

    4. With large-volume aerosols (ultrasonic nebulizers), a face mask should be used.

    5. With small-volume nebulizers, a mouthpiece is normally used. However, the patient's mouth should be opened widely about the mouthpiece.

    6. Exhalation should be relaxed and normal.

    7. Coughing should be encouraged if secretion mobilization occurs and at the completion of treatment.

  C. Attempts should be made to have all patients receiving aerosol therapy assume the ventilatory pattern described.

IV. Clearance of Aerosols

• Inhaled particles are removed from the respiratory tract by three mechanisms:

  A. Primary mechanism: Mucociliary escalator, which moves about 100 ml of secretions to the oropharynx per day (see Chapter 3, section I–C).

  B. Normal cough mechanism.

  C. Phagocytosis by type III alveolar cells.

V. Indications for Aerosol Therapy

  A. Retained secretions.

  B. The need for a vehicle to administer bronchodilators and other pharmacologic agents directly on the respiratory mucosa.

  C. Humidification of the inspired gas of patients acutely requiring short-term artificial airways.

  D. Patients presenting with the following conditions:

    1. Retained secretions

    2. Asthma and other reactive airway diseases

    3. Bronchitis or emphysema

    4. Cystic fibrosis

    5. Severe laryngitis, trachetitis, or croup

    6. Bronchiectasis

    7. Smoke inhalation or chemical trauma to the airways

    8. Physical trauma to the upper airway

    9. Postextubation therapy to prevent laryngeal edema

  E. Aerosol therapy may also be necessary for sputum induction.

VI. General Goals of Aerosol Therapy

  A. Improve bronchial hygiene

    1. Hydrate dried retained secretions.

    2. Improve efficiency of cough mechanism

    3. Restore and maintain normal function of mucociliary escalator.

  B. Humidify gases delivered to patients with artificial airways.

  C. Deliver medications.

VII. Hazards of Aerosol Therapy
   A. Precipitation of bronchoconstriction
      1. Is most common in asthmatic patients.
      2. May follow administration of certain drugs (e.g., acetylcysteine or bland aerosol).
      3. May result in hypoxemia.
   B. Increased airway obstruction because of swelling of dried retained secretions
      1. Is a problem more frequently with ultrasonic nebulizers than with mechanical aerosols.
      2. Is seen primarily in debilitated patients with a poor cough mechanism.
      3. May result in hypoxemia.
   C. Systemic fluid overload
      1. Is a problem primarily with neonates and infants.
      2. Is associated more frequently with the use of ultrasonic nebulizers than with the use of mechanical nebulizers.
   D. Cross-contamination
   E. When administering bronchodilators, one should be cautious of the side effects associated with bronchodilator therapy (see Chapter 40).
VIII. Mechanical Aerosol Generators
   A. These generators use jet mixing (see Chapter 2) to produce an aerosol and entrain a second gas.
   B. A system of baffles is utilized to impact large particles out of suspension.
   C. These generators are commonly used in delivery of medications and for humidification of inspired gases.
   D. Heating increases water content of delivered gas.
IX. Ultrasonic Aerosol Generators
   A. Ultrasonic nebulizers function by transforming standard household current into ultrasonic sound waves.
   B. The frequency range (1–2 megacycles/sec) for ultrasonic sound waves of ultrasonic nebulizers is governed by the Federal Commerce Commission. All ultrasonic nebulizers produced and sold in the United States have preset frequencies in this range.
   C. The ultrasonic sound waves are applied to a quartz crystal or ceramic disk, causing it to vibrate at the same frequency as the ultrasonic waves. This is referred to as the *piezoelectric quality of the disk.*
   D. The crystal or disk transfers its vibratory energy to the fluid to be nebulized, creating an aerosol.
   E. These nebulizers incorporate an amplitude control that varies the intensity of ultrasonic waves, allowing varying aerosol (medication) outputs.
   F. Ultrasonic nebulizers are used principally in maintenance of bronchial hygiene.
X. Babington (Hydrosphere) Nebulizer
   A. This nebulizer consists of:
      1. A small hollow glass sphere.
      2. Medication reservoir.
      3. Pneumatic gas source.
      4. Baffles.
      5. Syphoning system.
   B. As pressurized gas enters the unit:
      1. It activates the syphoning system, bringing medication to the area directly above the glass sphere.
      2. The medication then drips over the surface of the sphere, creating a thin film.
      3. The pressurized gas exits the glass sphere via one or two small openings located on the lateral aspect of the sphere.

    4. As the gas exits, it strikes the fluid film, creating an aerosol.

    5. A circular baffle is placed in front of each gas exit port.

    6. Large aerosol particles strike the baffle and return to the medication reservoir.

XI. Comparison of Nebulizer Output

    A. Mechanical nebulizers: Up to 1 to 1.5 ml/min

    B. Ultrasonic nebulizers: Up to 6 ml/min

    C. Babington nebulizers: Up to 6 ml/min

XII. Comparison of Nebulizer Particle Size

    A. Mechanical nebulizers: 55% of particles produced fall in the therapeutic range of 1 to 5 μ.

    B. Ultrasonic nebulizers: 97% of particles produced fall in the therapeutic range of 1 to 5 μ.

    C. Babington nebulizers: 90% of the particles produced fall in the therapeutic range of 1 to 5 μ.

XIII. Humidifiers

    A. A humidifier is designed to increase the water vapor content of a dry gas.

    B. Generally, two types of humidifiers are utilized.

        1. Bubble-through

        2. Pass-over

    C. In addition, humidifiers are either heated or unheated.

    D. Unheated bubble-through humidifiers are normally used with simple oxygen therapy appliances.

        1. These units are intended to bring dry gas to about 40% relative humidity at body temperature.

        2. The humidification capacity of these units depends on:

            a. Temperature of atmosphere.

            b. Gas flow.

            c. Size of the bubble formed.

            d. Volume of water in the humidifier.

    E. In patients with artificial airways who are mechanically ventilated, heated humidifiers are normally used.

        1. Both bubble-through and pass-over humidifiers are available.

        2. Systems are usually heated to achieve 34°C to 37°C at the patient's airway.

        3. As a result of the temperature drop as a gas moves from the humidifier to the patient, excess water vapor condensates in the tubing.

        4. The use of heated ventilator circuits with some humidifier systems has greatly reduced condensate in circuits.

XIV. Hygroscopic Condenser Humidifiers

    A. These devices sequester some or most of the water vapor exhaled by the patient.

    B. On the subsequent inspiration, the sequestered water is used to humidify the next inspiration.

    C. Some of these units are also bacteria filters. Those capable of filtering bacteria are referred to as *heat and moisture exchanging filters.*

    D. These units are capable of maintaining adequate humidification for short-term (up to 72 hours) and periodic use (16–20/hours/day) in chronic patients.

    E. Their use may be contraindicated.

        1. They should not be used if V_{T}s are small because of the volume of deadspace (V_{D}) in some units. Care should be exercised to prevent increasing V_{D}/V_{T} ratios, especially in pediatric patients.

        2. The presence of copious amounts of secretions increases the likelihood of secretions occluding the unit and increasing resistance to gas flow.

        3. A very large V_{T}, greater than 1.0 to 1.2 L, may exceed the capacity of certain units to provide adequate humidity.

4. In the presence of large air leaks where inspired Vт is greater than exhaled Vт, an insufficient volume of water is sequestered during exhalation, resulting in inadequate humidification of inspired gas (uncuffed tracheostomy tubes).

F. The resistance to gas flow may be excessive for some spontaneously breathing patients.

BIBLIOGRAPHY

Bendixen HH, et al: *Respiratory Care*. St Louis, CV Mosby Co, 1965.

Brain J: Aerosol and humidity therapy. *Am Rev Respir Dis* 1980; 122:17–21.

Brain J, Valberg PA: Deposition of aerosol in the respiratory tract. *Am Rev Respir Dis* 1979; 120:1325–1373.

Brown JH, Cook KM, Ney FG, et al: Influence of particle size upon the retention of particulate matter in the human lung. *Am J Public Health* 1950; 40:450–458.

Burton GG, Gee GN, Hodgkin JE: *Respiratory Care: A Guide to Clinical Practice*, ed 2. Philadelphia, JB Lippincott Co, 1984.

Demers R: Humidification systems, in Kacmarek RM, Stoller JK (eds): *Current Respiratory Care*. Toronto, BC Decker, 1988.

Deshpande VM, Pilbeam SP, Dixon RJ: *A Comprehensive Review in Respiratory Care*. Norwalk, Conn, Appleton & Lange, 1988.

Garrett D, Donaldson W: *Physical Principles of Respiratory Therapy Equipment*. Madison, Wis, Ohio Medical Products, 1978.

Glover DW, Glover MM: *Respiratory Therapy: Basics for Nursing and the Allied Health Professions*. St Louis, CV Mosby Co, 1978.

Jackson EE: The administration of respiratory therapy: Aerosol therapy, techniques and equipment. *J Am Assoc Nurse Anesth* 1976; 44:373–389.

Klein E, Shah D, Shah N, et al: Performance characteristics of conventional and prototype humidifiers and nebulizers. *Chest* 1973; 64:690–696.

Krumpe PE, McNair R: Successful substitution of aerosol nebulization therapy for IPPB at a veterans administration medical center. *Milit Med* 1981; 146:689–692.

Litt M, Swift D: The Babington nebulizer: A new principle for generation of therapeutic aerosols. *Am Rev Respir Dis* 1972; 105:308–310.

McPherson SP: *Respiratory Therapy Equipment*, ed 3. St Louis, CV Mosby Co, 1989.

Miller W: Fundamental principles of aerosol therapy. *Respir Care* 1972; 17:295–302.

Morrow PE: Aerosol characterization and deposition. *Am Rev Respir Dis* 1974; 110:88–99.

Nelson EJ, Morton EA, Hunter PM: *Critical Care Respiratory Therapy: A Laboratory and Clinical Manual*. Boston, Little Brown & Co, 1983.

Newhouse MT: Principles of aerosol therapy. *Chest* 1982; 82 (suppl):39S–41S.

Op't Holt T: Aerosol generators and humidifiers, in Barnes TA (ed): *Respiratory Care Practice*. Year Book Medical Publishers, Chicago, 1988.

Rarey KP, Youtsey JW: *Respiratory Patient Care*. Englewood Cliffs, NJ, Prentice-Hall, 1981.

Safer P (ed): *Respiratory Therapy*. Philadelphia, FA Davis Co, 1965.

Shapiro BA, Harrison RA, Kacmarek RM, et al: *Clinical Application of Respiratory Care*, ed 3. Chicago, Year Book Medical Publishers, 1985.

Simonsson BG: Anatomical and pathophysiological considerations in aerosol therapy. *Eur J Respir Dis Suppl* 1982; 63:7–14.

Spearman CB, Sheldon RL, Egan DF: *Egan's Fundamentals of Respiratory Therapy*, ed 4. St Louis, CV Mosby Co 1982.

Stiksa GF: Indications for continuous aerosol therapy. *Eur J Respir Dis Suppl* 1982; 63:89–96.

Swift DL: Aerosols and humidity therapy: Generation and respiratory deposition of therapeutic aerosols. *Am Rev Respir Dis* 1980; 122:71–77.

Tabachnik E, Levison H: Clinical application of aerosols in pediatrics. *Am Rev Respir Dis* 1980; 122:97–103.

Young JA, Crocker D: *Principles and Practice of Respiratory Therapy*, ed 2. Chicago, Year Book Medical Publishers, 1976.

Chapter 31

Chest Physiotherapy

I. Definition
- Chest physiotherapy is a general term used in reference to a number of techniques designed to assist with bronchial hygiene or the mobilization of secretions and prevention or reversal of atelectasis. Specifically, the following modalities are included under this general heading:
  - A. Postural drainage (positioning)
  - B. Percussion
  - C. Vibration
  - D. Shaking
  - E. Cough assistance
  - F. Breathing instruction and retraining

II. Postural Drainage
  - A. Postural drainage is a method of removing pooled secretions by positioning the patient so as to allow gravity to assist in movement of secretions. Ideally, the patient is placed with the dependent lung segment uppermost and as vertical as possible.
  - B. Indications
    1. Acute or chronic pulmonary diseases in which secretions are poorly mobilized, resulting in excessive retention and accumulation of secretions.
    2. Atelectasis as a postoperative complication or as a result of poor distribution of ventilation.
    3. Prophylactic care of patients in the immediate postoperative period with a history of acute or chronic pulmonary problems and who have undergone an abdominal or thoracic surgical procedure.
  - C. Standard postural drainage positions for each of the lung segments
    1. *Apical segments of right and left upper lobes:* Patient in semi-Fowler's position with head of the bed raised 45 degrees (Fig 31–1).
    2. *Anterior segments of both upper lobes:* Patient supine with the bed flat (Fig 31–2).
    3. *Posterior segments of right upper lobe:* Patient one-quarter turn from prone with the right side up, supported by pillows, with head of the bed flat (Fig 31–3).
    4. *Apical-posterior segment of left upper lobe:* Patient one-quarter turn from prone with the left side up, supported by pillows, with head of the bed elevated 30 degrees (Fig 31–4).
    5. *Medial and lateral segments of right middle lobe:* Patient one-quarter turn from supine with right side up and foot of the bed elevated 12 in. (Fig 31–5).

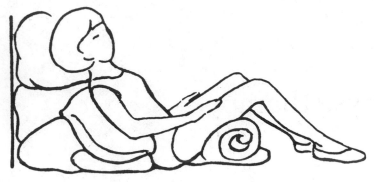

FIG 31–1.
Position for drainage of apical segments of upper lobes.

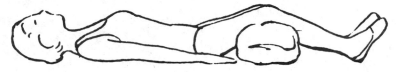

FIG 31–2.
Position for drainage of anterior segments of upper lobes.

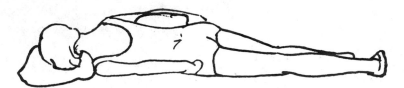

FIG 31–3.
Position for drainage of posterior segment of right upper lobe.

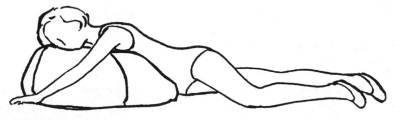

FIG 31–4.
Position for drainage of apical-posterior segment of left upper lobe.

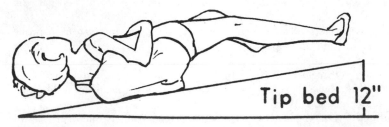

Tip bed 12"

FIG 31–5.
Position for drainage of medial and lateral segments of right middle lobe.

6. *Superior and inferior segments of lingula:* Patient one-quarter turn from supine with left side up and foot of the bed elevated 12 in. (Fig 31–6).
7. *Superior segments of both lower lobes:* Patient prone with head of the bed flat and pillow under abdominal area (Fig 31–7).
8. *Anteromedial segment of left lower lobe and anterior segment of right lower lobe:* Patient supine, with foot of the bed elevated 20 in. (Fig 31–8).
9. *Lateral segment of right lower lobe:* Patient directly on left side with right side up and foot of the bed elevated 20 in. (Fig 31–9).
10. *Lateral segment of left lower lobe and medial (cardiac) segment of right lower lobe:* Patient directly on right side, with left side up and foot of the bed elevated 20 in. (Fig 31–10).
11. *Posterior segment of both lower lobes:* Patient prone with foot of the bed elevated 20 in. (Fig 31–11).

D. Precautions should be taken when patients with the following conditions are positioned:
1. Empyema
2. Pulmonary embolus
3. Open wounds, skin grafts, burns
4. Untreated tension pneumothorax
5. Flail chest
6. Frank hemoptysis
7. Orthopedic procedures
8. Acute spinal cord injuries

E. Head-down positioning may be contraindicated in patients with the following conditions:
1. Unstable cardiac status
2. Hypertension
3. Head injuries
4. Thoracic surgery
5. Abdominal surgery
6. Diaphragmatic surgery
7. Tracheoesophageal surgery
8. Chronic obstructive pulmonary disease
9. Obesity
10. Recent meals or tube feeding

Note: If positioning the patient in the head-down position is necessary, care must be taken to carefully monitor the patient's cardiopulmonary status throughout the procedure.

III. Percussion
A. Percussion is a technique of rhythmically tapping the chest wall with cupped hands. It is designed to loosen secretions in the area underlying the percussion by the air pressure that is generated by the cupped hand on the chest wall. Percussion is performed during inspiration and expiration.
B. Indications (same as those for postural drainage, section II–B).
C. Percussion may be contraindicated in patients with the following conditions:
1. Cancer with known metastatic changes
2. Anticoagulant therapy
3. Tuberculosis
4. Petechiae
5. Osteoporotic changes
6. Empyema
7. Pulmonary embolus
8. Wounds, skin grafts, burns
9. Untreated tension pneumothorax

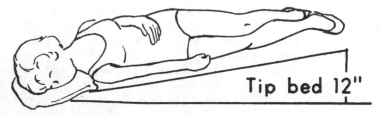

FIG 31–6.
Position for drainage of superior and inferior segments of lingula.

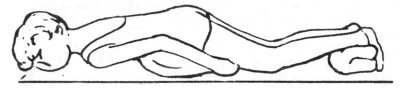

FIG 31–7.
Position for drainage of superior segments of both lower lobes.

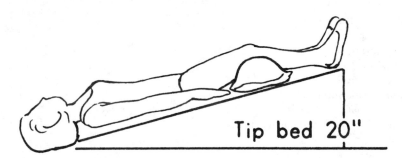

FIG 31–8.
Position for drainage of anteromedial segment of left lower lobe and anterior segment of right lower lobe.

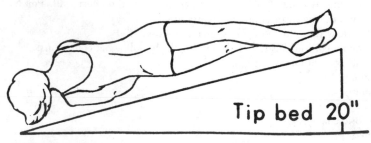

FIG 31–9.
Position for drainage of lateral segment of right lower lobe.

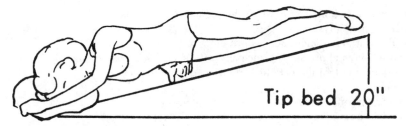

FIG 31–10.
Position for drainage of lateral segment of left lower lobe and medial segment of right lower lobe.

    10. Flail chest
    11. Frank hemoptysis
    12. Acute spinal cord injuries
    13. Limited patient tolerance
    14. Chest tubes
    15. Unstable cardiac status
    16. Thoracic surgery
    Note: If percussion is performed, care must be taken to carefully monitor the patient's cardiopulmonary status throughout the procedure.

IV. Vibrations
    A. Vibrations are performed by placing one hand on top of the other over the affected area and tensing the shoulders, keeping the arms straight and applying a vibrating action from shoulder to hand.
    B. Vibrations are intended to move secretions into larger airways.
    C. Vibrations are applied only during exhalation.
    D. Indications (same as those for postural drainage, section II–B).
    E. Possible contraindications are similar to those for percussion (see section III–C).

V. Shaking
    A. Shaking is a more vigorous form of vibration.
    B. The basic premise is that shaking dislodges resistant or thick secretions not moved by vibration.
    C. The combination of shaking and vibration may improve thoracic mobility.
    D. Possible contraindications are similar to those for percussion (see Section III–C)
    E. Indications
        1. Very thick retained secretions
        2. Emphysema with rib cage stiffness.

VI. General Hazards and Complications of Postural Drainage, Percussion, Vibration and Shaking
    A. Hypoxemia, particularly if the patient is positioned with affected areas dependent.

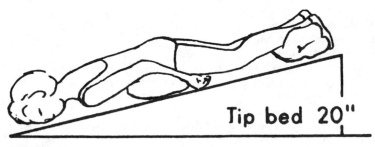

FIG 31–11.
Position for drainage of posterior segments of both lower lobes.

      B. Cardiovascular instability, primarily if the patient is positioned head down.

      C. Hemorrhage, hemoptysis.

      D. Fractured ribs if metastatic cancer is present.

      E. Increased intracranial pressure, principally with head-down positioning.

      F. Dyspnea, particularly if the patient is positioned head down.

VII. Cough Assistance

    A. Sequence of a normal cough

      1. A deep inspiration

      2. Closure of glottis

      3. Contraction of abdominal muscles, building up intrapulmonary pressure

      4. Opening of glottis and a rapid forceful exhalation

    B. Cough assistance is indicated in the patient who cannot develop a forceful cough.

    C. Cough assistance can be performed by:

      1. Applying pressure to the upper abdominal area during the compression and expiratory phase of the cough.

      2. In patients with an artificial airway, hyperinflating the lung with a manual ventilator, holding gas volume in the lung at end of inspiration, then rapidly releasing pressure, allowing exhalation, while an associate applies vigorous chest wall compression in an inward and downward fashion. Care should be taken to follow the normal anatomic movement of the chest.

    D. "Huffing" (in patients with ineffective cough): The patient is instructed to rapidly expel air through an open glottis. This technique is less painful and less stressful than coughing.

    E. "Panting": The patient is instructed to follow normal cough sequence, but the tongue is kept forward to prevent swallowing of secretions.

VIII. Breathing Instruction and Retaining

    A. These techniques are designed to assist patients with muscular weakness, postoperative pain, or chronic pulmonary disease to assume an efficient ventilatory pattern and effective cough.

    B. Goals

      1. To increase and improve ventilation.

      2. To strengthen respiratory musculature.

      3. To prevent development of atelectasis.

      4. To decrease work of breathing.

      5. To improve the effectiveness of cough.

    C. Specific techniques

      1. Diaphragmatic breathing exercises

        a. The therapist and patient locate the xiphoid process. The patient is instructed to "sniff" to determine the location of the diaphragm.

        b. The patient is relaxed, supported with a pillow, and directed to inspire by contracting the diaphragm slowly and completely to allow a normal inspiratory pattern.

          (1) Abdominal expansion

          (2) Lateral chest expansion

          (3) Upper chest expansion

        c. The patient is encouraged to exhale slowly, passively, and completely. The therapist may assist exhalation by exerting a slight inward and upward pressure below the xiphoid process.

      2. Lateral costal expansion exercises

        a. The therapist places his or her hands over the patient's lower rib cage with the thumbs just above the xiphoid process.

        b. The patient is encouraged to relax and inspire against a slight pressure exerted by the therapist's hands. The patient is instructed to try to expand area located under the therapist's hands.

TABLE 31–1.

General Guidelines for the Treatment of Specific Pathophysiologic Problems*

Pathophysiology	Goals	Techniques
Atelectasis	Reverse collapse	Postural drainage
		Percussion
		Vibration
Pneumonia	Remove excess secretions	Postural drainage
	Prevent or reverse collapse	Cough assistance
Adult respiratory distress syndrome	Maximize oxygenation	Postural drainage
	Mobilize secretions	Vibration
Emphysema	Decrease work of breathing	Breathing instructions
	Improve chest wall mobility	Shaking
		Cough assistance
Chronic bronchitis	Mobilize secretions	Postural drainage
		Percussion
		Vibration
		Breathing instructions
Asthma	Decrease work of breathing	Modified postural drainage
	Mobilize secretions	Vibration
		Cough assistance
Abscess	Mobilize secretions	Postural drainage
		Percussion
		Vibration
Spinal cord injury	Maximize ventilation	Breathing instructions
	Mobilize secretions	Cough assistance
		Postural drainage
		Vibration

*Significant variation may be necessary in specific patients.

    c. Exhalation should be passive but complete. The therapist can assist exhalation by applying an inward and downward pressure during exhalation.

  3. Localized expansion exercises designed to direct the gas flow to a specific area of the lung

    a. The therapist places his or her hands over the problem area and instructs the patient to inspire against a slight pressure exerted by the therapist.

    b. Exhalation should be passive, complete, and assisted by the therapist. The therapist exerts an inward and downward force during exhalation, following the natural movement of the rib cage.

BIBLIOGRAPHY

Bartlett RH, Gazzaniza AB, Gerahty TR: Respiratory maneuvers to prevent postoperative pulmonary complications. *JAMA* 1973; 22:1017–1019.

Bendixen HH, et al: *Respiratory Care.* St Louis, CV Mosby Co, 1965.

Breslin EH: Prevention and treatment of pulmonary complications in patients after surgery of the upper abdomen. *Heart Lung* 1981; 10:511–519.

Campbell AH, O'Connell JM, Wilson F: the effects of chest physiotherapy upon the FEV, in chronic bronchitis. *Med J Aust* 1975; 1:33–35.

Cherniak RM: Physical therapy. *Am Rev Respir Dis* 1980; 122:25–27.

Connors AF Jr, Hammon WE, Martin RJ, et al: Chest physical therapy: The immediate effect on oxygenation in acutely ill patients. *Chest* 1980; 78:559–564.

Dhainaut J-F, Bons J, Bricard C, et al: Improved oxygenation in patients with extensive unilateral pneumonia using the lateral decubitus position. *Thorax* 1980; 35:792–793.

Frownfelter DL: *Chest Physiotherapy and Pulmonary Rehabilitation*, ed 2. Chicago, Year Book Medical Publishers, 1987.

Gaskell DV, Webber BA: *The Brompton Hospital Guide to Chest Physiotherapy*. Philadelphia, JB Lippincott Co, 1974.

Harris JA, Jerry BA: Indications and procedures for segmental bronchial drainage. *Respir Care* 1975; 20:1164–1168.

Ingwersen U: *Respiratory Physical Therapy and Pulmonary Care*. New York, John Wiley & Sons, 1976.

Kigin CM: Chest physical therapy, in Kacmarek RM, Stoller JK [eds]: *Current Respiratory Care*. Toronto, BC Decker, 1988.

Lewis FR: Management of atelectasis and pneumonia. *Surg Clin North Am* 1980; 60:1391–1401.

Oulton JL, Hobbs GM, Hicken P: Incentive breathing devices and chest physiotherapy: A controlled study. *Can J Surg* 1981; 24:638–640.

MacKenzie DF, Ciesla W, Imle PC, et al (eds): *Chest Physiotherapy in the Intensive Care Unit*. Baltimore, Williams & Wilkins Co, 1981.

MacKenzie CF, Shin B, McAslan TC: Chest physiotherapy: The effect on arterial oxygenation. *Anesth Analg* 1978; 57:28–30.

Peters RM, Turnier E: Physical therapy indications for and effects in surgical patients. *Am Rev Respir Dis* 1980; 122:147–154.

Pierce AK, Robertson J: Pulmonary complications of general surgery. *Am Rev Med* 1977; 28:211–221.

Rarey KP, Youtsey JW: *Respiratory Patient Care*. Englewood Cliffs, NJ, Prentice-Hall, 1981.

Rigg JRA: Pulmonary atelectasis after anesthesia: Pathophysiology and management. *Can Anesth Soc J* 1981; 28:305–313.

Safar P (ed): *Respiratory Therapy*. Philadelphia, FA Davis Co, 1965.

Schmidt GB: Prophylaxis of pulmonary complications following abdominal surgery including atelectasis, ARDS, and pulmonary embolism. *Surg Annu* 1977; 9:29–73.

Schuppisser JP: Postoperative intermittent positive pressure breathing versus physiotherapy. *Am J Surg* 1980; 104:682–686.

Shapiro BA, Harrison RA, Kacmarek RM, et al: *Clinical Application of Respiratory Care*, ed 3. Chicago, Year Book Medical Publishers, 1985.

Shearer M, Joyce M, Banks BS: Lung ventilation during diaphragmatic breathing. *Am Phys Ther Assoc* 1972; 52:139–146.

Thacker EW: *Postural Drainage and Respiratory Control*. Chicago, Year Book Medical Publishers, 1973.

Tyler ML: Complications of positioning and chest physiotherapy. *Respir Care* 1982; 27:458–466.

Vraciu JK, Vraciu RA: Effectiveness of breathing exercises in preventing pulmonary complications following open heart surgery. *Phys Ther* 1977; 57:1367–1371.

Young JA, Crocker D: *Principles and Practices of Respiratory Therapy*, ed 2. Chicago, Year Book Medical Publishers, 1976.

Zack MB, Pontoppidantt Kazemi H: The effect of lateral positions on gas exchange in pulmonary disease: A prospective evaluation. *Am Rev Respir Dis* 1974; 110:49–55.

Chapter 32

Mechanical Aids to Intermittent Lung Expansion

I. Physiologic Basis of Mechanical Aids for Intermittent Lung Inflation in the Treatment or Prevention of Atelectasis
   A. Transpulmonary pressure (alveolar distending pressure) is equal to intra-alveolar pressure minus intrapleural pressure (see Chapter 4).
   B. Increases in lung volumes are accomplished only by increases in transpulmonary pressures.
      1. If intra-alveolar pressure increases more than pleural pressure, transpulmonary pressure increases, as does lung volume. (This occurs during intermittent positive pressure breathing [IPPB] and continuous positive pressure therapy).
      2. If intrapleural pressure decreases more than intra-alveolar pressure, transpulmonary pressure increases, as does lung volume. (This occurs during incentive spirometry and spontaneous breathing.)
      3. If intrapleural pressure increases more than intra-alveolar pressure, transpulmonary pressure decreases, as does lung volume. This occurs with blow bottles.
   C. For any lung expansion technique to be successful in overcoming or preventing atelectasis, it must increase transpulmonary pressures, thus increasing lung volume.
   D. This effect is most pronounced if the maneuver sustains inspiratory volume (slow deep breath with inflation hold).
II. Intermittent Positive Pressure Breathing (IPPB)
   A. The delivery of a slow, deep, sustained inspiration by a mechanical device providing a controlled positive pressure breath during inspiration.
   B. Physiologic effects on the respiratory system
      1. Positive pressure breathing reverses the normal intrathoracic and intrapulmonary pressure relationship. With IPPB, the mean intrathoracic pressure is most positive during inspiration and least positive during expiration. Figures 4–3 and 4–4 depict normal intrathoracic and intrapulmonary pressure curves. These pressure curves are considerably altered during IPPB and may cause decreases in venous return and cardiac output (Fig 32–1).
      2. Lung expansion is accomplished by increasing transpulmonary pressure gradients.

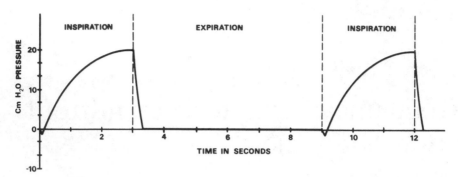

FIG 32–1.
Ideal intrapulmonary pressure curve associated with administration of IPPB.

3. Work of breathing with properly applied IPPB treatment may be significantly decreased. Since IPPB provides the ventilatory power, the work of the patient's ventilatory muscles is reduced.
   a. This allows the same degree of alveolar ventilation with far less expenditure of muscular energy.
   b. Decreased work of breathing occurs only during therapy, unless significant areas of atelectasis are reversed or a significant volume of secretions is mobilized.
   c. To ensure that work of breathing is decreased with IPPB, the ventilatory pattern established with the IPPB must match the patient's inspiratory demands and satisfy his or her ventilatory drive.
   d. One of the major reasons for failures in properly applying IPPB is patient-machine asynchrony.
4. Inspiratory: expiratory (I:E) ratios may be manipulated during properly applied IPPB treatment. This is accomplished by restoring a more efficient ventilatory pattern. Under most circumstances, this pattern is maintained only during therapy.
5. The tidal volume (V_T) may be increased by three to four times the patient's resting spontaneous tidal exchange during IPPB therapy.
6. Secretions are more effectively mobilized during IPPB treatment. This is accomplished by increasing lung volume and improving distribution of inspired gas.
7. The Po_2 normally is increased and the Pco_2 normally is decreased *during* IPPB treatment. Improved alveolar ventilation during therapy may result in better gas exchange during therapy.
C. Indications
   1. In general, IPPB is indicated only in patients who cannot voluntarily cough effectively and breathe deeply. Specifically, IPPB *may be* indicated if a patient's vital capacity is *less than* 15 ml/kg of ideal body weight.
      a. Therapeutic
         (1) Atelectasis unresponsive to simple therapy (e.g., incentive spirometry, chest physiotherapy)
         (2) Retained secretions
         (3) Temporary relief of hypoventilation
      b. Prophylactic: Following thoracic or abdominal surgery in patients with chronic or acute pulmonary disease
D. Goals
   1. To provide a significantly deeper breath with more physiologic I:E ratios than patient can produce with spontaneous ventilation

2. To improve and promote cough mechanism
    a. Optimal peripheral distribution of air through a slow, deep, sustained inspiration with an end-inspiratory pause.
    b. Mechanical provision of necessary power.
3. To improve distribution of ventilation
    a. Ventilation distribution is improved in patients with ventilation/perfusion inequalities.
    b. The incidence of postoperative atelectasis and pneumonia is potentially decreased, and already atelectatic alveoli may be reexpanded.
4. To deliver medication
    a. It should be used only if no means other than IPPB (e.g., hand-held nebulizer) can safely and conveniently deliver the medication. The mechanical advantages of IPPB have been overshadowed by its use to deliver medication.
E. Administration
    1. The efficacy of IPPB treatments is greatly dependent on the therapist.
    2. Prerequisites for ideal administration of effective IPPB treatments are:
        a. Knowledgeable, well-trained therapist completely familiar with operation, maintenance, and clinical application of equipment.
        b. Relaxed, informed, cooperative patient.
        c. Concise concept of therapeutic goals by physician, therapist, and patient.
        d. Pressure-limited machine.
        e. Appropriate cough and breathing instruction.
        f. Honest appraisal by therapist of benefits from therapy for particular patient.
F. Hazards
    1. Hyperventilation
        a. Incorrect administration of IPPB often causes rapid, deep ventilation leading to acute alveolar hyperventilation with the following possible results:
            (1) Dizziness
            (2) Loss of consciousness
            (3) Tetany
            (4) Paresthesia
        b. Decreased cerebrovascular P_{CO_2} during hyperventilation causes vasoconstriction and decreased cerebral blood flow.
    2. Excessive oxygenation
        a. When driven with oxygen, pneumatically powered, pressure-limited machines give excessively high oxygen concentrations. These high concentrations are potentially harmful to chronic obstructive pulmonary disease (COPD) patients who are breathing on a "hypoxic drive."
        b. The high oxygen concentration can be avoided by using machines powered by air compressors or by using a compressed air source.
    3. Increased air trapping (auto-PEEP)
        a. Excessive ventilation of partially obstructed areas in patients with severe COPD.
        b. Insufficient time available to allow complete exhalation of the increased V_T.
        c. Potential decrease in venous return and cardiac output.
        d. Posttreatment increase in difficulty of ventilation due to increased functional residual capacity.
    4. Decreased cardiac output
        a. Spontaneous ventilation normally facilitates venous return. Increasingly negative intrathoracic pressure on inspiration widens the pressure gradient between abdominal viscera and thoracic cavity. This enhances venous return via inferior vena cava and is called the *thoracoabdominal pump*.

    b. Intermittent positive pressure breathing ablates the thoracoabdominal pump by causing a less negative or possibly positive mean intrathoracic pressure during inspiration.

    c. Proper I:E ratios in conjunction with minimal airway pressure helps to minimize this.

    d. Clinical signs of decreased cardiac output

      (1) Systemic hypotension

      (2) Tachycardia

      (3) Dyspnea

      (4) Distended neck veins

      (5) Anxiety

  5. Increased intracranial pressure

    a. Cranial venous drainage is potentially impeded by increased mean intrathoracic pressure.

    b. This results in an increase in intracranial pressure, since more blood is contained in the cranium and the volume of the cranium is fixed.

  6. Pneumothorax

    a. Intermittent positive pressure breathing mouth pressures of 20 cm H_2O seldom result in excessive alveolar pressures. These pressures by themselves normally are not high enough to cause a "bleb" to rupture.

    b. Intermittent positive pressure breathing may result in better distribution of ventilation and gas entering poorly ventilated lung areas (e.g., a bleb) during IPPB treatment. The overdistention of diseased lung areas with the application of high transpulmonary pressure may result in a pneumothorax.

    c. Possible complaints of chest pain with or after coughing should be anticipated.

    d. If pneumothorax occurs, IPPB should be discontinued until chest decompression is accomplished.

  7. Hemoptysis

    a. May occur due to an increase in cough effectiveness that follows IPPB.

    b. Is usually the result of bronchial venous bleeding; may be secondary to a tumor or to blood vessel rupture.

  8. Gastric distention

    a. The pressure used in IPPB may result in the movement of air into the stomach.

    b. Some patients actually swallow air during IPPB treatments.

    c. The potential for distention increases when IPPB is administered to a semi-alert or comatose patient via mask.

  9. Increased airway resistance

    a. Intermittent positive pressure breathing may increase bronchospasm in patients with chronic asthma.

  10. Psychologic dependence

    a. Patients with COPD receiving IPPB may develop psychologic dependence because of the subjective benefit they receive from IPPB.

  G. Absolute contraindication

    1. Untreated tension pneumothorax

      a. Tension is increased with positive pressure due to the one-way check-valve mechanism.

      b. Intermittent positive pressure breathing treatment should not be initiated until chest decompression is performed.

III. Mask Continuous Positive Airway Pressure (CPAP) Therapy

  A. Continuous positive airway pressure therapy is the application of a constant supra-atmospheric pressure to the airway.

B. Technically it is accomplished with a continuous flow of gas or a demand valve.

C. When it is applied, resting lung volume is increased by increasing the transpulmonary pressure.

D. It is usually used on a continuous basis for the treatment of hypoxemia.

E. It is frequently employed in the management of postoperative atelectasis in the thoracic surgical patient.

F. It is used to recruit collapsed lung areas.

G. It is applied via a standard face mask for 20 to 30 min, as often as necessary, to maintain expansion.

H. See Chapter 3 for details on the effects of positive end-expiratory pressure and CPAP.

IV. Incentive Spirometry

A. This is a technique using visual feedback to encourage patients to take slow, deep, sustained inspirations.

B. The apparatus acts purely as a visual motivator encouraging patient effort and compliance.

C. Expansion to a specific lung volume is not guaranteed with the use of an incentive spirometer.

D. Indications

1. Treatment of atelectasis

a. For the treatment to be effective, the patient must be capable of taking a deep breath.

b. In general, a vital capacity of greater than 15 ml/kg of ideal body weight is necessary for effective use.

2. Prevention of atelectasis: It is specifically indicated if:

a. The patient has just undergone thoracic or upper abdominal surgery, and

b. There is a history of chronic or acute pulmonary disease.

E. For maximum effectiveness the technique should be performed hourly for approximately 10 breaths.

F. The ideal breathing pattern is slow, deep, sustained inspiration.

G. Types of incentive spirometers

1. Flow-oriented

a. The patient's inspiratory flow rate causes a float or ball to rise in a cannister. The float or ball remains suspended for a sustained period of time.

b. The patient should maintain an inspiratory flow that slowly elevates the float.

c. A rapid inspiration will cause the float to rise quickly but will not maintain it in a suspended position.

d. Slow inspirations do not generate sufficient flow to raise the float.

2. Volume-oriented

a. The patient inspires until a preset volume of gas is inhaled.

b. Indicators are used to motivate patients and indicate when desired volume is achieved.

c. Most systems are designed to require a sustained inspiration before the achieved volume indicator is activated.

H. Possible complications (nondocumented)

1. Hyperventilation

2. Barotrauma

V. Rebreathing Devices

A. A rebreathing device is any tube or cannister designed to increase the depth of breathing by accumulating a patient's exhaled CO_2 and forcing rebreathing.

B. Normally an increase in respiratory rate is noted with very little increase in VT.

C. These devices do nothing to control inspiratory flow rates and do not provide for development of an inspiratory pause.

D. They are not effective in reversing alveolar collapse.

E. They are rarely used either prophylactically or therapeutically for the treatment of postoperative pulmonary complications.

F. No specific indication exists for the use of these devices in modern respiratory care.

G. Hypoxemia due to small patient VT in relation to the deadspace volume of the device is a common complication that can be prevented by bleeding oxygen into the system.

VI. Blow Bottles

A. Blow bottles are defined as devices in which fluid is moved from one container to another by means of pressure created by the patient during exhalation.

B. These devices provide a threshold load to exhalation.

C. Proper use requires a deep inspiration prior to any exhalation.

1. The deep inspiration is necessary to increase static distending pressures.

2. If static distending pressures are not increased, no benefit is derived from the use of the device.

3. The emphasis on exhalation diminishes the likelihood of consistent deep inspirations.

D. Indications

1. Prevention of postoperative atelectasis

2. Treatment of postoperative atelectasis

E. Complications

1. Atelectasis if exhalation is started at normal VT and continued to residual volume

2. Hyperventilation

BIBLIOGRAPHY

Bartlett RH: Respiratory therapy to prevent pulmonary complications of surgery. *Respir Care* 1984; 29:667–679.

Burton GG, Gee GN, Hodgkin JE: *Respiratory Care: A Guide to Clinical Practice* ed 2. Philadelphia, JB Lippincott Co, 1984.

Douce FH: Incentive spirometry and aids to lung inflation, in Barnes TA (ed): *Respiratory Care Practice*. Chicago, Year Book Medical Publishers, 1988.

Gale GD, Sanders DE: The Barlett-Edwards incentive spirometer. *Can Anesth Soc J* 1977; 27:408–416.

Gale GD, Sanders DE: Incentive spirometry: Its value after cardiac surgery. *Can Anaesth Soc J* 1980; 27:475–480.

Hudson LD: Is IPPB Effective? A controversy in respiratory therapy. *Primary Care* 1978; 5:529–542.

Ingram RH: Mechanical aids to lung expansion. *Am Rev Respir Dis* 1980; 123:23–24.

Iverson LIG, Ecker RR, Fox HE, et al: A comparative study of IPPB, the incentive spirometer, and blow bottles: The prevention of atelectasis following cardiac surgery. *Ann Thorac Surg* 1978; 25:197–200.

Jung R, Wight J, Nusser R, et al: Comparison of three methods of respiratory care following upper abdominal surgery. *Chest* 1980; 78:31–35.

Krastins ERB, Corey ML, McLeod A, et al: An evaluation of incentive spirometry in the management of pulmonary complications after cardiac surgery in a pediatric population. *Crit Care Med* 1982; 10:525–528.

Lewis FR: Management of atelectasis and pneumonia. *Surg Clin North Am* 1980; 60:1391–1401.

Martin RJ, Rogers RM, Gray GA: Mechanical aids to lung expansion: The physiologic basis for the use of mechanical aids to lung expansion. *Am Rev Respir Dis* 1980; 122:105–107.

Miller WF: Intermittent positive pressure breathing (IPPB), in Kacmarek RM, Stoller S (eds): *Current Respiratory Care*. Toronto, BC Decker, 1988.

Murray JF: Indications for mechanical aids to assist lung inflation in medical patients. *Am Rev Respir Dis* 1980; 122:121–125.

O'Donohue WJ: Maximum volume IPPB for the management of pulmonary atelectasis. *Chest* 1976; 76:683–687.

Oulton JL, Hobbs GM, Hicken P: Incentive breathing devices and chest physiotherapy: A controlled trial. *Can J Surg* 1981; 24:638–640.

Paul WL, Downs JB: Postoperative atelectasis: Intermittent positive pressure breathing, incentive spirometry and face-mask positive end-expiratory pressure. *Arch Surg* 1981; 116:861–863.

Pierce AK, Robertson J: Pulmonary complications of general surgery. *Annu Rev Med* 1977; 28:211–221.

Pontoppidan H, Mechanical aids to lung expansion in non-intubated surgical patients. *Am Rev Respir Dis* 1980; 122:109–119.

Schuppisser JP, Brandli O, Meili U: Postoperative intermittent positive pressure breathing versus physiotherapy. *Am J Surg* 1980; 104:682–686.

Shapiro BA, Harrison RA, Kacmarek RM, et al: *Clinical Application of Respiratory Care,* ed 3. Chicago, Year Book Medical Publishers, 1985.

Shapiro BA, Peterson J, Cane RD: Complications of mechanical aids to intermittent lung inflation. *Respir Care* 1982; 27:467–470.

Smith RA: Masked and nasal continuous positive pressure breathing, in Kacmarek RM, Stoller J (eds): *Current Respiratory Care.* Toronto, BC Decker, 1988.

Spearman CB, Sheldon RL, Egan DF: *Egan's Fundamentals of Respiratory Therapy,* ed 4. St Louis, CV Mosby Co, 1982.

Torres G, Lyons HA, Emerson P: The effects of intermittent positive pressure breathing on the intrapulmonary distribution of inspired air. *Am J Med* 1960; 29:946–954.

Welch MA, Shapiro BJ, Mercuiro P, et al: Methods of intermittent positive pressure breathing. *Chest* 1980; 78:463–467.

Wiezalis CP: Intermittent positive-pressure breathing, in Barnes TA (ed): *Respiratory Care Practice.* Chicago, Year Book Medical Publishers, 1988.

Wojciechowski WV: Incentive spirometers and secretion evacuation devices, in Barnes TA (ed): *Respiratory Care Practice.* Chicago, Year Book Medical Publishers, 1988.

Chapter 33

Analyzers

I. Oxygen Analyzers
  A. Analyzers that use Pauling's principle of paramagnetic susceptibility of oxygen (Beck-man D–2)
    1. The principle of operation is based on the ability of oxygen to be attracted by a magnetic field and cause displacement of nitrogen from the field.
    2. A *dry* gas is drawn into a chamber containing a magnetic field.
      a. The gas is dried by passing through anhydrous (blue) silica gel crystals.
      b. The gas must be dried because water vapor causes interference in the magnetic field and exerts a partial pressure.
    3. Since oxygen is paramagnetic, it is drawn to the strongest portion of the magnetic field. In doing so, oxygen displaces nitrogen, which is diamagnetic, from the field. Displacement occurs by rotation of the nitrogen-filled dumbbell that is suspended by a quartz fiber within the magnetic field.
    4. Attached to the dumbbell is a mirror, which reflects a beam of light that indicates the degree of rotation of the dumbbell.
    5. Degree of rotation is directly related to partial pressure of oxygen in the system and is indicated on a scale in millimeters of mercury of Po_2 and the percentage of oxygen.
    6. Since the analyzer measures partial pressure of oxygen, the millimeters of mercury scale is accurate at all altitudes.
    7. The percent oxygen scale is accurate only at sea level unless it is recalibrated with changes in altitude.
    8. The analyzer accurately measures oxygen partial pressure in all respiratory gas mixtures.
  B. Analyzers that use the thermal conductivity of oxygen
    1. The principle of operation is based on the ability of oxygen to cool an electric wire more so than air.
    2. The cooler the electric wire, the less resistant the wire is to flow of electrons and the greater the current passing through the wire.
    3. The analyzer uses an electric circuit referred to as the *Wheatstone bridge.*
    4. The Wheatstone bridge has two reference chambers on one side that contain room air. A constant cooling (thermoconductive) effective by the room air maintains current at a specific constant level.

5. On the other side of the bridge is one measuring chamber and a second chamber, which is a calibrating potentiometer.
6. The two sides of the bridge are connected in the middle by a voltmeter (galvanometer), which measures the electrical potentials of each side of the circuit.
7. The potential difference is converted to the percent oxygen of the sample gas.
8. This analyzer actually measures oxygen concentration.
   a. Cooling ability of the sample gas is always compared to the constant thermoconductive effect of room air with about 21% oxygen and 79% nitrogen.
   b. Thus, no matter what the altitude, there is always a comparison to a fixed oxygen/nitrogen concentration.
9. Only oxygen nitrogen gas mixtures can be analyzed because the cooling effect of sampled gas is always compared to a reference oxygen nitrogen mixture.
10. In most units, gas entering the sample chamber must contain water vapor (some units require a dry sample).
    a. Water vapor is added by using hydrated (pink) silica gel crystals.
    b. The gas is saturated to prevent buildup of a static charge in the system.
11. These analyzers cannot be used with a flammable gas mixture because of the electric circuitry.

C. Analyzers operating on the polarographic principle (Clark electrode) (Figs 33–1 and 33 2)
   1. The basic overall chemical reaction occurring in electrode system is:

$$O_2 + 2H_2O + 4 \text{ electrons} \rightarrow 4OH^- \tag{1}$$

   2. The analyzer is composed of two electrodes immersed in a potassium chloride electrolyte solution.
      a. At the silver anode, oxidation of chloride ion to silver chloride takes place. This reaction releases electrons, developing a current.
      b. At the platinum cathode, oxygen is reduced to form OH^- ions, thus consuming electrons produced from the anode.

P_{O_2} ELECTRODE:

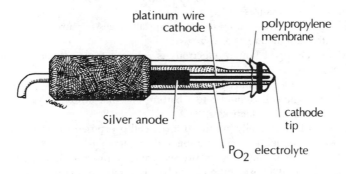

FIG 33–1.
The Clark electrode. See Figure 33–2 for specifics. (From Shapiro BA, Harrison RA, Walton JR: *Clinical Application of Arterial Blood Gases,* ed 3. Chicago, Year Book Medical Publishers, 1982. Used by permission.)

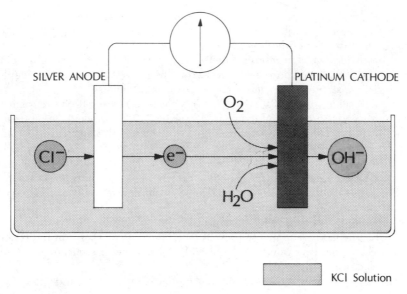

FIG 33–2.
The basic principle of the polarographic electrode. The chloride ion will react with the silver anode to form silver chloride—an oxidation reaction that produces electrons. Oxygen will react with platinum and water, utilizing electrons (a reduction reaction). The flow of electrons can be measured as a current. The greater the concentration of oxygen in solution, the greater the current used. (From Shapiro BA, Harrison RA, Walton JR: *Clinical Application of Arterial Blood Gases,* ed 3. Chicago, Year Book Medical Publishers, 1982. Used by permission.)

3. In solution, the greater the partial pressure of oxygen, the greater the current produced and used.
4. A -0.6-V polarizing voltage is applied to the anode.
   a. This voltage is needed to maintain direction of current from anode to cathode through the electrolyte solution.
   b. At -0.6 V, oxygen is the only respiratory gas that will be readily reduced.
5. The tip of the Clark electrode is covered with a polypropylene membrane that allows slow diffusion of oxygen from blood or gas being analyzed.
6. This analyzer type directly measures partial pressure of the gas. For this reason the analyzer must be carefully calibrated at varying altitudes and to changing atmospheric pressures.
7. The analyzer must be used in all respiratory gas mixtures and is the type incorporated into blood gas analyzer systems.
8. Measurement of flow of electrons is referred to as an *amperometric measurement.*
D. Analyzers using a galvanic cell
   1. The galvanic cell is similar to a battery cell that utilizes oxygen to create a current between its electrodes.
   2. Current is continually produced if the cell is exposed to oxygen; thus, the life of the cell is dependent on duration and frequency of use.
   3. The analyzer is composed of two electrodes immersed in an alkali metal hydroxide solution. Generally the electrolyte is potassium hydroxide, but some models use cesium hydroxide.
      a. A lead anode, in the presence of oxygen, produces a current as a result of an oxidation reaction with the hydroxide compound.

   b. A gold cathode, in the presence of oxygen, produces the following reaction:

$$O_2 + 2H_2O + 4 \text{ electrons} \rightarrow 4OH^- \tag{2}$$

      (*Note:* Overall reactions for galvanic cell and polarographic analyzers are the same.)

   4. The current is measured from anode to cathode, which allows completion of an electric circuit.

   5. The greater the partial pressure of oxygen, the greater the measured current.

   6. As with the polarographic analyzer, the galvanic cell measures the partial pressure of oxygen and consequently must be carefully calibrated at varying altitudes and atmospheric pressure.

II. pH (Sanz) Electrode (Figs 33–3 and 33–4)

  A. The electrode is composed of two half-cells connected via a potassium chloride electrolyte bridge.

    1. A reference half-cell composed of mercury–mercurous chloride (calomel)

    2. A measuring half-cell composed of silver–silver chloride

  B. The measuring half-cell has two chambers separated by pH-sensitive glass, which allows measurement of voltage differences across the glass.

    1. The enclosed buffer chamber with a buffer of a constant pH surrounds the pH-sensitive glass capillary tube.

    2. The sample chamber capillary tube allows blood to be in contact with the pH-sensitive glass.

  C. The reference half-cell is immersed in potassium chloride solution, which allows completion of the basic electrical circuit while providing constant reference voltage.

  D. As a result of electric activity on the pH-sensitive glass, a potential difference can be measured.

  E. The potential difference is measured on a voltmeter calibrated in pH units.

  F. This type of system comparing voltage measurements is termed *potentiometric*.

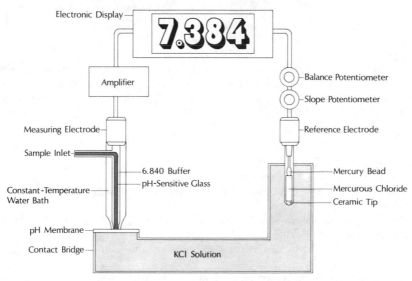

FIG 33–3.

The complete Sanz (pH) electrode. See Figure 33–4 for specifics. (From Shapiro BA, Harrison RA, Walton JR: *Clinical Application of Arterial Blood Gases,* ed 3. Chicago, Year Book Medical Publishers, 1982. Used by permission.)

(a)

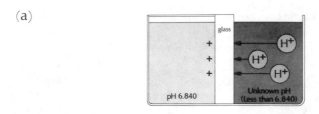

(b)

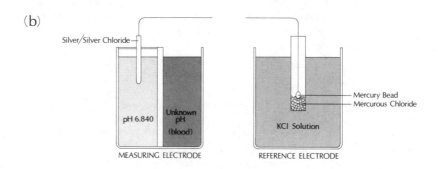

(c)

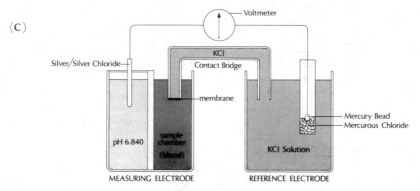

FIG 33–4.
Basic principles of the pH electrode. **A,** voltage is developed across pH-sensitive glass when the hydrogen ion concentration is unequal in the two solutions. **B,** chemical half-cell is used as the measuring electrode and another half-cell is the reference electrode. **C,** the basic principle of the modern pH electrode. (From Shapiro BA, Harrison RA, Walton JR: *Clinical Application of Arterial Blood Gases,* ed 3. Chicago, Year Book Medical Publishers, 1982. Used by permission.)

III. P_{CO_2} (Severinghaus) Electrode (Fig 33–5)
    A. The P_{CO_2} electrode is a modified pH electrode.
    B. The P_{CO_2} is measured indirectly by determining the change in pH of an $NaHCO_3$ solution.
    C. The electrode is composed of two half-cells, each composed of silver–silver chloride.
    D. Functioning of electrode
        1. Carbon dioxide diffuses across a silicon membrane into an $NaHCO_3$ electrolyte solution.
        2. After the solution is entered, carbon dioxide reacts with water to form hydrogen and bicarbonate ions:

$$CO_2 + H_2O \rightarrow H_2CO_3 \rightarrow H^+ + HCO_3^- \tag{3}$$

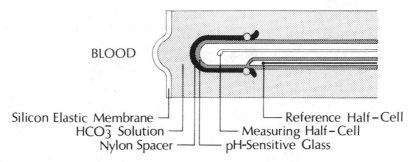

BLOOD

Silicon Elastic Membrane ┘
HCO₃⁻ Solution ┘
Nylon Spacer ┘

Reference Half–Cell
Measuring Half–Cell
pH-Sensitive Glass

FIG 33–5.
A typical Severinghaus (Pco_2) electrode. (From Shapiro BA, Harrison RA, Walton JR: *Clinical Application of Arterial Blood Gases,* ed 3. Chicago, Year Book Medical Publishers, 1982. Used by permission.)

3. The H^+ formed sets up a potential difference across the pH-sensitive glass in the measuring half-cell.
E. All other aspects of the electrode are consistent with the pH electrode.
F. The potential difference is measured on a voltmeter and reflected as millimeters of mercury of carbon dioxide.
(*Note:* The PO_2 (Clark) electrode for blood gas analyzers is covered in section I–C.)
IV. Transcutaneous Po_2 (TcPo_2) and Pco_2 (TcPco_2) Monitoring
A. Both of these techniques make use of miniaturized blood gas (Clark and Severinghaus) electrodes.
B. TcPo_2 monitoring
1. Oxygen molecules diffusing through the skin diffuse through the semipermeable membrane covering the Clark electrode.
2. To facilitate diffusion and arterialize blood, the skin surface under the electrode is heated to about 42°C.
3. Normally, electrodes are placed on flat surfaces of the chest and abdomen.
4. This electrode is reasonably accurate if perfusion is normal and the skin over which it is placed is thin.
5. As a result, it is used almost exclusively in infants.
C. TcPco_2 monitoring
1. The skin under the electrode is heated to about 44°C.
2. Heating of the skin increases diffusion, allowing more carbon dioxide to diffuse, but may increase local metabolism and carbon dioxide production.
3. Electrodes are placed on the chest and abdomen.
4. As long as perfusion is adequate and diffusion is normal, TcPco_2 accurately tracks Pco_2.
D. Both TcPo_2 and TcPco_2 electrodes should be changed every 4 hours to prevent first- and second-degree burns.
V. Spectrophotometric Analyzers
A. A spectrophotometer is an apparatus that determines the light absorbence of matter in solution by the quantity of light absorbed in passing through the fluid.
1. Molecules of a substance in solution can absorb light waves. Various substances absorb differing spectra.
2. Spectrophotometers create light waves specific to the substance to be measured.
3. Light waves of specific spectra are passed through a sample and measured.
4. Since the amount of input light waves is constant, measuring the output waves allows determination of the amount of light absorption by the sample.
5. Finally, according to *Beer's law,* the absorption of light by a solution is a function of the concentration of the solute and the absorption depth of the solution. The

greater the sample absorption, the greater the concentration of the substance being measured since the absorption depth is a constant determined by the sample
chamber.
  B. Functional components of spectrophotometers
    1. Light source of known intensity
    2. Sample chamber of known depth
    3. Light collector (photomultiplier)
    4. Readout display
  C. Types of units commonly used
    1. Pulse oximeters
      a. These units use two wavelengths of light: red and infrared.
      b. The absorption of light by oxyhemoglobin and reduced hemoglobin is com-
         pared.
      c. Both require a pulsating arterial bed for operation. Typical measurement sites
         are:
        (1) The finger.
        (2) The ear.
        (3) The bridge of the nose.
      d. The emitter and detector are placed on each side of the capillary bed.
      e. Most units fail to function if a pulse is not noticeable.
      f. These units measure oxyhemoglobin saturation with an accuracy of ±2% in
         the 80% to 100% saturation range.
      g. They are frequently used on all sizes of patients in all clinical settings to mon-
         itor oxyhemoglobin saturation.
    2. CO-oximeter
      a. It uses light wave spectra specific to:
        (1) Oxyhemoglobin.
        (2) Reduced hemoglobin.
        (3) Carboxyhemoglobin.
        (4) Methemoglobin.
      b. In addition, total hemoglobin readout is provided.
    3. Flame photometer
      a. Atomizes blood sample and measures light absorption from a propane flame.
      b. Measures potassium, sodium, and lithium using lithium or cesium as a control.
    4. Capnography (end-tidal CO_2 monitoring)
      a. This device utilizes the radioabsorptive quality of CO_2 (Fig 33–6).
      b. Energy from an infrared source is passed through two parallel cells (sample
         and reference cells).
      c. It then passes into two halves of a detector cell, which are divided by a thin
         metal diaphragm located close to an electrically isolated fixed plate.
      d. Both sides of the detector half-cell contain gas of similar makeup.
      e. Infrared radiation reaching the detector half-cell causes the gases therein to
         vibrate, but as long as the CO_2 concentrations in the detector half-cells are
         the same, the metal diaphragm remains stationary.
      f. When CO_2 is introduced into the sample cell, the top portion of the detector
         half-cell vibrates more than the bottom half of the detector cell, indicating in-
         creased CO_2 levels.
      g. These units accurately measure exhaled CO_2 but can be affected by:
        (1) Moisture.
        (2) Barometric pressure.
        (3) Temperature.
        (4) Vibration.
      h. In addition, end-tidal CO_2 readings are altered by any factor affecting dead-
         space.

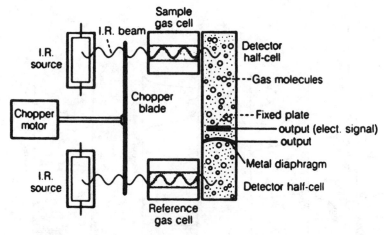

FIG 33–6.
A typical infrared CO_2 analyzer. (From Beauchamp RK: Pulmonary function testing procedures, in Barnes T [ed]: *Respiratory Care Practice*. Chicago, Year Book Medical Publishers, 1988. Used by permission.)

　　i. The greater the deadspace, the poorer the correlation of end tidal CO_2 with Pa_{CO_2}.
　　j. A normal capnogram tracing is depicted in Figure 33–7.
　　　　(1) From point a to b, gas is exhaled from the anatomic deadspace; no CO_2 is present.
　　　　(2) From point b to c, there is a changeover from deadspace to alveolar gas, and the amount of exhaled CO_2 rapidly increases.
　　　　(3) From point c to d, gas is exhaled entirely from alveolar. In this stage a gently sloping plateau should be established.
　　　　(4) From point d to e, inspiration begins, which continues into point a.
　　k. Many variations in the normal capnogram are noticed clinically (Fig 33–8).
　　　　(1) Pulsing of exhaled gas caused by cardiac oscillations is noted in Figure 33–8,A.
　　　　(2) Hyperventilation is noted in Figure 33–8,B. The percent of exhaled CO_2 is normally decreased.

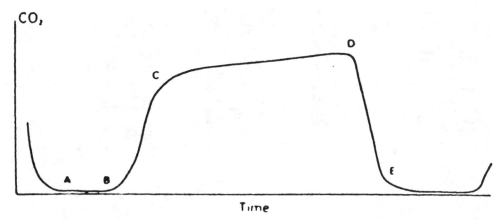

FIG 33–7.
Normal capnogram end-tidal CO_2 percent tracing. See text for discussion. (From Swedlow DB: Capnometry and capnography: The anesthesia disaster early warning system. *Semin Anesth* 1986; 5:194–202. Used by permission.)

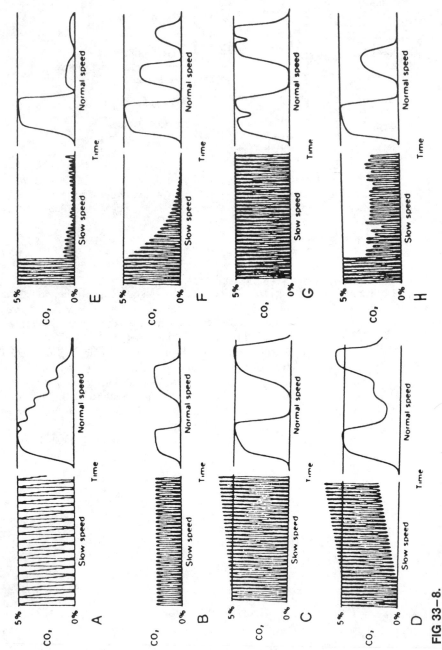

FIG 33–8.
Variations in normal capnograms during clinical setting (see text for discussion). (From Swedlow DB: Capnometry and capnography: The anesthesia disaster early warning system. *Semin Anesth* 1986; 5:194–202. (Used by permission.)

(3) The beginning of hypoventilation is noted in Figure 33–8,C. Carbon dioxide levels start to increase.

(4) Rebreathing of CO_2 results in the baseline CO_2 level increasing above zero (see Fig 33–8,D).

(5) Ventilator disconnect or apnea in spontaneous ventilation is indicated by a sudden loss of the capnogram (see Fig 33–8,E).

(6) A rapid progressive decay in the plateau is noted during cardiac arrest or severely developing hypotension. Because of loss of perfusion, deadspace markedly increases and CO_2 decreases (see Fig 33–8,F).

(7) Spasmodic contraction of the diaphragm or the interruption of exhalation by an incomplete breath is illustrated in Figure 33–8,G.

(8) A periodic decrease in CO_2 level and a loss of plateau are associated with same ineffective tidal breaths or poor sampling (see Fig 33–8,H).

BIBLIOGRAPHY

Adams A, Hahn C: *Principles of Blood Gas Analysis,* ed 2. New York, Churchill-Livingstone, 1982.

Bageant R: Oxygen analyzers. *Respir Care* 1976; 21:410–416.

Beauchamp GG: Pulmonary function testing procedures, in Barnes T (ed): *Respiratory Care Practice.* Year Book Medical Publishers, Chicago, 1988.

Beyerl D: Noninvasive measurement of blood oxygen levels. *Am J Med Technol* 1982; 48:355–359.

Biox Product Literature: *On Ear Oxymetry and Biox Ear Oximeter, #112 M2000 B 7/14/ 82, 109 M1000 D 6/11/82.* Boulder, Colo, Biox Technology, 1982.

Critikon Product Literature: *Transcutaneous Gas Monitors.* Tampa, Fla, Critikon, 1982.

Degn H, Balsleu I, Brook R (eds): *Measurement of Oxygen.* New York, Elsevier Scientific Co, 1976.

Duffin J: *Physics for Anesthetists.* Springfield, Ill, Bannerstone House, 1976.

Hicks GH (ed): *Problems in Respiratory Care: Applied Noninvasive Monitoring.* Philadelphia, JB Lippincott Co, 1989; 2:78–96.

McPherson SP: *Respiratory Therapy Equipment,* ed 2. St Louis, CV Mosby Co, 1981.

Mindt W: *Skin Sensors for Monitoring Oxygen Tension of Newborns.* Product literature. Basel, Switzerland, Hoffmann-LaRoche, 1980.

Nuzzo P: Capnography in infants and children. *Perinatol Neonatal* May–June 1978; 3:186–194.

Paloheima M, Valli M, Ahjopalo H: A guide to CO_2 monitoring. Finland, Datex Instumen Tarklum Oy, 1983.

Shapiro BA, Harrison RA, Walton JR: *Clinical Application of Blood Gases,* ed 3. Chicago, Year Book Medical Publishers, 1982.

Spearman CB, Sheldon RL, Egan DF: *Egan's Fundamentals of Respiratory Therapy,* ed 4. St Louis, CV Mosby Co, 1982.

Swedlow DB: Capnometry and capnography: The anesthesia disaster early warning system. *Semin Anesth* 1986; 5:194–202.

Young JA, Crocker D: *Principles and Practice of Respiratory Therapy,* ed 2. Chicago, Year Book Medical Publishers, 1976.

Chapter 34

Fluidics

I. General Characteristics of Fluidic Gas Flow Systems
   A. Fluidic systems possess a basic logic by design.
      1. This basic logic is referred to as the *fluidic logic* or *fluidic element*.
      2. The logic determines the direction of gas flow.
   B. These systems normally do not require moving parts for proper function.
   C. Changes in direction of flow are accomplished by:
      1. Backpressure.
      2. Subatmospheric (negative inspiratory) pressure.
      3. Amplification (cycling pressure).
         a. Amplification is the control of the direction of a large flow of gas by a small momentary flow of gas (Fig 34–1).
         b. Normally, amplification flow enters the system perpendicular to the main gas flow.
         c. By acting on the main gas flow, the amplification flow causes the main gas flow to alter its direction.
         d. Amplification allows adjustment of sensitivity and cycling pressure.
   D. The basic phenomenon responsible for the overall fluidic mechanism is the *Coanda effect* (Fig 34–2; see also Fig 34–1).
      1. The Coanda effect is based on the fact that a free-flowing gas system creates a subatmospheric pressure at its periphery.
      2. If a wall is placed near the source of gas, the stream of gas adheres to the wall. Adherence is caused by subatmospheric pressure.
      3. When this phenomenon is incorporated in a fluidic system, it is referred to as a *wall attachment fluidic element* and may be used to alter direction of gas flow.
      4. Once wall attachment has been achieved, a bond between the wall and the gas flow is developed and maintained unless affected by:
         a. Backpressure.
         b. Subatmospheric pressure.
         c. Amplification.
      5. The creation of the Coanda effect and the strength of its bond are predictable.
         a. The greater the driving pressure, the stronger the bond.
         b. The design of the system's logic can strengthen the bond.
            (1) If an "outcropping" (see Fig 34–1) is designed into the system, the Coanda effect is intensified. The outcropping creates an area of low pressure called a *vortex*. The larger the outcropping, the lower the pressure and the stronger the resulting bond.

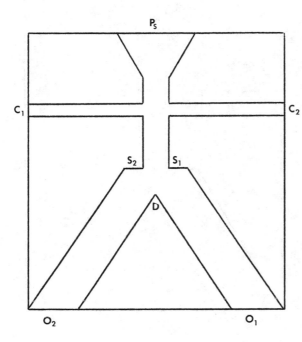

FIG 34–1.
Symmetric bistable fluidic logic. P_S is the gas source. S_1 and S_2 are "outcroppings." O_1 and O_2 are exit ports, and D is the separator. A vortex is created at S_2 or S_1. C_1 and C_2 are amplification ports. Momentary gas flow from amplification port C_1 would direct gas flow to exit port O_1. Momentary gas flow from C_2 would direct gas flow to exit port C_1.

(2) The addition of a *foil* (see Fig 34–2) also strengthens the bond. A foil is a curvilinear narrowing on one wall of the system and acts similar to the wing of an aircraft. As gas moves over the foil, gas velocity increases, creating a negative pressure downstream that enhances wall attachment.

II. Asymmetric Fluidic Logic (Fig 34–3)
   A. Gas powering the logic enters at P_S in Figure 34–3.
   B. Point A is a constriction in the gas entry port designed to accelerate gas velocity.
   C. Lateral to point B is where the Coanda effect begins to appear.

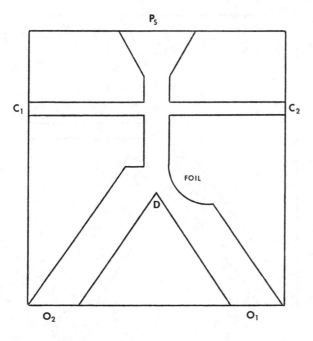

FIG 34–2.
Bistable fluidic logic incorporating a foil. Point D is the separator, O_1 and O_2 are exit ports, and C_1 and C_2 are amplification ports. The foil creates a negative pressure, enhancing wall attachment.

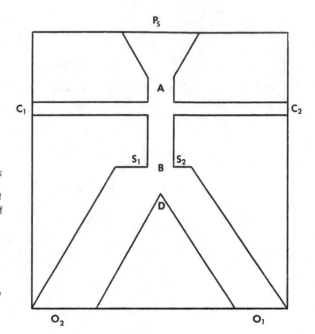

FIG 34–3.
Asymmetric bistable fluidic logic. P_S is a gas source. Point *A* represents initial constriction of system. Point *B* indicates location of development of Coanda effect. Point *D* is the separator. C_1 and C_2 are amplification ports, S_1 and S_2 are outcroppings, and O_1 and O_2 are exit ports. Although the system is bistable, the larger outcropping at S_1 results in a stronger attachment down exit port O_2.

    D. Outcroppings are represented by S_1 and S_2. Since S_1 is larger than S_2, the wall attachment bond at S_1 would be greater than S_2.

    E. Point *D* is referred to as the *separator*. The location of the separator determines the type of logic. If the separator is directly midline, the logic is bistable (see section III). If the separator is not midline, the system is monostable (see section V).

    F. Amplification ports are represented by C_1 and C_2.

FIG 34–4.
Monostable fluidic logic. P_S is gas source. Point *D* is the separator. O_1 and O_2 are exit ports, and C_2 is an amplification port.

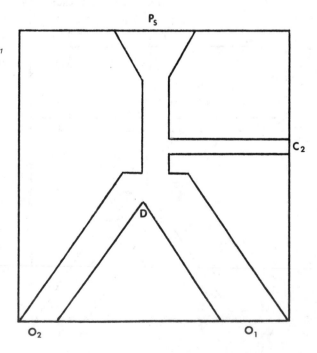

III. Symmetric Bistable Fluidic Logic (see Fig 34–1)
   A. Gas entering the element at P_S is stable in either leg (exit port) of the system, O_1 or O_2. Both exit ports in the system are symmetric in design.
   B. Once gas enters a leg of the system, it will remain stable in that leg until acted on by an external force.
   C. Amplification may occur from C_1 (or C_2), causing flow to move from O_2 to O_1 (or O_1 to O_2).
   D. A subatmospheric (negative inspiratory) pressure created at O_1 also will cause gas to move in a stable manner down that exit port.
   E. As pressure begins to increase at O_1 to a predetermined level (based on design), it will then direct the flow to O_2 and remain stable there until it is acted on by an external force.
   F. All bistable logics may be referred to as a *flip-flop valve with a memory*.
IV. Asymmetric Bistable Fluidic (see Fig 34–3)
   A. In an asymmetric bistable system, the two exit ports of the system (O_1 and O_2) are not designed similarly; however, the separator is midline.
   B. As in a symmetric bistable system, once gas flow enters either leg, it is stable in that leg unless acted on by an external force.
   C. Because of the asymmetric design (S_1 greater in size than S_2) wall attachment is stronger in one leg (O_2) than the other (O_1); however, it is stable in both.
 V. Monostable Fluidic Logic (Fig 34–4)
   A. This system is asymmetric in design.
   B. The asymmetric design is a result of positioning one of the system's exit ports off center. This is accomplished by the location of the separator (point D).
   C. Gas will normally proceed from P_S to O_1 as a result of the separator. Gas flow will be stable in O_1 until an external force causes movement to leg O_2.
   D. As gas moves to O_1, additional gas will be entrained from O_2, thus increasing the volume exiting at O_1. (Air entrainment is possible in any fluidic logic system.)
   E. Gas flow will move to leg O_2 only under the following circumstances:
      1. Backpressure were generated at O_1 great enough to overcome wall attachment.

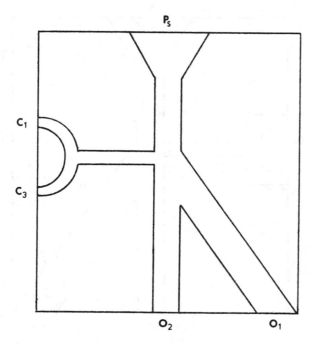

FIG 34–5.
AND/NAND fluidic logic. Flow is normally stable form P_S to O_2. For flow to be diverted to O_1, simultaneous amplification must originate from both C_1 and C_3.

TABLE 34–1.

Truth Table for AND/NAND System

Line	C_1	C_3	O_1	O_2
1	0	0	0	X
2	X	0	0	X
3	0	X	0	X
4	X	X	X	0

    2. If amplification were to occur at point C_2, the main flow of gas would be directed down leg O_2
       a. The flow from C_2 needs to be directed perpendicular to the main gas flow.
       b. The amplification flow must enter the system on a side opposite to that where it is directing the main gas flow.
  F. Once the backpressure is removed and the amplification flow is stopped, the main flow will return to its original path. O_1,

VI. AND/NAND Fluidic Logic (Fig 34–5 and Table 34–1)
  A. The flow is always stable from P_S to O_2 unless it is acted on by an external force (monostable element).
  B. For flow to move from O_2 to O_1, simultaneous amplification must occur from both C_1 and C_3.
  C. If gas were to enter only from C_1, it would exit at C_3 without affecting the main gas flow. The same type of situation occurs if gas enters only from C_3.
  D. Once amplification flow is stopped, flow will revert to O_2 and again remain stable.
  E. The truth table (see Table 34–1) accompanying Figure 34–5 is used to explain the direction that flow will take in response to the forces acting on it.
    1. A zero (0) in Table 34–1 indicates no flow from the particular source.

FIG 34–6.
OR/NOR fluidic logic. Flow is normally stable from P_S to O_2. Flow may be diverted from O_2 to O_1 with amplification from either C_1 or C_3, or both.

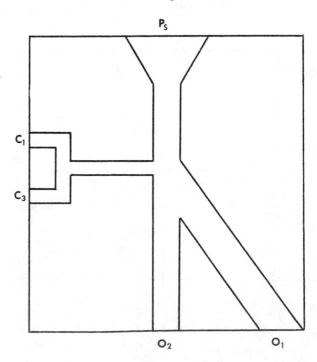

TABLE 34–2.

Truth Table for OR/NOR System

Line	C_1	C_3	O_1	O_2
1	0	0	0	X
2	X	0	X	0
3	0	X	X	0
4	X	X	X	0

    2. An X in the table indicates flow.

    3. For example, in line 1, there is no flow from C_1 or C_3; thus, gas flows only to O_2.

VII. OR/NOR Fluidic Logic (Fig 34–6 and Table 34–2)

    A. The flow is always stable from P_s to O_2 unless acted on by an external force (monostable logic).

    B. For flow to move from O_2 to O_1, amplification must occur from C_1 or C_3, or both.

    C. Once amplification is stopped, flow will revert to O_2 and again remain stable.

VIII. Proportional Amplifier (Fig 34–7)

    A. This is basically a symmetric bistable logic system in which directional flow change occurs by amplification alone.

    B. Flow always enters the system from C_1 and C_2.

    C. Gas moves toward O_1 or O_2, depending on whether amplification is greater at C_1 or C_2.

    D. Points A and B are adjustable valves. These valves may be incorporated and used to function as sensitivity or pressure cycling regulators.

        1. If a patient were connected at point O_1, valve A would act as a sensitivity control. Thus, gas flow from O_2 to O_1 would depend on amplification from A and patient subatmospheric pressure at O_1.

        2. In the situation described, B would act as a peak pressure (cycling pressure) control. Gas movement from O_1 to O_2 would depend on backpressure at O_1 and amplification at C_2.

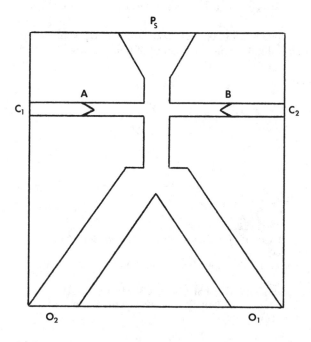

FIG 34–7.

Proportional amplifier. P_S is the gas source. A and B are adjustable valves. C_1 and C_2 are amplification ports, and O_1 and O_2 are exit ports.

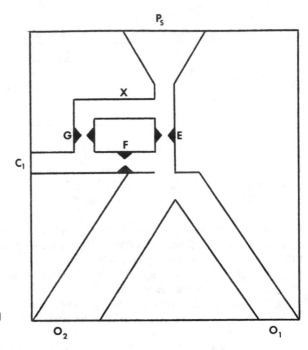

FIG 34–8.
Backpressure switch. P_S is the gas source. Points E, F, and G are restrictors. X is shunt for main flow gas. C_1 is an amplification port, and O_1 and O_2 are exit ports.

IX. Backpressure Switch (Fig 34–8)
  A. This is a modified monostable logic. Gas is stable in leg O_2.
  B. As gas enters the system, a portion of it is shunted through X because of the restriction at point E.
  C. The gas entering X moves through the restriction at point G and out C_1.
  D. If C_1 is blocked, gas from X moves through the restriction at point F and acts as amplification on the system. As a result, gas is forced from O_2 to O_1.
  E. Opening and closing of C_1 can be governed by a microprocessor-controlled solenoid switch.
  F. If a patient were connected at point O_1, the opening and closing of C_1 would act as a time cycling mechanism that is determining the amount of time gas would flow to O_1.

X. Ventilators Incorporating Fluidic Logics
  A. Retec X70/IPPB
  B. Mine Safety Appliance IPPB
  C. Ohio 550
  D. Monaghan 225
  E. Sechrist IV-100B

BIBLIOGRAPHY

Angrist S: Fluid control devices. *Sci Am* 1964; 211:80.
Deshpande VM, Pibeam SP, Dixon RJ: *A Comprehensive Review in Respiratory Care.* Norwalk, Conn, Appleton & Lange, 1988.
Garrett DF: *Physical Principles of Respiratory Therapy Equipment.* Madison, Wis, Ohio Medical Products, 1978.
McPherson SP: *Respiratory Therapy Equipment,* ed 2. St Louis, CV Mosby Co, 1981.
Monaghan Product Information: *Fluidics and Monaghan Volume Ventilators.* Schaumburg, Ill, Monaghan Co, Division of Sandoz, 1973.

Mushin WW: *Automatic Ventilation of the Lungs*, ed 3. Boston, Blackwell Scientific Publications, 1980.

Reba I: Application of the Coanda effect. *Sci Am* 1966; 214:84.

Respiratory Products Bulletin, Retec X70/IPPB. Portland, Ore, Retec Development Laboratory, 1975.

Spearman CP, Sheldon RL, Egan DF: *Egan's Fundamentals of Respiratory Therapy*, ed 4. St Louis, CV Mosby Co, 1982.

Chapter 35 _____

Technical Aspects
of Mechanical Ventilators

I. Classification of Mechanical Ventilators
- This chapter discusses the technical characteristics of conventional intensive care unit mechanical ventilators. Information on home care ventilators is presented in Chapter 23, and information on high-frequency ventilators is presented in Chapter 38.
- To present this material in a logical manner, the following 13-point system is used to classify ventilators.
  A. Positive or negative pressure
      1. Positive pressure ventilators make use of a supra-atmospheric pressure applied to the airway to deliver tidal volumes.
      2. Negative pressure ventilators make use of a subatmospheric pressure applied to the thorax to deliver tidal volumes.
  B. Powering mechanism
      1. Physical energy source that provides the power for ventilator function
      2. Available powering mechanisms
          a. Electric: Normally uses 120-V electrical current.
          b. Pneumatic: Normally uses a 40 to 60 pounds per square inch (psi) gas source.
          c. Combined electric/pneumatic: Both of which must be activated for proper machine function.
  C. Driving mechanism
      1. Provides the mechanical force that produces the flow of gas necessary for delivery of tidal volumes
      2. Characteristic types of driving systems
          a. Pneumatic systems: Driven by a compressed gas source (either internal or external to ventilator) regulated by electronic, fluidic, or mechanical devices inside the ventilator.
              (1) Pneumatic clutches and valves
              (2) Electronic servo-mechanisms
              (3) Electronic and mechanical solenoids
              (4) Preset and adjustable regulators
              (5) Fluidic regulation
          b. Piston systems: Driven by devices exhibiting:
              (1) Linear motion.

472

(2) Rotary motion (i.e., exponential or logarithmic acceleration/deceleration).

   c. Bellows systems: Driven by a compressed gas source (either internal or external to ventilator) generated by a:
   (1) Compressor (e.g., turbine).
   (2) Fluidic system.
   (3) Pneumatic system.

D. Maintenance of gas flow pattern
   1. The ability of a ventilator to maintain a consistent gas flow pattern is dependent on the driving mechanism of the ventilator and the total patient resistance to ventilation.
   2. If the maximum pressure generated by the driving force of a ventilator is at least five times the highest system pressure developed during gas delivery, the ventilator is considered a *flow generator*. These machines can maintain their gas flow patterns despite increasing backpressure.
   3. If the driving mechanism generates a force considerably less than five times the highest system pressure, the ventilator is referred to as a *pressure generator*. These ventilators demonstrate significant variations in gas flow patterns as resistance to ventilation changes (e.g., increased airway resistance, decreased compliance, or both).
   4. Constant flow vs. constant pressure generators
      a. Constant flow generators: Driving pressures maintained are greater than 4,000 cm H_2O. *There is little or no variation in gas flow pattern.*
      b. Nonconstant flow generators: Driving pressures are normally greater than 4,000 cm H_2O, and there is a reproducible gas flow pattern that does not vary with alterations in patient resistance to ventilation. *Although the pattern of gas flow is the same breath after breath, the rate of gas delivery during each breath varies.*
      c. Modified constant flow generators: Driving pressures are considerably less than 4,000 cm H_2O. *Gas flow patterns may change significantly with changes in resistance to ventilation.*
      d. Constant pressure generators: Driving pressures are less than 100 cm H_2O. *There may be a continual modification of gas flow pattern during the inspiratory phase in response to changes in resistance to ventilation.*
   5. As a result of the servo-controlled flow valves in the microprocessor-controlled ventilators and the speed with which feedback can be provided, this group of ventilators is better capable of ensuring a consistent delivered gas flow pattern on a breath-by-breath basis.

E. Number of circuits
   1. A circuit is the path the gas flow follows inside the ventilator.
   2. A single circuit ventilator has one pressurized gas volume. This pressurized gas volume is the same as that delivered to the patient (i.e., the same gas flow that is produced by the ventilator's driving mechanism is delivered to the patient).
   3. A double circuit ventilator has two separate pressurized gas volumes. One gas volume is used to compress the second gas. This latter compressed gas is the volume delivered to the patient (i.e., one gas powers the driving mechanism and the other gas is delivered to the patient). Two distinct gas flow systems are involved in tidal volume delivery.

F. Gas flow and airway pressure patterns
   1. The gas flow pattern developed during inspiration is dependent on the driving mechanism employed and the ability of the machine to maintain flow despite increasing backpressure.

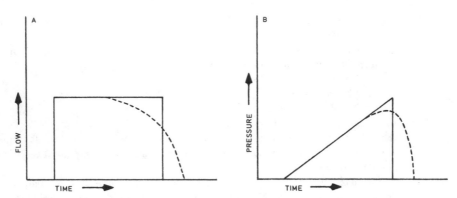

FIG 35−1.
A, square wave flow pattern. *Dotted line* represents normal flow tapering. **B,** rectilinear pressure pattern. *Dotted line* represents the effect of a flow taper.

2. The pressure pattern is dependent on the gas flow pattern and total resistance to ventilation (pressure = gas flow × resistance).
3. Specific pressure patterns are always associated with a particular gas flow pattern. However, this may not hold true if the patient fights the ventilator.
4. Characteristic gas flow and pressure patterns
   a. Square wave flow and rectilinear pressure patterns: A constant flow is maintained throughout the inspiratory phase. This tends to result in a constant pressure change per unit of time, or a rectilinear pressure pattern (Fig 35−1). However, few ventilators are capable of maintaining a constant flow. The dotted lines in Figure 35−1 demonstrate the effect of backpressure on flow rate and pressure patterns. If this flow taper effect (decelerating flow pattern) develops, inspiratory time is lengthened. These flow and pressure patterns are characteristic of modified constant flow generators.
   b. Sine wave flow and sigmoidal pressure patterns: Normally they are produced by logarithmically accelerating/decelerating (rotary) piston-driving mechanisms. Flow begins slowly, then accelerates until the middle of inspiration, then decreases toward the end of inspiration. One half of a sine wave is produced, resulting in a sigmoidal pressure pattern (Fig 35−2). This is the most common example of a nonconstant flow generator.

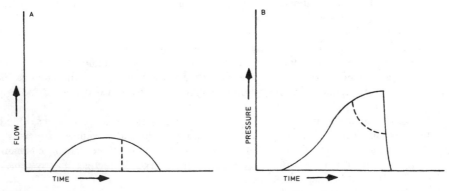

FIG 35−2.
A, sine wave flow pattern. *Dotted line* represents a modified sine wave flow pattern. **B,** sigmoidal pressure pattern. *Dotted line* represents the pressure curve seen with a modified sine wave flow pattern.

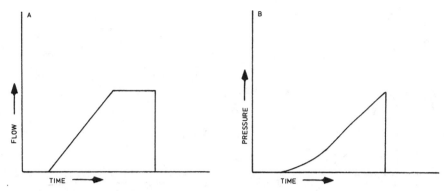

FIG 35–3.
A, accelerating flow pattern. **B,** nonlinearly increasing pressure pattern.

    c. Accelerating flow and nonlinearly increasing pressure patterns: Flow progressively increases during inspiration until a preset limit is reached, at which time the flow plateaus to a square wave (Fig 35–3). A nonlinearly increasing pressure pattern develops. These curves are produced by nonconstant flow generators.

    d. Decelerating flow and parabolic pressure patterns. Gas flow begins at a maximum and at some preset point during the inspiratory phase the flow rate begins to decrease until the end of inspiration. Two basic patterns exist, a flow taper (Fig 35–4) and a decaying flow pattern (Fig 35–5). These flow patterns result in parabolic pressure patterns that may be initially linear but terminally the rate of pressure change diminishes. Figure 35–4 is an example of a modified constant flow generator, and Figure 35–5 is an example of a constant pressure generator.

  G. Cycling parameter

    1. The physical parameter that, when reached, will result in termination of the mechanical inspiratory phase.

    2. Four basic parameters are involved in the delivery of gas to any patient. One (or more) of these is always the cycling parameter.

      a. Volume

      b. Pressure

      c. Time

      d. Flow

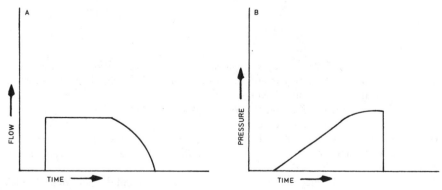

FIG 35–4.
A, square wave flow with flow taper (decelerating flow). **B,** parabolic pressure pattern.

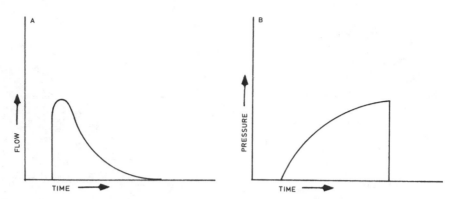

FIG 35–5.
A, decaying flow pattern (decelerating flow). **B,** parabolic pressure pattern.

       3. A primary cycling parameter does *not* activate an audiovisual or audio alarm when reached.
          a. An alarm being activated with each inspiration normally indicates an inappropriate condition for continuous mechanical ventilation.
          b. Limiting parameters (see section I–H) may function as secondary cycling mechanisms. When attained, these parameters normally activate an alarm.
    H. Limit
       1. A limit is a physical parameter (flow, time, pressure, volume) that cannot be exceeded but is not the primary cycling mechanism. Limiting parameters may be divided into three categories:
          a. Limits that are preset but adjustable. *Examples:*
            (1) Peak flow control on the Puritan-Bennett 7200
            (2) Normal pressure limit control on the Intermed Bear 5
            (3) Pressure relief on the Emerson Post-Op
          b. Limits that are the result of two preset adjustable parameters. *Examples:*
            (1) Inspiratory time on the Bird 6400 ST

$$\text{Inspiratory time} = \frac{\text{Tidal volume}}{\text{Flow}}$$

            (2) Volume on the Siemens Servo 900C:

$$\text{Tidal volume} = \frac{\text{Minute Volume}}{\text{Rate}}$$

          c. Limits that also may serve as a secondary means of ending inspiration. All limiting factors that end inspiration should have simultaneous audio or audiovisual alarms. *Examples:*
            (1) Pressure limit on the Puritan-Bennett 7200
            (2) I/E ratio limit on the Bear 3
II. Modes of ventilation: The term mode is used to represent the manner in which gas is delivered, regardless of whether the tidal volume is pressurized or not (see Chapter 36 for greater detail).
       1. Control: The machine is responsible for initiation and delivery of each tidal volume. Volume limit or pressure limit may be used.

2. Assist: The patient is totally responsible for initiation of the inspiratory phase, but the ventilator delivers the tidal volume.

3. Assist/control: The machine functions in the assist mode unless the patient's respiratory rate falls below a present level, at which time the machine converts to the control mode.

4. Intermittent mandatory ventilation (IMV): The patient is allowed to breathe spontaneously from an external high-flow system or from the ventilator via a demand valve, and at preset intervals the machine functions in the control mode.

5. Synchronized intermittent mandatory ventilation (SIMV): The patient is allowed to breathe spontaneously from the ventilator via a demand valve, and at preset intervals the machine functions in the assist/control mode.

6. Mandatory minute ventilation (MMV): A minimum minute volume delivery is set on the machine. The patient may receive this volume (1) breathing totally spontaneously, (2) while being mechanically ventilated, or (3) a combination of 1 and 2. If the patient's spontaneous minute volume falls below the minimum level, mandatory positive pressure breaths make up the difference. It may be used in conjunction with inspiratory pressure support (IPS).

7. Continuous positive airway pressure (CPAP): The patient breathes spontaneously via a demand valve or high-flow system (no positive pressure breaths are delivered.) Positive end-expiratory pressure (PEEP) can be maintained at any level.

8. Inspiratory pressure support (IPS): During spontaneous ventilation, the ventilator functions as a constant pressure generator.
   a. Pressure develops rapidly in the ventilator system and remains at that level until spontaneous inspiratory flow rates decrease to 25% of peak inspiratory flow (or a specific flow rate).
   b. The mode may be used:
      (1) Independently.
      (2) In conjunction with CPAP.
      (3) In conjunction with SIMV.

9. Airway pressure release ventilation (APRV) or bilevel positive airway pressure (BiPAP): Alternating levels of CPAP are used in the "spontaneous" breathing patient.
   a. A baseline CPAP level is set, normally at 2 to 10 cm H_2O.
   b. A secondary CPAP level is set to ensure a pressure-assisted tidal volume, normally at 10 to 30 cm H_2O.
   c. The rate is dependent on the level of ventilation required.
   d. The expiratory time is kept short to prevent collapsing of alveoli.
   e. Frequently a reversal of the inspiratory: expiratory (I:E) ratio is used.
   f. At each level of CPAP the patient may breathe spontaneously.

J. Inspiratory airway maneuvers (see Chapter 36 for a discussion of the physiologic effects and clinical use of these maneuvers):
   1. Sigh: The periodic delivery of a mechanical tidal volume that is greater (commonly 50%) than the patient's set mechanical tidal volume.
   2. Inflation hold (inspiratory hold, inspiratory pause): The incorporation of a static phase at the end of inspiration. This can be achieved by holding the delivered tidal volume within the patient's airway or by maintaining a constant pressure at the patient's airway.
   3. Flow taper: The gradual reduction of delivered flow rate during inspiration. Flow tapers may be adjusted to modify flow, beginning at any point during inspiration.

K. Expiratory airway maneuvers (see Chapter 36 for a discussion of the physiologic effects and clinical use of these maneuvers):
   1. Expiratory retard: Establishment of a resistance to exhalation, decreasing expiratory gas flow and hence lengthening the time it takes peak airway pressure to reach baseline.
   2. Positive end expiratory pressure (PEEP): The maintenance of airway pressure above atmospheric at end-exhalation.
   3. Negative end-expiratory pressure (NEEP): The maintenance of airway pressure below atmospheric at end-exhalation.
L. Ventilator alarm systems: Standard alarms incorporated into the ventilation system that indicate malfunction in gas delivery, oxygen concentration, machine function, or patient status.
M. Monitoring of patient variables: Many of the microprocessor units monitor numerous functions related to gas delivery.

II. Specific Mechanical Ventilators
   • The following commonly used ventilators are classified according to the 13-point classification scheme presented earlier, in their factory-delivered stock condition. Many can be significantly modified from that which is presented.
   A. Bird Mark 7 and 8
      1. Pressure: Positive
      2. Powering mechanism: Pneumatic
      3. Driving mechanism: Pneumatic system regulated by a Venturi device with a pneumatic clutch and peak flow needle valve
      4. Maintenance of gas flow pattern: Modified constant pressure generator
      5. Circuit: single
      6. Gas flow and airway pressure patterns
         a. Airmix setting: Decelerating flow and parabolic pressure pattern
         b. 100% setting: Square wave flow and rectilinear pressure pattern
      7. Cycling parameter: Pressure
      8. Limit: Flow (preset)
      9. Modes
         a. Assist
         b. Assist/control
         c. Control
      10. Inspiratory airway maneuvers: None
      11. Expiratory airway maneuvers: Mark 7, none; Mark 8, NEEP
      12. Alarms: None standard
   B. Bennett PR series
      1. Pressure: Positive
      2. Powering mechanism: Pneumatic
      3. Driving mechanism: Pneumatic system regulated by pressure-reducing valve (diluter-regulator)
      4. Maintenance of gas flow pattern: Modified constant pressure generator
      5. Circuit: Single
      6. Gas flow and airway pressure patterns: Decelerating flow and parabolic pressure patterns
      7. Cycling parameters
         a. Flow (primary)
         b. Time
      8. Limit: Pressure (preset)
      9. Modes
         a. Assist
         b. Assist/control

    10. Inspiratory airway maneuvers: None
    11. Expiratory airway maneuvers: NEEP (PR-2 only)
    12. Alarms: None standard
C. Emerson 3-PV Post-Operative
    1. Pressure: Positive
    2. Powering mechanism: Electric
    3. Driving mechanism: Rotary piston system driven by electric motor
    4. Maintenance of gas flow pattern: Nonconstant flow generator
    5. Circuit: Single
    6. Gas flow and airway pressure patterns: Sine wave and sigmoidal pressure patterns
    7. Cycling parameter: Time
    8. Limits (preset)
      a. Volume (preset)
      b. Pressure (relief/pop-off)
      c. Flow (resultant of time and volume)
    9. Modes
      a. Control
      b. Assist/control (option)
      c. IMV (option)
      d. CPAP (option)
    10. Inspiratory airway maneuvers: Sigh (optional)
    11. Expiratory airway maneuvers: PEEP
    12. Alarms (option)
      a. High pressure
      b. Loss of PEEP
      c. Failure to cycle
D. Emerson 3-MV (IMV ventilator)
    1. Pressure: Positive
    2. Powering mechanism: Electric/pneumatic (pneumatic source required for spontaneous breathing in IMV mode)
    3. Driving mechanism: Rotary piston system driven by an electric motor
    4. Maintenance of gas flow pattern: Nonconstant flow generator
    5. Circuit: Single
    6. Gas flow and airway pressure patterns: Sine wave flow and sigmoidal pressure patterns
    7. Cycling parameter: Time
    8. Limits (preset)
      a. Pressure (relief/pop-off)
      b. Volume (preset)
      c. Flow (result of time and volume)
    9. Modes
      a. Control
      b. IMV
      c. CPAP
    10. Inspiratory airway maneuvers: None
    11. Expiratory airway maneuvers: PEEP
    12. Alarms (option)
      a. High pressure
      b. Loss of PEEP
      c. Failure to cycle
E. Bennett MA-1
    1. Pressure: Positive

2. Powering mechanism: Electric
3. Driving mechanism: Bellows system driven by gas from electric compressor
4. Maintenance of gas flow pattern: Modified constant flow generator
5. Circuit: Double
6. Gas flow and airway pressure patterns: Square wave flow with taper; rectilinear to parabolic pressure pattern
7. Cycling parameters
   a. Volume (primary)
   b. Pressure
8. Limits
   a. Flow (preset)
   b. Pressure (preset)
   c. Time (result of volume and flow)
9. Modes
   a. Control
   b. Assist/control
   c. Assist
   d. IMV (option)
   e. SIMV (option)
   f. CPAP (option)
10. Inspiratory airway maneuvers: Sigh
11. Expiratory airway maneuvers
    a. PEEP (option)
    b. NEEP (option)
    c. Expiratory retard
12. Alarms
    a. Patient alarms
       (1) High inspiratory pressure
       (2) Low exhaled tidal volume, disconnect, or both
       (3) I/E ratio
    b. Machine alarms
       (1) Oxygen system failure
F. Bennett MA-2, MA-2 + 2
   1. Pressure: Positive
   2. Powering mechanism: Electric
   3. Driving mechanism: Bellows system driven by gas from an electric compressor
   4. Maintenance of gas flow pattern: Modified constant flow generator
   5. Circuit: Double
   6. Gas flow and airway pressure patterns: Square wave flow with taper; rectilinear to parabolic pressure pattern
   7. Cycling parameters
      a. Volume (primary)
      b. Pressure
   8. Limits
      a. Pressure (preset)
      b. Flow (preset)
      c. Time (result of volume and flow)
   9. Modes
      a. Control
      b. Assist
      c. Assist/control
      d. IMV (option)
      e. SIMV
      f. CPAP

10. Inspiratory airway maneuvers
    a. Sigh
    b. Inflation hold
11. Expiratory airway maneuvers
    a. PEEP
12. Alarms
    a. Patient alarms
       (1) High airway pressure
       (2) Low inspiratory pressure
       (3) Loss of pressure
       (4) Low PEEP/CPAP
       (5) Low exhaled tidal volume
       (6) I:E ratio
       (7) Fail to cycle
    b. Machine alarms
       (1) Oxygen/compressed air system failure
       (2) High gas temperature
       (3) High/low $F_{I_{O_2}}$ (option)
13. Montors: Exhaled tidal volume
G. Bear I
    1. Pressure: Positive
    2. Powering mechanism: Electric
    3. Driving mechanism: Pneumatic system regulated by solenoids and regulators
    4. Maintenance of gas flow patterns: Modified constant flow generator
    5. Circuit: Single
    6. Gas flow and airway pressure patterns: Square wave flow with taper; rectilinear to parabolic pressure pattern
    7. Cycling parameters
       a. Volume (primary)
       b. Pressure
       c. Time (via I:E ratio limit)
    8. Limits
       a. Pressure (preset)
       b. Flow (preset)
       c. Time (result of volume and flow)
    9. Modes
       a. Control
       b. Assist/control
       c. SIMV
       d. CPAP
    10. Inspiratory airway maneuvers
        a. Sigh
        b. Inflation hold
        c. Flow taper
    11. Expiratory airway maneuvers: PEEP
    12. Alarms
        a. Patient alarms
           (1) High/low inspiratory airway pressure
           (2) Low PEEP/CPAP
           (3) Low exhaled tidal volume
           (4) I:E ratio
           (5) Apnea
        b. Machine alarms
           (1) Oxygen/compressed air system failure

        (2) Ventilator inoperative

        (3) Electric failure

    13. Monitors

      a. Exhaled minute volume

      b. Total respiratory rate

H. Bear 2 and Bear 3

    1. Pressure: Positive

    2. Powering mechanism: Electric

    3. Driving mechanism: Pneumatic system operated by solenoids and regulators

    4. Maintenance of gas flow pattern: Modified constant flow pattern

    5. Circuit: Single

    6. Gas flow and airway pressure patterns: Square wave flow with taper; rectilinear to parabolic pressure pattern

    7. Cycling parameters

      a. Volume (primary)

      b. Pressure

      c. Time (via I:E ratio limit)

    8. Limits

      a. Pressure (preset)

      b. Flow (preset)

      c. Time (result of volume and flow)

    9. Modes

      a. Control

      b. Assist/control

      c. SIMV

      d. CPAP

      e. IPS (Bear 3 only)

    10. Inspiratory airway maneuvers

      a. Sigh

      b. Inflation hold

      c. Flow taper

    11. Expiratory airway maneuvers: PEEP

    12. Alarms

      a. Patient alarms

        (1) High/low inspiratory pressure

        (2) Low PEEP/CPAP

        (3) Low exhaled tidal volume

        (4) I:E ratio

        (5) Apnea

        (6) High respiratory rate

      b. Machine alarms

        (1) Oxygen/compressed air system failure

        (2) Ventilator inoperative

        (3) High gas temperature

        (4) Electric failure

    13. Monitors

      a. Exhaled minute volume

      b. Total respiratory rate

I. Veriflo CV 2000

    1. Pressure: Positive

    2. Powering mechanism: Pneumatic

    3. Driving mechanism: Pneumatic system regulated by pneumatic relays and balanced diaphragm mechanism

4. Maintenance of gas flow pattern: Constant flow generator
5. Circuit: Single
6. Gas flow and airway pressure patterns: Square wave flow and rectilinear pressure patterns
7. Cycling parameter: Time
8. Limits
   a. Pressure (relief/pop-off)
   b. Flow (preset)
   c. Volume (result of time and flow)
9. Modes
   a. Control
   b. Assist/control
   c. SIMV
   d. CPAP
10. Inspiratory airway maneuvers: Sigh
11. Expiratory airway maneuvers: PEEP
12. Alarms
    a. Patient alarms: High/low inspiratory pressure
    b. Machine alarms: Oxygen/compressed air system failure
J. Siemens Servo 900, 900B, 900C, and 900E
   1. Pressure: Positive
   2. Powering mechanism: Combined electric/pneumatic
   3. Driving mechanism: Pneumatic system regulated by servo-mechanisms
   4. Maintenance of gas flow pattern: Modified constant flow and nonconstant flow generator
   5. Circuit: Single
   6. Gas flow and pressure patterns
      a. Square wave flow with taper; rectilinear to parabolic pressure pattern (modified constant flow)
      b. Accelerating flow and nonlinearly increasing pressure pattern (nonconstant flow)
   7. Cycling parameters
      a. Time (primary)
      b. Pressure
   8. Limits
      a. Pressure (preset)
      b. Volume (preset)
      c. Volume (result of time and volume)
   9. Modes
      a. Control
      b. Assist/control
      c. SIMV (900B, 900C, and 900E; lower rate limit 4 breaths/min with the 900E)
      d. CPAP
      e. Pressure support (900C and 900E)
      f. Pressure control (900C only): The ventilator functions as a time-cycled pressure-limited unit. Sufficient flow is provided to allow pressure to be reached rapidly and held for the remainder of the inspiratory time. In this mode the unit functions as a near-constant pressure generator.
   10. Inspiratory airway maneuvers
       a. Sigh
       b. Inflation hold (pause time percent)
       c. Accelerating flow pattern

    11. Expiratory airway maneuvers
       a. PEEP
       b. NEEP (option)
       c. Expiratory retard
    12. Alarms
       a. Patient alarms
          (1) High inspiratory pressure
          (2) High/low expired minute volume (pediatric minute volume alarm scale not available on the 900E)
          (3) Apnea (900C and 900E)
       b. Machine alarms
          (1) Power failure
          (2) Oxygen/compressed air system failure (900C, 900E)
          (3) Ventilator inoperative (900C, 900E)
          (4) High/low oxygen percent (900C and 900E)
    13. Monitors:
       a. Exhaled minute volume and tidal volume
       b. Total respiratory rate
       c. Peak, plateau, and mean pressure
       d. PEEP
       e. $F_{I_{O_2}}$
       f. Inspired tidal volume
       g. Auto-PEEP level

K. Engström 300
    1. Pressure: Positive
    2. Powering mechanism: Electric
    3. Driving mechanism: Piston system driven via rotary motion by electric motor
    4. Maintenance of gas flow pattern: Nonconstant flow generator
    5. Circuit: Double
    6. Gas flow and pressure pattern: Modified sine wave flow and modified sigmoidal pressure patterns
    7. Cycling parameter: Time (fixed I:E ratio, 1:2)
    8. Limits (preset)
       a. Pressure (relief/pop-off)
       b. Volume
    9. Modes
       a. Control
       b. IMV (option)
    10. Inspiratory airway maneuvers: Inflation hold, variable but mandatory
    11. Expiratory airway maneuvers
       a. PEEP
       b. NEEP
       c. Expiratory retard
    12. Alarms
       a. Patient alarms: Low inspiratory pressure
       b. Machine alarms: Power failure

L. Engstöm Erica
    1. Pressure: Positive
    2. Powering mechanism: Combined electric/pneumatic
    3. Driving mechanism: Modified bellows system driven by electronically regulated compressed gases
    4. Maintenance of gas flow pattern: Constant and nonconstant flow generator

   5. Circuit: Double
   6. Gas flow and pressure pattern:
      a. Square wave flow and rectilinear pressure pattern (constant flow)
      b. Accelerating flow and nonlinearly increasing pressure patterns (nonconstant flow)
      c. Decelerating flow and parabolic pressure patterns (nonconstant flow)
   7. Cycling parameters
      a. Volume (primary)
      b. Time
      c. Pressure
   8. Limits (preset)
      a. Time
      b. Pressure
      c. Flow
   9. Modes
      a. Control
      b. Assist/control
      c. SIMV
      d. Extended MMV (same as MMV)
      e. Pressure assist
      f. CPAP
  10. Inspiratory airway maneuvers
      a. Sigh
      b. Inflation hold
      c. Flow taper
  11. Expiratory airway maneuvers: PEEP
  12. Alarms
      a. Patient alarms
         (1) High/low inspiratory pressure
         (2) High/low minute volume
         (3) Apnea
      b. Machine alarms
         (1) Oxygen/compressed air system failure
         (2) Electrical failure
  13. Monitors
      a. Minute volume
      b. Total respiratory rate
M. Monaghan 225 and 225/SIMV
   1. Pressure: Positive
   2. Powering mechanism: Pneumatic
   3. Driving mechanism: Bellows system driven by compressed gas source
   4. Maintenance of gas flow pattern: Constant flow generator
   5. Circuit: Double
   6. Gas flow and pressure pattern: Square wave flow and rectilinear pressure patterns
   7. Cycling parameters
      a. Volume (primary)
      b. Pressure
      c. Time
   8. Limits (preset)
      a. Pressure
      b. Time
      c. Flow

9. Modes
    a. Control
    b. Assist
    c. Assist/control
    d. SIMV
    e. CPAP
10. Inspiratory airway maneuvers: None
11. Expiratory airway maneuvers: PEEP
12. Alarms (visual only)
    a. Patient alarms
        (1) High inspiratory pressure
        (2) I:E ratio
    b. Machine alarms: None

N. Biomed Devices IC-5
1. Pressure: Positive
2. Powering mechanism: Combined electric/pneumatic
3. Driving mechanism: Microprocessor controlled pneumatic system
4. Maintenance of gas flow pattern: Constant flow generator
5. Circuit: Single
6. Gas flow and pressure patterns: Square wave flow and rectilinear pressure patterns
7. Cycling parameters
    a. Time (primary)
    b. Pressure
8. Limits (preset)
    a. Pressure
    b. Volume
    c. Flow
9. Modes
    a. Assist/control
    b. SIMV
    c. CPAP
10. Inspiratory airway maneuvers
    a. Sigh
    b. Inflation hold
11. Expiratory airway maneuvers: PEEP
12. Alarms
    a. Patient alarms
        (1) High/low inspiratory pressure
        (2) High/low mean airway pressure
        (3) High/low PEEP
        (4) High/low tidal volume
        (5) High/low minute volume
        (6) High/low $F_{I_{O_2}}$
    b. Machine alarms
        (1) Oxygen/compressed air system failure
        (2) Fail to cycle
        (3) High/low gas temperature

O. Baby Bird (neonatal and pediatric)
1. Pressure: Positive
2. Powering mechanism: Pneumatic
3. Driving mechanism: Pneumatic system adjustable reducing valve
4. Maintenance of gas flow pattern: Constant flow generator

   5. Circuit: Single
   6. Gas flow and pressure patterns: Square wave flow and rectilinear pressure patterns
   7. Cycling parameter: Time
   8. Limits (preset)
       a. Pressure (does not cycle)
       b. Flow
   9. Modes
       a. IMV
       b. CPAP
   10. Inspiratory airway maneuvers: Inflation hold (via pressure limit setting)
   11. Expiratory airway maneuvers
       a. PEEP
       b. NEEP
   12. Alarms
       a. Patient alarms: Inspiratory time
       b. Machine alarms
          (1) Low source gas pressure
          (2) Oxygen/compressed air system failure

Note: When used as a pressure-limited, time cycled unit, the machine functions essentially as a constant pressure generator.

P. Baby Bird 2A (neonatal and pediatric)
   1. Pressure: Positive
   2. Powering mechanism: Combined electric/pneumatic
   3. Driving mechanism: Pneumatic system regulated by a microprocessor
   4. Maintenance of gas flow pattern: Constant flow generator
   5. Circuit: Single
   6. Gas flow and pressure patterns: Square wave flow and rectilinear pressure patterns
   7. Cycling parameter: Time
   8. Limits (preset)
       a. Pressure (does not cycle)
       b. Flow
   9. Modes
       a. IMV
       b. CPAP
   10. Inspiratory airway maneuvers: Inflation hold (via pressure limit)
   11. Expiratory airway maneuvers: PEEP
   12. Alarms
       a. Patient alarms
          (1) Short expiratory time
          (2) Long inspiratory time
       b. Machine alarms
          (1) Low source gas pressure (air/O_2)
          (2) Power failure

Note: When used as a pressure-limited, time cycled unit, the machine functions essentially as a constant pressure generator.

Q. Bourns LS 104-150 (neonatal and pediatric)
   1. Pressure: Positive
   2. Powering mechanism: Electric
   3. Driving mechanism: Linear motion piston system driven by electric motor
   4. Maintenance of gas flow pattern: Constant flow generator
   5. Circuit: Single

6. Gas flow and pressure patterns: Square wave flow and rectilinear pressure patterns
7. Cycling parameters
   a. Volume (primary)
   b. Pressure
8. Limits
   a. Flow (preset)
   b. Pressure (relief/pop-off or ends inspiration)
   c. Time (resultant of volume and flow)
9. Modes
   a. Control
   b. IMV
   c. Assist/control
   d. Assist
10. Inspiratory airway maneuvers: None
11. Expiratory airway maneuvers: PEEP
12. Alarms: Machine alarms
    a. Low airway pressure
    b. High airway pressure
    c. Apnea

R. Bourns BP200 (neonatal and pediatric)
1. Pressure: Positive
2. Powering mechanism: Combined electric/pneumatic
3. Driving mechanism: Pneumatic system regulated by solenoids and regulators
4. Maintenance of gas flow pattern: Constant flow generator
5. Circuit: Single
6. Gas flow and pressure pattern: Square wave flow and rectilinear pressure pattern
7. Cycling parameters: Time
8. Limits (preset)
   a. Pressure (does not cycle)
   b. Flow
9. Modes
   a. IMV
   b. CPAP
10. Inspiratory airway maneuvers: Inflation hold (via pressure limit)
11. Expiratory airway maneuvers: PEEP
12. Alarms
    a. Patient alarms: Insufficient expiratory time
    b. Machine alarms
       (1) Low source gas pressure (air/O_2)
       (2) Power failure
Note: When used as a pressure-limted, time-cycled unit, the machine functions essentially as a constant pressure generator.

S. Bear Cub Infant Ventilator BP 2001 (neonatal and pediatric)
1. Pressure: Positive
2. Positive mechanism: Combined electric/pneumatic
3. Driving mechanism: Servo-operated pneumatic system
4. Maintenance of gas flow pattern: Constant flow generator
5. Circuit: Single
6. Gas flow and pressure pattern: Square wave flow and rectilinear pressure pattern
7. Cycling parameter: Time

8. Limits (preset)
   a. Pressure (does not cycle)
   b. Flow
9. Modes
   a. IMV
   b. CPAP
10. Inspiratory airway maneuvers: Inflation hold (via pressure limit)
11. Expiratory airway maneuvers: PEEP
12. Alarms
    a. Patient alarms
       (1) Low inspiratory pressure
       (2) Low PEEP/CPAP
       (3) I:E ratio
       (4) High pressure
    b. Machine alarms
       (1) Low source gas pressure (air/O_2)
       (2) Ventilator inoperative
       (3) Electrical failure or disconnect
       (4) Rate/time incompatibility (expiratory time must be at least 0.25 second)

Note: When used as a pressure-limited, time cycled unit, the machine functions essentially as a constant pressure generator.

T. Sechrist IV-100B (neonatal and pediatric)
   1. Pressure: Positive
   2. Powering mechanism: Combined electric/pneumatic
   3. Driving mechanism: Pneumatic, controlled by a microprocessor and fluidic system
   4. Maintenance of gas flow pattern: Constant flow generator
   5. Circuit: Single
   6. Gas flow and pressure pattern: Square wave flow and rectilinear pressure pattern
   7. Cycling parameter: Time
   8. Limit (preset)
      a. Pressure (does not cycle)
      b. Flow
   9. Modes
      a. IMV
      b. CPAP
   10. Inspiratory airway maneuvers: Inflation hold (via pressure limit)
   11. Expiratory airway maneuvers: PEEP
   12. Alarms
       a. Patient alarms
          (1) Low airway pressure
          (2) Prolonged inspiratory time or expiratory time
          (3) Apnea
       b. Machine alarms: Ventilator disconnect

Note: When used as a pressure-limited, time-cycled unit, the machine functions essentially as a constant pressure generator.

U. Healthdyne 105 (neonatal and pediatric)
   1. Pressure: Positive
   2. Powering mechanism: Combined electric/pneumatic
   3. Driving mechanism: Pneumatic system regulated by microprocessors
   4. Maintenance of gas flow pattern: Constant flow generator
   5. Circuit: Single

6. Gas flow and pressure pattern: Square wave flow and rectilinear pressure pattern
7. Cycling parameter: Time
8. Limits (preset)
   a. Pressure (does not cycle)
   b. Flow
9. Modes
   a. IMV
   b. CPAP
10. Inspiratory airway maneuvers: Inflation hold (via pressure limit)
11. Expiratory airway maneuvers: PEEP
12. Alarms
   a. Patient alarms
      (1) High/low inspiratory pressure
      (2) I:E ratio
      (3) Short expiratory time
      (4) Disconnect
   b. Machine alarms
      (1) Low source gas pressure (air/O_2)
      (2) Electrical failure

Note: When used as a pressure-limited, time-cycled unit, the machine functions essentially as a constant pressure generator.

V. McGaw CV200 (neonatal and pediatric)
1. Pressure: Positive
2. Powering mechanism: Pneumatic
3. Driving mechanism: Pneumatic system regulated by relays and a balanced diaphragm
4. Maintenance of gas flow pattern: Constant flow generator
5. Circuit: Single
6. Gas flow and pressure pattern: Square wave flow and rectilinear pressure pattern
7. Cycling parameter: Time
8. Limits (preset)
   a. Pressure (does not cycle)
   b. Flow
9. Modes
   a. Control
   b. Assist/control
   c. IMV
   d. CPAP
10. Inspiratory airway maneuvers: Inflation hold (via pressure limit)
11. Expiratory airway maneuvers
   a. PEEP
   b. NEEP
12. Alarms
   a. Patient alarms
      (1) High/low inspiratory pressure
      (2) Low PEEP/CPAP
      (3) Apnea
      (4) Patient disconnect
   b. Machine alarms
      (1) Oxygen/compressed air system failure
      (2) Power failure

W. Sechrist Volume Ventilator
1. Pressure: Positive
2. Powering mechanism: Electric
3. Driving mechanism: Piston driven by microprocessor in a linear or nonlinear fashion
4. Maintenance of gas flow pattern: Selectable constant or nonconstant flow generator
5. Circuit: Single
6. Gas flow and pressure patterns: Capable of consistently producing square wave, square wave and taper, accelerating and square or sine wave flow patterns producing rectilinear, rectilinear and parabolic, accelerating and rectilinear, or sigmoidal pressure patterns, respectively
7. Cycling parameters
   a. Time (primary)
   b. Pressure
8. Limits (preset)
   a. Pressure (relief/pop-off)
   b. Volume
   c. Flow
9. Modes
   a. Control
   b. Assist/control
   c. SIMV
   d. MMV
   e. CPAP
10. Inspiratory airway maneuvers
    a. Sigh
    b. Inflation hold
    c. Selectable flow wave forms
       (1) Square
       (2) Square to taper
       (3) Accelerate to square
       (4) Sine wave
11. Expiratory airway maneuver: PEEP
12. Alarms
    a. Patient alarms
       (1) High/low tidal volume
       (2) High/low minute volume
       (3) High/low pressure
       (4) High/low respiratory rate
    b. Machine alarms
       (1) Low source gas pressures (O_2/air)
       (2) Electrical disconnect
       (3) High temperature
13. Monitors
    a. Tidal volume
    b. Minute volume
    c. Respiratory rate
X. Puritan-Bennett 7200, 7200a, and 7200sp
1. Pressure: Positive
2. Powering mechanism: Electric
3. Driving mechanism: Pneumatic sources regulated by microprocessors operating proportional solenoid valves

4. Maintenance of gas flow patterns: Constant or nonconstant flow generator
5. Circuit: Single
6. Gas flow and pressure patterns: Capable of producing consistently square, tapered, or sine wave flow patterns that produce rectilinear, parabolic or sigmoidal pressure patterns, respectively
7. Cycling parameters
    a. Volume (primary)
    b. Pressure
8. Limits (preset)
    a. Pressure
    b. Flow
    c. Time (resultant of flow pattern and volume)
9. Modes
    a. Control (volume, pressure 7200a only option)
    b. Assist/control
    c. SIMV
    d. CPAP
    e. Pressure support
    f. Flow by (option 7200a)
    g. Apnea
    h. Backup ventilation
10. Inspiratory airway maneuvers
    a. Sigh
    b. Inflation hold
    c. Selectable flow wave forms
        (1) Square
        (2) Tapered
        (3) Sine
11. Expiratory airway maneuvers: PEEP
12. Alarms
    a. Patient alarms
        (1) High/low pressure
        (2) Low tidal volume
        (3) Low minute volume
        (4) Low PEEP/CPAP pressure
        (5) High respiratory rate
        (6) Apnea (activates backup ventilation)
        (7) I:E ratio
    b. Machine alarms
        (1) Low source gas pressure (O_2/air)
        (2) Low battery
        (3) Exhalation valve leak during inspiration
        (4) Ventilator inoperative
13. Monitors
    a. Exhaled minute volume and tidal volume
    b. Total respiratory frequency
    c. Peak, plateau, and mean airway pressure
    d. PEEP
    e. Spontaneous minute volume
    f. Pressure and flow wave form (option)
    g. Compliance and resistance (option)
    h. Peak flow and negative inspiratory force (option)

Y. Ohmeda CPU-1
   1. Pressure: Positive
   2. Power mechanism: Combined electric/pneumatic
   3. Driving mechanism: Pneumatic source controlled by microprocessor operated valves
   4. Maintenance of gas flow patterns: Constant flow generator
   5. Circuit: Single
   6. Gas flow and pressure patterns: Square wave flow and rectilinear pressure pattern
   7. Cycling parameters
     a. Time (primary)
     b. Pressure (primary)
   8. Limits (preset)
     a. Volume (result of flow and inspiratory time)
     b. Flow
   9. Modes
     a. IMV
     b. SIMV
     c. MMV
     d. Pressure-cycled IMV
     e. Pressure-cycled SIMV
     f. CPAP
  10. Inspiratory airway maneuver: Sigh
  11. Expiratory airway maneuver: PEEP
  12. Alarms
     a. Patient alarms
       (1) High pressure
       (2) Low tidal Volume
       (3) I:E ratio
       (4) Apnea
       (5) Circuit disconnect and leaks
     b. Machine alarms
       (1) Source gas disconnect
       (2) Electrical disconnect or failure
       (3) Flow transducer failure
       (4) Microprocessor failure
  13. Monitors
     a. Exhaled tidal volume
     b. Total respiratory rate
     c. Exhaled minute volume

Z. Ohmeda Advent
   1. Pressure: Positive
   2. Powering mechanism: Electric and pneumatic
   3. Driving mechanism: Pneumatic/electric via a series of nine electrically controlled solenoid valves
   4. Maintenance of gas flow pattern: Functions as both a constant flow and constant pressure generator
   5. Circuit: Single
   6. Gas flow and pressure patterns: Square wave flow with rectilinear pressure pattern or decelerating flow with plateau pressure pattern
   7. Cycling
     a. Time (primary)
     b. Flow (secondary)

8. Limits
   a. Volume
   b. Pressure
   c. Time
9. Modes
   a. Control (volume and pressure)
   b. Assist/control
   c. SIMV
   d. IPS
   e. CPAP
   f. MMV
   g. Apnea ventilation
10. Inspiratory airway maneuvers: None
11. Expiratory airway maneuvers: PEEP
12. Alarms
    a. Patient
       (1) High/low airway pressure
       (2) Low minute volume
       (3) Low spontaneous exhaled tidal volume
       (4) High respiratory rate
       (5) Apnea
       (6) Inverse ratio
    b. Machine
       (1) Low gas pressure
       (2) Power failure
       (3) Ventilation inoperative
13. Patient monitors
    a. Exhaled tidal volume and minute volume
    b. Total respiratory rate
    c. PEEP, peak, plateau, and mean airway pressure
    d. Spontaneous respiratory rate and minute volume
    e. Circuit temperature
    f. Auto-PEEP level
    g. Peak flow
    h. Pressure wave form (option)
    i. Compliance and resistance (option)
AA. Hamilton Veolar and Amadeus
    1. Pressure: Positive
    2. Powering mechanism: Electric and pneumatic
    3. Driving mechanism: Pneumatic/electric via a microprocessor-controlled flow valve
    4. Maintenance of gas flow patterns: Functions as both a constant flow and constant pressure generator
    5. Circuit: Single
    6. Gas flow and pressure patterns: Square wave flow with rectilinear pressure pattern and decelerating flow with plateau pressure pattern (both units); sine wave flow with sigmoidal pressure pattern, accelerating flow with nonlinearly increasing pressure pattern and decelerating flow with parabolic pressure pattern Veolar only
    7. Cycling
       a. Volume (primarily)
       b. Flow (secondary)
       c. Time (secondary)

8. Limits
   a. Flow
   b. Time
   c. Pressure
9. Modes
   a. Control (volume and pressure (Veolar only))
   b. Assist/control
   c. SIMV
   d. CPAP
   e. IPS
   f. MMV (Veolar only)
   g. Apnea ventilation
10. Inspiratory airway maneuvers: None
11. Expiratory airway maneuvers: PEEP
12. Alarms
    a. Patient
       (1) High pressure
       (2) High/low minute volume
       (3) High respiratory rate
       (4) Apnea
       (5) Inverse I:E ratio (Amadeus only)
       (6) High/low $F_{I_{O_2}}$
    b. Machine
       (1) Turn flow sensor
       (2) Power failure
       (3) Low gas pressure
       (4) Ventilator inoperative
13. Patient monitors
    a. Exhaled minute volume and tidal volume
    b. Total respiratory frequency
    c. Peak and plateau airway pressure
    d. Mean airway pressure (Veolar)
    e. PEEP
    f. Spontaneous respiratory frequency
    g. $F_{I_{O_2}}$
    h. Inspiratory tidal volume (Veolar)
    i. Compliance and resistance
    j. Peak flow (Veolar)

BB. Bird 6400 ST
1. Pressure: Positive
2. Powering mechanism: Electric and pneumatic
3. Driving mechanism: Pneumatic/electric via regulators and a stepper motor-operated flow valve under microprocessor control
4. Maintenance of gas flow pattern: Functions as both a constant flow and constant pressure generator
5. Circuits: Single
6. Gas flow and pressure patterns: Square wave flow with rectilinear pressure pattern, decelerating flow with parabolic pressure pattern, and decelerating flow with plateau pressure pattern
7. Cycling
   a. Volume (primary)
   b. Flow (secondary)

8. Limits
   a. Volume
   b. Pressure
   c. Time
9. Modes
   a. Control
   b. Assist/control
   c. CPAP
   d. IPS
10. Inspiratory airway maneuvers: None
11. Expiratory airway maneuvers: PEEP
12. Alarms
    a. Patient
       (1) High/low airway pressure
       (2) High/low minute volume
       (3) Low PEEP
       (4) Low inspiratory tidal volume
       (5) Apnea
       (6) Inverse I:E ratio
    b. Machine
       (1) Low inlet gas pressure
       (2) Ventilator inoperative
       (3) Pressure transducer malfunction
       (4) Mode/waveform discrepancy
13. Monitors
    a. Total minute volume
    b. Total respiratory rate
    c. Inspiratory tidal volume

CC. Intermed Bear 5
   1. Pressure: Positive
   2. Powering mechanism: Electric
   3. Driving mechanism: Electric via a compressor with microprocessor-controlled stepper motor-operated flow valve
   4. Maintenance of gas flow pattern: Functions as both a constant flow and constant pressure generator
   5. Circuit: Single
   6. Gas flow and pressure patterns: Square wave flow with rectilinear pressure pattern, sine wave flow with sigmoidal pressure pattern, decelerating flow with parabolic pressure pattern, and decelerating flow with plateau pressure pattern
   7. Cycling
      a. Volume (primary)
      b. Flow (secondary)
   8. Limits
      a. Volume
      b. Pressure
      c. Time
   9. Modes
      a. Control
      b. Assist/control
      c. SIMV
      d. CPAP
      e. IPS
      f. MMV
      g. Continuous flow in CPAP

10. Inspiratory airway maneuvers: Inflation hold
11. Expiratory airway maneuvers: Expiratory retard
12. Alarms
    a. Patients
       (1) High/low pressure
       (2) High/low minute volume
       (3) Low exhaled mechanical and spontaneous tidal volume
       (4) High respiratory rate
       (5) Low CPAP
       (6) Inverse ratio
    b. Machine
       (1) Low oxygen pressure
       (2) Low air pressure
       (3) Ventilator inoperative
13. Monitors
    a. Exhaled minute volume and tidal volume
    b. Total respiratory rate
    c. Peak and mean airway pressure
    d. PEEP
    e. Circuit temp
    f. Pressure and flow wave form
    g. Compliance and resistance

DD. PPG (Drager) IRISA
1. Pressure: Positive
2. Powering mechanism: Electric and pneumatic
3. Driving mechanism: Pneumatic/electric via proportional solenoids and pressure regulators
4. Maintenance of gas flow pattern: Functions as both a constant flow and constant pressure generator
5. Circuits: Single
6. Gas flow and pressure patterns: Square wave flow with rectilinear pressure pattern or decelerating flow with plateau pressure pattern
7. Cycling
   a. Time (primary)
   b. Flow (secondary)
   c. Pressure (secondary)
8. Limits
   a. Volume
   b. Pressure
   c. Time
9. Modes
   a. Control (volume or pressure)
   b. Assist/control
   c. CPAP
   d. SIMV
   e. IPS
   f. MMV
   g. Apnea ventilation
10. Inspiratory airway maneuvers: Inflation hold
11. Expiratory airway maneuvers: PEEP
12. Alarms
    a. Patient
       (1) High/low pressure
       (2) High/low minute volume

(3) High total respiratory rate
(4) Apnea
(5) High/low $F_{I_{O_2}}$
  b. Machine
(1) Low gas pressure
(2) Machine failure
(3) Ventilator inoperative
13. Monitor
  a. Exhaled minute volume and tidal volume
  b. Total respiratory rate
  c. Peak, plateau, and mean airway pressure
  d. PEEP
  e. Spontaneous respiratory rate and minute volume
  f. Circuit temperature
  g. $F_{I_{O_2}}$
  h. Pressure and flow wave form
  i. Compliance and resistance
EE. Infrasonics Adult Star
  1. Pressure: Positive
  2. Powering mechanism: Pneumatic and electric
  3. Driving mechanism: Electric via a compressor and proportional solenoid valves under microprocessor control
  4. Maintenance of gas flow pattern: Functions as both a constant flow and constant pressure generator
  5. Circuit: Single
  6. Gas flow and pressure patterns: Square wave flow with rectilinear pressure pattern, sine wave flow with sigmoidal pressure pattern, decelerating flow with parabolic pressure pattern, decelerating flow with plateau pressure pattern, and accelerating flow with nonlinearly increasing pressure pattern
  7. Cycling
    a. Volume (primary)
    b. Pressure (secondary)
  8. Limits
    a. Volume
    b. Pressure
    c. Time
  9. Modes
    a. Control
    b. Assist/control
    c. CPAP
    d. IPS
  10. Inspiratory airway maneuvers: Inflation hold
  11. Expiratory airway maneuvers: Expiratory hold
  12. Alarms
    a. Patient
      (1) High/low pressure
      (2) Low minute volume
      (3) Low exhaled mechanical tidal volume
      (4) Low spontaneous exhaled tidal volume
      (5) High respiratory rate
      (6) Low PEEP
      (7) Apnea
      (8) Inverse I:E ratio

    b. Machine
      (1) Low oxygen pressure
      (2) Low air pressure
      (3) Low internal battery
      (4) Machine failure
13. Monitors
    a. Exhaled minute volume and tidal volume
    b. Total respiratory frequency
    c. Peak, plateau, and mean airway pressure
    d. PEEP
    e. Spontaneous minute volume
    f. Pressure, flow, and volume wave forms

BIBLIOGRAPHY

Adult Star Operating Manual. San Diego, Infrasonic, no 9910142 1989.

Advent Ventilator Technical Manual. Madison, Wis, Ohmeda Corp, 1989.

Air-Shields: *Manufacturer's Literature: Healthdyne Model 105 Infant/Pediatric Ventilator.* Hatboro, Pa, Healthdyne.

Amadeus Operating Manual. Reno, Nev, Hamilton Medical, 1989.

Bennett Medical Equipment. *Operating Instructions: Bennett Model PR1 Respiration Unit.* Los Angeles, Puritan-Bennett Corp.

Bennett Medical Equipment: *Operating Instructions: Bennett Model PR-2 Respiration Unit.* Los Angeles, Puritan-Bennett Corp.

Bio-med Devices: *Instruction Manual: Bio-med Devices 1C-5 Ventilator.* Stamford, Conn, Bio-med Devices.

Bird Products/3M: *Manufacturer's Literature: Baby Bird.* St Paul, Minn, Bird Products/3M.

Bird Products/3M: *Manufacturer's Literature: Baby Bird 2A.* St Paul, Minn, Bird Products/3M.

Bird Corporation: *Instruction Manual: Bird Mark 7 Respirator.* Palm Springs, Calif, Bird Corporation/3M.

Bird Corporation: *6400 ST Volume Ventilator Instruction Manual.* Palm Springs, Calif, Bird Products Corp, 1988.

Bourns Medical Systems: *Instruction Manual: Bourns LS 104-150D Ventilator.* Riverside, Calif, Bourns Medical System.

Dupuis YG: *Ventilator's Theory and Clinical Application.* St Louis, CV Mosby Co, 1986.

JH Emerson Company: *Manufacturer's Literature: Emerson IMV 3MV Ventilator.* Cambridge, Mass, JH Emerson Co.

JH Emerson Company: *Manufacturer's Literature: Emerson Post-Op 3PV Volume Ventilator.* Cambridge, Mass, JH Emerson Co.

Engström Medical AB: *Manufacturer's Literature: Engström 300 Ventilator.* Bromma, Sweden, Engström Medical AB.

Engström Medical AB: *Reference Manual: Engström Erica.* Bromma, Sweden, Engström Medical AB.

Hamilton Medical: *Hamilton Veolar Ventilator Operator's Manual, part no 610131.* Reno, Nev, Hamilton Medical, 1985.

Intermed Bear Medical Systems: *Instruction Manual: Bear 1 Adult Volume Ventilator.* Riverside, Calif, Bear Medical Systems.

Intermed Bear Medical Systems: *Instruction Manual: Bear 2 Adult Volume Ventilator.* Riverside, Calif, Bear Medical Systems.

Intermed Bear Medical Systems: *Instruction Manual: Bear 3 Adult Volume Ventilator.* Riverside, Calif, Bear Medical Systems.

Intermed Bear Medical Systems: *Instruction Manual: Bear Cub Infant Ventilator Model BP2001.* Riverside, Calif, Bear Medical Systems.

Intermed Bear Medical Systems: *Instruction Manual: Infant Ventilator Model BP200.* Riverside, Calif, Bear Medical Systems.

Intermed Bear Medical Systems: *Instructional Manual: Bear 5 Ventilator*. Riverside, Calif, Bear Med Systems.

IRISA Ventilator Operating Manual no 23504069-001A. Lenexa, Kan, PPG Biomedical Systems, 1988.

Kacmarek RM, Meklaus G: New generation of mechanical ventilators, in Tobin MJ (ed): *Mechanical Ventilation. Critical Care Clinics*. Philadelphia, WB Saunders Co (in press).

Kacmarek RM, Meklaus G: Microprocessor controlled mechanical ventilators, in Banner MJ (ed): *Positive Pressure Ventilation. Problems in Critical Care*. Philadelphia, JB Lippincott Co (in press).

Kacmarek RM, Spearman CB: New generation mechanical ventilators: Seimens Servo 900C. *Respir Times* 1987; 2(8):7–8.

Kacmarek RM, Spearman CB: New generation mechanical ventilators: The Puritan-Bennett 7200/7200a. *Respir Times* 1988; 3(3):7–9.

Kacmarek RM, Spearman CB: The new generation mechanical ventilators: The Hamilton Medical Veolar. *Respir Times* 1988; 3(5):8–9.

Life Products: *Operation Manual: Model LP5 Volume ventilator*. Boulder, Colo, Life Products.

McGaw Respiratory Therapy: *Manufacturer's Literature: CV200 Neonatal Ventilator*. Carlsbad, Calif, AHSC/International Export.

McGaw Respiratory Therapy: *Manufacturer's Literature: Monaghan 225/SIMV Volume Ventilator*. Plattsburgh, NY, Monaghan Medical Corp.

McPherson SP: *Respiratory Therapy Equipment*, ed 3. St Louis, CV Mosby Co, 1985.

Mushin WW, et al: *Automatic Ventilation of the Lungs*, ed 3. Boston, Blackwell Scientific Publications, 1980.

Newport Medical Instructions: *Manufacturer's Literature: The E100 Ventilator*. Newport Beach, Calif, Newport Medical Instruments.

Ohio Medical Products: *Manufacturer's Literature: CPU1 Ventilator*. Madison, Wis, Ohio Medical Products.

Puritan-Bennett Corporation: *Operating Instructions: MA-1 Ventilator*. Kansas City, Mo, Puritan-Bennett Corp.

Puritan-Bennett Corporation: *Operating Instructions: MA2 and MA2 + 2 Ventilators*. Kansas City, Mo, Puritan-Bennett Corp.

Puritan-Bennett Corporation: *Manufacturer's Literature: 7200 Microprocessor Ventilator*. Kansas City, Mo, Puritan-Bennett Corp.

Sechrist Industries: *Operational Instructions Manual: Model IV-100B Infant Ventilator*. Anaheim, Calif, Sechrist Industries, Medical Products Division.

Sechrist Industries: *Operational Instructions Manual: Sechrist Volume Ventilator*. Anaheim, Calif, Sechrist Industries, Medical Products Division.

Siemens-Elema AB: *Operating Manual: Servo Ventilator 900/900B*. Solona, Sweden, Siemens-Elema AB.

Siemens-Elema AB: *Training Instructions: Servo Ventilator 900C*. Solona, Sweden, Siemens-Elema AB.

Smith RA, Desautels DA, Kirby RR: Mechanical ventilators, in Kirby RR, Smith RA, Desautels DA (eds): *Mechanical Ventilation*. New York, Churchill-Livingstone, 1985.

Vandine JD: Mechanical ventilators, in Barnes TA (ed): *Respiratory Care Practice*. Chicago, Year Book Medical Publishers, 1988.

Chapter 36 _____

Continuous Mechanical Ventilation

I. Physiologic Effects of Positive Pressure in Relation to Continuous Mechanical Ventilation
   A. Increased mean airway pressure
      1. Normally mean airway pressure is about zero (or atmospheric) (see Fig 4–4).
      2. Since positive pressure ablates the normal mechanisms for gas movement, intrapulmonary pressures are always supraatmospheric (see Fig 32–1).
      3. The extent that intrapulmonary pressure is increased is dependent on:
         a. Tidal volume (V_T).
         b. Inspiratory time (T_i).
         c. Inspiratory: expiratory (I:E) ratio.
         d. Respiratory rate (RR).
         e. Airway resistance (R_{AW}).
         f. Pulmonary and thoracic compliance.
   B. Increased mean intrathoracic pressure (Fig 36–1)
      1. Transmission of intrapulmonary pressure to the intrathoracic space is dependent on pulmonary and thoracic compliance. In general, the stiffer the lung, the lower the amount of pressure transmitted from the intrapulmonary to the intrathoracic space. In contrast, the stiffer the thorax, the greater the amount of pressure transmitted to the intrathoracic space.
      2. In most patients requiring mechanical ventilation, *the mean intrathoracic pressure changes from negative to positive.*
   C. Decreased venous return (see Fig 36–1)
      1. Since intrathoracic pressures become positive with the application of mechanical ventilation, the thoracic pump mechanism assisting venous return is eliminated.
      2. As a result, the pressure gradient favoring venous flow to the right side of the heart is decreased, and right ventricular filling is impaired.
      3. Frequently the decreased transmural pressure across the vena cava is large enough to require fluid therapy to maintain appropriate right ventricular filling.

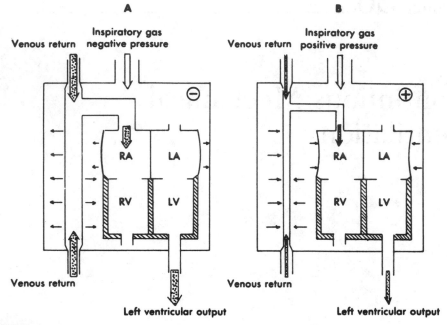

FIG 36–1.
A, effect of spontaneous ventilation or negative pressure ventilation on intrathoracic pressure and cardiac output. **B,** effect of positive pressure on intrathoracic pressure and cardiac output. (From Spearman CB, Sheldon RL, Egan DF: *Egan's Fundamentals of Respiratory Therapy,* ed 4. St Louis, CV Mosby Co, 1982. Used by permission.)

4. Most patients are hypoxemic, acidotic, and hypercarbic prior to the institution of mechanical ventilation, which causes an increased sympathetic tone. The normalization of acid-base balance, the relief of hypoxemia, and the decrease in work of breathing results in a marked decrease in sympathetic tone. This may result in:
   a. Decreased vascular tone and relative hypovolemia.
   b. Decreased heart rate.
   c. Decreased force of myocardial contraction.
D. Decreased cardiac output
   1. Since venous return and sympathetic tone are decreased, there is some decrease in cardiac output.
   2. With appropriate fluid therapy and pharmacologic support, adequate cardiac output can be maintained.
E. Increased intracranial pressure
   1. Since venous return is decreased, blood will pool in the periphery and in the cranium.
   2. The increased volume of blood in the cranium will increase intracranial pressure.
F. Decreased urinary output
   1. Decreased cardiac output results in decreased renal blood flow, which alters renal filtration pressures and diminishes urine formation.
   2. Decreased venous return and decreased right atrial pressures are interpreted as a decrease in overall blood volume. As a result, antidiuretic hormone levels are increased and urine formation is decreased (see Chapters 9 and 15).

G. Decreased work of breathing (WOB)
  1. Since the force necessary to ventilate is provided by the ventilator, the patient's WOB decreases.
  2. The amount of work performed by the ventilator and the amount performed by the patient vary, depending on the approach used to ventilate (see section IV).
H. Mechanical bronchodilation
  1. Positive pressure causes a mechanical dilation of all conducting airways.
  2. The transmural pressure gradients affecting the airways are always greater than during normal spontaneous ventilation.
I. Increased deadspace ventilation
  1. Since positive pressure distends conducting airways and inhibits venous return, the portion of the V_T that is deadspace increases.
  2. In addition, there is an alteration of normal distribution of ventilation. A greater percentage of ventilation goes to the apices and less to the bases than in spontaneous ventilation.
  3. Normal deadspace/V_T ratios are 0.20 to 0.40; however, mechanical ventilation will cause these ratios to increase to 0.40 to 0.60 in the normal individual.
J. Increased intrapulmonary shunt
  1. With positive pressure ventilation, gas distribution and pulmonary perfusion are altered.
  2. Ventilation to the most gravity-dependent aspects of the lung is decreased, whereas blood flow to these areas is increased.
  3. Normal intrapulmonary shunts are about 2.0% to 5.0%; however, mechanical ventilation may increase the shunt fraction to about 10% in the normal individual.
  4. Allowing some level of spontaneous ventilation (partial ventilatory support; see section IV) minimizes the ventilation/perfusion mismatch.
K. Manipulation of level of ventilation: Hyperventilation or hypoventilation may be induced by inappropriate setting of parameters.
L. Respiratory rate, V_T, I_T, and flow rate may all be manipulated.
M. Effect on gastrointestinal (GI) tract: The stress produced by positive pressure ventilation may lead to increased gastric secretion, resulting in the development of stress ulcers.
N. Effect on psychologic status: The continued stress associated with mechanical ventilation may result in:
  1. Insomnia.
  2. Anxiety.
  3. Frustration.
  4. Depression.
  5. Apprehension.
  6. Fear.
II. Indications for Mechanical Ventilation
  • Numerous pathophysiologic conditions may necessitate mechanical ventilation. However, each may be categorized into one of the following general indications:
A. Apnea: The cessation of breathing
B. Acute ventilatory failure: A P_{CO_2} of more than 50 mm Hg along with a pH less than 7.30.
C. Impending acute ventilatory failure
  1. This is a clinical prognosis based on serial laboratory data and clinical findings indicating that the patient is progressing toward ventilatory failure.
  2. Clinical problems frequently resulting in impending acute ventilatory failure may be categorized as:

     a. Primary pulmonary abnormalities, such as:
       (1) Respiratory distress syndrome (RDS).
       (2) Pneumonia.
       (3) Pulmonary emboli.
     b. Abnormalities associated with the mechanical ability of the lung to move air, such as:
       (1) Ventilatory muscle fatigue.
       (2) Nutritional deficiencies.
       (3) Chest injury.
       (4) Thoracic abnormalities.
       (5) Pleural disease.
       (6) Myoneural disease.
       (7) Neurologic disease.
3. Clinical evaluation of the patient in impending acute ventilatory failure
     a. Vital signs: With increased cardiopulmonary stress, pulse and blood pressure typically increase. If bacterial infection is present, temperature also increases.
     b. Ventilatory parameters: As WOB increases:
       (1) The V_T decreases.
       (2) The RR increases.
       (3) Accessory muscle use increases.
     c. Paradoxical breathing may occur.
     d. Retractions may be noted.
     e. Ventilatory reserve is decreased.
       (1) If vital capacity (VC) decreases acutely below 10 ml/kg of ideal body weight, ventilatory failure may be imminent.
       (2) If maximum inspiratory pressure is less than -20 cm H_2O in 20 seconds, ventilatory failure may be imminent.
       (3) As V_T becomes a greater percentage of VC, the likelihood of the development of ventilatory failure increases.
     f. Development of impending acute ventilatory failure may demonstrate, for example:
       (1) Progressive muscle weakness in patients with neuromuscular or neurologic diseases.
       (2) Continued progress of pulmonary or plural infections.
       (3) *Increasing fatigue* associated with any cardiorespiratory disease. Fatigue can be the primary factor precipitating impending acute ventilatory failure in any disease state.
       (4) Serial blood gases demonstrating a trend toward acute ventilatory failure. *For example:*

	9 A.M.	10 A.M.	11 A.M.	12 P.M.
pH	7.58	7.53	7.46	7.38
P_{CO_2} (mm Hg)	22	28	35	42
HCO_3^- (mEq/L)	21	22	23	24
P_{O_2} (mm Hg)	60	55	50	43

       Along with these results, the patient's RR, heart rate, and blood pressure continue to increase while the V_T decreases.
       (a) Without intervention to break this trend, a blood gas value measured at 1 P.M. may show a pH of 7.33 and a P_{CO_2} of 48 mm Hg, whereas at 2 P.M. the pH may be 7.28 and the P_{CO_2} 53 mm Hg.

(b) As a result, the decision may be made at 12 noon to institute mechanical ventilation because the patient is in impending acute ventilatory failure.

Note: None of the material just presented discussed oxygenation, because oxygenation is not a direct indication for ventilation. However, the increased WOB associated with attempting to maintain a normal oxygenation state may precipitate impending acute ventilatory failure. *It is ventilatory problems that require mechanical ventilation, not oxygenation problems.* Oxygenation problems are treated with oxygen therapy, positive end-expiratory pressure (PEEP), or cardiovascular stabilization.

III. Ventilator Commitment
  A. Ventilate with bag and mask, then establish an artificial airway.
  B. Manually support ventilation.
    1. Reverse hypercarbia and acidosis.
    2. Decrease WOB.
    3. Slowly alter patient's ventilatory pattern to pattern desired during mechanical ventilation.
  C. Stabilize cardiovascular system
    1. Prior to manual ventilation, the patient's sympathetic tone is pronounced because of:
      a. Hypercarbia.
      b. Acidosis.
      c. Hypoxemia.
      d. Generalized increased stress.
    2. Since manual ventilation and mechanical ventilation inhibit venous return and theoretically reverse hypercarbia, acidosis, and hypoxemia, a decreased sympathetic tone results. *This may result in hypotension when manual or mechanical ventilation is instituted.*
    3. The use of narcotics may also add to the hypotensive state.
    4. Fluid therapy may be essential during ventilator commitment (see Chapter 15).
    5. In addition, some patients may require the use of sympathomimetics for beta-one effects (see Chapter 40).
  D. Record baseline values for:
    1. Vital signs.
    2. Blood gases.
  E. Institute appropriate cardiovascular and pulmonary monitors.
    1. Electrocardiogram
    2. Arterial line
    3. Central venous line
    4. Pulmonary artery line
  F. Determine settings on the ventilator (see section IV).
  G. Sedate and/or paralyze patient, if indicated.
  H. Attach patient to ventilator. Transition should be smooth, orderly, and controlled.
IV. Determination of Settings on the Mechanical Ventilator
  A. Modes (technical)
    1. Control (Fig 36–2)
      a. Patient is unable to control any aspect of gas delivery.
      b. All WOB is taken over by the ventilator.
      c. Sedation is typically required.
      d. The use of the technical mode setting of control is discouraged, because if the patient sedation wears off, fighting of the ventilator frequently results.

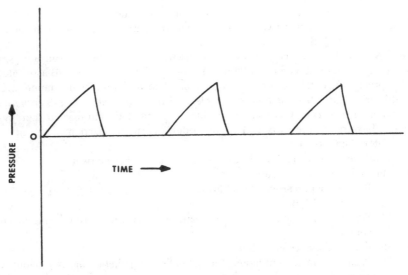

FIG 36–2.
Ventilator system pressure curve developed during control mode ventilation. No negative deflections should be noted.

  e. Control mode ventilation can be "mimicked" with assist/control, intermittent mandatory ventilation (IMV), or synchronized IMV (SIMV), by giving proper sedation.
  f. Control mode ventilation is useful:
    (1) During the first 24 to 48 hours of initiation of mechanical ventilation to ensure rest.
    (2) During severe adult RDS (ARDS), especially if high levels of PEEP are required, or the I:E ratio is reversed.
    (3) During the early postoperative mechanical ventilatory period if prolonged ventilation is required.
2. Assist (Fig 36–3)
  a. The patient is able to control the ventilatory rate.
  b. The machine performs the vast majority of the WOB.
  c. *This mode should not be used for continuous ventilation because if the patient becomes apneic, ventilation stops.*
3. Assist/control (Fig 36–4)
  a. The patient is able to control the ventilatory rate as long as the spontaneous rate is greater than the machine backup rate; if not, the machine goes into control mode.
  b. The machine performs the majority of the WOB.
  c. Because the patient controls the ventilatory rate, wide swings in acid-base status may occur. This is particularly true with central nervous system (CNS) disturbances and bulbar involvement.
  d. As the patient-initiated ventilatory rate increases, the mean intrapulmonary pressure increases and normally results in an increased mean intrathoracic pressure, a decrease in venous return, and air trapping with auto-PEEP. (See Section V.G.)
  e. Sedation is frequently required to prevent hyperventilation.
  f. Assist/control is useful during the early phases of ventilatory support where rest is required. Careful setting of the peak flow and inspiratory time T_I is essential to ensure minimal effort. See subsequent sections.

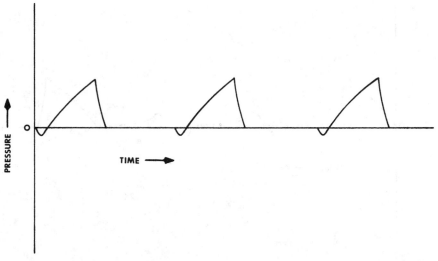

FIG 36-3.
Ventilator system pressure curve developed during assist mode ventilation. The negative deflection prior to inspiration is the patient triggering the breath.

    g. It is useful for long-term maintenance of patients not yet ready to wean.
    h. It is useful during rest periods in patients being weaned, in patients using a T piece, or in continuous positive airway pressure (CPAP) trials.
  4. Intermittent mandatory ventilation (IMV) (Fig. 36-5)
    a. Positive pressure ventilation is provided by a control mode breath on a periodic basis.
    b. In between positive pressure breaths, the patient breathes spontaneously.
    c. Gas flow during spontaneous ventilation is provided by an external continuous gas flow system or an internal demand valve.

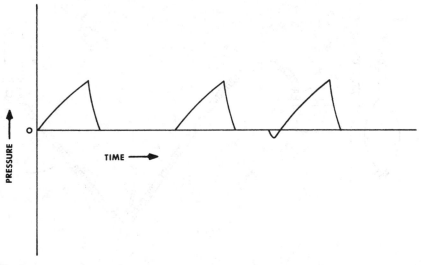

FIG 36-4.
Ventilatory system pressure curve developed during assist/control mode ventilation. Assist breaths are mixed with control breaths. The negative deflection prior to inspiration is the patient triggering the assist breath.

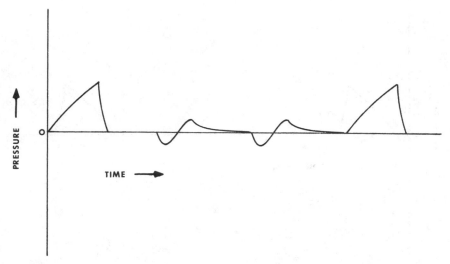

FIG 36−5.
Ventilator system pressure curve developed during IMV mode ventilation. The positive pressure breaths are always control breaths.

(1) Demand trigger sensitivity must be set to prevent increased WOB. Many of today's mechanical ventilators provide small levels of inspiratory pressure support (IPS) (1−3 cm H_2O) during demand system breathing. Inappropriate humidifier selection, water condensate in tubing, and preventive maintenance of equipment affect imposed WOB.

(2) Continuous gas flow systems should always be of the *closed rather than the open type* (Fig 36−6).

(a) At least four times the patient's measured spontaneous minute volume should be entering the system (60−90 L/min).

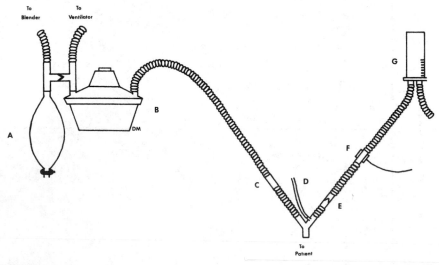

FIG 36−6.
Continuous flow IMV circuit. **A,** 5-L reservoir attached to ventilator's inspiratory limb via one-way valve; **B,** large-volume humidifier; **C,** temperature probe; **D,** proximal system pressure manometer attachment; **E,** optional one-way valve in expiratory limb; **F,** exhalation valve; **G,** Emerson water column PEEP valve.

(b) Throughout the spontaneous breathing phase, gas should be continuously leaving the exhalation valve.

(c) A 3- to 5-L reservoir attached proximal to the system humidifier should be used.

(d) System pressure fluctuations should not exceed ±2 cm H_2O.

d. Sedation may be necessary.

e. Intermittent mandatory ventilation is useful during the early phases of ventilatory support where rest of ventilatory muscles is required. Careful setting of peak flow and T_I is essential to reduce work of breathing. Sedation usually required.

f. It is useful for long-term maintenance of patients not yet ready to wean (same concerns as in no. 4e).

g. It is used as a weaning technique in *short-term* ventilator-dependent patients without ventilatory muscle dysfunction.

h. It is useful during rest periods in patients being weaned, in patients using a T piece, or in CPAP trials. It ensures a high enough IMV rate to allow rest (8–12 breaths/min (bpm)).

5. Synchronized intermittent mandatory ventilation (Fig 36–7)

a. Positive pressure ventilation is provided by a periodic assist/control breath.

b. In between positive pressure breaths, the patient is allowed to breathe spontaneously.

c. Gas flow during spontaneous ventilation is provided by a demand system (Fig 36–8). If the system is a true SIMV system, a demand valve must be used. Continuous flow would interfere with the patient's triggering of the positive pressure breath. Some ventilators (e.g., Bear 5 and CPU 1) do use low-level bias flows. Patient trigger may be adversely affected in these situations.

Note: Because many of the demand valves may respond poorly and cause an increased WOB, it is not advisable to use the SIMV mode at rates of 4 bpm or less or to use the CPAP mode on these ventilators. Under these circumstances, the system should be transformed to or replaced by an IMV system or a continuous flow CPAP system (see Chapter 37) or IPS should be provided.

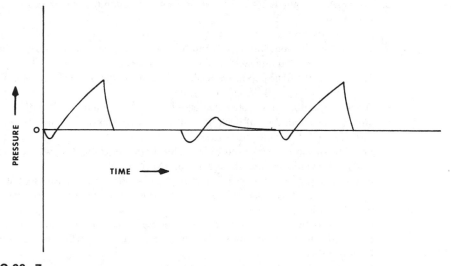

FIG 36–7.
Ventilator system pressure curve developed during SIMV mode ventilation. The positive pressure breaths are normally assist breaths.

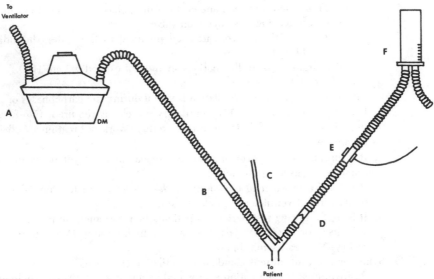

FIG 36–8.
SIMV circuit. **A,** large-volume humidifier; **B,** temperature probe; **C,** proximal demand valve probe attachment; **D,** one-way valve expiratory limb; **E,** exhalation valve; **F,** Emerson water column PEEP valve.

    d. Sedation may be necessary.
    e. Synchronized intermittent mandatory ventilation is useful during the early phase of ventilatory support where rest of ventilatory muscles is required. (Careful setting of peak flow and T_I is essential to reduce WOB. Sedation is usually required.)
    f. It is useful for long-term maintenance of patients not yet ready to wean (same concerns as in no. 5e).
    g. It is used as a weaning technique in *short-term* ventilator-dependent patients without ventilatory muscle dysfunction.
  6. Inspiratory pressure support (IPS) (Fig 36–9)
    a. The ventilator functions as a constant pressure generator during patient assist ventilation.
      (1) A positive pressure is set.
      (2) Once the patient initiates inspiration, a predetermined pressure is rapidly established and held at the patient's airway.
    b. The patient ventilates spontaneously, establishing his or her own rate, V_T, T_I, peak inspiratory flow, and I:E ratio.
    c. When inspiratory flow rates decreased to a designated level (with most units this is about 25% of peak flow), the positive pressure returns to baseline, allowing the patient to exhale.
    d. Pressure support can be used independently or in conjunction with CPAP, SIMV, or mandatory minute ventilation (MMV).
    e. Inspiratory pressure support is a pure assist mode; thus, it is essential to ensure an intact ventilatory drive. Some ventilators have backup ventilation available during IPS.
    f. It may be indicated to reduce the work imposed by ventilator demand systems and endotracheal tubes. Usually 5 to 20 cm H_2O IPS are necessary for this indication.
    g. It has been frequently used as a weaning technique.
      (1) A set IPS_{max} (12 ml/kg V_T) is achieved by adjusting the IPS level, then slowly reducing the IPS as clinical status improves.

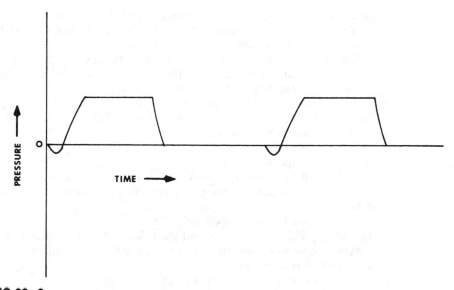

FIG 36–9.
Ventilator system pressure curve developed during pressure support. The negative deflection indicates patient triggering.

(2) Two IPS levels are alternately used to work and rest the ventilatory muscles, one level being IPS_{max} (for rest) and a secondary level being a lower level of IPS, producing a normal patient V_T.

(3) Inspiratory pressure support is used to maintain a normal V_T along with SIMV. High SIMV rates (8–12 bpm) are used to rest with IPS. No SIMV is given during work periods.

(4) Assist/control is used to rest with IPS levels to establish normal V_{TS} during work

(5) Low levels of CPAP 3 to 7 cm H_2O are frequently used with IPS.

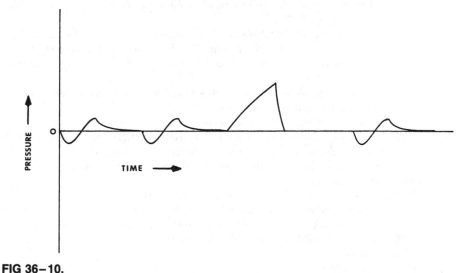

FIG 36–10.
Ventilator system pressure curve developed during MMV. Positive pressure breaths are delivered only if the patient's spontaneous minute volume is not at or above the mandatory level.

       (6) Inspiratory pressure support combined with MMV improves safety, since a decrease in ventilatory drive results in an activation of an MMV volume–limited breath.

       (7) The use of continuous flow in-line nebulizer therapy with IPS may result in an inability to trigger the IPS breath and hypoventilation. The use of a backup SIMV rate is usually necessary.

7. Mandatory minute ventilation (MMV) (Fig 36–10)
    a. The desired minute volume (MV) is set on the ventilator.
    b. The patient may receive this volume:
       (1) Entirely as positive pressure MV.
       (2) Entirely as spontaneous MV.
       (3) As a varying combination of spontaneous and positive pressure MV.
    c. As long as the patient's MV exceeds the set MV, no mechanical breaths are delivered.
    d. Both CPAP and IPS can be used with MMV.
    e. The major problem with the present algorithms for MMV is that a rapid shallow ventilatory pattern may satisfy the set MV even though the ventilatory pattern is inappropriate.

8. Pressure control inverse ratio ventilation (PC-IRV) (Fig 36–11)
    a. Pressure-limited plateau inspiration is used with T_I exceeding expiratory time.
    b. Patients must be sedated and paralyzed during the use of PC-IRV.
    c. Peak airway pressures are greatly reduced with this mode.
    d. Usually, auto-PEEP is developed as expiratory time is decreased. Unless auto-PEEP's presence is monitored, it is frequently overlooked.
    e. The improved Po_2 appears to be a result of the high level of PEEP (applied + auto-PEEP).
    f. Primary problems are hemodynamic compromise and barotrauma.
    g. Contraindicated in the presence of dynamic airflow limitation.

9. Airway pressure release ventilation (APRV) (Fig 36–12)
    a. It is very similar to PC-IRV except that the patient is allowed to breathe spontaneously during the plateau pressure (P_{plat}) inspiration and expiration.
    b. All systems available are homemade continuous flow systems establishing two levels of CPAP.
    c. The high level of CPAP is established in relationship to oxygenation. Normally it is high enough to keep the $F_{I_{O_2}}$ below 0.50 (10–30 cm H_2O).
    d. The low level is set between 0 and 10 cm H_2O simply to maintain airways open.
    e. The rate of pressure dropped to the lower level of CPAP is dependent on the need for ventilatory assistance.
    f. Usually an inverse I:E ratio is maintained.
    g. Airway pressure release ventilation is used in ARDS, noncardiogenic pulmonary edema, and postoperative ventilatory management.
    h. It is contraindicated in the presence of dynamic airflow limitation.

B. Full ventilatory support
    1. The ventilator provides the vast majority of the WOB.
    2. Full ventilatory support is defined arbitrarily as a positive pressure rate of 8 bpm or more without significant spontaneous ventilation.
    3. It can be accomplished in the following modes:
       a. Control
       b. Assist/control
       c. IMV

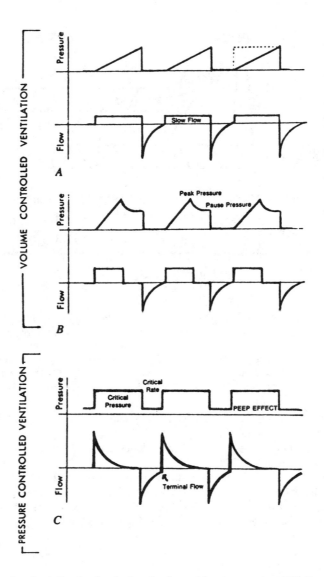

FIG 36–11.
Methods of inversing the I:E ratio. **A,** slowing the flow while at a constant RR allows the inspiratory phase to encroach onto the expiratory period. This wastes the early portion of inspiration because many unstable lung units may still be continuing to empty, despite being in the inspiratory portion of the cycle *(dotted area).* **B,** progressive prolongation of an end-inspiratory pause results in eventual reversal of the I:E ratio. This results in peak pressure that can overinflate more compliant regions before dropping to a pause (static pressure), which may be below the critical pressure necessary to maintain unstable lung units open. **C,** rapid insufflation with a decelerating flow maintains a preset pressure throughout inspiration. The critical rate is determined by setting each new breath to begin just prior to terminal flow returning to zero. Appropriate selection of I:E ratio and RR results in the desired PEEP effect (auto-PEEP). (From Gurevitch MJ: Selection of inspiratory-expiratory ratios, in Kacmarek RM, Stoller JK [eds]: *Current Respiratory Care.* Toronto, BC Decker, 1988. Used by permission.)

       d. SIMV
       e. MMV
       f. IPS (high-pressure IPS_{max})
       g. PC-IRV
       h. APRV

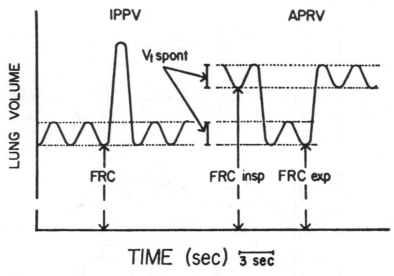

FIG 36–12.
Theoretic spirometoric tracing depicting change in lung volume that occurs in a patient with a mechanical IPPV breath compared with the change that would occur with an APRV breath. Inspiratory lung volume is the lung volume during spontaneous inspiration with CPAP during APRV. Expiratory lung volume is the lung volume during release of P_{AW} during APRV (i.e., lung volume after mechanical expiration). Expiratory lung volume is similar to functional residual capacity *(FRC)* during IPPV. (From Stock MC, Downs JB, Frolicher DA: *Crit Care Med* 1987; 15:462–466. Used by permission.)

    4. Most patients require full ventilatory support for the first 24 to 48 hours of ventilatory support.

    5. Regardless of the mode chosen, sedation is usually needed.

C. Partial ventilatory support

    1. The patient performs a significant portion of the WOB.

    2. Partial ventilatory support is defined arbitrarily as a positive pressure rate of 7 bpm or less where the patient is contributing significantly to the WOB.

    3. It can be accomplished in only the following modes:

      a. IMV

      b. SIMV

      c. IPS

      d. MMV

      e. APRV

    4. It may be indicated in the majority of patients after 24 to 48 hours of ventilatory support.

    5. Advantages

      a. Ventilation is provided in a more normal physiologic manner.

      b. Mean intrathoracic pressures are lower than with full ventilatory support.

      c. The distribution of gas is more normal than with full ventilatory support.

      d. The efficacy of PEEP is generally increased.

D. Tidal volume and ventilatory rate (Table 36–1)

    1. Large Vts with slow ventilatory rates are used in preference to small Vts and rapid rates because:

      a. Alveolar ventilation is increased.

      b. Distribution of inspired gas is improved.

      c. Mean intrathoracic pressure is reduced.

      d. Compressible volume is present in the ventilatory circuit.

TABLE 36-1.

Respiratory Rates and Tidal Volumes

Patient Type	Rate (bpm)	V_T (ml/kg)
Average patient with normal lungs	8-12	12-15
COPD	≤ 8-10 Lengthy expiratory time	12-15
chronic pulmonary restriction	>12-20	≤10
Severe, acute lung injury	>12-20	≤10

  e. Oxygenation is improved.
  f. Ventilation is improved.
  g. Sense of dyspnea is decreased.
 2. Tidal volume settings in adults range between 10 and 20 ml/kg of *ideal* body weight. Normally, initial V_Ts are calculated at 12 to 15 ml/kg of ideal body weight.
 3. Ventilatory rates in adults normally range between 4 and 12 bpm. However, patients with very stiff lungs may require much higher rates.
 4. This V_T–ventilatory rate relationship is indicated in all patients except those with severe acute or chronic restrictive pulmonary disease.
  a. In these patients small volumes and rapid rates are used because of the decrease in lung volumes associated with the disease.
  b. Tidal volume values in the range of 5 to 10 ml/kg of ideal body weight and RR of 20 to 30 bpm or more may be necessary.
E. Inspiratory time
 1. In most adults T_Is are maintained between 0.75 and 1.25 seconds.
 2. An estimate of T_I can be made by using the following formula:

$$T_I = \frac{V_T}{\text{Flow}} \tag{1}$$

where T_I is in seconds, V_T is in liters, and flow is in liters per second.

  Thus, if the V_T were 1.0 L and the flow rate 60 L/min, or 1 L/sec, the T_I would be 1 second:

$$T_I = \frac{1.0 \text{ L}}{1 \text{ L/sec}} = 1 \text{ second}$$

  a. This estimate may be slightly on the low side because most ventilators are incapable of maintaining a constant flow.
  b. This estimate can be used only if the ventilator is designed to deliver a square wave flow pattern.
  c. If the flow pattern is nonconstant, a stopwatch may be used to estimate T_I.
 3. Many patients fight positive pressure breaths because the time over which the breath is delivered is too lengthy. Decreasing the T_I until the positive pressure T_I equals the spontaneous breathing T_I normally decreases fighting of the delivered breath.

   4. If T_Is and peak flow rates do not correspond to patients' spontaneous levels, WOB may be equal to that during spontaneous breathing and, as a result, excessive (Fig 36–13).
   5. Inspiratory time is of concern because of its effect on mean intrathoracic pressure. The greater the T_I, the higher the mean intrathoracic pressure. This is usually true even if the peak airway pressure (PAP) is increased when the T_I is decreased. The length of time pressure is applied to the airway has a greater effect on mean airway pressure than does PAP.
F. Flow rate
   1. In most adult patients, flow rates are set between 40 and 80 L/min.
   2. The flow rate settings used are dependent on the desired T_I and the V_T, as in equation 1.
   3. Inadequate flows result in patients fighting the delivered breath and potentially working as hard as they were breathing spontaneously (see Fig 36–13).
   4. Most ventilators that are designed to provide a square wave flow pattern are actually incapable of maintaining a constant flow throughout inspiration. That is, the flow rate tapers toward the end of inspiration.
   5. A flow taper setting is available on many ventilators. Activation of the flow taper setting is used to improve the distribution of inspired gas.
G. Intermittent mandatory ventilation, CPAP systems, and continuous flow
   1. At least four times the patient's measured minute volume should enter the system (60–90 L/min).
   2. Gas should leave the system throughout the patient's spontaneous ventilatory cycle. Flow should be measurable leaving the exhalation valve during peak spontaneous inspiration.
   3. If flows are not sufficient to meet the patient's peak inspiratory demands, the WOB may markedly increase.
H. Inflation hold (Fig 32–14)
   1. Inflation hold is the maintenance of the delivered V_T or of a fixed pressure in the airway at the terminal portion of inspiration.

FIG 36–13.

Top, theoretical relationship between actual and ideal airway pressure curve during assisted mechanical breaths (assist/control or SIMV). No difference should exist between control breath and assisted breath. *Bottom,* actual airway pressure curve differences. The *hatched area* represents work performed by the patient during an assisted volume limited breath. If inspiratory flows and inspiratory times are inappropriate, patient WOB during assisted breathing may equal that during spontaneous breathing. (From Marini JJ, Rodriguez RM, Lamb V: *Am Rev Respir Dis* 1986; 134:902–909. Used by permission.)

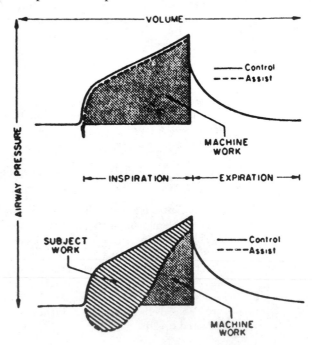

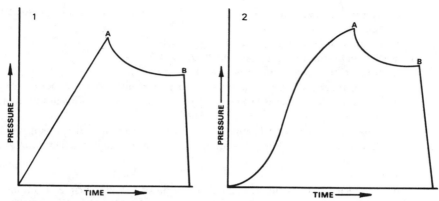

FIG 36–14.
Ideal pressure curves for square wave flow pattern with inflation hold **(1)** and sine wave flow pattern with inflation hold **(2).** The pressure drop from **A** to **B** indicates equilibrium between mouth and alveolar pressure during inflation hold period.

　　2. It improves the distribution of inspired gas in situations where regional variations in airway resistance and compliance cause ventilation/perfusion mismatch.

　　3. The length of time an inflation hold is activated is normally between 0.1 and 1.0 second.

　　4. When an inflation hold is used, it extends the *total inspiratory time* and thus may adversely affect mean intrathoracic pressure.

　　5. If an inflation hold is used, an increase in flow rate may be necessary to keep the total inspiratory time between 0.75 and 1.25 seconds, unless pharmacologic control ventilation is used.

　　6. Use of an inflation hold and lengthy inspiratory time normally result in fighting of the ventilator and increased WOB in the spontaneously breathing patient.

　I. Expiratory retard (Fig 36–15)

　　1. Expiratory retard is the application of a fixed resistance during exhalation.

　　2. This increases the length of time it takes for PAP to return to baseline during exhalation.

　　3. Expiratory retard is used to prevent premature closure of small airways during exhalation.

　　4. This maneuver is used primarily with obstructive pulmonary disease.

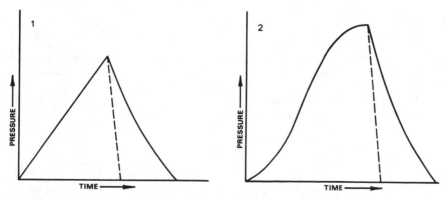

FIG 36–15.
Ideal pressure curves for square wave flow pattern with expiratory retard **(1)** and sine wave flow pattern with expiratory retard **(2).** *Dotted line* denotes "normal" return of pressure to baseline.

      5. The extent that expiratory retard is used is dependent on the severity of air trapping.

      6. Mean intrathoracic pressure may be increased.

  J. Positive end-expiratory pressure (see Chapter 37)

  K. Negative end-expiratory pressure (NEEP) (Fig 36–16)

      1. This is the maintenance of a subatmospheric airway pressure at end-exhalation.

      2. Theoretically it is used to prevent a significant increase in mean intrathoracic pressure.

      3. This maneuver is not recommended because it promotes air trapping and pulmonary edema and has not been demonstrated to clinically affect intrathoracic pressure.

  L. Sigh

      1. The sigh breath is the periodic delivery of a VT approximately 1.5 times the set VT.

      2. A sigh breath is used to prevent the patchy microatelectasis that may develop during continuous control or assist/control ventilation with small VTs.

      3. The use of large VTs and the development of IMV and SIMV have eliminated the need for sigh breaths. However, some recommend its use in the control and assist/control modes of ventilation.

V. Monitoring the Patient/Ventilator System

  A. Monitoring the functions of the system should be performed as frequently as the clinical situation dictates. In general, most patient/ventilator systems should be evaluated every 2 to 4 hours. However, the highly unstable patient may require hourly evaluation, whereas the chronic ventilator patient may require evaluation only every 4 hours.

      1. Drain all system tubing of condensate.

      2. Verify ventilator parameters are set as ordered.

      3. Independently measure exhaled tidal volumes ($V_{T_E}s$) to verify volumes ordered are actually delivered.

         a. Exhaled tidal volumes are measured because inhaled VTs may not indicate the volume of gas the patient is actually receiving, especially if a system leak is present.

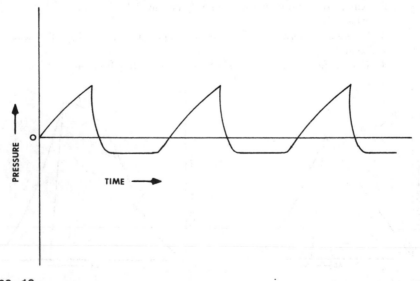

FIG 36–16.
Ventilator system pressure curve developed with the use of NEEP in the control mode.

      b. Correcting the V_{T_E} for compressible volume loss can also be done.

        (1) Compressible volume loss is the quantity of gas compressed in the system that is not delivered to the patient.

        (2) For most systems, this is about 3 to 4 ml/cm H_2O peak airway pressure (PAP). However, individual system values should be determined for each system used.

        (3) The use of this correction in determining V_{T_E} is not essential in adults because the magnitude of the compressible volume will be relatively consistent with every evaluation.

        (4) If correction is to be done, it should be done consistently, or conflicting V_{T_E} will be recorded.

    4. Time the ventilator rate to ensure appropriate calibration.

    5. Time the inspiratory phase as accurately as possible.

    6. Independently analyze the delivered FI_{O_2}.

    7. Measure the IMV continuous flow and the FI_{O_2} delivered by this system.

    8. Check the temperature and function of the humidifying system.

    9. Evaluate the function of the cuff on the artificial airway.

B. The patient's response to mechanical ventilation should be monitored at the same time the technical function of the machine is evaluated.

    1. Determine spontaneous RR and heart rate.

    2. Measure blood pressure.

    3. If hemodynamic monitoring is being utilized, record all available parameters.

    4. Record peak pressure and P_{plat} (Fig 36–17).

    5. Measure spontaneous V_T. Ideally, measure for 10 breaths and calculate the average.

    6. Measure and record vital capacity and maximum inspiratory pressure at least daily, if indicated.

    7. Determine patient/ventilator system compliance.

      a. Patient/ventilator system compliance is referred to as *effective static compliance* (C_{ES}) to differentiate it from true compliance calculated in the pulmonary function laboratory.

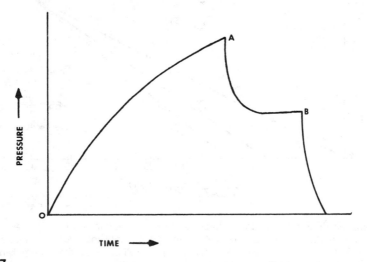

FIG 36–17.
A, PAP, **B,** P_{plat}. **A – B,** approximate pressure necessary to overcome R_{AW}. **B,** approximate pressure necessary to overcome total patient/ventilator system compliance.

b. Effective static compliance is determined by dividing the V_{T_E} by the P_{plat} minus applied PEEP ($PEEP_A$) minus auto-Peep ($PEEP_I$). Ideally, P_{plat} should be measured as close to the patient's airway as possible:

$$C_{ES} = \frac{V_{T_E}}{P_{plat} - PEEP_A - PEEP_I} \qquad (2)$$

c. If $PEEP_A$ and $PEEP_I$ are not considered in the C_{ES} determination, grossly different compliance values may be determined (Fig 36–18).

d. Exhaled tidal volume is used because it most closely reflects the volume of gas in the airway at end-inspiration.
   (1) The V_{T_E} can be corrected for the patient/system compressible volume loss.
   (2) This correction, however, is not necessary because the same level of error is included in each determination, and specific C_{ES} values are not as important as the change in this variable over time.

e. Plateau pressure is used because it is an equilibration pressure that reflects the airway pressure under the most static conditions attainable in the patient/ventilator system.

f. Peak airway pressure is not used because it reflects the amount of pressure necessary to overcome airway resistance as well as elastic resistance.

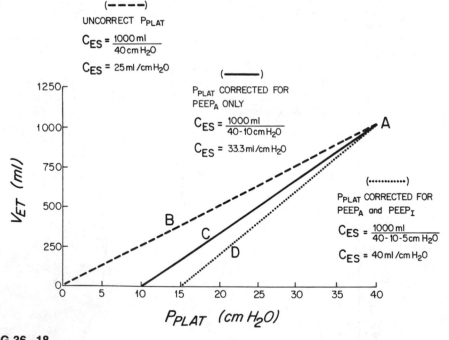

FIG 36–18.
Effects of applied PEEP *(PEEP$_A$)* and Auto-peep *(Peep$_I$)* on determination of C_{ES}. **A** = P$_{PLAT}$; **B** = atm pressure; **C** = PEEP$_A$ level; and **D** = PEEP$_I$ level. *BA* compliance curve without correction for PEEP$_A$ or PEEP$_I$. *CA* = compliance curve with correction for PEEP$_A$ only. *DA* = compliance curve for corrections for PEEP$_A$ and PEEP$_I$. (From Kacmarek RM: Noninvasive monitoring techniques in the ventilated patient, in Kacmarek RM, Stoller JK [eds]: *Current Respiratory Care.* Toronto, BC Decker, 1988. Used by permission.)

    g. Positive end-expiratory pressure levels *must* be subtracted from the P_{plat} because the amount of pressure necessary to maintain the V_T in the patient's airway is the increase in pressure from baseline levels.

    h. Effective static compliance in most adults is much lower than total compliance (C_{TOT}) because of existing disease and the crude conditions under which the determination is made.

    i. Normal C_{ES} for most adults is about 40 to 60 ml/cm H_2O.

    j. The use of C_{ES} is limited by the ability to obtain a true static P_{plat}.

        (1) If the patient is ventilating spontaneously, inspiratory efforts will prevent a true P_{plat} from being obtained.

        (2) However, with conscious patient cooperation or control mode ventilation, P_{plat} can generally be obtained.

    k. Effective static compliance reflects the "stiffness" of the lung-thorax/ventilator system.

8. Determination of dynamic compliance (C_{dyn})

    a. Dynamic compliance is a reflection of the total ventilatory system impedance, compliance plus resistance.

    b. It is determined from the PAP:

$$C_{dyn} = \frac{V_{T_E}}{PAP - PEEP_A - PEEP_I} \tag{3}$$

    c. Not as useful a valve to monitor as C_{ES} or airway resistance. (R_{AW}).

9. Determination of R_{AW} (see Fig 36–17)

    a. An estimate of R_{AW} can be obtained by dividing the difference between the PAP and P_{plat} by the flow rate ($\dot{V}$) in liters per second or liters per minute:

$$R = \frac{PAP - P_{plat}}{\dot{V}} \tag{4}$$

        (1) Since PAP is the maximum pressure developed in the system and P_{plat} is the static system pressure, the difference between these two values reflects the amount of pressure necessary to maintain gas flow.

        (2) For a reasonable estimate of R_{AW} to be made, $\dot{V}$ should be constant (square wave flow pattern).

        Example:

$$PAP = 60 \text{ cm } H_2O$$
$$P_{plat} = 40 \text{ cm } H_2O$$
$$\dot{V} = 60 \text{ L/min or 1 L/sec}$$

$$R_{AW} = \frac{(60 \text{ cm } H_2O) - (40 \text{ cm } H_2O)}{60 \text{ L/min}}$$

$$R_{AW} = 0.33 \text{ cm } H_2O/L/min$$

or

$$R_{AW} = \frac{(60 \text{ cm } H_2O) - (40 \text{ cm } H_2O)}{1 \text{ L/sec}}$$

$$R_{AW} = 20 \text{ cm } H_2O/L/sec$$

      b. In spontaneously ventilating patients, the accuracy of the P_{plat} determination and the stability of the PAP limit the accuracy of R_{AW} determinations.

C. Arterial blood gas analysis should be performed whenever *a change in the patient's clinical status or ventilator settings occur.*

      1. Ideally, critically ill patients should have an arterial line in place to permit rapid access to arterial blood.

      2. Routine blood gas analysis is usually necessary on only an 8-hour basis in critically ill patients and less frequently as the patient's condition improves.

D. Determination of intrapulmonary shunt on a daily basis provides information on the extent of the patient's pulmonary pathophysiology (see Chapter 12).

E. Hemodynamic monitoring on a regular basis is crucial to the care of critically ill mechanically ventilated patients. The data should be tabulated with other patient/ventilator system data to ensure the unwanted cardiovascular changes associated with ventilator adjustments or changes are identified.

F. Careful monitoring of fluid and electrolyte balance is also essential to the overall care of the ventilator patient (see Chapter 15).

G. Determination of auto-PEEP

      1. Auto-PEEP is the development of an alveolar end-expiratory pressure not measurable in the ventilator circuit unless an expiratory hold is applied at the moment the next positive pressure breath is to be delivered and that breath delivery delayed (Fig 36–19). This method is useful only in nonspontaneously breathing patients.

      2. In spontaneously breathing patients, the simultaneous measurement of esophageal pressure (reflection of pleural pressure) change and gas flow at the mouth is necessary. The baseline esophageal pressure change required to initiate flow at the airway is the auto-PEEP level.

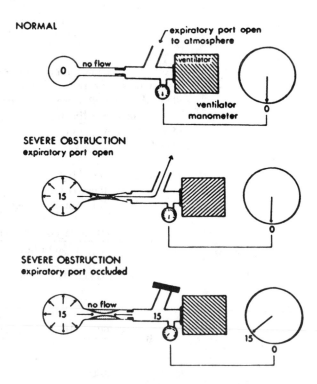

FIG 36–19.
Measurement of auto-PEEP by expiratory port occlusion. Normally *(top)* alveolar pressure is atmospheric at the end of passive exhalation. With severe airflow obstruction *(middle)*, alveolar pressure remains elevated and slow flow continues, even at the end of the set exhalation period. The ventilator manometer senses negligible pressure because it is open to atmosphere through large-bore tubing and downstream from the site of flow limitation. With gas flow stopped by occlusion of the expiratory port at the end of the set exhalation period *(lower)*, pressure equilibriates throughout the lung ventilator system and is displayed on the ventilator manometer. (From Pepe PE, Marini JJ: *Am Rev Respir Dis* 1982; 126:166–170. Used by permission.)

3. The existence but not the magnitude of auto-PEEP can be established by monitoring exhaled flow; if exhaled flow does not stop before the initiation of the next breath, auto-PEEP is present.
4. The physiologic effects of auto-PEEP are the same as applied PEEP. However, the presence of auto-PEEP is frequently overlooked, and thus its detrimental effects on hemodynamics are attributed to other causes.
5. Specifically, auto-PEEP:
   a. Affects hemodynamic measurement in the same manner as applied PEEP (see Chapter 37).
   b. Affects the calculation of C_{ES}, rendering a low determination.
   c. Increases the work of breathing by forcing decompression of the auto-PEEP before gas can enter the lungs.
   d. Increases the likelihood of barotrauma.
6. Auto-PEEP is a result of insufficient expiratory time.
   a. If compliance is multiplied by resistance, the result is time:

$$C_{ES} \times R_{AW} = \text{Time} \tag{5}$$
$$0.060 \text{ L/cm H}_2\text{O} \times 20 \text{ cm H}_2\text{O/L/sec} = 1.2 \text{ seconds}$$

   b. The value 1.2 seconds is the pulmonary time constant. This value varies from individual to individual and from clinical setting to clinical setting.
   c. During passive exhalation, at least three time constants are necessary for complete exhalation (3.6 seconds). If this time is not available, air trapping and auto-PEEP result (Fig 36–20).
7. Auto-PEEP normally develops in healthy lungs if exhalation is passive and rates exceed 20 bpm.

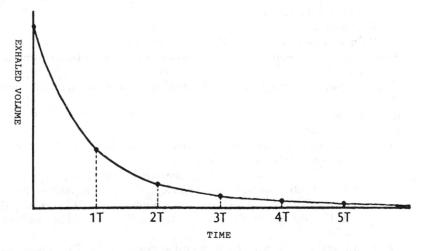

FIG 36–20.
The percentage of V$_T$ exhaled *passively* per unit of time is an exponentially decaying curve based on the length of the pulmonary time constant *(T)*. In one time constant, 63% of V$_T$ is exhaled, 86.5% in two time constants, 95% in three time constants, 98.2% in four time constants, and 99.3% in five time constants. The greater the length of the pulmonary time constant, the longer the total passive exhalation. If exhalation is active, a shorter expiratory time is required. (From Shapiro BA, Harrison RA, Trout CA: *Clinical Application of Respiratory Care.* Chicago, Year Book Medical Publishers, 1975. Used by permission.)

8. Auto-PEEP normally develops in chronic obstructive pulmonary disease (COPD) patients, if exhalation is passive and rates exceed 12/min.
9. Auto-PEEP almost always develops during high-frequency ventilation and PC-IRV.
10. Auto-PEEP can be decreased by:
    a. Slower RRs.
    b. Shorter T_Is.
    c. Longer expiratory times.
    d. Larger VTs.
    e. Less compliant ventilator circuits.
    f. Appropriate bronchial hygiene techniques to modify compliance and resistance.
11. If Auto-PEEP is a result of dynamic airway compression, as noted in COPD patients, the use of low levels of applied PEEP (3–7 cm H_2O) is helpful (after all of the rest of the list has been employed) in reducing WOB.
    a. If applied PEEP is helpful, the P_{plat} and the PAP should not significantly increase when applied.
    b. The applied PEEP level should never exceed the auto-PEEP level.
    c. When it is applied appropriately, alveolar and central airway pressure equilibrate and:
       (1) Work of breathing decreases.
       (2) Peak expiratory flow increases.
       (3) Expiratory resistance decreases.
VI. Ventilator Alarm Systems
    A. Every volume ventilator must incorporate at least the following ventilator alarm systems for safe function.
       1. Patient/system leak or disconnect: This alarm may be either:
          a. Low V_{T_E}.
          b. Low system pressure.
       2. High inspiratory pressure.
       3. If PEEP is used, a loss of PEEP alarm is necessary.
    B. Many of the newer ventilators are overalarmed, and frequent false positive alarms are sounded.
    C. Proper setting of alarm limits is essential to prevent frequent false positive alarms.
VII. Ventilator Maintenance
    A. Eucapneic ventilation
       1. Most patients who are mechanically ventilated should be maintained at a P_{CO_2} within a range of *their normal values*.
          a. For most patients, that is a Pa_{CO_2} between 30 and 50 mm Hg.
          b. In COPD patients who retain CO_2, Pa_{CO_2} should be maintained in a range that provides a normal acid-base status resulting in a pH between 7.35 and 7.40. If a previous baseline Pa_{CO_2} is known, Pa_{CO_2} should be maintained at that level.
       2. In patients with increased intracranial pressure (ICP), Pa_{CO_2} is frequently maintained at 25 to 35 mm Hg.
          a. When ICP is acutely increased, the patient should be further hyperventilated. This constricts cerebral vasculature and decreases cerebral vascular volume, resulting in a decreased ICP.
             (1) Constant hyperventilation is effective in decreasing ICP for only short periods of time (approximately 12–24 hours).
             (2) After this period, cerebral vascular tone and blood volume return toward normal despite continued hyperventilation.

(3) For this reason, hyperventilation is encouraged during initial stabilization but not for prolonged periods of time. If low to normal Pa_{CO_2} values are maintained, the patient can be easily hyperventilated if ICP should spike acutely.
3. Chronic hyperventilation results in:
   a. Electrolyte imbalances, decreased HCO_3^-, K^+, and Cl^-.
   b. Increased potential for cardiac arrhythmias.
   c. Altered hepatorenal function.
   d. Decreased cerebral blood volume.
   e. Altered autonomic receptor response to pharmacologic agents.
4. *The ventilator should be used to correct metabolic acid-base disturbances for only short periods of time.*
   a. The source of the disturbances should be identified and appropriately treated.
   b. If mechanical hypoventilation or hyperventilation is used to normalize a metabolic acid-base disturbance, when the metabolic disturbance is finally corrected, the patient is frequently in a state of chronic respiratory acidosis or alkalosis.
   c. In addition, mechanical hypoventilation or hyperventilation will mask the metabolic problem and may interfere with its identification and final resolution.
5. Hypoventilation with the administration of HCO_3^- is frequently indicated in severe ARDS, status asthmaticus, and any other disturbance requiring high minute ventilation to maintain normal Pco_2 levels.
   a. This technique is used increasingly to prevent having to increase minute ventilation, mean airway pressure, and PAP in the severely ill.
   b. Allowing CO_2 to rise minimizes the likelihood of barotrauma from continual increases in minute ventilation.
   c. As the patient's status begins to improve, the Pco_2 can be gradually returned to normal.
   d. Pco_2 values as high as 65 mm Hg are frequently allowed.
   e. Normally, sedation and paralysis are required if the Pco_2 is allowed to rise.
B. Fighting the ventilator
   1. Patients generally fight the ventilator or ventilate out of phase with the ventilator secondary to technical or clinically related inadequacies.
   2. The most common cause is the *technical* setup of the ventilator system.
      a. Inadequate IMV system flow
      b. Insensitive demand valves
      c. Lengthy T_Is as a result of inadequate positive pressure inspiratory flow rates.
   3. If the problem is not technical, an assessment of the patient's clinical status should be made.
      a. Level of ventilation
      b. Level of oxygenation
      c. Cardiovascular stability
      d. Metabolic rate
      e. Electrolyte imbalance
      f. Breath sounds
   4. If the cause of the problem can be identified, it should be corrected. If a cause is not immediately identifiable or the patient is simply agitated, sedation, paralysis, or both may be indicated.
C. Pharmacologic support (see Chapter 40 for details)
   1. Most patients require some level of pharmacologic support during the initial phase of mechanical ventilation.

2. If a patient is fighting the ventilator, pharmacologic intervention may be indicated.

3. When patients are maintained on *full ventilatory support,* pharmacologic support is needed if the control mode is used and is frequently necessary if the assist/control, IMV, or SIMV mode is used.

4. The ideal pharmacologic agent for use in maintaining patients receiving ventilatory support must:
   a. Be a potent CNS depressant.
   b. Have minimal cardiovascular side effects.
   c. Be a potent euphoric.
   d. Be a strong analgesic.
   e. Be *totally reversible.*

5. Morphine sulfate most closely fits the description of the ideal agent.
   a. It is a potent CNS depressant.
   b. It does cause some hypotension because of:
      (1) Decreased venous tone.
      (2) Histamine release.
   c. The hypotension is usually easily correctable with fluid therapy.
   d. It is a potent euphoric and analgesic.
   e. It is totally reversible with naloxone hydrochloride (Narcan).
   f. Initial morphinizing dosage is 0.2 to 0.3 mg/kg.
   g. Maintenance dosage is 0.05 to 0.1 mg/kg every hour.
   h. Hypotensive side effects are greatly minimized if patients are kept totally sedated. In patients in whom sedation is allowed to "wear off," hypotension may develop with each morphinizing dose.
   i. Other narcotics may also be used (see Chapter 40).

6. Diazepam (Valium)
   a. It has minimal cardiovascular side effects.
   b. It is a euphoric.
   c. It is *not* an analgesic.
   d. It has variable and unpredictable CNS depressant effects.
   e. It is *not* reversible.
   f. Other sedatives/hypnotics have similar effects (see Chapter 40).

7. Paralyzing agents
   a. For ventilator maintenance, nondepolarizing neuromuscular blocking agents are the drugs of choice.
      (1) *d*-Tubocurarine (Curare)
      (2) Pancuronium bromide (Pavulon)
   b. Since these agents do not affect a patient's mental state, morphine sulfate or some other sedative should *always be used* in conjunction with paralyzing agents.
   c. See Chapter 40 for more detail and other agents.

D. Bronchial hygiene
   1. Many patients requiring mechanical ventilation also require bronchial hygiene therapy.
   2. Aerosol therapy may be provided in-line with the ventilator circuit.
   3. Postural drainage, chest percussion, and chest vibration may be performed.
   4. Fiberoptic bronchoscopy may also be indicated.
   5. The trachea should be suctioned frequently.
   6. Manual ventilation (hyperinflation) may be used.
   7. Aerosolized bronchodilator therapy may be used.

E. Adjustment of ventilator settings
   1. In general, one ventilator parameter should be adjusted at a time, followed by cardiovascular assessment and arterial blood gas measurement in 10 to 15 min.

2. Simultaneous adjustment of ventilator parameters is encouraged only when significant and detrimental variations from expected blood gas values exist.
   Example:

   Blood gas results are:
   pH   7.28 HCO_3^- 26 mEq/L
   Pa_{CO_2} 56 mm Hg Pa_{O_2} 40 mm Hg

   a. Clearly this patient is being mechanically hypoventilated and is severely hypoxemic.
   b. Because of the severity of the abnormality, both ventilation and F_{IO_2} or PEEP should be increased as rapidly as possible.
3. When parameters are adjusted simultaneously, it is occasionally difficult to determine a precise cause and effect relationship if expected outcomes are not realized.

F. Approaches to maintaining proper Pa_{CO_2} levels
   1. In general, all adjustments in level of ventilation should be made only after careful consideration of the cardiovascular consequence of each adjustment.
   2. The adjustment of choice is generally the one resulting in the least cardiovascular embarrassment.
   3. Use of mechanical deadspace is appropriate only if a patient is being ventilated in the control mode.
      a. Increasing deadspace will increase Pa_{CO_2}.
      b. Decreasing deadspace will decrease Pa_{CO_2}.
      c. In the control mode, mechanical deadspace is recommended only when very large mechanical VTs are required to satisfy a patient's sense that he or she is being adequately ventilated. Typically, only patients mechanically ventilated for nonpulmonary disease require the use of deadspace.
         (1) Neuromuscular diseases
         (2) Neurologic diseases
      d. If deadspace is used in other modes, it simply increases the patient's ventilatory drive, increasing the WOB.
   4. Control mode
      a. To correct increased Pa_{CO_2}:
         (1) Increase VT (first).
         (2) Increase rate.
      b. To correct decreased Pa_{CO_2}:
         (1) Decrease rate (first).
         (2) Decrease VT.
   5. Assist/control mode
      a. To correct increased Pa_{CO_2}:
         (1) Increase VT (first).
         (2) Increase rate.
      b. To correct decreased Pa_{CO_2}:
         (1) Because the patient has control over the frequency of ventilation, decreasing the machine rate or the VT may have no effect on the level of ventilation.
         (2) Patients mechanically hyperventilating in the assist/control mode frequently require pharmacologic intervention to decrease the ventilatory drive.
   6. IMV/SIMV modes
      a. To correct increased Pa_{CO_2}:
         (1) Increase VT (first).
         (2) Increase rate.

b. To correct decreased Pa_{CO_2}:
  (1) Decrease rate (first).
  (2) Decrease V_T.
7. Extended mandatory minute ventilation
  a. To correct increased Pa_{CO_2}, increase mandatory minute ventilation.
  b. To correct decreased Pa_{CO_2}, decrease mandatory minute ventilation.
8. Pressure support
  a. To correct increased Pa_{CO_2}:
    (1) Increase pressure support level.
    (2) Implement SIMV breaths if this mode is not already being used or increase the number of SIMV breaths.
    (3) Change to some other mode guaranteeing a specific level of ventilation.
  b. To correct decreased Pa_{CO_2}, decrease pressure support level.
9. When considering changes in V_T, remember that for most patients, V_T should remain in the 10- to 20-ml/kg range. Ideally, V_Ts are about 12 to 15 ml/kg.
10. Changes in the rate should be considered in connection with changes in the V_T.
Example A:

| Pa_{CO_2}: | 52mm Hg | Rate: | 4 bpm |
| Mode: | IMV | V_T: | 15 ml/kg |

In this situation the rate should be increased because the V_T is large but greater ventilation is required and the rate is slow.
Example B:

| Pa_{CO_2}: | 52 mm Hg | Rate: | 10 bpm |
| Mode: | Control | V_T: | 10 ml/kg |

Here, the V_T should be increased because the rate is adequate, yet increased ventilation is required and the V_T is relatively small. Always make the change that will correct hypoventilation but also cause the least increase in mean intrathoracic pressure.

G. Approaches to maintaining proper arterial oxygenation
1. The most crucial variable determining oxygen *content* is the hemoglobin value, which should be maintained as close to normal as possible.
2. If the hemoglobin value is normal, a Pa_{O_2} of 60 mm Hg will normally result in an oxyhemoglobin percent saturation of 90%.
3. If hypoxemia is primarily responsive, alter the $F_{I_{O_2}}$ to keep the Pa_{O_2} greater than 60 mm Hg.
4. If the responsive hypoxemia is a result of noncardiogenic pulmonary edema, 5 to 15 cm H_2O PEEP may be helpful.
5. If the hypoxemia is refractory, higher levels of PEEP therapy may be indicated (see Chapter 37).
6. Tissue oxygenation is also dependent on:
  a. Acid-base status.
  b. Tissue perfusion.
7. Patients who fight the ventilator increase their oxygen consumption and may develop hypoxemia. Use appropriate sedation or technical modification to reduce fighting.
VIII. Ventilator Discontinuance
  A. Criteria for ventilator discontinuance
    1. *Reversal of pathophysiologic condition necessitating ventilatory support*

2. No active acute pulmonary disease process
3. Stable vital signs
   a. Fever even if not of pulmonary origin:
      (1) Increases oxygen consumption
      (2) Increases carbon dioxide production
   b. Tachycardia and hypertension, indicative of increased level of stress
   c. Bradycardia and hypotension, possibly indicating a lack of myocardial reserves and poor peripheral perfusion
4. Optimal nutritional status (see Chapter 19)
   a. This is of particular concern if patients have been ventilated for a lengthy period of time and have a chronic underlying disease process.
   b. If a patient is receiving hyperalimentation, it may be preferable to delay ventilator discontinuance until hyperalimentation is complete.
      (1) This is particularly true if all nonprotein calories are administered as carbohydrates.
      (2) When lipids are not administered, the respiratory quotient for the conversion of carbohydrates to lipids is greater than 8.0.
      (3) As a result, the patient's carbon dioxide production is markedly increased.
      (4) Patients with marginal cardiopulmonary reserves may not be able to meet the demands of ventilator discontinuance when coupled with an increased carbon dioxide load.
5. Adequate cardiovascular reserves
   a. Normal pulse and blood pressure
   b. No arrhythmias
   c. Good peripheral perfusion
   d. If a pulmonary artery catheter is in place:
      (1) Stable and relatively normal hemodynamic values
      (2) Normal cardiac output
      (3) Normal mixed venous P_{O_2} level and arteriovenous oxygen content difference
6. Normal renal function
7. Intact CNS
8. Normally functioning GI tract
9. Proper electrolyte and fluid balance (see Chapter 15)
   a. Electrolyte abnormalities may result in muscular weakness. Specifically, the following electrolytes should be normal:
      (1) K^+
      (2) Cl^-
      (3) Ca^{+2}
      (4) PO_4^{-3}
      (5) Mg^{+2}
   Note: Any electrolyte, fluid, or major organ system malfunction results in an increase in physiologic stress. This, coupled with the added stress of spontaneous ventilation, may be enough to cause a patient to fail and require ventilatory support.
10. Adequate gas exchange capabilities
   a. Acceptable arterial blood gas values
      (1) Pa_{CO_2} at patient's normal level
         (a) For most patients, this is about 40 mm Hg.
         (b) For COPD patients, it may be at some elevated Pa_{CO_2} level.
      (2) Normal pH
      (3) Pa_{O_2} greater than 60 mm Hg but not above the normal level

      b. Intrapulmonary shunt fraction less than 20% to 25%

      c. No indication of increased deadspace

  11. Adequate ventilatory capability: Even if all these variables are acceptable, if the patient's ventilatory capabilities are diminished, he or she may not be able to sustain spontaneous ventilation.

      a. Vital capacity should be greater than or equal to 10 to 15 ml/kg of ideal body weight.

      b. If the vital capacity cannot be determined, there should be a maximum inspiratory pressure of at least -20 to -25 cm H_2O in 20 seconds.

      c. Spontaneous V_T should be 2 to 3 ml/kg of ideal body weight.

      d. Spontaneous RR should be less than 30 bpm.

      Note: If patients have been maintained on full ventilatory support, their stimulus to ventilate spontaneously may be diminished. As a result, when ventilatory capabilities are evaluated, values less than the levels indicated may be obtained. If this occurs, a well-monitored trial off the ventilator may produce the stimulus necessary for the patient to exhibit acceptable ventilatory abilities.

B. Psychologic preparation

  1. The transition from mechanical ventilation to spontaneous ventilation produces a great deal of anxiety in most patients. This is particularly evident in patients ventilated for more than several days.

  2. To relieve some of this anxiety:

      a. Carefully explain the procedure in detail.

      b. Attempt to develop the patient's confidence by reinforcing the improvement noted in the disease process.

      c. Assure patients that they will be continually monitored throughout the time they are ventilating spontaneously and that you will stay with them.

      d. *Do not tell patients they will never need the ventilator again.*

        (1) If this is done and ventilatory support must be reestablished, it is not uncommon for patients to lose confidence in themselves and the medical team caring for them.

        (2) It is more appropriate to inform patients that their capability of ventilating spontaneously is going to be evaluated. If they are ventilating adequately, they will be allowed to continue; however, if they deteriorate clinically, mechanical ventilation will be reinstituted.

C. Complete discontinuance

  1. In some 70% to 80% of patients maintained on ventilatory support, support can be totally discontinued without a gradual weaning phase if:

      a. Physiologic preparation is adequate.

      b. The ventilatory course was short.

      c. There is no need for psychologic support.

  2. Discontinuance procedure

      a. Manually ventilate with a high F_{IO_2} (0.70+).

        (1) This allows a gradual transition from ventilatory support to spontaneous ventilation.

        (2) The F_{IO_2} is increased to avoid any increased stress from an inappropriate oxygenation status.

        (3) However, patients functioning on a hypoxic drive must be maintained at their maintenance F_{IO_2}.

      b. Over a 5- to 10-min period, gradually allow the patient to assume a greater role in ventilation.

c. After the transition is complete, administer an aerosol via a Briggs T piece at an $F_{I_{O_2}}$ 0.10 higher than the ventilator $F_{I_{O_2}}$. (Do not elevate the $F_{I_{O_2}}$ in patients functioning on a hypoxic drive.) Ensure a high flow system is used (see Chapter 28).

d. Monitor the patient's clinical presentation, vital signs, and WOB.

e. Obtain an arterial blood gas in 10 to 15 min.

f. Normal Pa_{CO_2} levels rise during initial discontinuance period.

   (1) If a patient is apneic with a normal metabolic rate, the arterial Pa_{CO_2} will increase about 6 mm Hg in the first minute and about 3 mm Hg every minute thereafter.

   (2) A small increase in the Pa_{CO_2} is expected during the first 10 to 15 min to establish a stimulus to maintain spontaneous ventilation. After this the Pa_{CO_2} should return to the patient's normal level.

   (3) In general a 3- to 5-mm Hg increase in Pa_{CO_2} may occur in the initial period.

      (a) If this increase is *not* accompanied by significant cardiovascular and pulmonary stress, allow spontaneous ventilation to continue.

      (b) If pulse, blood pressure, and RR are markedly elevated, arrhythmias develop, and the patient becomes diaphoretic and makes extensive use of accessory muscles, reinstitute mechanical ventilation.

g. Reassess blood gases and clinical status 15 min later. If the patient is stable, continue.

h. Repeat frequent reassessment of status.

i. Once the patient is stabilized, return the $F_{I_{O_2}}$ to an appropriate level.

j. When you are satisified that ventilatory support will not need to be reinstituted, evaluate for extubation (see Chapter 29).

D. Gradually decreasing the IMV or SIMV rate

  1. About 15% to 20% of patients receiving mechanical ventilation require a gradual discontinuance of ventilatory support.

  2. In the majority of these patients, ventilatory support can be discontinued over 6 to 8 hours.

  3. If the process is extended over days, the patient's ventilatory capabilities should be reevaluated.

  4. A gradual decrease in IMV/SIMV rate is necessary if:

    a. Physiologic preparation is questionable.

    b. Ventilatory course is prolonged.

    c. An underlying chronic disease exists in any organ system.

    d. Psychologic support is necessary.

  5. Procedure

    a. Convert to the IMV or SIMV mode at a rate of 8 to 10 bpm.

    b. Evaluate cardiopulmonary status.

    c. If this is tolerated, decrease the rate by 2 bpm every 1 to 2 hours, followed by evaluation of cardiopulmonary status.

    d. Discontinue support when the rate is decreased to 2 bpm. Follow the procedure outlined in section VIII–C, 2.

    e. Low levels of pressure support are frequently used to decrease the imposed WOB. Patients may be extubated from 3 to 7 cm H_2O IPS if the IPS is used to reduce imposed WOB.

    f. The MMV mode may be used in place of the gradual decrease in IMV rate. However, as stated earlier, concern about inappropriate ventilatory patterns may modify this approach.

g. Maximum IPS (10–12 ml/kg V$_T$) may be used as a means of gradually decreasing ventilatory support as patients demonstrate greater and greater capability of breathing spontaneously.

E. Periodic discontinuance
1. A small population of patients (approximately 3%–5%) require a very lengthy weaning phase.
2. Most patients in this group have severe COPD, ventilatory muscle dysfunction or neuromuscular or neurologic dysfunction.
3. This approach gradually increases the patients' physiologic and psychologic assets but also permits their ventilatory muscles to rest while they are being ventilated.
4. This procedure involves lengthy periods of rest interspaced with periods of work.
   a. Work periods should avoid the development of fatigue (see Chapter 18).
5. During rest periods, full ventilatory support should be maintained.
   a. Assist/control
   b. SIMV
   c. SIMV with IPS
   d. IPS
   e. Low levels of CPAP (3–7 cm H$_2$O), are usually used with each approach
6. The following approaches are commonly used during work periods:
   a. T piece
   b. CPAP
   c. IPS
   d. IPS with CPAP
   e. Low level SIMV
   f. Low-level SIMV with IPS
   g. Low-level SIMV with IPS and CPAP
7. The length of time for each work period is gradually increased. At the start, only 5 to 10 min may be tolerated.
8. No magical approach is definable. Whatever works is appropriate.
9. It is important that patients are rested in full ventilatory support at night.

F. The difficult-to-wean patient
1. There is always an underlying reason why ventilatory support cannot be discontinued in a patient.
2. Many such patients have pathophysiologic conditions that prevent them from ventilating spontaneously and as a result become chronic ventilator patients.
3. However, many are not prepared to assume the increased stress associated with spontaneous ventilation.
4. If support cannot be discontinued, this protocol may be followed:
   a. Evaluate the technical setup used during the work phase.
      (1) The work required to activate demand systems may be excessive.
      (2) The gas flow through the high-flow system used may be inadequate.
   b. Reassess the patient's physiologic preparation for discontinuance, paying particular attention to:
      (1) Acid-base status.
      (2) Oxygenation status.
      (3) Nutritional status.
      (4) Fluid and electrolyte balance.
   c. Determine if a psychologic dependence has developed.
      (1) If this occurs, it may be necessary to transfer the patient to another area of the hospital or institution where the patient's confidence in the medical staff is not a factor.

5. Most patients within this group are:
   a. Improperly maintained patients, either from a ventilatory or a general medical perspective.
   b. COPD patients with:
      (1) Poor physiologic preparation.
      (2) Psychologic dependence on the ventilator.
   c. Patients with spinal cord injuries.
6. Many of these patients end up as chronic ventilator patients.

BIBLIOGRAPHY

Agusti AGN, Torres A, Estopa R, et al: Hypophosphatemia as a cause of failed weaning: The importance of metabolic factors. *Crit Care Med* 1982; 12:142–143.

Benson MS, Pierson DJ: Auto-PEEP during mechanical ventilation of adults. *Respir Care* 1988; 33:557–568.

Bergman NA: Intrapulmonary gas trapping during mechanical ventilation at rapid frequencies. *Anesthesiology* 1972; 37:626–633.

Benzer H: The value of intermittent mandatory ventilation [editorial]. *Intensive Care Med* 1982; 8:267–268.

Berry AJ: Respiratory support and renal failure. *Anesthesiology* 1981; 55:655–667.

Bone RC: Complications of mechanical ventilation and positive end-expiratory pressure. *Respir Care* 1982; 27:402–407.

Brochard L, Harf A, Lorino H, et al: Inspiratory pressure support prevents diaphragmatic fatigue during weaning from mechanical ventilation. *Am Rev Respir Dis* 1989; 139:513–521.

Brochard L, Rua F, Lorino H, et al: The extra work of breathing due to endotracheal tube is abolished during inspiratory pressure support breathing. *Am Rev Respir Dis* 1987; 137:64.

Brown Dg, Pierson DJ: Auto-PEEP is common in mechanically ventilated patients: A study of incidence, severity and detection. *Respir Care* 1986; 31:1069–1073.

Burton GG, Hodgkin JE: *Respiratory Care: A Guide to Clinical Practice*, ed 2. Philadelphia, JB Lippincott Co, 1984.

Cartwright DW, Willis MM, Gregory GA: Functional residual capacity and lung mechanics at different levels of mechanical ventilation. *Crit Care Med* 1984; 12:422–427.

Civetta JM: Intermittent mandatory ventilation and positive end-expiratory pressure in acute ventilatory insufficiency. *Int Anesthesiol Clin* 1980; 18:123–141.

Civetta JM, Banner M: Nursing assessment of intermittent mandatory ventilation. *Int Anesthesiol Clin* 1980; 18:143–177.

Dhingra S, Solven F, Wilson A, et al: Hypomagnesemia and respiratory muscle power. *Am Rev Respir Dis* 1984; 129:497–498.

Downs JB, Douglas MF: Intermittent mandatory ventilation and weaning. *Int Anesthesiol Clin* 1980; 18:81–95.

DuPuis YG: *Ventilators: Theory and Clinical Application*. St Louis, CV Mosby Co, 1986.

Eross B, Powner D, Greenvik A: Common ventilatory modes: Terminology. *Int Anesthesiol Clin* 1980; 18:11–22.

Fairley HG: Critique of intermittent mandatory ventilation. *Int Anesthesiol Clin* 1980; 18:179–189.

Fernandez A, de la Cal MA, Esteban A, et al: Simplified method for measuring physiologic V_D/V_t in patients on mechanical ventilation. *Crit Care Med* 1983; 11:823.

Gibney RTN, Wilson RS, Pontoppidan H: Comparison of work of breathing on high gas flow and demand valve continuous positive airway pressure systems. *Chest* 1982; 82:692–695.

Gjerde GE, Katz JA, Kraemer RW: Inspiratory work and airway pressure with continuous positive airway pressure delivery systems, abstract. *Crit Care Med* 1984; 12:272.

Graybar CB, Smith RA: Apparatus and techniques for intermittent mandatory ventilation. *Int Anesthesiol Clin* 1980; 18:53–79.

Henry WC, West GA, Wilson RS: A comparison of the oxygen cost of breathing between a continuous-flow CPAP system and a demand-flow CPAP system. *Respir Care* 1983; 28:1273–1281.

Hylkema BS, Barkmeijer-Degenhart P, van der Mark TW, et al: Central venous versus esophageal pressure changes for calculation of lung compliance during mechanical ventilation. *Crit Care Med* 1983; 11:271–275.

Kacmarek RM: Mechanical ventilatory rates and tidal volumes. *Respir Care* 1987; 32:466–478.

Kacmarek RM: The role of pressure support ventilation in reducing the work of breathing. *Respir Care* 1988; 33:99–120.

Kacmarek RM, Dimas S, Reynolds J, et al: Technical aspects of positive end-expiratory pressure (PEEP): part II. PEEP with positive-pressure ventilation. *Respir Care* 1982; 27:1490–1504.

Katz JA, Kraemer RW, Gjerde GE: Inspiratory work and airway pressure with continuous positive airway pressure delivery system. *Chest* 1985; 88:519–526.

Lindahl S: Influence of an end inspiratory pause on pulmonary ventilation, gas distribution and lung perfusion during artificial ventilation. *Crit Care Med* 1979; 7:540–546.

Marini JJ, Capps JS, Culver BH: The inspiratory work of breathing during assisted ventilation. *Chest* 1985; 87:612–618.

Marini JJ, Smith TC, Lamb VJ: External work output and force generation during synchronized intermittent mandatory ventilation. *AM Rev Respir Dis* 1988; 138:1169–1179.

Marquez JM, Douglas ME, Downs JB, et al: Renal function and cardiovascular responses during positive airway pressure. *Anesthesiology* 1979; 50:393–398.

Mathru M, Venus B: Ventilator-induced barotrauma in controlled mechanical ventilation versus intermittent mandatory ventilation. *Crit Care Med* 1983; 11:359–361.

McIntyre NR: Respiratory function during pressure support ventilation. *Chest* 1986; 89:677–683.

Millbern SM, Downs JB, Jumper LC, et al: Evaluation of criteria for discontinuing mechanical ventilatory support. *Arch Surg* 1978; 113:1441–1443.

Nishimura M, Tabnaka N, Takezawa J, et al: Oxygen cost of breathing and inspiratory work of breathing as weaning monitor in critically ill. *Crit Care Med* 1984; 12:2–58.

Pepe PE, Marini JJ: Occult positive end-expiratory pressure in mechanically ventilated patients with airflow obstruction. *Am Rev Respir Dis* 1982; 126:166–170.

Rasanen J, Nikki P, Heikkila J: Acute myocardial infarction complicated by respiratory failure: The effects of mechanical ventilation. *Chest* 1984; 85:21–28.

Rau JL: Continuous mechanical ventilation: part I. *Crit Care Update* 1981; 8:10–29.

Rau JL: Continuous mechanical ventilation: part II. *Crit Care Update* 1981; 8:5–19.

Rivara D, Artucio H, Arcos J, et al: Positional hypoxemia during artificial ventilation. *Crit Care Med* 1984; 12:436–438.

Robotham JL, Cherry D, Mitzner W, et al: A re-evaluation of the hemodynamic consequences of intermittent positive pressure ventilation. *Crit Care Med* 1983; 11:783–793.

Schachter EN, Tucker D, Beck GL: Does intermittent mandatory ventilation accelerate weaning? *JAMA* 1981; 246:1210–1214.

Shapiro BA, Harrison RA, Kacmarek RM, et al: *Clinical Application of Respiratory Care*, ed 3. Chicago, Year Book Medical Publishers, 1985.

Smith TC, Marini JJ: Impact of PEEP on lung mechanics and work of breathing in severe airflow obstruction. *J Appl Physiol* 1988; 65:1488–1499.

Spearman CB, Sheldon RL, Egan DL: *Egan's Fundamentals of Respiratory Therapy*, ed 4. St Louis, CV Mosby Co, 1982.

Viale JP, Annat G, Bertrand O: Additional inspiratory work in intubated patients breathing with continuous positive airway pressure systems. *Anesthesiology* 1985; 63:536–539.

Weisman IM, Rinaldo JE, Rogers RM, et al: Intermittent mandatory ventilation. *Am Rev Respir Dis* 1983; 127:641–647.

_____

Chapter 37

Positive End-Expiratory Pressure

I. Definition of Terms
   A. Positive end-expiratory pressure (PEEP): The establishment and maintenance of a preset airway pressure greater than ambient at end-exhalation.
   B. Continuous positive airway pressure (CPAP): The application of PEEP therapy to the spontaneously breathing patient. Both inspiratory and expiratory airway pressures are supra-atmospheric.
   C. Continuous positive pressure ventilation (CPPV): The application of PEEP therapy to a patient receiving positive pressure ventilation. It is applied regardless of mode of ventilation used on the ventilator (control, assist/control, intermittent mandatory ventilation [IMV], etc.).
   D. Additional terminology
      1. IMV + CPAP: The application of PEEP therapy to the patient being ventilated in the IMV mode.
      2. Synchronized IMV (SIMV) + CPAP: The application of PEEP therapy to the patient being ventilated in the SIMV mode.
      3. Expiratory positive airway pressure (EPAP): The application of PEEP therapy to the spontaneously breathing patient. Positive pressure is maintained only during exhalation; a subatmospheric pressure must be developed during inspiration.
         a. This approach of applying PEEP to the spontaneously breathing patient parallels the development of CPAP.
         b. However, it has been demonstrated that the work of breathing with EPAP may be *four times* as great as when CPAP is delivered via a continuous flow system at the same PEEP level.
         c. This technical approach of applying PEEP *is not recommended*.
II. Physiologic Effects of Positive End-Expiratory Pressure
   A. Effects on intrapulmonary pressures
      1. Figure 37–1 depicts intrapulmonary pressure curves during spontaneous breathing, CPAP, EPAP, CPPV, IMV or SIMV with CPAP, and IMV or SIMV with EPAP.
      2. With CPAP, CPPV, and IMV or SIMV with CPAP, the shape of the curve is not altered; only the baseline pressure from which the patient is ventilated changes. Therefore, the dynamics of air movement are not directly affected.

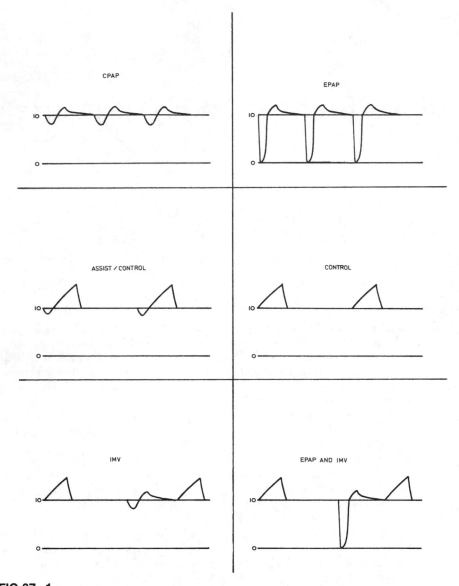

FIG 37–1.
Theoretical airway pressure curves with the application of PEEP to various modes of ventilation.

  3. With EPAP and IMV or EPAP and SIMV there is a significant alteration in the airway pressure curve during spontaneous ventilation. Therefore, the dynamics of gas movement are grossly affected, causing large increases in the work of breathing. In general, EPAP systems are not used today.
B. Effects on intrapleural (intrathoracic) pressures
  1. Positive end-expiratory pressure increases intrapleural pressures.
  2. The extent of the increase is determined by:
    a. The amount of PEEP applied.
    b. The stiffness of the individual's lung.
      (1) The greater the individual's pulmonary compliance, the greater the transmission of PEEP to the intrapleural space and the greater the increase in intrapleural pressure.

(2) In patients with normal lungs, PEEP therapy causes a significant increase in intrapleural pressure.

(3) In patients with a generalized diffuse pulmonary disease process resulting in decreased compliance, a given level of PEEP may not cause a significant increase in intrapleural pressure.

(4) Patients with localized pulmonary disease (e.g., pneumonia, atelectasis) demonstrate a similar increase in intrapleural pressure as patients with normal pulmonary compliance.

(5) The effects of PEEP are most marked in COPD patients with increased pulmonary compliance.

c. Changes in thoracic compliance.

(1) If thoracic compliance is decreased, more pressure than normal will be transmitted to the intrapleural space because overall expansion of the lung-thorax system is inhibited.

(2) An increase in thoracic compliance will allow the system to expand and usually results in less of an increase in intrapleural pressure when compared to normal.

C. Effects on functional residual capacity (FRC)

1. Regardless of the condition of the lung at the time of application PEEP therapy causes an increase in FRC.

2. Functional residual capacity is increased by:

a. Increasing the transpulmonary pressure gradient (Fig 37–2). This occurs in all individuals.

b. Recruiting collapsed alveoli.

(1) In patients with a decreased FRC as a result of alveolar collapse due to surfactant instability, PEEP maintains alveoli inflated.

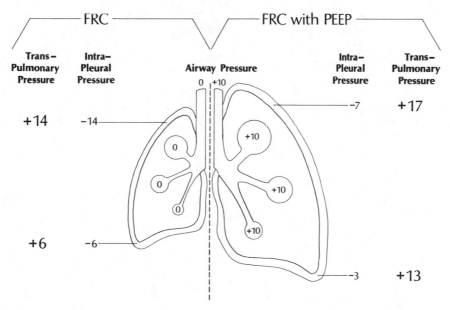

FIG 37–2.
Transpulmonary pressure gradients vary from the apex to the base of the lung. In ARDS the magnitude of these gradients increase because of the increased elastance of the lung. Applying PEEP increases the FRC by increasing the transpulmonary pressure gradient. Note that the gradient is normally increased most in the most gravity-dependent area of the lung. (From Shapiro BA, Harrison RA, Kacmarek RA, et al: *Clinical Application of Respiratory Care,* ed 3. Chicago, Year Book Medical Publishers, 1985. Used by permission.)

(2) This is accomplished by PEEP maintaining a backpressure exceeding the force of surface tension and lung elastance, which tend to collapse alveoli.

(3) The actual reexpansion of alveoli is accomplished by the force of normal inspiration or positive pressure. Positive end-expiratory pressure simply maintains the alveoli open once they are reexpanded.

D. Effect on pulmonary compliance
  1. Since PEEP therapy increases FRC, it may alter pulmonary compliance.
  2. In the normal lung the increased FRC may move alveoli from the steep portion to the flat portion of their compliance curve, thus decreasing compliance (Fig 37–3).
  3. In patients with adult respiratory distress syndrome (ARDS), the application of PEEP therapy increases compliance (Fig 37–4).
    a. As ARDS develops, the compliance curve shifts to the right and downward.
    b. As PEEP therapy is applied, the compliance curve shifts upward and to the left.
    c. With appropriate application of PEEP, a near-normal compliance curve can be reestablished.
  4. The monitoring of effective static compliance (see Chapter 36) can be used to determine the "optimal" or most appropriate PEEP level.
    a. The highest compliance is thought to coincide with the most appropriate PEEP level.
    b. The major problem associated with the use of compliance as a means of determining optimal PEEP is the difficulty in determining compliance in patients ventilated in anything but the control mode. With other modes, a reliable measurement of effective static compliance is often difficult because of active movement of the chest wall by the patient, preventing equilibration.

E. Effect of PEEP on deadspace
  1. Since PEEP increases FRC by distending alveoli, deadspace is usually increased in:
    a. Those with normal lungs.

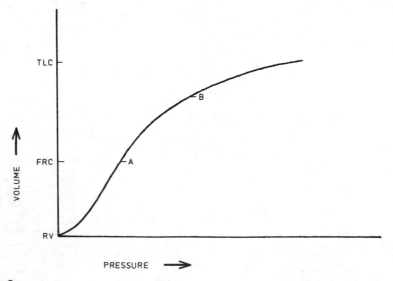

FIG 37–3.
Total compliance curve of the lung-thorax system. **A,** normal pressure-volume point (FRC) in a healthy individual, **B,** the application of PEEP in the normal lung increases the FRC and may move the pressure-volume point at FRC to the steep portion of the curve, decreasing total compliance.

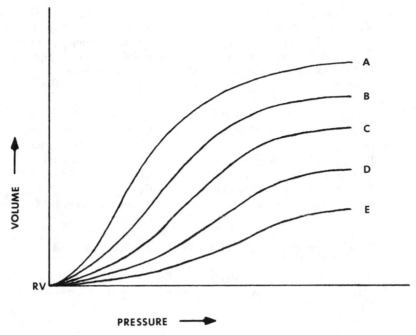

FIG 37–4.
A, normal total compliance curve. **B,** through **E,** total compliance curves with increasing acute restrictive lung disease (ARDS). The application of PEEP, by recruiting alveoli and increasing transpulmonary pressure gradients, can alter the compliance curve, moving the curve from **E** to **D** or from **D** to **B,** and ideally returning the pressure-volume relationship back to normal **(A).**

      b. Patients with COPD.
      c. Patients with a nonuniform disease process.
    2. In patients with generalized acute lung injury because of recruitment of collapsed alveoli, appropriate PEEP levels usually decrease deadspace. Some have proposed monitoring deadspace as an indication of appropriate PEEP level.
F. Effect of PEEP on the cardiovascular system
    1. Since PEEP therapy increases intrapleural pressure, it can decrease venous return and thus decrease cardiac output.
    2. The greater the increase in intrapleural pressure, the greater the potential detrimental effect on cardiac output.
    3. Positive end-expiratory pressure therapy causes a decrease in cardiac output by:
      a. Decreasing venous return (decreased preload) as a result of increased mean intrapulmonary pressures.
      b. Increasing right ventricular afterload by increasing pulmonary vascular resistance.
        (1) Right ventricular end-diastolic volume (RVEDV) is increased.
        (2) However, in the healthy individual, right ventricular ejection fraction (RVEF) is unchanged until high levels of PEEP are applied if flow is adequate.
        (3) In patients with right ventricular failure, RVEF decreases.
      c. Decreasing left ventricular distensibility (intraventricular septal shift).
        (1) The elevated RVEDV shifts the intraventricular septum to the left and decreases left ventricular volume and distensibility.
        (2) This is also a direct result of the increased intrathoracic pressure.

4. When the effect of PEEP on cardiac output is evaluated, it is important to place the decreased cardiac output into proper perspective. Following are two examples of the effect of PEEP on cardiac output. In example A, the patient is young and has excellent cardiovascular reserves, whereas in example B, the patient is older and has very limited cardiovascular reserves.
Example A:

A 25-year-old man with ARDS*:

Pa_{O_2}	48 mm Hg	Pulse	130 beats min
pH	7.53	BP	160/100 mm Hg
Pa_{CO_2}	27 mm Hg	CO	13.5 L/min
HCO_3^-	22 mEq/L	CI	7.7 L/min/sq m
Spon. RR	35 breaths/min (bpm)	$F_{I_{O_2}}$	0.8
V_T	350 ml	No mechanical ventilation support	

With the application of PEEP, the following data are obtained:

Pa_{O_2}	75 mm Hg	Pulse	85 beats/min
pH	7.43	BP	130/80 mm Hg
Pa_{CO_2}	38 mm Hg	CO	6.6 L/min
HCO_3^-	24 mEq/L	CI	3.7 L/min/sq m
Spon. RR	20 bpm	$F_{I_{O_2}}$	0.8
V_T	350 ml	CPAP at 10 cm H_2O	

In this example the patient's cardiac output dropped 7 L, but his cardiac index returned to normal. This occurred because the original cardiac output of 13.5 L/min was a result of cardiopulmonary stress. With the application of PEEP, oxygenation improved and cardiopulmonary stress decreased. Thus, the cardiac output and cardiac index returned to normal. This reduction in cardiac output and cardiac index is both dramatic and desirable.
Example B:

A 60-year-old man with ARDS:

Pa_{O_2}	48 mm Hg	Pulse	130 beats/min
pH	7.48	BP	140/90 mm Hg
Pa_{CO_2}	32 mm Hg	CO	5.5 L/min
HCO_3^-	23 mEq/L	CI	3.6 L/min/sq m
Spon. RR	35 bpm	$F_{I_{O_2}}$	0.6
V_T	300 ml	No mechanical ventilation support	

With the application of PEEP, the following data are obtained:

Pa_{O_2}	68 mm Hg	Pulse	150 beats/min
pH	7.47	BP	90/60 mm Hg
Pa_{CO_2}	33 mm Hg	CO	3.5 L/min
HCO_3^-	23 mEq/L	CI	2.3 L/min/sq m
Spon. RR	28 bpm	$F_{I_{O_2}}$	0.6
V_T	300 ml	CPAP at 10 cm H_2O	

*Spoon. RR = spontaneous respiratory rate: V_T = tidal volume; BP = blood pressure; CO = cardiac output; CI = cardiac index.

In this example the patient's cardiac output dropped only 2 L/min, but the cardiac index is now well below normal. A cardiac output of 3.5 L/min is clearly inappropriately low for this patient, and either fluid therapy or pharmacologic support is required to return the cardiac output to an acceptable level. The reduction in cardiac output is small but places the patient at increased risk.

    a. The drop in cardiac output was appropriate in example A but clearly inappropriate in example B.

    b. The patient's complete clinical presentation must be evaluated to determine if PEEP therapy had a detrimental effect on cardiac output.

5. Hemodynamic effects of PEEP therapy (see Chapter 14)

    a. Since PEEP therapy decreases venous return and cardiac output, a decrease in systemic blood pressure is normally noted as PEEP is applied.

        (1) Usually the decrease is minimal or moves the blood pressure to a more acceptable level.

        (2) However, with PEEP levels that significantly interfere with cardiac output, systemic blood pressure may drop precipitously.

    b. As PEEP therapy increases intrapleural pressure, it abates the thoracic pump mechanism. As a result, the pressure gradient distending intrathoracic blood vessels decreases, thereby increasing resistance to blood flow. This causes:

        (1) A decrease in the volume of blood returning to the right ventricle.

        (2) An alteration in pressure measured within the intrathoracic vessels.

    c. If the increased intrapleural pressure *does not significantly* alter flow, hemodynamic readings taken within the thoracic cavity *increase slightly.*

        (1) Increase in central venous pressure) ($\uparrow$ CVP)

        (2) Increase in mean pulmonary artery pressure ($\uparrow$ $\overline{\text{PAP}}$)

        (3) Increase in pulmonary wedge pressure ($\uparrow$ PWP)

    d. If, on the other hand, the increased intrapleural pressure *does significantly* alter flow, hemodynamic readings taken within the thoracic cavity *will decrease.* The extent of the decrease is a result of the interrelationship among myocardial capabilities, vascular volume, and intrapleural pressure.

        (1) $\downarrow$ CVP

        (2) $\downarrow$ $\overline{\text{PAP}}$

        (3) $\downarrow$ PWP

    e. If pulmonary hemodynamic values drop with the application of PEEP, then fluid therapy, pharmacologic support, or a decrease in PEEP level is indicated.

    f. The following example is designed to illustrate the effects of PEEP on hemodynamics values:

	No PEEP		
Pulse	160 beats/min	CVP	12 cm H_2O
BP	150/100 mm Hg	$\overline{\text{PAP}}$	26 mm Hg
		PWP	10 mm Hg

	5 cm H_2O PEEP		
Pulse	158 beats/min	CVP	13 cm H_2O
BP	148/92 mm Hg	$\overline{\text{PAP}}$	27 mm Hg
		PWP	11 mm Hg

10 cm H_2O PEEP

Pulse	140 beats/min	$\overline{CVP}$	15 cm H_2O
BP	142/96 mm Hg	$\overline{PAP}$	29 mm Hg
		PWP	13 mm Hg

15 cm H_2O PEEP

Pulse	126 beats/min	$\overline{CVP}$	16 cm H_2O
BP	130/84 mm Hg	$\overline{PAP}$	30 mm Hg
		PWP	14 mm Hg

20 cm H_2O PEEP

Pulse	154 beats/min	$\overline{CVP}$	6 cm H_2O
BP	90/60 mm Hg	$\overline{PAP}$	22 mm Hg
		PWP	5 mm Hg

The application of 5, 10, and 15 cm H_2O PEEP was appropriately tolerated from a hemodynamic perspective. However, with the application of 20 cm H_2O PEEP, the hemodynamic values decreased sharply, indicating inability of the cardiovascular system to tolerate 20 cm H_2O PEEP at its present status. If this patient receives proper fluid therapy, pharmacologic support or both, the following profile may be achieved:

20 cm H_2O PEEP

Pulse	124 beats/min	$\overline{CVP}$	18 cm H_2O
BP	120/84 mm Hg	$\overline{PAP}$	32 mm Hg
		PWP	16 mm Hg

Note: In actual clinical practice, hemodynamic values should also be correlated with the patient's clinical presentation, signs of adequate tissue perfusion (e.g., urinary output, sensorium, skin temperature), and cardiac output.

  G. Effects of PEEP on lung water
1. Positive end-expiratory pressure *does not* decrease overall pulmonary vascular volume.
2. Normally, PEEP causes a redistribution of lung water.
3. Fluid generally moves from the intrapulmonary to the interstitial space.
4. This movement assists in improving oxygenation, increasing compliance, and decreasing shunting.

  H. Effect of PEEP therapy on Pa_{O_2}
1. Since PEEP therapy causes a minor increase in the partial pressure of oxygen in the lung, a small increase in Pa_{O_2} may be noted even in the healthy lung.
2. In the patient with ARDS, Pa_{O_2} levels also demonstrate only a small increase as the PEEP level is increased and will not markedly rise until a significant number of alveoli have been recruited. When appropriate numbers of alveoli have been recruited, Pa_{O_2} values may increase 20 to 40 mm Hg or more. The following examples illustrate how Pa_{O_2} may change as PEEP is applied:

PEEP (cm H_2O)	Pa_{O_2} (mm Hg)
0	45
5	48
10	53
15	56
20	110

3. The Pa_{O_2} values may continue to increase slightly, remain the same, or decrease if the PEEP levels inhibit cardiac output.
    a. A continual increase in PEEP will eventually affect cardiac output. However, the blood that is capable of perfusing the lung will still be oxygenated and its oxygenation state may continue to improve slightly as cardiac output decreases.
    b. When appropriateness of PEEP therapy is monitored, Pa_{O_2} must be evaluated; however, Pa_{O_2} provides no indication of the adequacy of cardiovascular function or of systemic oxygen delivery (see section II–L).
I. Effects on intrapulmonary shunt
    1. Increasing PEEP levels results in a decrease in intrapulmonary shunt.
    2. As alveoli are recruited, ventilation/perfusion matching improves and shunting decreases.
    3. As with Pa_{O_2}, intrapulmonary shunt may continue to decrease even when cardiac output is significantly decreased.
        a. This occurs because any blood that is presented to the lung may be better oxygenated.
        b. When the appropriateness of PEEP therapy is monitored, intrapulmonary shunt should be evaluated; however, the intrapulmonary shunt provides no indication of adequacy of cardiovascular function or systemic oxygen delivery (see section II–L).
J. Mixed venous Po_2 ($P\bar{v}_{O_2}$) (see Chapter 14)
    1. $P\bar{v}_{O_2}$ is a variable affected by:
        a. Cardiac output.
        b. Tissue perfusion.
        c. Oxygen content.
        d. Metabolic rate.
    2. A decreased cardiac output, a decrease in oxygen content, a decrease in tissue perfusion, or an increase in metabolic rate can cause a decrease in $P\bar{v}_{O_2}$.
    3. In cardiopulmonary-stressed patients with ARDS, the $P\bar{v}_{O_2}$ is normally decreased.
        a. The extent of this decrease is *most* dependent on the cardiovascular reserves of the patient.
        b. In patients with good cardiovascular reserves, the $P\bar{v}_{O_2}$ will be decreased only slightly (35–40 mm Hg) because these patients can increase their cardiac outputs significantly in response to stress.
        c. However, in patients with limited cardiovascular reserves, the $P\bar{v}_{O_2}$ may be significantly decreased (30–35 mm Hg or lower) because these patients cannot increase their cardiac outputs in response to stress.
    4. As PEEP therapy is applied, the $P\bar{v}_{O_2}$ should increase if the cardiac output is not adversely affected. This occurs because oxygen delivery increases.
    5. If excessive PEEP is applied, the $P\bar{v}_{O_2}$ will decrease because of the effect of PEEP on cardiac output, thus decreasing oxygen delivery:

PEEP (cm H_2O)	$P\bar{v}_{O_2}$ (mm Hg)	CO (L/min)
0	36	12.5
5	36	12.3
10	38	9.6
15	40	8.9
20	43	7.2
25	35	4.8

At PEEP levels from 5 to 20 cm H_2O, the $P\bar{v}_{O_2}$ increased appropriately, but at 25 cm H_2O the PEEP inhibited cardiac output significantly, resulting in a drop in the $P\bar{v}_{O_2}$. Fluid therapy, pharmacologic support, or a decrease in PEEP level is indicated to support cardiovascular function and optimize $P\bar{v}_{O_2}$.

K. Arteriovenous oxygen content difference ($a-\bar{v}DO_2$) (see Chapter 14)
   1. $a-\bar{v}DO_2$ is dependent on:
      a. Arterial oxygen content.
      b. Venous oxygen content.
      c. Metabolic rate.
      d. Cardiac output.
   2. In patients with ARDS, $a-\bar{v}DO_2$ varies from normal, depending on the cardiovascular reserves of the patient.
   3. In the patient with good cardiovascular reserves, decreased arterial oxygen content results in an increase in cardiac output.
      a. If the patient's metabolic rate is constant and cardiac output is increased, the volume of oxygen extracted per volume of blood decreases.
         (1) As a result, the venous oxygen content of the patient will not be significantly decreased, and
         (2) $a-\bar{v}DO_2$ will decrease.
         (3) Since the tissue is extracting less oxygen per given volume of blood, the difference between the arterial and venous contents becomes smaller, regardless of the actual contents of each.
   4. In patients with poor cardiovascular reserves, a decrease in arterial oxygen content may not affect cardiac output.
      a. If the patient's metabolic rate and cardiac output are constant but arterial oxygen content is decreased, then $a-\bar{v}DO_2$ will increase.
      b. If the patient's metabolic rate is constant and the cardiac output and arterial oxygen content are decreased, then $a-\bar{v}DO_2$ will also increase.
   5. With the appropriate application of PEEP, the $a-\bar{v}DO_2$ should return toward normal levels.
      a. If PEEP is applied and $a-\bar{v}DO_2$ levels increase beyond acceptable limits, cardiovascular reserves are questionable. Fluid therapy or pharmacologic support may be indicated.
      b. If, with the application of PEEP, $a-\bar{v}DO_2$ values increase appropriately but then exceed upper limits, PEEP therapy is beginning to adversely affect cardiac output. Fluid therapy, pharmacologic support, or a decrease in PEEP level may be indicated:

PEEP (cm H_2O)	$a-\bar{v}DO_2$ (vol %)	CO (L/min)
0	2.8	12.2
5	3.0	10.5
10	3.3	9.0
15	3.6	7.5
20	4.0	6.0
25	5.6	3.5

In this table, it is assumed the patient's cardiovascular reserves are good. The application of 5 to 20 cm H_2O PEEP resulted in appropriate increases in $a-\bar{v}DO_2$. However, with the application of 25 cm H_2O PEEP, cardiac output was adversely affected, causing $a-\bar{v}DO_2$ to increase significantly toward the upper limits of normal. Fluid therapy, pharmacologic support, or decreasing PEEP is indicated.

L. Effect of PEEP on oxygen transport
1. Oxygen transport is defined as cardiac output times arterial oxygen content:

$$O_2 \text{ transport} = CO \times Ca_{O_2} \qquad (1)$$

2. With the development of ARDS, oxygen transport normally decreases because of the decrease in Ca_{O_2}.
3. As PEEP is applied and Ca_{O_2} is increased, oxygen transport improves.
4. With excessive application of PEEP, oxygen transport may decrease because of the effect of PEEP on cardiac output. If this occurs, fluid therapy, pharmacologic support, or decreasing PEEP is indicated.

M. Effects of PEEP on closing volume.
1. Closing volume is that point in a forced vital capacity maneuver at which gravity-dependent airways close.
2. The point at which gravity-dependent airways close may become a larger percentage of the forced vital capacity and possibly exceed FRC in anesthetized individuals, postoperative patients, and obese patients.
3. Positive end-expiratory pressure therapy may have the effect of decreasing closing volume and improving oxygenation in the patients defined; however, no conclusive data supporting this are available.

N. Effect on intracranial pressure
1. Since PEEP impedes venous return, it can be expected to increase intracranial pressure by causing blood to pool in the cranium.
2. If PEEP therapy is required in patients with an increased intracranial pressure, elevation of the head of the patient's bed a distance equal to the amount of PEEP applied can minimize the effects of PEEP on intracranial pressure.

O. Barotrauma and PEEP
1. Any time positive pressure is applied to the lung, the likelihood of barotrauma is increased.
2. However, barotrauma normally occurs when patients simulate a cough, fight the ventilator, or engage in any activity that markedly increases intrapulmonary pressure.
3. When high levels of PEEP are applied, careful monitoring for barotrauma must be maintained. This is necessary because the lung requiring high levels of PEEP is significantly diseased, and any increase in airway pressure may result in barotrauma.

P. The effects of PEEP therapy on renal, gastrointestinal, and endocrine function are the same as those of all forms of positive pressure (see Chapter 32).

III. Indications for Positive End-Expiratory Pressure Therapy
A. The primary indications for PEEP therapy is ARDS.
1. Positive end-expiratory pressure is truly indicated only in patients with a generalized diffuse acute restrictive disease process characterized by:
   a. Decreased pulmonary compliance.
   b. Decreased FRC.
   c. Refractory hypoxemia.
   d. Increased intrapulmonary shunting.
2. It does not correct the refractory hypoxemia associated with a localized disease process such as:
   a. Pneumonia.

   b. Pleural effusion.
   c. Localized atelectasis.
B. Other indications for PEEP include the treatment of noncardiogenic pulmonary edema or early ARDS. The capillary endothelial changes associated with the early phase:
   1. Are diffuse.
   2. Are generalized.
   3. Cause a decrease in FRC; however, this decrease is minimal.
   4. Include hypoxemia, which is normally somewhat responsive to oxygen therapy.
C. Positive end-expiratory pressure therapy has also been recommended for the following pathophysiologic conditions:
   1. Chest trauma: It stabilizes the chest wall internally and prevents atelectasis.
   2. Pulmonary edema from left-sided heart failure: It helps to stabilize the pressure gradient across the alveolar capillary membrane, prevents further transudation of fluid, and improves gas exchange. It does not by itself decrease overall lung water (see section II–G).
IV. Physiologic Positive End-Expiratory Pressure
   A. This is the application of 3 to 5 cm H_2O PEEP to replace the glottic mechanism.
   B. The placement of a foreign body between the vocal cord results in a reflexive decrease in FRC.
   C. This occurs in all individuals but has been demonstrated to be clinically significant in only two populations.
      1. Neonatal and pediatric patients: *This group should not have a short-term artificial airway in place without 3 to 5 cm H_2O PEEP.* If extubation is indicated, they are extubated from 3 to 5 cm H_2O PEEP rather than from atmospheric pressure.
      2. Patients with severe COPD: Again, establishment of an artificial airway under acute conditions results in a significant decrease in the FRC causing hypoxemia. It is advisable to maintain 5 cm H_2O PEEP in these patients until extubation.
      3. Positive end-expiratory pressure of 3 to 5 cm H_2O is often used in the average patient requiring a short-term artificial airway. The efficacy of such treatment has not been established, nor have any adverse reactions been documented.
V. Prophylactic Positive End-Expiratory Pressure
   A. Positive end-expiratory pressure has been used to prevent ARDS or postoperative pulmonary complications.
   B. No definitive data for or against this application of PEEP are available.
VI. Inadvertent Positive End-Expiratory Pressure
   A. Inadvertant PEEP is PEEP applied externally that registers on the system manometer but is undesirable.
   B. It is seen with:
      1. High continuous gas flow systems.
      2. Some PEEP devices.
   C. It has the same effects of any applied PEEP.
VII. Auto or Intrinsic Positive End-Expiratory Pressure
   A. This is PEEP developed at the lung parenchymal level as a result of air flow limitations (COPD) or insufficient expiratory time (rapid rates).
   B. This PEEP is not noticed on the system manometer unless equilibration of total system pressure occurs at end-exhalation.
   C. See Chapter 36 for details.
   D. Auto-PEEP has the same effects as any applied PEEP.

VIII. Clinical Goals of Positive End-Expiratory Pressure
    A. The end point of PEEP therapy is defined by:
        1. Adequate arterial oxygenation.
        2. Minimal $F_{I_{O_2}}$.
        3. Adequate cardiovascular function.
    B. Adequate arterial oxygenation:
        1. Is defined as a P_{O_2} greater than 50 to 60 mm Hg. This normally results in an 87% to 90% oxyhemoglobin percent saturation if there is no significant shift in the oxyhemoglobin dissociation curve (Fig 37–5).
        2. Has normal hemoglobin content.
    C. Minimal $F_{I_{O_2}}$
        1. The specific $F_{I_{O_2}}$ that is "safe" to inspire over a period of time has not been determined.
        2. Most suspect that an $F_{I_{O_2}}$ greater than 0.50 may cause pulmonary epithelial damage.
        3. Positive end-expiratory pressure therapy should be titrated until an $F_{I_{O_2}}$ less than 0.50 is achieved. Maintaining the $F_{I_{O_2}}$ below 0.40 is ideal.
    D. Adequate cardiovascular function:
        1. Entails maintaining appropriate cardiac index and cardiac output for the particular patient.
        2. Entails maintaining adequate tissue perfusion.
           a. Normal skin temperature
           b. Normal urinary output
           c. Intact sensorium
           d. Normal $P\bar{v}_{O_2}$
           e. Normal $a-\bar{v}DO_2$

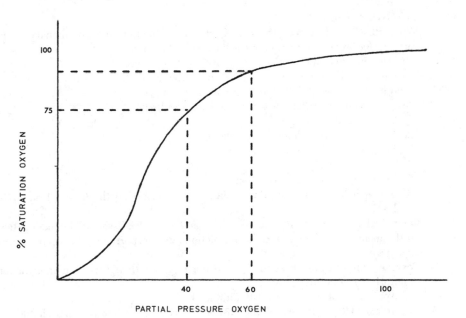

FIG 37–5.
At a Pa_{O_2} of 60 mm Hg the hemoglobin is approximately 90% saturated with oxygen. Because the curve is relatively flat beyond the 90% saturation level, the Pa_{O_2} must be significantly increased to effect a significant change in hemoglobin saturation, whereas increasing the Pa_{O_2} from 40 to 60 mm Hg increases the hemoglobin saturation by about 15%.

IX. Monitoring Positive End-Expiratory Pressure Therapy
  A. With the application of PEEP or the alteration of PEEP levels, extensive monitoring of the patient's cardiopulmonary status must be performed.
  B. Monitoring should be done 10 to 20 min after each PEEP adjustment and periodically thereafter.
  C. Gas exchange should be monitored.
    1. Arterial blood gases
    2. Oxyhemoglobin percent saturation
    3. Intrapulmonary shunt if accessible
  D. Pulmonary mechanics should be monitored.
    1. Evaluation of V_T, RR, and work of breathing, if appropriate.
    2. Effective static compliance if patient is in control mode or not spontaneously ventilating
  E. Cardiovascular function should be monitored.
    1. Pulse and blood pressure
    2. Skin color
    3. Skin turgor
    4. Skin temperature
    5. Urinary output
    6. Sensorium
    7. Cardiac output
    8. Cardiac index
    9. $\overline{PAP}$
    10. CVP
    11. PWP
    12. $P\bar{v}_{O_2}$
    13. $a-\bar{v}DO_2$
    14. Oxygen transport
  F. When PEEP level exceeds 15 cm H_2O, it is advisable to insert a pulmonary artery catheter for proper evaluation of cardiovascular function.
X. Periodic Discontinuation of Positive End-Expiratory Pressure
  A. The periodic discontinuation of PEEP should be avoided. This is particularly true when higher levels of PEEP are employed.
  B. Discontinuation of PEEP on a periodic basis results in:
    1. Significant decreases in Pa_{O_2}.
    2. Increase in intrapulmonary shunt.
    3. Possible increased venous return.
    4. Decreased FRC.
    5. Decreased pulmonary compliance.
    6. A complete reversal of the changes accomplished with the application of PEEP.
  C. Once PEEP levels reach or exceed 15 cm H_2O, PEEP should be maintained on the manual ventilators used during suctioning, transport, and chest physiotherapy.
  D. Positive end-expiratory pressure *should not be discontinued* when hemodynamic monitoring is being performed.
XI. Clinical Application of Positive End-Expiratory Pressure
  A. Regardless of the severity of the disease process, all adult patients should be started on 5 cm H_2O PEEP. Pediatric and neonatal patients should be started on 2 to 3 cm H_2O PEEP.
  B. Positive end-expiratory pressure levels should be increased in 3 to 5 cm H_2O increments in adults, in 2 to 3 cm H_2O increments in neonatal and pediatric patients, followed by complete monitoring of the effects of PEEP.

C. If an increase in PEEP results in adverse cardiovascular effects, fluid therapy, pharmacologic support, or both should be used to stabilize cardiovascular function before the PEEP level is again increased.

D. As PEEP is applied, a significant increase in Pa_{O_2} should be noted. If a 20 to 40 mm Hg increase in Pa_{O_2} is not seen, the optimal level to PEEP for that patient may not have been attained.

E. Once the Pa_{O_2} has shown a reasonable increase and the patient is stabilized cardiovascularly, attempt to decrease the $F_{I_{O_2}}$.
   1. If the $F_{I_{O_2}}$ is more than 0.5, a 0.05 to 0.2 decrease in $F_{I_{O_2}}$ followed by arterial blood gas measurement is indicated.
   2. If the $F_{I_{O_2}}$ is at or less than 0.5, decrease the $F_{I_{O_2}}$ by 0.05, followed by arterial blood gas measurement.

F. When one is weaning the patient from PEEP and $F_{I_{O_2}}$, the variable decreased depends on the $F_{I_{O_2}}$ level.
   1. If the $F_{I_{O_2}}$ is more than 0.5, always decrease the $F_{I_{O_2}}$ before the PEEP.
   2. If the $F_{I_{O_2}}$ is 0.5 or less, decrease the PEEP to 5 to 10 cm H_2O before further decreasing the $F_{I_{O_2}}$.

G. The previous sequence is used in patients with severe ARDS. If the patient has noncardiogenic pulmonary edema or early ARDS, 5 to 15 cm H_2O may be sufficient to maintain Pa_{O_2} at a low (less than 0.5) $F_{I_{O_2}}$. *Since no significant intrapulmonary shunting from atelectasis normally exists, a marked increase (20–40 mm Hg) in the Pa_{O_2} may not be noted.*

H. Generally, patients may be extubated from 2 to 5 cm H_2O PEEP, since this is normally considered physiologic PEEP.

XII. Technical Application of Positive End-Expiratory Pressure
   A. Devices used to apply PEEP are classified as three types.
      1. Orificial resistors: These devices generate PEEP by developing a resistance to gas flow (Fig 37–6).
         a. Ohm's law, or the law of flow, describes how PEEP is developed:

$$\text{Resistance (R)} = \frac{\text{Pressure (P)}}{\text{Flow (}\dot{V}\text{)}} \tag{2}$$

If equation 2 is solved for pressure, the relationship becomes:

$$\text{Pressure} = \text{Resistance} \times \text{Flow} \tag{3}$$

         b. Thus, with a fixed resistance, the level of PEEP generated is dependent on the flow through the system.
            (1) Higher flow creates more PEEP.
            (2) Lower flow creates less PEEP.
         c. The major problem with orificial resistors is that PEEP levels are altered if flow through the system changes.
         d. In adults, inadvertently high levels of PEEP can develop during forced exhalation if orificial resistors are used.
         e. These PEEP devices are used only in pediatric and neonatal patients, in whom expiratory flows are minimal.
      2. Threshold resistors: These devices are capable of maintaining a constant, predictable, and quantifiable PEEP level.
         a. All commonly used adult PEEP devices are normally listed as threshold resistors.

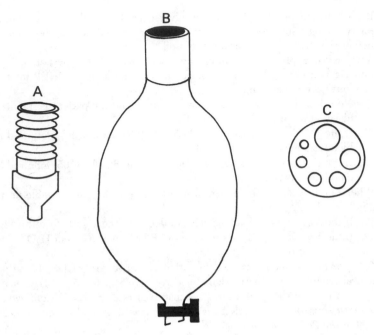

FIG 37–6.
Schematic representation of three common types of orificial resistors. **A,** endotracheal tube adapter attached to flex tube; **B,** screw clamp and reservoir bag; **C,** variable orificial plate. (From Kacmarek RM, Dimas S, Reynolds J, et al: *Respir Care* 1982; 27:1478–1488. Used by permission.)

      b. However, all threshold resistors have some orificial properties. If the area across which exhalation occurs is less than the cross-sectional area of the large-bore tubing leading to the device, gas flow resistance develops.

      c. It appears that the Emerson water column (Fig 37–7) offers the least resistance to gas flow.

      d. The most commonly used threshold resistor is the balloon-type exhalation valve on ventilator circuits (Fig 37–8).

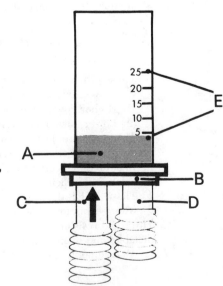

FIG 37–7.
Emerson water column PEEP device. **A,** water reservoir; **B,** flexible diaphragm; **C,** entrance port; **D,** exit port to atmosphere; **E,** calibrated scale in cm H_2O. (From Kacmarek RM, Dimas S, Reynolds J, et al: *Respir Care* 1982; 27:1478–1488. Used by permission.)

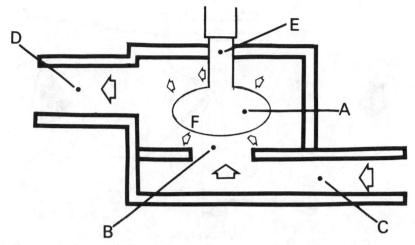

FIG 37-8.
Balloon-type exhalation PEEP valve. *Arrows* represent gas flow. **A,** balloon valve; **B,** outlet orifice; **C,** inlet port; **D,** exit port to atmosphere; **E,** gas nipple; **F,** inferior surface of balloon valve that may occlude outlet orifice. (From Kacmarek RM, Dimas S, Reynolds J, et al: *Respir Care* 1982; 27:1478–1488. Used by permission.)

        (1) Many of the disposable circuits utilizing this type of valve offer significant resistance to gas flow.

        (2) Frequent increases in expiratory pressure are noted with forced exhalation.

        (3) Many produce an expiratory retard with or without PEEP.

    e. Other commonly used threshold resistors with significant orificial properties are:

        (1) Weighted ball valves.

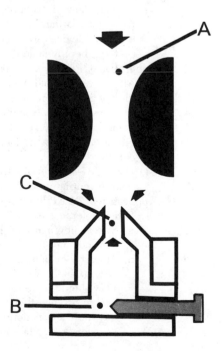

FIG 37-9.
Bourns opposing-flow exhalation PEEP valve. **A,** exhalation outlet; **B,** Venturi jet source gas; **C,** Venturi jet. Thumb screw adjusts Venturi source gas flow. *Small arrows* represent gas entrainment; *large arrows* indicate patient's exhalation. (From Kacmarek RM, Dimas S, Reynolds J, et al: *Respir Care* 1982; 27:1478–1488. Used by permission.)

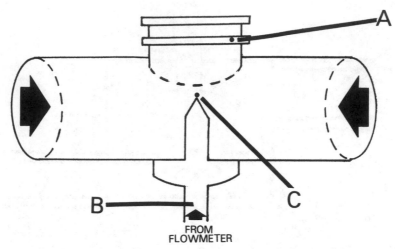

FIG 37–10.
Glazener PEEP device, used in adults for transport or for short-term therapy. *Arrows* represent gas entrainment. **A,** exhalation outlet; **B,** Venturi jet source gas; **C,** Venturi jet. (From Kacmarek RM, Dimas S, Reynolds J, et al. *Respir Care* 1982; 27:1478–1488. Used by permission.)

        (2) Spring-loaded valves.

        (3) Magnetic valves.

    f. In spite of their limitations, threshold resistors are the devices of choice in the adult. However, care must be taken to evaluate the appropriate function of each of these valves.

    g. In general, ventilator systems develop PEEP at the exhalation valve by a threshold resistor mechanism.

  3. Opposing flow devices: These devices are similar to threshold resistors in their ability to maintain a constant, predictable, and quantifiable PEEP level by directing a flow of gas opposing patient exhalation (Figs 37–9 and 37–10).

    a. Minimal orificial resistance is noted with these devices.

    b. These devices are used either in pediatrics and neonatology or for short-term therapy in adults.

B. Application of PEEP during positive pressure ventilation

  1. All of the threshold devices discussed can be easily applied to the expiratory limb of positive pressure ventilators.

  2. The most commonly and easily used of these devices is the balloon-type exhalation valve in the ventilator circuit.

  3. However, the most reliable of these devices appears to be the Emerson water column.

  4. Figures 37–11 and 37–12 illustrate approaches to the application of PEEP to manual ventilators.

C. Application of PEEP to the spontaneously breathing patient (Fig 37–13)

  1. Patient tolerance of a CPAP system is most directly related to system flow.

    a. System flow must be high enough to meet the patient's peak inspiratory demands (60–90 L/min).

    b. At least four times the patient's measured minute volume should enter the system.

    c. Flow should leave the system at all times, even at peak inspiration.

    d. A 3- to 5-L anesthesia bag, used as a reservoir, is included on the inspiratory limb. For patients who have very high peak inspiratory flows, two reservoir bags may be included.

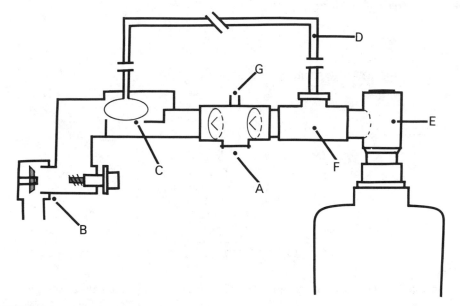

FIG 37–11.
Schematic representation of Universal PEEP system for manual ventilators. **A,** patient T piece with one-way valves; **B,** threshold-resistor PEEP device; **C,** balloon-type exhalation valve; **D,** pressure line to exhalation valve; **E,** manual ventilator gas-collecting head; **E,** T piece with pressure-line tap off; **G,** manometer nipple. (From Kacmarek RM, Dimas S, Reynolds J, et al: *Respir Care* 1982; 27:1490–1504. Used by permission.)

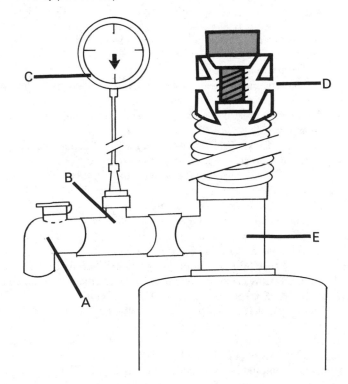

FIG 37–12.
PEEP system for manual ventilators with single exit port gas-collecting head. **A,** patient connection; **B,** T piece with manometer tap-off; **C,** manometer; **D,** threshold resistor PEEP device; **E,** single exit port gas-collecting head. (From Kacmarek RM, Dimas S, Reynolds J, et al: *Respir Care* 1982; 27:1490–1504. Used by permission.)

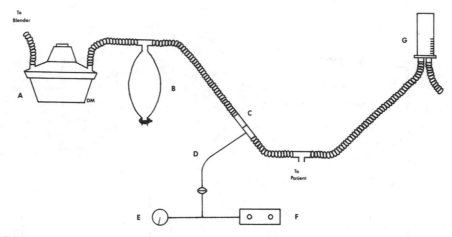

FIG 37–13.
Continuous flow CPAP system. **A,** large volume humidifier; **B,** 5-L reservoir bag; **C,** attachment of high/low pressure alarm and manometer to inspiratory limb; **D,** small-bore tubing to alarm and manometer; **E,** pressure manometer; **F,** high/low pressure alarm; **G,** water column PEEP device.

     e. A high/low pressure alarm and a pressure manometer are included in the system to monitor pressure changes.
     f. A properly set up and functioning system should demonstrate no more than a ± 2 cm H_2O fluctuation in pressure about PEEP level.
     g. A screw clamp is attached to the open tail of the reservoir bag to allow pressure relief if the system becomes obstructed.
  2. A typical EPAP system is depicted in Figure 37–14.
     a. This system is *not* a constant flow system.
     b. The patient must reduce system pressure to less than atmospheric to inspire.
     c. The work of breathing with this system is four times as great as the work of breathing with a CPAP system.
     d. The use of EPAP systems to deliver PEEP to the spontaneously breathing patient is discouraged secondary to the excessive work of breathing involved.
  3. Mask vs. artificial airway for the application of CPAP
     a. Mask CPAP can be used for short-term application of PEEP therapy if PEEP levels do not exceed about 10 cm H_2O.
     b. Patients in whom mask CPAP is used must:
       (1) Be alert, oriented, and cooperative.
       (2) Have good control of their airway.
     c. A nasogastric tube should be placed to prevent abdominal distention.
     d. Mask CPAP is useful in patients with noncardiogenic pulmonary edema or early ARDS for periods of about 12 to 36 hours.
     e. The vast majority of patients requiring CPAP also require an artificial airway.
  4. Nasal CPAP
     a. Nasal CPAP is used in the treatment of sleep apnea of either the obstructive or combined obstructive and central type.
     b. The CPAP forces the soft palate and the base of the tongue forward for a seal of the airway and to relieve the obstruction.
     c. Nasal CPAP is applied only during sleep.
     d. The CPAP system used is markedly simplified from standard CPAP systems.

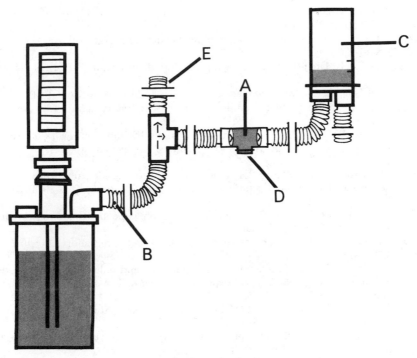

FIG 37–14.
EPAP system. **A,** volume requiring decompression; **B,** constant flow aerosol system; **C,** threshold resistor PEEP device; **D,** patient T piece with one-way valves; **E,** aerosol system reservoir. (From Kacmarek RM, Dimas S, Reynolds J, et al: *Respir Care* 1982; 27:1505–1518. Used by permission.)

BIBLIOGRAPHY

Albert RK: Non-respiratory effects of positive end-expiratory pressure. *Respir Care* 1988; 33:464–471.

Annest SJ, Gottlieb M, Paloski WH, et al: Detrimental effects of removing end-expiratory pressure prior to intubation. *Ann Surg* 1980; 191:539–546.

Benson MS, Pierson DJ: Auto-PEEP during mechanical ventilation of adults. *Respir Care* 1988; 33:557–568.

Bourns Inc. Life Systems Division: *Instruction Manual: Bourns Infant Ventilator Model LS-104-105 and Model BP 200.* Riverside, Calif, Bourns Medical Systems.

Bramson RD: PEEP without endotracheal intubation. *Respir Care* 1988; 33:598–612.

Bredenberg CE, Kazui T, Webb WR: Experimental pulmonary edema: The effect of positive end-expiratory pressure on lung water. *Ann Thorac Surg* 1978; 26:62–70.

Chapin C, Downs JB, Douglas ME, et al: Lung expansion and airway pressure transmission with positive end-expiratory pressure. *Arch Surg* 1979; 114:1193–1197.

Chomka CM: Cardiopulmonary effects of positive end expiratory pressure, in Shapiro RA, Cane RA (eds): *Positive Airway Pressure Therapy: PPV and PEEP. Anesth Clin North Am* 1987; 5:777–788.

Civetta JM, Barnes TA, Smith LO: "Optimal PEEP" and intermittent mandatory ventilation in the treatment of acute respiratory failure. *Respir Care* 1975; 20:551–557.

Craig DB, McCarthy DS: Airway closure and lung volumes during breathing with maintained airway positive measures. *Anesthesiology* 1972; 36:540–546.

Demling RH, Staub NC, Edmonds LH: Effect of end-expiratory airway pressure on accumulation of extravascular lung water. *J Appl Physiol* 1975; 38:907–915.

Douglas ME, Downs JB: Cardiopulmonary effects of PEEP and CPAP [letter]. *Anesth Analg* 1978; 57:347–350.

Emerson postoperative ventilator operating instructions. Cambridge, Mass, JH Emerson Co.

Falke KJ: Do changes in lung compliance allow the determination of "Optimal PEEP"? *Anesthetist* 1980; 29:165–169.

Gallagher TJ, Civetta JM: Goal-directed therapy of acute respiratory failure. *Anesth Analg* 1980; 59:831–836.

Fields A, Sterling D: Open-system IMV with PEEP [letter]. *Respir Care* 1979; 24:394–398.

Garg GP, Hill GE: The use of spontaneous continuous positive pressure (CPAP) for reduction of intrapulmonary shunting in adults with acute respiratory failure. *Can Anaesth Soc J* 1975; 22:284–290.

Gherini S, Peters RM, Virgilio RW: Mechanical work on the lungs and work of breathing with positive end-expiratory pressure and continuous positive airway pressure. *Chest* 1979; 76:251–256.

Gregory GA, Kitterman JA, Phibbs RH, et al: Treatment of the idiopathic respiratory distress syndrome with continuous positive airway pressure. *N Engl J Med* 1971; 284:1333–1340.

Hall JR, Rendleman DC, Downs JB: PEEP devices: Flow dependent increases in airway pressure [abstract]. *Crit Care Med* 1978; 6:100.

Hess D: The use of PEEP in clinical settings other than acute lung injury. *Respir Care* 1988; 33:581–597.

Hobelmann CF, Smith DE, Virgilio RW, et al: Left atrial and pulmonary artery wedge pressure differences with positive end-expiratory pressure: The contribution of the pulmonary vasculature. *J Trauma* 1975; 15:951–957.

Hobelmann CF, Smith DE, Virgilio RW, et al: Mechanics of ventilation with positive end-expiratory pressure. *Ann Thorac Surg* 1977; 24:68–74.

Hopewell PC, Murray JF: Effect of continuous positive pressure ventilation in experimental edema. *J Appl Physiol* 1976; 40:568–570.

Hudson LD, Weaver LJ, Haisch CE, et al: Positive end-expiratory pressure: Reduction and withdrawal. *Respir Care* 1988; 33:613–619.

Jardin F, Farcot J, Boisante L, et al: Influence of positive end-expiratory pressure on left ventricular performance. *N Engl J Med* 1981; 304:387–392.

Kacmarek RM, Dimas S, Reynolds J, et al: Technical aspects of positive end-expiratory pressure: Parts 1–3. *Respir Care* 1982; 27:1478–1518.

Kacmarek RM, Goulet RL: PEEP devices, in Shapiro RA, Cane RA (eds): *Positive Airway Pressure Therapy: PPV and PEEP. Anesthesiol Clin North Am* 1987; 5:757–776.

Katz JA, Ozanne GH, Zinn SE, et al: Time course and mechanisms of lung volume increases with PEEP in acute pulmonary failure. *Anesthesiology* 1981; 59:9–14.

Kirby RR: Best PEEP: Issues and choices in the selection and monitoring of PEEP levels. *Respir Care* 1988; 33:569–580.

Kirby RR, Downs JB, Civetta JM, et al: High level positive end-expiratory pressure (PEEP) in acute respiratory insufficiency. *Chest* 1975; 67:156–161.

Liebman PR, Patten MT, Manny J, et al: Humorally medicated alterations in cardiac performance as a consequence of positive end-expiratory pressure (PEEP). *Surgery* 1978; 83:594–599.

Lutch JS, Murray JF: Continuous positive-pressure ventilation: Effects of systemic oxygen transport and tissue oxygenation. *Ann Intern Med* 1972; 76:193–201.

Lysak SZ, Prough DS: Monitoring for patients receiving airway pressure therapy, in Shapiro RA, Cane RA (eds): *Positive Airway Pressure Therapy: PPV and PEEP. Anesth Clin North Am* 1987; 5:821–842.

Manny J, Justice R, Hechtman HB: Abnormalities in organ blood flow and its distribution during positive end-expiratory pressure. *Surgery* 1979; 85:425–431.

Marotta J, Greenbaum DM: PEEP attachment for puritan manual resuscitator. *Respir Care* 1976; 21:862–864.

Mathru M: The therapeutic application of positive end expiratory pressure, in Shapiro RA, Cane RA (eds): *Positive Airway Pressure Therapy: PPV and PEEP. Anesth Clin North Am* 1987; 5:789–796.

McCarthy GS, Hedenstierna G: Arterial oxygenation during artificial ventilation: The effect of airway closure and its prevention by positive end-expiratory pressure. *Acta Anaesthesiol Scand* 1978; 22:563–571.

Mitzner W, Batra G, Goldberg H: Lung inflation and extracellular fluid accumulation. *Circulation* 1976; 54(suppl II):14–19.

Nunn JF: *Applied Respiratory Physiology*, ed 2. Stoneham, Mass, Butterworth Publishing Co, 1977.

Op't Holt TB: Work of breathing and other aspects of patient interactions. *Respir Care* 1988; 33:444–453.

Pepe PE, Stager MA, Maunder RJ, et al: Early application of PEEP in patients at risk for ARDS [abstract] *Am Rev Respir Dis* 1983; 127(suppl):97.

Perel A, Eimerl D, Grossberg M: A PEEP device for a manual bag ventilator. *Anesth Analg* 1976; 55:745.

Petty TL, Nett LM, Ashbaugh DG: Improvement in oxygenation in the adult respiratory distress syndrome by positive end-expiratory pressure (PEEP). *Respir Care* 1976; 16:173–176.

Pierson DJ: Alveolar rupture during mechanical ventilation: Role of PEEP, peak airway pressure and distending pressure. *Respir Care* 1988; 33:472–486.

Quist J, Pontoppidan H, Wilson RS, et al: Hemodynamic responses to mechanical ventilation with PEEP. *Anesthesiology* 1975; 42:45–52.

Rose DM, Downs JB, Heenan TJ: Temporal responses of functional residual capacity and oxygen tension to changes in positive end-expiratory pressure. *Crit Care Med* 1981; 9:79–82.

Shoemaker WC, Thompson L (eds): *Critical Care: State of the Art*. Fullerton, Calif, Society of Critical Care Medicine, 1981, vol 2.

Smith RA: Physiologic PEEP. *Respir Care* 1988; 33:620–629.

Smith RA, Kirby RR, Gooding DO, et al: Continuous positive airway pressure (CPAP) by face mask. *Crit Care Med* 1980; 8:483–485.

Spearman CB: Positive end-expiratory pressure: Terminology and technical aspects of PEEP devices and systems. *Respir Care* 1988; 33:434–443.

Spearman CB, Sheldon RL, Egan DE: *Egan's Fundamentals of Respiratory Therapy*, ed 4. St Louis, CV Mosby Co, 1982.

Stoller JK: Respiratory effects of positive end expiratory pressure. *Respir Care* 1988; 33:454–463.

Sturgeon CI, Douglas ME, Downs JB, et al: PEEP and CPAP: Cardiopulmonary effects during spontaneous ventilation. *Anesth Analg* 1977; 56:633–639.

Suter PM, Fairley HB, Isenberg MD: Optimum end-expiratory airway pressure in patients with acute pulmonary failure. *N Engl J Med* 1975; 292:284–290.

Shapiro BA, Harrison RA, Kacmarek RM, et al: *Clinical Application of Respiratory Care*, ed 3. Chicago, Year Book Medical Publishers, 1985.

Shapiro BA, Cane RD, Harrison RA: Positive end-expiratory pressure therapy in adults with special reference to acute lung injury: A review of the literature and suggested clinical correlations. *Crit Care Med* 1984; 12:127–141.

Shapiro BA, Cane RD, Harrison RA: Positive end-expiratory pressure in acute lung injury. *Chest* 1983; 83:558–563.

Toung TJK, Saharia P, Mitzner WA, et al: The beneficial and harmful effects of positive end-expiratory pressure. *Surg Gynecol Obstet* 1978; 147:518–523.

Vender JS: Complications and physiologic alterations of positive airway pressure therapy, in Shapiro RA, Cane RA (eds): *Positive Airway Pressure Therapy: PPV and PEEP. Anesth Clin North Am* 1987; 5:807–820.

Venous B, Jacobs HK, Lim L: Treatment of the adult respiratory distress syndrome with continuous positive airway pressure. *Chest* 1979; 76:257–261.

Walkinshaw M, Shoemaker WC: Use of volume loading to obtain preferred levels of PEEP: A preliminary study. *Crit Care Med* 1980; 8:81–86.

Wiegett JA, Mitchell RA, Snyder WH III: Early positive end-expiratory pressure in the adult respiratory distress syndrome. *Arch Surg 1979; 114:497.*

Zamost BG, Alfery DD, Johanson I, et al: Description and clinical evaluation of a new continuous positive airway pressure device. *Crit Care Med* 1981; 9:109–113.

Zarins CK, Virgilio RW, Smith DE, et al: The effect of vascular volume on positive end-expiratory pressure induced cardiac output depression and left atrial wedge pressure discrepancy. *Surg Res* 1977; 23:348–355.

Chapter 38

High-Frequency Ventilation

I. Definitions
   A. High-frequency ventilation (HFV) is a form of mechanical ventilation that employs small tidal volumes (Vts) (approaching deadspace volume or less) and high respiratory rates (more than 60 beats/min [bpm]).
   B. Three different types of high-frequency models have been used.
      1. High-frequency positive pressure ventilation (HFPPV)
         a. Respiratory rate is 60 to 150 bpm.
         b. Tidal volume is 3 to 5 ml/kg
         c. Inspiratory:expiratory (I:E) ratios are about 0.3.
         d. The $F_{I_{O_2}}$ and Positive end-expiratory pressure (PEEP) are variable.
         e. Technically HFPPV is applied via conventional ventilators or pneumatic valve systems with bulk gas flow.
         f. With all systems, exhalation is passive.
         g. No additional gas is entrained.
      2. High-frequency jet ventilation (HFJV)
         a. Respiratory frequency is 60 to 1,600 bpm.
         b. Tidal volume is 2 to 5 ml/kg.
         c. The I:E ratio is about 0.3.
         d. The $F_{I_{O_2}}$ and PEEP are variable.
         e. All systems are specifically designed for HFJV.
         f. Each employs a 14- to 18-gauge small-bore injector where gas is periodically introduced at high pressure (15–50 pounds per square inch [psi]) into a specially designed endotracheal tube adapter (Fig 38–1).
         g. Gas is also entrained from a secondary source, mixing with the injector flow to establish VT (Fig 38–2).
         h. Exhaled gas leaves via a separate route (see Fig 38–2).
         i. Gas flow through the injector is interrupted at clinician-set intervals by pneumatic, fluid, or electronically controlled solenoid valves.
         j. With all systems, exhalation is passive.
         k. The jet flow is humidified by water dripped in front of the injector. The entrained gas is normally humidified (see Fig 38–1).
      3. High-frequency oscillation (HFO)
         a. Respiratory rates are 60 to 3,600 bpm (1–60 Hz). (One Hertz equals 60 cycles/min.)
         b. Tidal volume is 1 to 3 ml/kg.
         c. The I:E ratio is about 0.3.

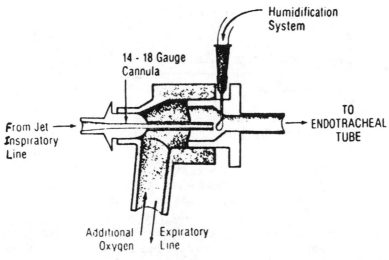

FIG 38–1.
Schematic representation of the injector cannula and endotracheal tube adapter with humidification system used during HFJV. (From Carlon GC, Miodownik S, Ray C Jr, et al: *Crit Care Med* 1981; 9:47–50. Used by permission.)

    d. The $F_{I_{O_2}}$ and PEEP are variable.
    e. All systems are specifically designed for HFO.
    f. Generally, systems provide to-and-fro movement of gas with a piston pump, hi-fi speaker, or ball-valve system (Fig 38–3).
    g. In contrast to HFPPV and HFJV, with HFO exhalation is active. Gas is drawn from the patient during the back stroke of the system.
    h. All gas entering the system is humidified.
    i. Exhalation is via a separate port.

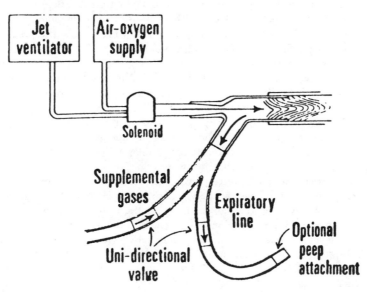

FIG 38–2.
Schematic diagram depicting HFJV circuit and flow of jet stream and entrained and expiratory gases. (From Carlon GC, Howland WS, Ray C, et al: *Chest* 1983; 9:47–50. Used by permission.)

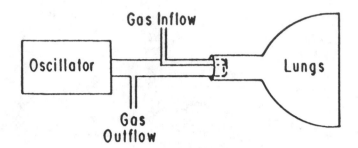

FIG 38–3.
Schematic diagram of HFO system, highlighting oscillator, bias flow, and expiratory ports. (From MacIntyre H: *Clin Chest Med* 1988; 9:50–65. Used by permission.)

II. Gas Movement
   A. Gas movement and carbon dioxide elimination become a more complex phenomenon as we move from conventional mechanical ventilation (CMV) to HFPPV, HFJV, and HFO.
   B. With CMV, HFPPV, and HFJV, bulk gas flow or convection accounts for the majority of gas movement, with diffusion being responsible for gas movement at the lung parenchyma.
   C. However, the smaller the V_T, the greater the number of additional factors that must be considered to explain gas movement.
   D. During HFO, and to a limited extent during HFJV, the following have been considered contributory factors to gas movement and CO_2 elimination:
      1. Pendelluft gas movement: Since neighboring gas units have varying compliance and resistance, filling of lung units is uneven (underventilation of some and overventilation of others); thus, gas exchange can occur by gas moving from one lung unit to another.
      2. Asymmetric velocity profiles: Gas in the center of a column moves faster than gas at the periphery. Thus, gas can move to a greater depth in the lung than predicted by the V_T delivered. There is also coaxial or bidirectional gas movement. At the center of the airway, gas (O_2) moves into the lung while at the periphery, gas (CO_2) moves to the mouth.
      3. Taylor dispersion (augmented dispersion): High-velocity gas movement enhances the development of turbulence in the conducting airways, causing eddies and swirling gas movement. This movement encourages dispersion of gas, both laterally and centrally.
      4. Cardiogenic oscillation: The oscillations of the circulatory system assist gas movement especially at high ventilatory frequencies.
      5. The lung may be considered in three zones with reference to HFV (Fig 38–4).
         a. Zone 1 is the large airways where flow is turbulent. Here convection and Taylor dispersion are responsible primarily for gas movement.
         b. Zone 2 is the lower airways, where flow is laminar. Here, gas movement is primarily by coaxial flow and asymmetric velocity profiles.
         c. Zone 3 is lung parenchyma where no bulk movement occurs. Here, gas movement is primarily by cardiac oscillations, pendelluft, and molecular diffusion.
      6. In general, gas movement in the upper airway seems to be the major limiting factor in HFV.
III. Oxygenation
   A. In general, it appears that HFV is somewhat more efficient in CO_2 removal in the normal lung and in acute lung injury than CMV.
   B. However, HFV shows no advantage over CMV in the area of oxygenation.

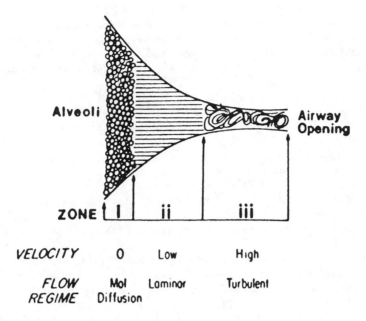

FIG 38–4.
Schematic illustration depicting gas flow characteristics and velocities as gas is transported from airway opening to alveolar region *(left)* during HFV. Slutsky AS: *Crit Care Med* 1984; 12:713–717. Used with permission.)

   C. In both CMV and HFV, mean airway pressure essentially determines oxygenation.
   D. Mean airway pressure in HFV is dependent on:
      a. Respiratory rate
      b. V_T.
      c. I:E ratio.
      d. PEEP applied.
      e. Auto-PEEP developed.
      f. Driving pressure in HFJV.
 IV. Manipulation of Ventilation and Oxygenation in High-Frequency Jet Ventilation
   A. Carbon dioxide elimination can be directly affected by:
      1. Driving pressure.
      2. Inspiratory time.
      3. Respiratory rate.
   B. Oxygenation can be directly affected by:
      1. $F_{I_{O_2}}$.
      2. PEEP.
      3. Inspiratory time.
   C. With HFPPV, oxygenation and ventilation are controlled in the same manner as in CMV.
   D. No universally accepted algorithms for manipulation of oxygenation and ventilation have been established for HFO.
  V. Respiratory and Cardiovascular Effects of High-Frequency Ventilation
   A. High-frequency ventilation maintains the lung in a state of hyperinflation. This is more pronounced the greater the compliance of the lung. However, even with acute lung injury (adult respiratory distress syndrome), auto-PEEP develops.
   B. High-frequency ventilation does not appear to alter surfactant production to the same extent CMV does. Compliance decreases over time with CMV but does not seem to be altered with HFV.

C. As long as P_{CO_2} is maintained at a normal or below normal level, apnea is common with the use of HFV. Although spontaneous breathing does develop during rapid eye movement sleep, it is believed that inhibition of phrenic activity via the vagus nerve and activation of mechanoreceptors inhibit breathing at other times.

D. The frequency of barotrauma is equivalent to that of CMV.

E. Hemodynamic compromise is similar to that with CMV.

F. The other overall respiratory and cardiovascular effects of HFV are similar to CMV.

VI. Clinical Application

  A. Upper airway surgery and bronchoscopy

    1. Both HFPPV and HFJV are preferred over CMV in these clinical settings.

    2. Both are capable of providing more efficient gas exchange than CMV.

  B. Bronchopulmonary fistula

    1. Initially HFV was considered superior to CMV in the presence of a large air leak.

    2. At least theoretically, gas distribution with CMV is dependent primarily on compliance, whereas as rate increases, gas distribution becomes more dependent on airway resistance.

    3. Recent data indicate CMV and HFV are equally capable of ventilating in the presence of a bronchopulmonary fistula if acute lung injury is also present.

    4. With major air leaks without acute lung injury, HFV may ventilate more effectively.

  C. Acute lung injury

    1. In the adult population, HFV provides no advantage over CMV.

    2. In the neonatal population, HFO has been used with success in infants with perpherial interstitial emphysema (PIE).

VII. Safety

  A. Extreme care must be taken with the use of HFV systems because of the potential for tremendous increases in airway pressure in a short period of time.

  B. In addition to alarms, mechanisms to abort gas delivery must be included.

VIII. Humidification

  A. A major problem with HFJV is humidification. No efficient mechanism to appropriately humidify the 20 to 60 L of gas delivered per minute during HFJV is available.

  B. As a result of insufficient humidification, necrotizing tracheobronchitis and squamous metaplasia of the bronchial mucosa with submucosal inflammatory cell infiltration are common.

REFERENCES

Butler WJ, Bohn DJ, Bryan AC, et al: Ventilation by high frequency oscillation in humans. *Anesth Analg (Cleve)* 1980; 59:577–584.

Carlon GC, Howland WS, Ray C, et al: High-frequency jet ventilation. A prospective randomized evaluation. *Chest* 1983; 84:551–559.

Carlon GC, Miodownik S, Ray C Jr, et al: Technical aspects and clinical implications of high frequency jet ventilation with a solenoid valve. *Crit Care Med* 1981; 9:47–50.

Carlon GC, Ray C Jr, Klain M, et al: High-frequency positive pressure ventilation in management of a patient with bronchopleural fistula. *Anesthesiology* 1980; 52:160–162.

Forese AB, Bryan AC: High frequency ventilation. *Am Rev Respir Dis* 1987; 135:1363–1374.

Glenski J, Crawford M, Rehder K: High-frequency, small volume ventilation during thoracic surgery. *Anesthesiology* 1986; 64:211–214.

The HIFI Study Group: High-frequency oscillatory ventilation compared with conventional mechanical ventilation in the treatment of respiratory failure in preterm infants. *N Engl J Med* 1988; 320:88–93.

Holzapfel L, Perrin RF, Gaussorgues P, et al: Comparison of high-frequency jet ventilation to conventional ventilation in adults with respiratory distress syndrome. *Intensive Care Med* 1987; 13:100–105.

Klain M, Smith RB: High frequency percutaneous transtrachel jet ventilation. *Crit Care Med* 1977; 5:280–287.

MacIntyre N: New forms of mechanical ventilation in the adult. *Clin Chest Med* 1988; 9:50.

Nevin M, Van Besouw JP, Williams CW, et al: A comparative study of conventional versus high frequency jet ventilation with relation to the incidence of postoperative morbidity in thoracic surgery. *Ann Thorac Surg* 1987; 44:625–627.

Ray C, Miodownik S, Carlon G, et al: Pneumatic-to-electric analog for high frequency jet ventilation of disrupted airways. *Crit Care Med* 1984; 12:711–712.

Rossing TH, Slutsky AS, Lehr JL, et al: Tidal volume and frequency dependence of carbon dioxide elimination by high-frequency ventilation. *N Engl J Med* 1981; 305:1375–1379.

Schuster DP, Klain M, Snyder J: Comparison of high frequency jet ventilation to conventional mechanical ventilation during severe acute respiratory failure in humans. *Crit Care Med* 1982; 10:624–630.

Slutsky AS: Mechanisms affecting gas transport during high frequency oscillation. *Crit Care Med* 1984; 12:713–717.

Slutsky AS, Drazen JM, Ingram RH Jr, et al: Effective pulmonary ventilation with small-volume oscillations at high frequency. *Science* 1980; 209:609–611.

Standiford TJ, Morgan Roth ML: High-frequency ventilation. *Chest* 1989; 96:1381–1389.

Chapter 39 _____

Ventilatory Support of the Neonatal and Pediatric Patient

I. Types of Positive Pressure Ventilators
   A. Volume-cycled
      1. A preset tidal volume (V_T) is delivered.
      2. Inspiration ends when the volume is delivered.
      3. Delivery of the V_T is terminated if the preset pressure limit is met.
      4. It is the ventilator of choice with changing lung compliance.
   B. Pressure-cycled
      1. A maximum plateau pressure is met.
      2. Delivery of the V_T is terminated when the preset pressure is met.
      3. Inspiration ends when the preset pressure is reached.
      4. The V_T is the result of preset pressure, flow, and lung compliance.
      5. The ventilator of choice when peak airway pressures need to be limited
   C. Time-cycled
      1. The inspiratory time (T_I) is set.
      2. A continuous gas flow system is commonly employed.
      3. Inspiration ends when the T_I is complete.
      4. Tidal volume is the result of T_I, pressure gradient, flow rate, and compliance of the patient's lungs.
      5. Manipulation of T_I changes V_T.
      6. Time-cycled positive pressure ventilators are frequently employed with a pressure limit to minimize peak airway pressure and maintain T_I.
II. Ventilator Modes
   A. Intermittent mandatory ventilation/synchronized intermittent mandatory ventilation
      1. This mode allows the patient to play a role in regulating the Pa_{CO_2}.
      2. Newborn ventilators commonly use a continuous gas flow system. However, some employ a demand flow.
   B. Continuous positive airway pressure (CPAP)
      1. Continuous positive airway pressure is administered with nasal prongs, endotracheal tube, or face mask.

2. Goals
   a. Increase FRC
   b. Reduce the work of breathing
   c. Improve oxygenation
3. Indications
   a. Pa_{O_2} less than 60 mm Hg at an $F_{I_{O_2}}$ more than 0.40
   b. Respiratory distress (grunting, retractions, nasal flaring)
   c. Pa_{CO_2} less than 50 mm Hg
4. Continuous positive airway pressure is initiated at 4 to 6 cm H_2O to maintain a Pa_{O_2} at more than 50 mm Hg.
5. An increase in the Pa_{CO_2} may occur from:
   a. Ineffective alveolor ventilation.
   b. Increased work of breathing and fatigue.
6. A decrease in the Pa_{O_2} may occur from:
   a. Ineffective alveolar ventilation (shunting).
   b. Excessive PEEP (overdistention of alveoli) resulting in increased shunting and deadspace.
7. The Pa_{CO_2} is monitored to determine effective ventilation and patient fatigue.
8. A Pa_{CO_2} greater than 50 mm Hg normally initiates ventilatory failure and requires mechanical ventilation.
9. An infant developing metabolic acidosis may require assisted ventilation.

III. Ventilator Controls
A. Peak inspiratory pressure (PIP)
   1. An increase in PIP normally results in:
      a. Increased V_T.
      b. Increased alveolar ventilation.
      c. Decreased Pa_{CO_2}.
      d. Increased mean airway pressure (MAP).
      e. Increased Pa_{O_2}.
   2. High PIP (more than 30 cm H_2O) may increase the incidence of pulmonary air leaks, barotrauma, and bronchopulmonary dysplasia.
B. Mechanical rate
   1. Changes in the mechanical rate alter alveolar ventilation and the Pa_{CO_2}.
   2. Increasing the mechanical rate normally should:
      a. Increase minute ventilation.
      b. Lower the Pa_{CO_2}.
      c. Raise the pH.
   3. The potential effects of high PIP may be reduced by employing high rates. This will allow the PIP to be reduced while minute ventilation is maintained.
   4. The expiratory time (T_E) may be markedly shortened by high rates leading to air trapping and increased FRC.
   5. High rates may be indicated to induce respiratory alkalosis for persistent pulmonary hypertension. The alkalosis helps reduce the pulmonary vascular resistance, improve oxygenation, and close the patent ductus arteriosus (PDA).
C. T_I, T_E, inspiratory:expiratory [I:E] ratio
   1. Total cycling time is equal to T_I plus T_E.
   2. For adequate pressure to be delivered to create a volume change, T_I normally is 0.4 second or more.
   3. The time necessary for lungs to inflate and deflate depends on compliance and resistance.
   4. Normal pulmonary compliance is 0.003 to 0.006 L/cm H_2O.
   5. Normal airway resistance is 20 to 40 cm H_2O/L/sec.

6. Compliance and airway resistance can be used to determine the time necessary to maintain airway pressure or deliver V_T.
7. The time constant is a resultant of compliance and resistance, multiples of which establish the time required for passive exhalation:

$$\text{Time constant (seconds)} = \text{Compliance} \times \text{Airway resistance} \qquad (1)$$

8. If a normal newborn has a compliance of 0.004 L/cm H_2O and an airway resistance of 30 cm H_2O/L/sec, the time constant is:

$$0.004 \text{ L/cm } H_2O \times 30 \text{ cm } H_2O/L/sec = 0.12 \text{ seconds}$$

9. One time constant is necessary for 63% of V_T to be passively exhaled.
10. Four time constants are necessary for complete exhalation ($5 \times 0.12 = 0.6$ seconds).
11. Incomplete expiration may occur if T_E is less than four time constants, which may lead to an increase in FRC and inadvertent auto-PEEP.
12. To ensure passive distribution of ventilation, the inspiratory phase should be at least four time constants in length.
13. Ineffective tidal volume may result during pressure-cycled or time-cycled, pressure-limited ventilation if T_I is short.
14. With recovery and improvement of compliance and airway resistance, time constants change and require alterations in T_I and T_E to prevent air trapping.
15. Tidal volume may be estimated during pressure-limited, time-cycled ventilation:
   a. $V_T = \dot{V}$ (ml/sec) $\times T_I$ (seconds)
   b. $V_T = 8$ L/min $\times 0.6$ second

$$\frac{8,000 \text{ ml/min}}{60 \text{ sec/min}} = 133 \text{ ml/sec}$$

   c. 133 ml/sec $\times 0.6$ sec $= 80$ ml
16. Estimation of T_I during volume-limited ventilation
   a. Ventilator settings
      (1) Respiratory rate: 25 breaths/min (bpm)
      (2) PIP: 50 cm H_2O
      (3) Flow rate: 8 L/min
      (4) V_T: 80 ml
   b. $T_I = \dfrac{V_T}{\dot{V}}$
   c. $T_I = \dfrac{80 \text{ ml}}{8 \text{ L/min}}$
   d. 8 L/min equals 133 ml/sec:
   e. $\dfrac{80 \text{ ml}}{133 \text{ ml/sec}} = 0.6$ seconds T_I
   f. If total cycling time is 1.5 seconds, then:

$$1.5 - 0.6 = 0.9 \text{ sec } T_E$$

   g. I:E ratio:

$$0.6{:}0.9 = 1{:}1.5$$

D. Flow rate
   1. Flow rate and T_I are inversely related.
   2. In general, the shorter the T_I, the higher the flow rate needed to maintain the V_T delivered.
   3. Inspiratory flow should be high enough to deliver the desired V_T and still create a pressure plateau.
   4. If inspiratory flow is not high enough for a given respiratory rate, the PIP may not be reached until the end of inspiration.
   5. Flow rates must be high enough to meet the patient's inspiratory demand.
E. PEEP
   1. Benefits
      a. Maintain FRC
      b. Prevent collapse of alveoli
      c. Optimize oxygenation (increases MAP)
   2. Disadvantages
      a. Reduced venous return
      b. Decrease in compliance due to excessive PEEP
      c. Increase in deadspace
   3. An indication for PEEP is a Pa_{O_2} less than 50 mm Hg on an $F_{I_{O_2}}$ of more than 0.60.
   4. It is instituted at 3 to 5 cm H_2O.
   5. Both $F_{I_{O_2}}$ and PEEP are titrated to maintain a Pa_{O_2} of 50 to 70 mm Hg.
   6. An increase of PEEP may result in an increase in Pa_{CO_2} if PIP is not increased (ventilating pressure = PIP − PEEP). That is, if PIP is constant, the pressure gradient establishing V_T is decreased.
   7. Hyperinflation and CO_2 retention may occur with PEEP levels of more than 10 cm H_2O.
F. $F_{I_{O_2}}$
   1. It is adjusted to maintain a Pa_{O_2} of 50 to 70 mm Hg.
   2. Generally it is adjusted upward to 0.60 or 0.70 prior to increasing the PEEP level.
   3. It is decreased in 1% or 2% increments, maintaining the Pa_{O_2} at more than 50 mm Hg.
G. MAP
   1. Average airway pressure maintained throughout the ventilatory cycle (Fig 39–1)
   2. Oxygenation is affected primarily by MAP.
   3. High MAP may markedly reduce venous return and cardiac output (MAP more than 14 cm H_2O).
   4. It is affected by:
      a. PIP
         (1) Increasing PIP increases MAP.
         (2) Peak inspiratory pressures of more than 25 cm H_2O have been associated with barotrauma and pulmonary air leaks.
      b. PEEP
         (1) Increasing PEEP increases MAP.
         (2) Levels more than 10 cm H_2O may cause hyperinflation and increasing CO_2 levels.
      c. I:E ratio
         (1) Higher I:E ratios (more than 1:2) increase MAP.
         (2) Reversing I:E ratios (more than 1:1) markedly increases MAP.
      d. Pressure waveform
         (1) The longer the pressure plateau, the greater the MAP.

Mean Airway Pressure

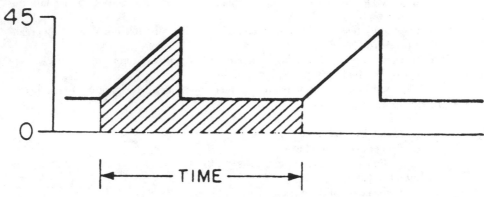

FIG 39–1.

Mean airway pressure is calculated from the *shaded area* that represents the inspiratory and expiratory proximal airway pressure waveforms. (From Thibeault D, Gregory G: *Neonatal Pulmonary Care,* ed 2. Norwalk, Conn, Appleton-Century-Crofts, 1986. Used by permission.)

      e. Calculation of MAP during pressure-limited time-cycled ventilation

        (1) $\dfrac{PEEP + (PIP - PEEP \times T_I)}{T_I + T_E}$

        Example:

        (a) Ventilator settings

            i. PIP: 25 cm H_2O

            ii. PEEP: 5 cm H_2O

            iii. T_I: 1.0 second

            iv. T_E: 1.0 second

        (b) $\dfrac{5 + (25 - 5 \times 1.0)}{1.0 + 1.0}$

        (c) $\dfrac{5 + 20}{2}$

        (d) $\dfrac{25}{2}$ = 12.5 cm H_2O

      f. Optimum MAP between 10 and 14 cm H_2O

IV. Initiation of Mechanical Ventilation

  A. Indications

    1. Marked hypoxia

      a. Pa_{O_2} less than 50 mm Hg at an FI_{O_2} more than 0.80

    2. Increase in Pa_{CO_2} to more than 50 mm Hg, pH less than 7.20

    3. Frequent apnea unresponsive to other forms of therapy (CPAP)

    4. Premature infants less than 1,000 gm with asphyxia or respiratory distress. These infants look well initially but may develop hypotension, apneic spells, acidosis, and intraventricular hemorrhage within hours after birth.

  B. Ventilator parameters: Initial settings

    1. Newborn with compliant lungs

      a. PIP: Less than 20 cm H_2O

      b. Respiratory rate: 15 to 20 bpm

      c. PEEP: 3 to 5 cm H_2O

      d. Flow rate: 7 to 10 L/min

      e. T_I: 0.4 to 0.8 second

      f. FI_{O_2}: Titrated to maintain Pa_{O_2} at more than 50 mm Hg

  2. Newborn with noncompliant lungs (respiratory distress syndrome [RDS])

      a. PIP: More than 20 cm H_2O

      b. Respiratory rate: 25 to 45 bpm

      c. PEEP: 4 to 8 cm H_2O

      d. Flow rate: 7 to 10 L/min

      e. T_I: 0.4 to 0.8 second

      f. FI_{O_2}: Titrated to maintain Pa_{O_2} at more than 50 mm Hg

  3. Parameter changes

      a. Each parameter should be changed in small increments and followed with blood gas analysis.

      b. Generally the following increment changes can be employed:

        (1) FI_{O_2}: Increase by 5% to 10%; decrease by 1% to 2%.

        (2) PIP: Increase and decrease by 1 to 2 cm H_2O.

        (3) PEEP: Increase and decrease by 1 cm H_2O.

        (4) Respiratory rate: Increase by 2 to 3 bpm; decrease by 1 to 2 bpm.

      c. To increase Pa_{O_2}:

        (1) Increase the FI_{O_2} up to 0.60.

        (2) Increase the PEEP if it is not already more than 5 cm H_2O.

        (3) Increase the PIP up to 25 cm H_2O by increments of 1 to 2 cm H_2O.

        (4) Increase the respiratory rate. This rate adjustment may require T_I to be shortened to maintain T_E and prevent air trapping.

        (5) If the Pa_{O_2} is still unacceptable, continue increasing the FI_{O_2} and PIP in appropriate increments.

      d. To increase ventilation:

        (1) Increase the PIP to 25 cm H_2O in appropriate increments.

        (2) Increase the respiratory rate (upper limit of 45 bpm may be used) in appropriate increments.

        (3) If there is no change in the ventilatory status, increase the PIP to more than 25 cm H_2O in appropriate increments.

        (4) Next, depending on the T_E, adjust the PIP or respiratory rate in appropriate increments.

      e. To decrease ventilation:

        (1) Reduce the PIP if it is more than 25 cm H_2O by 1 to 2 cm H_2O.

        (2) If the PIP is less than 25 cm H_2O, reduce respiratory rate by 1 to 2 bpm.

        (3) If the rate is adjusted, the T_I may require adjustment to maintain the proper I:E ratio.

V. Weaning From Mechanical Ventilation

  A. Ventilator settings are adjusted to maintain acceptable arterial blood gas levels.

    1. pH: More than 7.30

    2. Pa_{CO_2}: 35 to 45 mm Hg

    3. Pa_{O_2}: 50 to 70 mm Hg

    4. Sa_{O_2}: More than 90%

  B. Once the newborn's blood gases are stable, the following ventilator adjustments can be initiated.

    1. FI_{O_2} level decreased by 2%: Some neonatal conditions may require a smaller FI_{O_2} change such as persistent pulmonary hypertension.

    2. Peak inspiratory pressure is reduced by 1 to 2 cm H_2O.

    3. The ventilatory rate is reduced by 2 bpm.

    4. Positive end-expiratory pressure is reduced to 3 to 5 cm H_2O. This level is maintained to ensure alveolar stability.

5. These parameter changes are continued as tolerated by the patient. Each change is followed by an arterial blood gas evaluation.
6. Continuous positive airway pressure may be instituted when minimal ventilator settings have been achieved. Generally, assisted ventilation may be terminated when the following settings have been achieved:
   a. PIP: 15 cm H_2O
   b. PEEP: 3 to 5 cm H_2O
   c. Respiratory rate: Less than 10 bpm
   d. $F_{I_{O_2}}$: Less than 0.40
7. If CPAP is instituted, 10% higher $F_{I_{O_2}}$ is administered with 3 to 5 cm H_2O.
8. Some patients (less than 2,000 gm) may not tolerate CPAP through an endotracheal tube. These patients may do better extubated in a head hood with 10% higher $F_{I_{O_2}}$ than with an endotracheal tube.
9. Respiratory monitoring and vital signs should be done every 15 to 30 min within the first hour following discontinuance of ventilation.
10. Watch for fatigue and increased work of breathing.
11. Symptoms include:
    a. Increased heart rate.
    b. Retractions.
    c. Nasal flaring.
    d. Increased Pa_{CO_2}.
    e. Increased respiratory rate.
    f. Seesaw breathing.
    g. Tracheal tug.

VI. Extracorporeal Membrane Oxygenation (ECMO)
   A. Description
      1. Extracorporeal membrane oxygenation allows lung recovery by providing cardiopulmonary support and minimizing harmful effects from high pressure mechanical ventilation.
      2. The newborn can be supported with low oxygen concentration, low ventilatory pressures, and low respiratory rates.
      3. Extracorpeal membrane oxygenation is provided via a modified heart-lung machine normally for 4 to 10 days.
   B. Candidates for ECMO
      1. Full-term infants with retractible respiratory disease such as:
         a. Meconium aspiration syndrome.
         b. RDS.
         c. Persistent pulmonary hypertension or PDA.
         d. Pneumonia.
      2. Congenital diaphragmatic hernia
      3. Weight greater than 2 kg
      4. Gestational age greater than 35 weeks
      5. Failure to respond to maximal medical management (100% oxygen, hyperventilation, tolazoline trial)
      6. No more than 7 days of assisted ventilation
      7. P $(A - a)_{O_2}$ 600 mm Hg or more for 8 to 12 hours at an $F_{I_{O_2}}$ 1.0
      8. PIP more than 38cm H_2O for 4 hours
   C. Contraindications
      1. Congenital heart disease
      2. Intracranial hemorrhage (greater incidence in newborns less than 35 weeks' gestational age)
      3. Postnatal age more than 7 days
      4. Severe coagulopathy

D. Equipment
  1. The setup consists of:
     a. An oxygen supply.
     b. Membrane lung for O_2 and CO_2.
     c. A servo-regulated pump.
     d. Heat exchanger to maintain proper temperature.
     e. Heparin infusion pump.
E. Bypass sites
  1. Either veno-arterial (VA) bypass or veno-venous (VV) may be utilized.
  2. The VA bypass requires a cannula entering the right internal jugular vein and a cannula entering the right common carotid artery. These are then passed into the right atrium and aortic arch, respectively (Fig 39–2).
  3. For VV bypass, a cannula is passed into the femoral artery and advanced into the right atrium by way of the inferior vena cava (Fig 39–3).
  4. A priming volume of 300 to 500 ml in the extracorporeal circuit is established with the necessary electrolyte, hematocrit, and platelet concentration added.
  5. The newborn is then attached to the oxygenator.
  6. Mechanical ventilator settings are adjusted downward to provide minimal support.
     a. PIP: 20 cm H_2O or less
     b. IMV: 10 bpm or less
     c. PEEP: 3 to 5 cm H_2O
     d. F_{IO_2}: 0.30 to 0.40
  7. The ECMO flow is titrated to maintain arterial oxygenation (60 mm Hg), blood pressure, and mixed venous oxygenation.

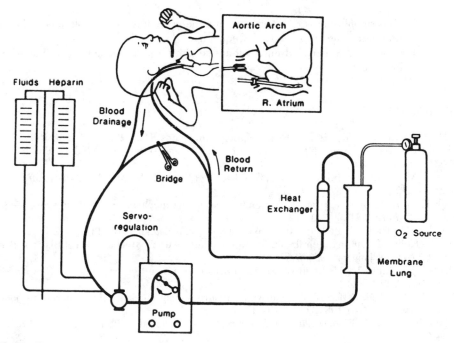

FIG 39–2.
Veno-arterial route for the provision of ECMO with illustrated circuit. (From Goldsmith J, Karokin E: *Assisted Ventilation of the Neonate,* ed 2. Philadelphia, WB Saunders Co, 1988. Used by permission.)

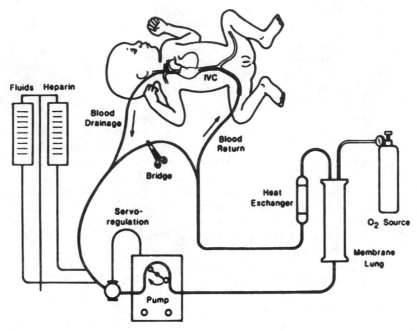

FIG 39–3.
Veno-venous route for the provision of ECMO with illustrated circuit. (From Goldsmith J, Karokin E: *Assisted Ventilation of the Neonate,* ed 2. Philadelphia, WB Saunders Co, 1988. Used by permission.)

8. Heparin infusion is maintained during the procedure, and whole blood clotting times are done at the bedside frequently.
9. Other medications and nutrition are administered as needed, as well as whole blood and platelets.

BIBLIOGRAPHY

Barlett R: Extracorporeal membrane oxygenation in neonates. *Hosp Pract* 1984; 10:139–151.

Carlo W, Chatburn R: *Neonatal Respiratory Care.* Chicago, Year Book Medical Publishers, 1988.

Carlo W, Marin R: Principles of neonatal assisted ventilation. *Pediatr Clin North Am* 1980; 33:221–237.

Ciszek T, et al: Mean airway pressure-significance during mechanical ventilation in neonates. *J Pediatr* 1981; 99:121–126.

Downes J, Raphaelly R: Pediatric intensive care. *Anesthesiology* 1975; 43:238–250.

Finer N, Kelly M: Optimal ventilation for the neonate, part 2. Mechanical ventilation. *Perinatol Neonatol* January 1983; 7:63–69.

Gallagher J, Banner M: Mean airway pressure as a determinant of oxygenation. *Crit Care Med* 1981; 8:244.

Glenski J, et al: Calculation of mean airway pressure during mechanical ventilation in neonates. *Crit Care Med* 1984; 12:642–644.

Goldsmith J, Karokin E: *Assisted Ventilation of the Neonate,* ed 2. Philadelphia, WB Saunders Co, 1988.

Kirby R: Mechanical ventilation of the newborn, pitfalls and practice. *Perinatology/Neonatology* 1981, 5:47–52.

Koff P, Eitzman D, Neu J: *Neonatal and Pediatric Respiratory Care.* St Louis, CV Mosby Co, 1988.

Lotze A, et al: Lung compliance as a measure of lung function in newborns with respiratory failure requiring extracorporeal membrane oxygenation. *Crit Care Med* 1987; 15:226–229.

Lough M, Doershuk C, Stern R: *Pediatric Respiratory Therapy*, ed 3. Chicago, Year Book Medical Publishers, 1985.

MacIntyre N, Hagus C: *Graphical Analysis of Flow, Pressure and Volume During Mechanical Ventilation*. Riverside, Calf, Bear Medical Systems, 1987.

Pirie G, Cain D: Options for ventilating the pediatric patient, part 1. *Perinatal Neonatol* November–December 1983; 7:62–71.

Pirie G, Cain D: Options for ventilating the pediatric patient, part 2. *Perinatal Neonatol* January–February 1984; 8:61–68.

Pollock E, et al: ECMO brings new dimensions in neonatal care. *AARTimes* 1986; 10:34–36.

Thibeault D, Gregory G: *Neonatal Pulmonary Care*, ed 2. Norwalk, Mass, Appleton-Century-Crofts, 1986.

Zwischenberger J, et al: The role of extracorporeal membrane oxygenation in the management of respiratory failure in the newborn. *Respir Care* 1986; 31:491–495.

Chapter 40

Pharmacology

I. General Information
   A. Definitions
      1. Pharmacology: The study of the interaction of drugs with the organism.
      2. Drug: Any chemical compound that may be administered to or used in an individual to aid in the diagnosis, treatment, or prevention of disease; to relieve pain; or to control or improve any physiologic disorder or pathologic condition.
      3. LD_{50}: The dosage of a drug that would be lethal to 50% of a test population.
      4. ED_{50}: The dosage of a drug that would have therapeutic effects for 50% of a test population.
      5. Therapeutic index (TI): The numerical ratio of the LD_{50} to the ED_{50} (LD_{50}/ED_{50}). This ratio shows how close the lethal and therapeutic doses of a drug are for a test population. Low indices mean the therapeutic and lethal doses are similar and the drug has a high potential for overdose or toxic side effects (Fig 40–1).
      6. Side effect: Any physiologic response other than that for which the drug was administered.
   B. Pharmacologic nomenclature
      1. Chemical name: Name illustrative of chemical structural formula of the drug.
      2. Code name: An investigational designation; usually alphanumeric.
      3. Generic name: An assigned name given for clinical investigation of a promising chemical.
      4. Official name: Usually the generic name after the drug is accepted for general use.
      5. Trade, brand, or proprietary name: The name under which the drug is marketed by a particular manufacturer.
      6. Example: Ipratropium bromide
         a. Code name: SCH 1000
         b. Chemical name: 8-Azoniabicyclo[3.2.1]octane, 3-(3-hydroxy-1-oxo-2-phenylpropoxy)-8-methyl-8-(l-methyl-ethyl)-, bromide
         c. Official name: Ipratropium bromide
         d. Generic name: Ipratropium bromide
         e. Trade name: Atrovent (Boehringer-Ingelheim)

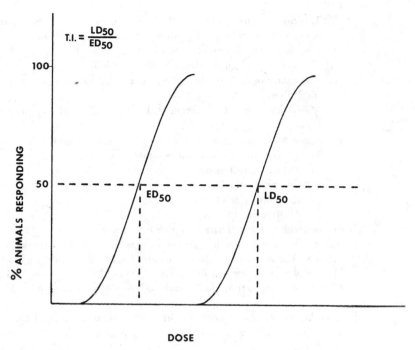

FIG 40–1.
Log-dose response curve demonstrating therapeutic index *(TI)* determination.

C. Principles of drug action
- There are three phases of drug action from initial dosing to pharmacologic effect. Each phase includes aspects of the pharmacology of the drug.
1. Pharmaceutical phase: Administering the drug.
   a. Dosage forms: Tablet, capsule, liquid, powder, or ointment.
   b. Route of administration (listed in order of speed in obtaining blood levels)
      (1) Intravenous (IV) injection
      (2) Via lung (aerosol)
      (3) Intramuscular (IM) injection
      (4) Subcutaneous (SC) injection
      (5) Sublingual and rectal absorption
      (6) Oral
      (7) Topical
      Note: Not all drugs may be administered by all routes listed, and the speed of absorption by route may also vary.
2. Pharmacokinetic phase: Entry into or elimination from the body. Generally, this phase includes absorption, distribution, metabolism, and elimination of a drug. These factors determine onset of action, peak plasma drug level, and duration of drug action.
   a. Absorption: Rate of absorption determined by the specific physical and chemical characteristics of a drug.
   b. Distribution: Movement of the drug to area of desired pharmacologic activity.
      (1) The primary mechanism for distribution is the circulatory system.

(2) Topical administration for effect on skin or mucous membrane decreases the likelihood of further undesired distribution.

  c. Metabolism: Actual inactivation of the drug by the body.

    (1) The primary organ for detoxification is the liver.

    (2) Secondary organs for detoxification are the kidneys and gastrointestinal tract.

    (3) Many drugs may be inactivated by the body's cells or plasma proteins.

  d. Excretion: Mechanism for elimination of the drug from the body.

    (1) Primary organ for excretion: Kidney

    (2) Secondary excretion sites

      (a) Gastrointestinal tract

      (b) Respiratory tract

      (c) All exocrine glands

3. Pharmacodynamic phase: Drug-receptor interaction.

  a. Affinity: Tendency of a drug to combine with a matching receptor.

  b. Potency: The activity of a drug per unit weight. A potent drug has a large biologic activity at a small unit dose (Fig 40–2).

  c. Efficacy: The maximum effect produced by a drug regardless of dose (Fig 40–3).

  d. Cumulation: A gradual rise in the body's total drug level that occurs when the administration rate of the drug is greater than the body's rate of removal.

  e. Tolerance: The body's ability to increase its metabolism of a drug. Increasing amounts of the drug are required to produce the same effect.

  f. Tachyphylaxis: The rapid development of tolerance.

D. Drug interactions

  1. Additive: Two drugs, when given together, produce an effect equal to the sum of their individual effects.

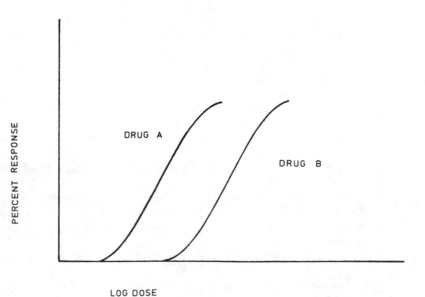

FIG 40–2.
Log-dose response curve comparing the potency of two drugs. The potency of *drug A* is greater than that of *drug B*.

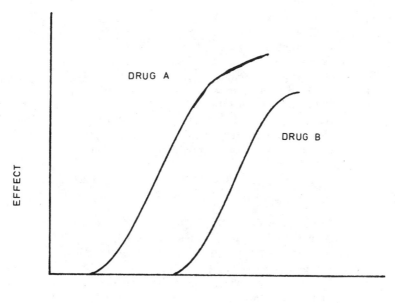

FIG 40-3.

Log-dose response curve comparing the efficacy of two drugs. A greater effect is caused by *drug A* than *drug B*. In addition, *drug A* is more potent than *drug B*.

2. Potentiation: Potentiation occurs when a drug active at a specific receptor site is given with a drug inactive at that receptor site, and the resulting effect is greater than that of the active drug alone $(1 + 0 = 3)$.
3. Synergism: Two drugs active at a receptor site, when given together, cause an effect greater than the sum of their individual effects $(1 + 2 = 6)$.
4. Antagonist: This is a drug with affinity *but no* efficacy (i.e., it blocks an effect).
   a. Competitive: An antagonist whose effects are directly related to dosage. A competitive antagonist decreases potency but does not affect efficacy of the other drug.
   b. Noncompetitive: An antagonist whose effects are not dose related. Both potency and efficacy of the other drug are decreased.
5. Agonist: This is a drug with affinity *and* efficacy (i.e., causes an effect).
 E. The prescription
   • This is the written order for a drug, composed of:
   1. The patient's name, the patient's address, and the date.
   2. Rx: "Take thou"; take and prepare the medication.
   3. Inscription: Name and quantity of the drug.
   4. Subscription: Directions (when applicable) to the pharmacist for compounding the drug.
   5. Sig: Transcription, "write"; instructions to the patient for taking the drug.
   6. Name of prescriber.
II. Administering Aerosolized Drugs (see Chapter 30 for details)
 A. Devices
   1. Ultrasonic nebulizers (not recommended for bronchodilators)
   2. Gas-powered small reservoir nebulizers, with or without intermittent positive pressure breathing (IPPB)
   3. Metered dose inhaler (MDI), with or without extension (spacer) device

B. Particle size and deposition
   1. Upper airway (above larynx): More than 5 μ
   2. Central airways: 2 to 5 μ
   3. Periphery: 1 to 2 μ
C. Basic protocol of administration
   1. Gas-powered small reservoir nebulizers
      a. Fill volume: 2.5 to 4.0 ml
      b. Nebulizing flow: 6 to 8 L/min (viscous antibiotics: 12 L/min)
      c. Slow, deep inspirations, with breath-hold
      d. Inspiratory nebulization only, if possible
   2. Metered dose inhaler
      a. Assemble, shake canister, and charge with one actuation.
      b. Hold 4 cm in front of open mouth or rest on mandibular teeth of open mouth.
      c. Exhale normally.
      d. Begin slow deep breath and activate MDI.
      e. Inspire to total lung capacity and hold breath at least 3 to 5 seconds.
      f. Exhale normally.
      g. Use of a spacer device is generally recommended.
   3. General notes regarding administration
      a. Bronchodilators: Wait 1 min, then take a second puff.
      b. Corticosteroids: Take after bronchodilators, hyperextending the neck while inhaling; rinse mouth and throat after dosing.
      c. Dry powder inhalers: These require rapid inspiration with high flow rates (60–120 L/min) for dispersion.
      d. Spacers or extensions with MDIs reduce the need for coordination and oropharyngeal impaction.

III. Wetting Agents and Diluents
A. Isotonic solution: A solution equivalent to a 0.9% weight/volume (W/V) solution of NaCl. Isotonic solutions are used in respiratory therapy primarily in small-volume nebulizers.
B. Hypertonic solution: A solution with a concentration greater than a 0.9% W/V solution of NaCl. Hypertonic solutions are used in respiratory therapy primarily for sputum induction.
C. Hypotonic solution: A solution with a concentration of less than a 0.9% W/V solution of NaCl. Hypotonic solutions are most commonly used in respiratory therapy in large-volume aerosol generators and seem to have less effect on increasing airway resistance than normal saline or water.
D. Distilled water: Used in respiratory therapy in all types of humidifiers.

IV. Mucolytics
A. Trade name: Mucomyst.
B. Generic name: Acetylcysteine (*N*-acetyl-L-cysteine).
C. Mechanism of action: Lyses disulfide bonds holding mucoproteins together, thus increasing fluidity of mucoid sputum.
D. Concentration: 10% or 20% W/V solution.
E. Dosage
   1. Standard dosage: 4 ml of 10% W/V or 2 ml 20% W/V solution with 2 ml H_2O.
   2. Maximum dosage: None specified.
F. Indications: Thick, retained mucoid or mucopurulent secretions.
G. Contraindications: Hypersensitivity.
H. Side effects and hazards
   1. Bronchospasm
   2. Excessive liquification of dried, retained secretions

        3. Stomatitis
        4. Hypersensitivity
        5. Nausea
        6. Rhinorrhea

  I. Comments
     1. Highly recommended that drug be administered in conjunction with bronchodilator.
     2. Should be refrigerated after opening.
     3. Should be used within 96 hours after opening.
     4. Reacts with rubber, some plastics, and iron.
     5. Foul smelling.
     6. Should be administered in glass, plastic, or nontarnishable metal container.
     7. Minimal effectiveness on predominantly purulent secretions.
     8. Supplied in 4-, 10-, and 30-ml vials.

V. Prophylactic Antiasthmatics
  A. Trade name: Intal.
  B. Generic name: Cromolyn sodium.
  C. Mechanism of action
     1. Inhibits release of histamine and slow-reacting substance of anaphylaxis (SRS-A) during allergic, IgE-mediated responses on pulmonary mast cells.
     2. Suppresses response of mast cell to antigen-antibody reaction.
  D. Concentration: 20-mg capsules (powder) or 20 mg/2 ml H_2O ampules (liquid).
  E. Standard dosage: 20 mg three or four times daily.
  F. Maximum dosage: 20 mg three or four times daily.
  G. Primary indications: Prophylactic maintenance in patients with severe bronchial asthma exercise-induced bronchospasm.
  H. Secondary indications: Result of the effect of cromolyn sodium on all mast cells.
     1. Allergic rhinitis
     2. Diarrhea in systemic mastocytosis
     3. Ulcers of the oral mucosa
     4. Nonspecific inflammatory bowel disease
  I. Contraindications: Hypersensitivity.
  J. Side effects and hazards
     1. Local irritation
     2. Bronchospasm
     3. Maculopapular rash
     4. Urticaria
     5. Cough
     6. Congestion
     7. Sneezing
     8. Epistaxis
  K. Comments
     1. Ineffective in acute asthmatic attack.
     2. Maximum effect seen after 4 weeks of continuous use.
     3. Sometimes effective in controlling exercise-induced asthma.

VI. Surface-Active Agent
  A. Trade name: Ethyl alcohol, ethanol.
  B. Generic name: Ethyl alcohol, ethanol.
  C. Mechanism of action
     1. It has a direct surfactant-like effect on surface tension of frothy, serum-like fluid developed in acute pulmonary edema.
     2. Breaking up of frothy secretions allows them to occupy a much smaller volume, improving distribution of ventilation.

D. Concentration: 20% to 80% solution.

E. Standard dosage

　　1. Standard

　　　　a. Intermittent: 4 to 10 ml of 50% solution.

　　　　b. Continuous: 500 ml of 50% solution over a 24-hour period.

F. Indication: Acute pulmonary edema.

G. Contraindications: Hypersensitivity.

H. Side effects and hazards

　　1. Airway irritation

　　2. Bronchospasm

　　3. Local dehydration

I. Comments: Should not be administered in heated aerosol or ultrasonic nebulizer.

VII. Sympathomimetics: General Considerations

A. General classification

　　1. Alpha effect: Constriction of vascular smooth muscle.

　　　　a. Alpha-1: Excitatory on postsynaptic receptors (e.g., peripheral blood vessels).

　　　　b. Alpha-2: Inhibitory on presynaptic peripheral sympathetic nerves, possible postsynaptic in the central nervous system (CNS).

　　2. Beta effect: Peripheral relaxation of vascular smooth muscle (minimal).

　　　　a. Beta-1: Positive inotropic and chronotropic cardiac effects.

　　　　b. Beta-2: Relaxation of nonvascular smooth muscle (bronchodilation).

B. Mechanism of action (Fig 40–4)

　　1. Alpha effect: Inhibits membrane-bound adenylcyclase from converting adenosine triphosphate (ATP) to cyclic 3'5'-adenosine monophosphate (3'5'-AMP).

　　2. Beta effect: Stimulates release of membrane-bound adenylcyclase, which increases formation of cyclic 3'5'-AMP from ATP and probably decrease in (Ca^{+2}).

C. General therapeutic uses of sympathomimetics

　　1. Treatment of generalized bronchoconstriction

　　2. Treatment of mucosal congestion

　　3. Treatment of allergic disorders

　　4. Control of hemorrhage

　　5. Treatment of hypotension

　　6. Cardiac stimulation

　　7. Treatment of heart block

　　8. Treatment of CNS disorders

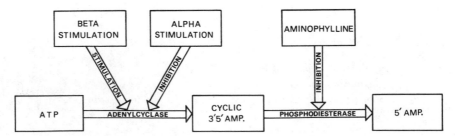

FIG 40–4.
Increased cyclic 3'5'-AMP levels result in bronchodilation. Beta stimulation increases cyclic 3'5'-AMP levels by release of adenylcyclase, whereas aminophylline increases cyclic 3'5'-AMP levels by inhibiting its metabolism by phosphodiesterase. Alpha stimulation inhibits adenylcyclase release and therefore decreases cyclic 3'5'-AMP levels.

    D. Contraindications
        1. Hyperthyroidism
        2. Hypertension
        3. Tachycardia
    E. Side effects and hazards
        1. Palpitations
        2. Tachycardia
        3. Hypertension
        4. Restlessness
        5. Fear
        6. Anxiety
        7. Tension
        8. Tremor
        9. Weakness
      10. Dizziness
      11. Pallor
    F. Comments
        1. Tolerance is frequently observed (tachyphylaxis).
        2. Synergistic effects may be seen.
        3. It is maximally administered every 2 to 3 hours.
        4. Normal duration of action is short, up to 3 hours, and may be as short as 1 to 1½ hours.
VIII. Specific Sympathomimetics (Table 40–1)
    A. Isoproterenol HCl
        1. Trade name: Isuprel.
        2. Generic name: Isoproterenol HCl.
        3. Concentration: 1:100 or 1:200 solution.
        4. Effects
            a. Alpha: None (0).
            b. Beta-1: Strong (+++).
            c. Beta-2: Strong (+++).
        5. Dosage (nebulizer)
            a. Standard
                (1) 0.5 ml of 1:200 solution in 4 ml of normal saline.
                (2) 0.25 ml of 1:100 solution in 4 ml of normal saline.
            b. Maximum
                (1) 1 ml of 1:200 solution in 4 ml of normal saline.
                (2) 0.5 ml of 1:100 solution in 4 ml of normal saline.
        6. Dosage (MDI)
                (1) Concentration: 131 µg/puff.
                (2) 1 to 2 puffs/Rx
    B. Racemic epinephrine
        1. Trade name: Vaponephrine, Micronephrine.
        2. Generic name: Racemic epinephrine.
        3. Concentration: 2.25% W/V solution.
        4. Effects
            a. Alpha: Medium (++).
            b. Beta-1: Weak (+).
            c. Beta-2: Medium (++).
        5. Dosage
            a. Standard: 0.5 ml of 2.25% W/V solution in 4 ml of normal saline.
            b. Maximum: 1 ml of 2.25% W/V solution in 4 ml of normal saline.

TABLE 40–1.

Comparison of Aerosolized Sympathomimetics*

Generic Name	Drug	Effects	Concentration	Dosage
Isoproterenol HCl	Isuprel	α 0 β_1 +++ β_2 +++	1:100; 1:200	0.5 ml 1:200 in 4 ml of NSS 0.25 ml 1:100 in 4 ml of NSS
Racemic epinephrine	Vaponephrine, Micronephrine	α ++ β_1 + β_2 ++	2.25% W/V	0.5 ml in 4 ml of NSS
Isoetharine	Bronkosol, Dilabron	α 0 β_1 + β_2 ++	1% W/V	0.5 ml in 4 ml of NSS
Epinephrine HCl	Adrenalin	α +++ β_1 +++ β_2 ++	1:100	0.2 ml in 4 ml of NSS 0.05 ml of 1:000, subq
Phenylephrine	Neo-Synephrine	α +++ β_1 0 β_2 0	0.25% W/V	0.2 ml in 4 ml of NSS
Metaproterenol sulfate	Alupent, Metaprel	α 0 β_1 ½+ β_2 +++	5% W/V 0.65 mg/spray	0.3 ml in 4 ml of NSS 2 sprays every 6 hr
Albuteral	Ventolin, Proventil	α 0 β_1 + β_2 +++	0.1 mg/spray 0.5% M/V	2 sprays every 6 hr 0.5 ml in 4 ml of NSS
Terbutaline sulfate	Bricanyl, Brethine, Brethaire	α 0 β_1 + β_2 +++	0.2% W/V 0.1% W/V	0.25–0.5 ml in 4 ml of NSS 2 sprays QID
Pirbuterol	Maxair	α 0 β_1 + β_2 ++	0.2 mg/puff	2 puffs every 4 hr
Bitolterol	Tornalate	α 0 β_1 + β_2 +++	0.37 mg/puff	2 puffs every 8 hr

*0 = none; + = weak; ++ = medium; +++ = strong; α = alpha; β_1 = beta-1; β_2 = beta-2; NSS = normal saline solution.

    C. Isoetharine
        1. Trade name: Bronkosol, Dilabron.
        2. Generic name: Isoetharine.
        3. Concentration: 1% W/V solution.
        4. Effects
            a. Alpha: None (0).
            b. Beta-1: Weak (+)
            c. Beta-2: Medium (++).
        5. Dosage
            a. Nebulizer
                (1) Standard: 0.5 ml in 4 ml of normal saline.
                (2) Maximum: 1 ml in 4 ml of normal saline.
            b. MDI
                (1) Concentration
                    (a) 0.34 mg/puff; 1 to 2 puffs/Rx.
                    (b) 0.2 mg/puff; 2 puffs/Rx.

D. Epinephrine HCl
   1. Trade name: Adrenalin.
   2. Generic name: Epinephrine HCl.
   3. Concentration: 1:100.
   4. Effects
      a. Alpha: Strong (+++).
      b. Beta-1: Strong (+++).
      c. Beta-two: Medium (++).
   5. Dosage
      a. Aerosol
         (1) Standard: 0.25 ml in 4 ml of normal saline.
         (2) Maximum: 0.50 ml in 4 ml of normal saline.
      b. Subcutaneous: 0.3 to 0.5 ml of a 1:1000 solution.
E. Phenylephrine
   1. Trade name: Neo-Synephrine.
   2. Generic name: Phenylephrine.
   3. Concentration: 0.25% W/V.
   4. Effects
      a. Alpha: Strong (+++).
      b. Beta 1: None (0).
      c. Beta-2: None (0).
   5. Dosage
      a. Standard: 0.2 ml in 4 ml of normal saline.
      b. Maximum: 0.5 ml in 4 ml of normal saline.
   6. Comment: Normally administered only as nasal decongestant by spray or drops.
F. Metaproterenol sulfate
   1. Trade name: Alupent, Metaprel.
   2. Generic name: Metaproterenol sulfate.
   3. Concentration
      a. Tablet: 10 and 20 mg (oral dosage).
      b. Metered mist: 0.65 mg/spray.
      c. Liquid: 5% W/V solution; 0.3 ml in 4 ml normal saline.
   4. Effects
      a. Alpha: None (0).
      b. Beta one: weak (+).
      c. Beta two: Medium (++).
   5. Dosage
      a. Standard
         (1) One tablet four times daily.
         (2) Two sprays every 4 to 6 hours.
         (3) 0.3 ml in 4 ml of normal saline via aerosol.
      b. Maximum
         (1) 0.6 ml in 4 ml of normal saline via aerosol.
   6. Comment: Duration of effect up to 6 hours.
G. Albuterol
   1. Trade name: Ventolin, Proventil.
   2. Generic name: Albuteral.
   3. Concentration: 90 mg/spray; 2-and 4-mg tablets.
   4. Effects: 0.5% W/V
      a. Alpha: None (0).
      b. Beta-1: Weak (+).
      c. Beta-2: Strong (+++).

     5. Dosage

       a. MDI: 90 μg/puff; 2 puffs/Rx.

       b. Nebulizer: 0.5 ml in 4 ml of normal saline.

     6. Comment: Duration of effect up to 6 hours.

  H. Terbutaline sulfate

     1. Trade name: Bricanyl, Brethine, Brethaire (MDI).

     2. Generic name: Terbutaline sulfate.

     3. Concentration: 0.1% W/V; 2.5- and 5-mg tablets.

     4. Effects

       a. Alpha: None (0).

       b. Beta-1: Weak (+)

       c. Beta-2: Strong (+++).

     5. Dosage

       a. Subcutaneous: 0.25 to 1.0 mg.

       b. Aerosol: 0.25 to 0.5 ml in 4 ml of normal saline solution.

       c. Tablets: 2.5 or 5.0-mg three times daily.

       d. MDI: 0.2 mg/puff; 2 puffs four times daily.

  I. Bitolterol

     1. Trade name: Tornalate.

     2. Generic name: Bitolterol.

     3. Concentration: 0.37 mg/puff.

     4. Effects

       a. Alpha: None (0)

       b. Beta-1: Weak (+).

       c. Beta-2: Medium (++).

     5. Dosage: 2 puffs every 8 hours.

  J. Pirbuterol

     1. Trade name: Maxair.

     2. Generic name: Pirbuterol.

     3. Concentration: 0.2 mg/puff.

     4. Effects

       a. Alpha: none (0).

       b. Beta-1: Weak (+)

       c. Beta-2: Strong (+++).

     5. Dosage: 2 puffs every 4 hours.

IX. Sympathomimetics Utilized for Their Effects on the Cardiovascular System

  A. Norepinephrine

     1. Trade name: Levophed, Noradrenalin.

     2. Generic name: Norepinephrine.

     3. Effects

       a. Alpha: Strong (+++).

       b. Beta-1: Weak (+).

       c. Beta-2: None (0).

     4. Indications: Hypotension.

     5. Administration: IV only.

  B. Dopamine HCl

     1. Trade name: Intropin, Dopastat.

     2. Generic name: Dopamine HC1.

     3. Effects: Dose dependent.

       a. Low dosages

         (1) Increased renal blood flow.

         (2) Mild increase in cardiac output.

 b. Moderate dosages
  (1) Increased renal blood flow.
  (2) Increased cardiac output.
 c. High dosages: Systemic vasoconstriction.
 4. Indications
  a. Hypotension
  b. Shock
  c. Renal failure
  d. Myocardial infarction
  e. Other hemodynamic problems
 5. Administration: IV only in appropriate dilution of nonalkaline solutions.
 6. Side effects and hazards
  a. Widening QRS interval
  b. Angina
  c. Conduction disturbances
  d. Tachycardia
C. Dobutamine
 1. Trade name: Dobutrex.
 2. Generic: Dobutamine.
 3. Effects
  a. Alpha: None (0).
  b. Beta-1: Moderate (+ +).
  c. Beta-2: None (0).
 4. Indications:
  a. Congestive heart failure
  b. Hemodynamic abnormalities
 5. Administration: IV only.
 6. Side effects and hazards
  a. Premature ventricular contractions
  b. Anginal pain
  c. Ishemic injury
 7. Comments
  a. Has inotropic selectivity (less increase in heart rate than other drugs).
  b. Decreases systemic vascular resistance.
  c. No increase in pulmonary or systemic blood pressure noted with administration.
D. Mephentermine sulfate
 1. Trade name: Wyamine sulfate.
 2. Generic name: Mephentermine.
 3. Effects
  a. Indirect: Releases norepinephrine (alpha).
  b. Direct: Stimulates cardiac beta-1 receptors.
 4. Indications
  a. Hypotension secondary to ganglionic blockade or spinal anesthesia.
  b. Emergency use for hypotension caused by hemorrhage until blood is available.
 5. Administration: IV preferred, IM possible.
 6. Side effects and hazards
  a. Anxiety
  b. Cardiac arrhythmias
  c. Hypertension

E. Metaraminol
 1. Trade name: Araminie.
 2. Generic name: Metaraminol.
 3. Effects: Primarily alpha-receptor-mediated peripheral vasoconstriction.
 4. Indications
  a. Acute hypotension caused by spinal anesthesia.
  b. Adjunctive treatment of hypotension due to hemorrhage.
  c. Hypotension due to surgery complications, reaction to medications, or brain damage caused by tumor or trauma.
 5. Administration: IM, SC, or IV (although IM and subq are rarely used).
 6. Side effects and hazards
  a. Sinus or ventricular tachycardia; reflex bradycardia or other arrhythmias
  b. Hypertension
  c. Headache
  d. Flushing
  e. Sweating
  f. Tremors
  g. Dizziness
F. Methoxamine HCl
 1. Trade name: Vasoxyl.
 2. Generic name: Methoxamine.
 3. Effects: Alpha-receptor stimulation increases peripheral vascular resistance.
 4. Indications: Blood pressure support during anesthesia.
 5. Administration: IM or IV.
 6. Side effects and hazards
  a. Hypertension
  b. Ventricular ectopic beats
  c. Nausea, vomiting
  d. Headache, anxiety
  e. Sweating
X. Noncatecholamines Affecting the Sympathetic Nervous System
 A. Ephedrine
  1. Trade name: Ephedrine.
  2. Generic name: Ephedrine.
  3. Mechanism of action: Causes release of epinephrine and norepinephrine stored throughout the body.
  4. Effects (lasting up to 6 hours)
   a. Bronchodilation
   b. Mild cardiac stimulation
   c. Peripheral vasoconstriction
   d. Mild CNS stimulation
  5. Indications
   a. Nonemergency allergic reactions
   b. Chronic asthma
   c. Nasal congestion
  6. Administration: Oral, intramuscular, or subcutaneous.
 B. Theophylline
  1. Trade name: Aminophylline.
  2. Generic name: Theophylline.
  3. Mechanism of action: Inhibits phosphodiesterase (see Fig 40–4) from converting cyclic 3'5'-AMP to inactive 5'-AMP.

4. Effects
   a. Bronchodilation
   b. Cardiac stimulation
   c. Coronary artery dilation
   d. Skeletal muscle stimulation
   e. Diuresis
   f. CNS stimulation
   g. Increased ventilatory drive
   h. Apnea of prematurity
5. Indications
   a. Acute and chronic asthma
   b. Abnormal respiratory patterns (e.g., Cheyne-Stokes)
   c. Sleep apnea (neonates)
6. Dosage: Sufficient quantity to maintain blood level in therapeutic range of 10 to 20 μg/ml of plasma.
7. Side effects (normally noted if therapeutic is level exceeded):
   a. Gastrointestinal irritation
   b. Headache
   c. Hyperactivity
   d. Dizziness
   e. Nausea
   f. Palpitation
   g. Chest pain
   h. Cardiac arrhythmias
   i. Seizures
8. Administration: Orally IM, IV, or by suppository.

XI. Parasympathomimetics
   A. Action: Enhance effects of parasympathetic nervous system.
   B. Classification of effects
      1. *Muscarinic:* Effect on parasympathetic postganglionic fibers, thus stimulating only the parasympathetic nervous system.
      2. *Nicotinic:* Effect on other sites where acetylcholine is the transmitter substance, thus stimulating sites outside the parasympathetic nervous system.
         a. Voluntary muscle
         b. Sympathetic nervous system
         c. CNS
         d. Adrenal medulla
   C. Classification of drug groups
      1. Choline esters (drugs with structure similar to acetylcholine)
         a. Primary effects: Muscarinic with limited nicotinic effects.
         b. Primary indications
            (1) Paroxysmal supraventricular tachycardia
            (2) Gastrointestinal disorders
            (3) Urinary bladder disorders
            (4) Bronchial provocation testing
         c. Representative drugs
            (1) Methacholine (Mecholyl)
            (2) Bethanechol (Urecholine)
      2. Naturally occurring alkaloids
         a. Primary effect: Almost exclusively at muscarinic sites.
         b. Primary indication: Glaucoma.
         c. Representative drug: Pilocarpine (generic and trade)

    3. Cholinesterase inhibitors
        a. Mechanism of action: Competitive inhibition of cholinesterase.
        b. Primary Effect: Strong stimulation at both nicotinic and muscarinic sites.
        c. Therapeutic uses
           (1) Paralytic ileus
           (2) Atony of urinary bladder
           (3) Glaucoma
           (4) Myasthenia gravis (symptomatic)
           (5) Atropine intoxication
           (6) Reversal of nondepolarizing neuromuscular blocking agents
    4. Representative drugs
        a. Neostigmine (Prostigmine)
        b. Pyridostigmine (Mestinon)
        c. Ambenonium (Mytelase)
        d. Edrophonium (Tensilon)
  D. Side effects associated with excessive stimulation of parasympathetic nervous system
    1. Gastrointestinal disorders
    2. Cardiovascular problems
    3. Excessive secretion by exocrine glands, (e.g., mucous, salivary)
XII. Parasympatholytics
  A. Action: Inhibition of parasympathetic nervous system.
  B. Mechanism of action: Competitive inhibition of acetylcholine at muscarinic sites only.
  C. Therapeutic uses
    1. CNS disorders
    2. Preanesthesia medication
    3. Ophthalmologic (pupil dilation)
    4. Upper airway allergies
    5. Gastrointestinal disorders
    6. Genitourinary tract disorders
    7. Common cold
    8. Over-the-counter sleeping pills
    9. Motion sickness, nausea and vomiting
   10. Cardiovascular problems
   11. Used with parasympathomimetics for reversal of neuromuscular blocking agents
   12. Bronchodilation
  D. Side effects
    1. Dry mouth
    2. Blurred vision
    3. Urinary retention
    4. Lightheadedness
    5. Fatigue
    6. Tachycardia
  E. Representative drugs
    1. *Atropa belladonna*, atropine
        a. Various solution concentrations.
        b. Dosage Nebulizer: 0.025 mg/kg three or four times daily.
    2. Ipratropium bromide (Atrovent)
        a. Dosage (MDI): 18 μg/puff; 2 puffs four times daily.

   3. Glycopyrrolate (Robinul)
      (1) Dosage Nebulizer: 0.1 mg/ml.
      (2) Tablets: 1.0 mg three or four times daily.
   4. Hyoscine (Scopolamine hydrobromide)
   5. Anticholinergics
      a. Parkinson's disease
         (1) Procyclidine (Kemadrin)
         (2) Trihexiphenidyl (Aphen, Artane, etc.)
         (3) Benztropine (Cogentin)
         (4) Biperiden (Akineton)
         (5) Ethopropazine (Pardisol)
         (6) Orphenadrine (Disipal)
         (7) Diphenhydramine (Benadryl and other formulations)
      b. Antispasmodic
         (1) L-Hyoscyamine (Anaspaz)
         (2) Clidinium (Quarzan)
XIII. Sympatholytics
   A. Action: Inhibition of the sympathetic nervous system.
   B. α-Adrenergic blocking agents
      1. Mechanism of action: Direct inhibitory affect at α-adrenergic receptor site.
      2. Effects
         a. Prevent excitatory responses of smooth muscle and exocrine glands.
         b. Can cause postural hypotension.
         c. Cause an increase in cardiac output and decrease in total peripheral resistance in normal recumbent subjects.
      3. Therapeutic uses
      4. Representative drugs
         a. Central activity
            (1) Methyldopa (Aldomet)
            (2) Clonidine (Catapres)
            (3) Guanabenz (Wytensin)
            (4) Guanfacine (Tenex)
         b. Peripheral activity
            (1) Reserpine (Serpasil)
            (2) Guanethidine (Ismelin)
            (3) Guanadrel (Hylorel)
            (4) Prazosin (Minipress)
            (5) Terazosin (Hytrin)
   C. β-Adrenergic blocking agents
      1. Action: Decrease beta-1 and beta-2 effects.
      2. Mechanism of action: Competitive inhibition at receptor site.
      3. Effects
         a. Negative inotropic and chronotropic effect on heart.
         b. Slight bronchoconstriction (contraindicated in asthmatics).
         c. Possibly partial agonist effect.
      4. Therapeutic uses
         a. Cardiac arrhythmias
         b. Angina pectoris
         c. Hypertension
         d. Migraine prophylaxis
         e. Glaucoma

5. Side effects and hazards
   a. Pulmonary edema
   b. Hypotension
   c. Heart block
6. Representative drugs
   a. Propranolol (Inderal)
   b. Metoprolol (Lopressor)
   c. Timolol (Bleocardin, Timolide)
   d. Nadolol (Corgard)
   e. Atenolol (Tenormin)
   f. Pindolol (Visken)
   g. Acebutolol (Sectral)
D. α- and β-Adrenergic blockers
   1. Representative drug: Labetalol (Normodyne, Trandate)

XIV. Steroids
   A. Adenocorticotropic hormone (ACTH) and adrenocorticosteroids
      1. Adenocorticotropic hormone (corticotropin) is produced and released from the adrenohypophysis (anterior pituitary).
      2. Physiology of steroid regulation
         a. Release of ACTH into the blood causes the adrenal cortex to release its steroids into the bloodstream.
         b. Release of ACTH is affected directly by corticotropin-releasing factor (CRF), which is secreted by the hypothalamus.
         c. Blood level of CRF is indirectly affected by blood steroid levels.
         d. Thus, there is a cyclic relation between ACTH, CRF, and steroid levels (Fig 40–5).
         e. An increase in steroid levels causes a decrease in CRF levels, which causes a decrease in ACTH levels. This results in a decrease in steroid levels, which causes an increase in CRF levels, and so forth, thus maintaining a normal equilibrium.
      3. Actions
         a. Stimulate glucose formation (i.e., increase blood glucose levels).
         b. Diminish glucose utilization.
         c. Promote storage of glucose in liver.
         d. Regulate rate of synthesis of proteins.

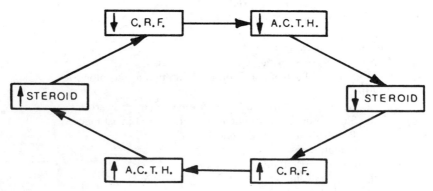

FIG 40–5.
There is a cyclic relationship of CRF, ACTH, and steroid levels. Normal steroid levels are maintained by this interrelationship. The CRF and ACTH levels are directly related; the ACTH and steroid levels are also directly related; the steroid and CRF levels are indirectly related.

e. Control distribution of body fat.
f. Regulate lipid metabolism.
g. Regulate reabsorption of sodium ions from kidney tubules.
h. Increase urinary excretion of both K^+ and H^+.
i. Maintain normal function of skeletal muscles.
j. Increase hemoglobin and red blood cell content of blood.
k. Maintain normal lymphoid tissue.
l. Prevent or suppress inflammatory responses caused by hypersensitivity.

4. Mechanisms of action
   a. Modification of cell function protein production and direct stimulation of tissue receptor sites to inhibit the complex mechanisms of inflammation.
   b. Allergic disorders: Has a catabolic effect on lymphoid tissue.
   c. Edema: Decreases capillary permeability by an unknown mechanism.

5. Therapeutic uses
   a. Allergic asthma
   b. Acute and chronic adrenal insufficiency
   c. Suppression of immune response in organ transplant patients
   d. Congenital adrenal hyperplasia
   e. Adrenal insufficiency secondary to anterior pituitary insufficiency
   f. Arthritis
   g. Rheumatic carditis
   h. Osteoarthritis
   i. Acute inflammatory diseases

6. Side effects
   a. Aerosol administration
      (1) Upper airway fungal infections
      (2) Hoarseness
      (3) Coughing
      (4) Dry mouth
      (5) Adrenal insufficiency following transfer from systemic steroids
   b. Systemic administration
      (1) Cushing's disease
         (a) Moon face
         (b) Hirsutism
         (c) Muscle wasting
         (d) Variable hypernatremia
         (e) Hypokalemia
      (2) Hypertension
      (3) Aggravation of diabetes mellitus (hyperglycemia)
      (4) Necrotizing arteritis in rheumatoid patients
      (5) Aggravation of peptic ulcer
      (6) Psychotic manifestations (mood changes)
      (7) Adrenal atrophy
      (8) Obesity
      (9) Growth suppression
      (10) Thinning of skin
      (11) Muscle wasting
      (12) Osteoporosis
      (13) Immunosuppression

7. Representative drugs (aerosolized drugs)
   a. Dexamethasone (Decadron)
      (1) Packaged in 10-ml vial with 4 mg/ml (0.4% W/V).

        (2) Administered by aerosol following extubation to diminish inflammation of larynx and trachea.

        (3) Dosage: 1 ml of dexamethasone, 0.5 mg of 2.25% racemic epinephrine, and 3 ml of normal saline.

    b. Beclomethasone dipropionate (Vanceril, Beclovent)

        (1) Supplied as metered mist (MDI) of 50 µg/inhalation.

        (2) Used for chronic treatment of bronchial asthma in patients in whom a corticosteroid is indicated.

        (3) Side effects

            (a) Localized (mouth, pharynx, larynx) infection with *Candida albicans* and *Aspergillus niger.*

            (b) Occasional deaths from ACTH suppression when beclomethasone has been used to replace previous therapies involving corticosteroids with strong systemic activity.

        (4) Dosage

            (a) Standard: Two inhalations three or four times daily.

            (b) Maximum: Twenty-two inhalations/day.

    c. Other aerosolized drugs

        (1) Triamcinolone acetonide (Azmacort); MDI, 100 µg/puff, 2 puffs three or four times daily.

        (2) Flunisolide (AeroBid); MDI, 250 µg/puff, 2 puffs two times daily.

  8. Representative drugs (systemic)

    a. Cortisone

    b. Hydrocortisone

    c. Prednisone

    d. Prednisolone

    e. Methylprednisolone

    f. Belamethasone

XV. Neuromuscular Blocking Agents

  A. Major action: Interruption of transmission of nerve impulse at skeletal neuromuscular junction, resulting in paralysis.

  B. Categories

    1. *Nondepolarizing* agents

      a. Mechanism of action: Competitive inhibition of acetylcholine at muscle postsynaptic receptor sites. The muscle tissue itself remains sensitive to external stimulation.

      b. Effects

        (1) Maximal effects are seen in about 3 to 4 min and persist 20 to 40 min.

        (2) Hypotension as a result of histamine release is seen occasionally with *d*-tubocurarine.

        (3) Bradycardia occasionally is seen with pancuronium.

        (4) Effects of this group of drugs may be reversed by cholinesterase-inhibiting agents (e.g., neostigmine).

      c. Representative drugs

        (1) Tubocurarine (*d*-tubocurarine)

        (2) Pancuronium (Pavulon)

        (3) Metocurine iodide (Metubine iodide)

        (4) Gallamine triethiodide (Flaxedil)

        (5) Atracurium besylate (Tracrium)

        (6) Vecuronium bromide (Norcuron)

    2. *Depolarizing* agents

      a. Mechanism of action

        (1) They cause persistent depolarization of muscle motor end-plates.

(2) As this wave of depolarization proceeds, a rippling of voluntary muscles occurs (muscle fasciculation), usually from the head downward. Since these agents are chemically similar to acetylcholine, they cause continual stimulation of the motor end-plate.

(3) This continual stimulation does not allow time for repolarization; therefore, the muscle develops a flaccid paralysis.

(4) With time, depolarizing agents are metabolized by pseudocholinesterase.

b. The muscle fiber itself is still sensitive to external stimulation.

(1) Effects are seen in about 30 to 40 seconds and persist 3 to 5 mins.

(2) They are irreversible.

c. Representative drugs

(1) Succinylcholine (Anectine, Quelicin, Sucostrin)

(2) Decamethonium (Syncurine)

XVI. Narcotics and Analgesics

A. Primary use (narcotics): Analgesia and relief of severe pain.

B. Mechanism of action: Unclear, but these drugs affect neurotransmission at specific CNS sites, affect autonomic nervous system transmission, and cause some histamine release.

C. General pharmacologic effects

1. Analgesic

a. Alters the perception of pain.

b. Interferes with the continuance of pain impulses in the spinal cord.

c. Alters the body's response to the pain stimulus.

d. May elevate the pain threshold.

2. Euphoric: Seen at therapeutic dosages.

3. Hypnotic: With increasing dosages, more subjective CNS depression.

4. Metabolic: Transient hyperglycemia.

5. Endocrine: Stimulates the release of antidiuretic hormone.

6. Pupil size: Miosis.

7. Gastrointestinal tract: Constipation because of decreased overall activity.

8. Nausea and vomiting: Direct stimulation of medullary control center.

9. Cardiovascular system

a. If patient is well oxygenated and in normal acid-base balance, there are no significant effects.

b. Cardiac arrhythmias may be seen with acid-base abnormalities.

c. Hypotension may result due to direct effect on venous smooth muscle and release of histamine.

10. Respiratory system

a. Direct depression of medullary respiratory center response to CO_2 changes.

b. Significant decrease in respiratory rate, tidal volume, and minute volume is seen with large dosages.

11. Cough reflex: Decreased as a result of direct depression of medullary cough center.

D. Therapeutic uses

1. Analgesia

2. Cough control

3. Emetic

4. Antidiarrhetic

5. Pulmonary edema

6. Control of patients on ventilators

E. Representative drugs
    1. High potency
        a. Morphine (generic and trade)
        b. Oxymorphone (Numorphan)
        c. Heroin
        d. Levorphanol (Levo-Dromoran)
        e. Methadone (Dolophine)
        f. Phenazocine (Prinadol)
    2. Intermediate potency
        a. Meperidine (Demerol)
        b. Alphaprodine (Nisentil)
        c. Pentazocine (Talwin)
        d. Anileridine (Leritine)
        e. Oxycodone (Percodan)
    3. Low potency
        a. Codeine (generic and trade)
        b. Diphenoxylate (Lomotil)

F. Non-narcotic analgesics and anti-inflammatory agents: All have analgesic properties and are normally used for mild or chronic pain.
    1. Salicylates
        a. Aspirin (acetylsalicytic acid)
        b. Methyl salicylate
        c. Diflunisal (Dolobid)
    2. Aniline derivatives
        a. Phenacetin
        b. Acetaminophen (Tempra, Tylenol)
    3. Pyrazole derivatives
        a. Antipyrine
        b. Amidopyrine
        c. Phenylbutazone (Butazolidin)
        d. Oxyphenbutazone (Oxalid)
    4. Central-acting agents
        a. Methotrimeprazine (Levoprome)
    5. Nonsteroidal anti-inflammatory drugs (NSAIDs)
        a. Indomethacin (Indocin)
        b. Ibuprofen (Motrin)
        c. Ketoprofen (Orudis)
        d. Fenoprofen (Nalfon)
        e. Naproxen (Naprosyn)
        f. Sulindac (Clinoril)
        g. Tolmetin (Tolectin)
        h. Mefenamic acid (Ponstel)
        i. Meclofenamate (Meclomen)
        j. Piroxicam (Feldene)

XVII. Narcotic Antagonists
A. Sole use: To reverse effects of narcotics.
B. Mechanism of action: Competitive displacement of agonist from receptor site.
C. Partial antagonists
    1. Cause narcotic-like effects in absence of a narcotic.
    2. Cause increased respiratory depression if administered in a nonnarcotic overdose (e.g., barbiturates).
    3. Representative drugs
        a. Nalorphine (Nalline)
        b. Levallorphan (Lorfan)

D. Pure antagonists: Have only narcotic antagonist properties.
 1. Will not increase respiratory depression in a nonnarcotic overdose.
 2. Representative drug: Naloxone (Narcan)
E. Duration of effect
 1. 45 to 60 min *(careful monitoring of overdosed patient must be maintained)*.
 2. Narcotic's effect may significantly outlast that of the narcotic antagonist.
XVIII. Sedative and Hypnotics
 A. Solid or liquid substances that cause a longer generalized depression of the CNS than do anesthetic gases.
 B. Mechanism of action: Selective depression of ascending reticular activating system at either the cellular or synaptic level, resulting in loss of consciousness.
 C. Physiologic effects
 1. Behavioral changes caused by increased dosages
 a. Sedation: Generalized decreased responsiveness
 b. Disinhibition: Impaired judgment and loss of self-control
 c. Relief of anxiety
 d. Ataxia and nystagmus
 e. Sleep (hypnosis)
 f. Anesthesia
 2. Electroencephalographic (EEG) pattern changes consistent with generalized CNS depression
 3. Poor analgesia
 4. Anticonvulsant: (phenobarbital the most effective)
 5. Withdrawal state with repeated long-term use and abrupt discontinuance
 6. Habit forming
 7. Voluntary muscle relaxation from spinal cord depression
 8. Depression of respiratory medullary center with larger doses
 9. Profound vasomotor depression and shock with larger doses
 10. No direct effect on myocardium
 D. Therapeutic uses
 1. Sleep induction
 2. Relief of anxiety (sedation)
 3. Treatment of neurotic anxiety
 4. Relief of depression
 5. Voluntary muscle relaxation
 6. Anticonvulsant
 E. Side effects
 1. Drowsiness
 2. Impaired performance and judgment
 3. Hangover
 4. Drug abuse
 5. Withdrawal state
 6. Overdose
 F. Contraindications
 1. Hypothyroidism
 2. Hypoadrenalism
 G. Types
 1. Barbiturates
 a. Ultra-short-acting: Anesthetic agents
 (1) Hexobarbital (Sombucaps)
 (2) Thiopental (Pentothal)
 (3) Thiamylal (Surital)
 b. Short-acting: Primarily for sleep induction
 (1) Pentobarbital (Nembutal)

          (2) Secobarbital (Seconal)

    c. Intermediate-acting: Relief of anxiety

          (1) Amobarbital (Amytal)

          (2) Butabarbital (Butisol)

          (3) Aprobarbital (Alurate)

          (4) Talbutal (Lotusate)

    d. Long-acting: Anticonvulsant

          (1) Phenobarbital (generic and trade)

          (2) Mephobarbital (Mebaral)

          (3) Metharbital (Gemonil)

2. Nonbarbiturate sedatives: Hypnotics

    a. Short-acting

          (1) Methaqualone (Quaalude)

          (2) Paraldehyde (generic and trade)

          (3) Chloral hydrate (generic and trade)

          (4) Flurazepam (Dalmane)

    b. Intermediate-acting

          (1) Meprobamate (Miltown, Equanil)

          (2) Glutethimide (Doriden)

          (3) Diazepam (Valium)

    c. Long-acting: Chlordiazepoxide (Librium)

3. Other antianxiety agents

    a. Acetylcarbromal (Paxarel)

    b. Ethinamate (Valmid)

    c. Propiomazine (Largon)

    d. Lorazepam (Ativan)

    e. Temazepam (Restoril)

    f. Triazolam (Halcion)

    g. Oxazepam (Serax)

    h. Clorazepate (Tranxene)

    i. Prazepam (Centrax)

    j. Halazepam (Paxipam)

    k. Alprazolam (Xanax)

    l. Buspirone (Buspar)

    m. Ethchlorvynol (Placidyl)

    n. Methyprylon (Noludar)

XIX. Antipsychotic Tranquilizers

  A. Action: Alter psychotic state without inducing sedation or hypnosis.

  B. Mechanism of action

    1. Decrease nervous input into the reticular activating system, thereby decreasing reticular activity.

    2. Enhance the breakdown of catecholamines.

    3. Indirectly decrease the formation of norepinephrine.

  C. Characteristics

    1. General effects are subjectively unpleasant.

    2. They are non–habit forming.

    3. They cause generalized increased electric activity (evidenced on EEG).

    4. Increasing dosages cause indifference, apathy, motor retardation, and convulsions.

    5. Patients remain arousable.

  D. Therapeutic uses

    1. Schizophrenia

    2. Mania

    3. Anxiety

        4. Anorexia

        5. Amphetamine intoxication

        6. Control of vomiting

    E. Representative drugs

        1. Chlorpromazine (Thorazine)

        2. Promazine (Sparine)

        3. Triflupromazine (Vesprin)

        4. Prochlorperazine (Compazine)

        5. Haloperidol (Haldol)

XX. Diuretics and Antihypertensive Agents

    A. Action: Increase rate of urine formation.

    B. Effects

        1. Most increase Na^+ excretion.

        2. Most cause an increased loss of K^+.

        3. Most are not affected by acid-base imbalances.

        4. Most can be administered in tablet form.

    C. Therapeutic uses

        1. Pulmonary edema

        2. Congestive heart failure

        3. Chronic or acute renal failure

        4. Systemic fluid overload

    D. Types

        1. Osmotic diuretics

           a. Mechanism of action

              (1) Cause osmotic gradient in urine tubular system, preventing reabsorption of fluid into bloodstream.

              (2) Cause osmotic movement of fluid from tissues into plasma.

           b. Characteristics

              (1) Filterable at the glomerulus

              (2) Poorly reabsorbed by the renal tubule

              (3) Pharmacologically inert

           c. Representative drugs

              (1) Mannitol

              (2) Urea

        2. Mercurial diuretics

           a. Mechanism of action

              (1) Prevent reabsorption of Na^+ and Cl^- in proximal convoluted tubule, thereby decreasing the volume of water reabsorbed.

              (2) Promote loss of K^+ and H^+ in distal convoluted tubules.

           b. Characteristics

              (1) May cause metabolic alkalosis with extended use.

              (2) Are ineffective in the presence of systemic metabolic alkalosis.

              (3) Are potentiated in the presence of metabolic acidosis.

           c. Contraindications

              (1) Renal insufficiency

              (2) Acute nephritis

           d. Characteristic drugs

              (1) Mercaptomerin sodium (Thiomerin)

              (2) Meralluride (Mercuhydrin)

              (3) Mersalyl (Salyrgan)

        3. Carbonic anhydrase inhibitors

           a. Mechanism of action: Inhibit effects of carbonic anhydrase in proximal convoluted tubule, thereby increasing the amount of HCO_3^- and the volume of urine excreted.

   b. Representative drugs
      (1) Acetazolamide (Diamox)
      (2) Dichlorphenamide (Daranide)
4. Thiazides
   a. Mechanism of action: Inhibit reabsorption of 5% to 10% of Na^+ and Cl^- at distal convoluted tubules.
   b. Characteristics
      (1) Cause an excessive loss of K^+.
      (2) Not affected by acid-base imbalances.
      (3) Can be administered in tablet form.
   c. Representative drugs
      (1) Chlorothiazide (Diuril)
      (2) Hydrochlorothiazide (Hydro-Diuril)
      (3) Hydroflumethiazide (Saluron)
      (4) Methyclothiazide (Enduron)
5. Loop of Henle diuretics
   a. Mechanism of action: Inhibit reabsorption of Na^+ and Cl^-, primarily at distal and proximal convoluted tubules, thereby increasing the volume of fluid passed as urine.
   b. Characteristics
      (1) Function independently of acid-base status.
      (2) Considered the most potent of all diuretics.
   c. Side effects and hazards
      (1) Loss of K^+ due to increased excretion
      (2) Development of metabolic alkalosis
      (3) Aggravation of diabetes mellitus due to impaired glucose tolerance
   d. Representative drugs
      (1) Ethacrynic acid (Edecrin)
      (2) Furosemide (Lasix)
E. Nondiuretic antihypertensives for reducing blood pressure below the hypertensive level (150/90 mm Hg)
   1. Antiadrenergic—central: These agents lower blood pressure by stimulating alpha-2 receptors in the CNS (brain stem–vasomotor center) to inhibit sympathetic outflow.
      a. Methyldopa (Aldomet)
      b. Clonidine (Catapres)
      c. Guanabenz (Wytensin)
      d. Guanfacine (Tenex)
   2. Antiadrenergic—peripheral: This group of drugs interferes with sympathetic activity at the neuroeffector, or terminal, junction.
      a. Reserpine (Serpasil)
      b. Guanethidine (Ismelin)
      c. Guanadrel (Hylorel)
      d. Prazosin (Minipress)
      e. Terazosin (Hytrin)
   3. β-Adrenergic blockade: These agents block beta-1 (cardiac) receptor sites to lower cardiac output and hence, blood pressure.
      a. Metoprolol (Lopressor)
      b. Atenolol (Tenormin)
      c. Acebutolol (Sectral)
      d. Nadolol (Corgard)
      e. Pindolol (Visken)

       f. Timolol (Blocadren)

       g. Propranolol (Inderal)

   4. α- and β-Adrenergic blockade: The combined action of alpha and beta block-ade inhibits alpha-mediated vasoconstriction and beta-1-induced cardiac out-put to lower blood pressure.

       a. Labetalol (Normodyne, Trandate)

   5. Vasolidation—direct-acting: These drugs vary in their action but generally stimulate receptor sites on vascular smooth muscle to cause vasodilation and to lower blood pressure.

       a. Hydralazine (Apresoline)

       b. Minoxidil (Loniten)

       c. Nitroglycerin

   6. Angiotensin-converting enzyme (ACE) inhibition: These agents inhibit the enzyme peptidyl dipeptidase, which is needed to convert angiotensin I to an-giotensin II. Angiotensin II is the active form that causes vasoconstriction and raises the body's blood pressure.

       a. Captopril (Capoten)

       b. Enalapril (Vasotec)

   7. Emergency (acute) antihypertensives: Nitroprusside and diazoxide directly dilate blood vessels by stimulating vascular receptors. Trimethaphan blocks ganglia, inhibiting sympathetic discharge, and also directly dilates peripheral blood vessels.

       a. Nitroprusside (Nipride)

       b. Diazoxide (Hyperstat)

       c. Trimethaphan (Arfonad)

   8. Miscellaneous agents

       a. Mecamylamine (Inversine) is a ganglionic blocker (similar to tri-methaphan).

       b. Pargyline is a monoamine oxidase inhibitor, which may either cause accumulation of false transmitters at the neuroeffector site or lead to norepinephrine stimulating alpha-2 receptors to inhibit sympathetic ac-tivity.

XXI. Anti-infective Agents

   • Anti-infective agents can be categorized as antibiotics, antibacterial chemicals such as sulfonamides, antifungals, antituberculosis agents, and antiviral agents, based on the type of microorganism they target.

  A. Antibiotics

   1. Penicillins

       a. Penicillin G

       b. Penicillin V

       c. Oxacillin (Prostaphlin)

       d. Cloxacillin (Tegopen)

       e. Methicillin (Staphcillin)

       f. Ampicillin (Omnipen)

       g. Amoxicillin (Polymox)

       h. Carbenicillin (Geopen)

       i. Ticarcillin (Ticar)

   2. Cephalosporins

       a. First-generation

          (1) Cefaclor (Ceclor)

          (2) Cephalexin (Keflex)

          (3) Cefadroxil (Duricef)

          (4) Cephalothin (Keflin)

            (5) Cephradine (Velosef)
            (6) Cefazolin (Ancef)
        b. Second-generation
            (1) Cefamandole (Mandol)
            (2) Cefoxitin (Mefoxin)
            (3) Cefonicid (Monocid)
        c. Third-generation
            (1) Cefoperazone (Cefobid)
            (2) Cefotaxime (Claforan)
            (3) Ceftizoxime (Cefizox)
            (4) Ceftazidime (Fortaz)
    3. Aminoglycosides
        a. Streptomycin
        b. Gentamicin (Garamycin)
        c. Tobramycin (Nebcin)
        d. Kanamycin (Kantrex)
        e. Amikacin (Amikin)
        f. Neomycin (Neosporin)
        g. Netilmicin (Netromycin)
    4. Tetracyclines
        a. Tetracycline (Achromycin)
        b. Oxytetracycline (Terramycin)
        c. Demeclocycline (Declomycin)
        d. Methacycline (Rondomycin)
        e. Doxycycline (Vibramycin)
        f. Minocycline (Minocon)
    5. Miscellaneous antibiotics
        a. Vancomycin (Vancocin)
        b. Chloramphenicol (Chloromycetin)
        c. Erythromycin (Erythrocin)
        d. Polymyxin B
        e. Polymyxin E (Colistin)
        f. Bacitracin
        g. Clindamycin (Cleocin)
        h. Lincomycin (Linococin)
        i. Metronidazole (Flagyl)
B. Antibacterial chemicals
    1. Sulfonamides
        a. Sulfisoxazole (Gantrisin)
        b. Sulfamethoxazole (Gantanol)
        c. Sulfadiozine
        d. Trimethoprim-sulfamethoxazole (TMP-SMZ, or Bactrim)
    2. Other agents
        a. Pentamidine isethionate (Pentam) (see Chapter 41)
        b. Nitrofurantoin (Furadantin)
C. Antifungal agents
    1. Amphotericin B
    2. Nystatin
    3. Griseofulvin
D. Antituberculosis agents
    1. Isoniazid (INH)
    2. Rifampin
    3. Streptomycin
    4. Ethambutol

    5. Pyrazinamide
    6. Ethionamide
    7. Cycloserine
    8. Capreomycin
  E. Antiviral agents
    1. Zidovudine, AZT (Retrovir)
    2. Ribavirin (Virazole)
    3. Amantadine (Symmetrel)
    4. Vidarabine (Vira-A)
    5. Acyclovir (Zovirax)
    6. Rimantadine (Flumadine)
    7. Ganciclovir (Cytovene)
  F. General principles of antibiotic therapy
    1. Clinical indications of infection should be present.
    2. The specific etiologic diagnosis must be formulated before antibiotic therapy is ordered.
    3. A specimen must be obtained for laboratory culture and sensitivity before therapy is begun.
    4. The most indicated antibiotic by sensitivity should be administered.
    5. The antibiotic should be correlated with the results of culture and sensitivity study.
    6. Patient must take full course of antibiotic therapy.
    7. Antibiotics, in general, are not effective against viruses.
XXII. Miscellaneous Drugs Affecting the Cardiovascular System
  A. Cardiac glycosides (digitalis)
    1. Action
      a. Exhibit a positive inotropic effect on the myocardium.
      b. Normally cause increased cardiac output.
      c. Indirectly cause increased renal blood flow and have a diuretic effect.
      d. Slow impulse conduction through the atrioventricular (AV) node and bundle of His.
      e. Exert a direct depressant effect on the sinoatrial (SA) node, causing decreased heart rate.
      f. Increase the refractory period of the AV node.
    2. Mechanism of action: Actions are mediated by vagal and extravagal means. One theory postulates that the drug may cause an increase in intracellular sodium that precipitates increased calcium mobilization. This leads to stronger myocardial contractions.
    3. Therapeutic use
      a. Used primarily in the treatment of congestive heart failure
      b. Atrial fibrillation
      c. Atrial flutter
      d. Paroxysmal atrial tachycardia
      e. Ventricular tachycardia
    4. Side effects and hazards
      a. Toxicity (therapeutic dose is one third of the lethal dose)
      b. Atrioventricular block
      c. Premature ventricular contractions
    5. Representative drugs
      a. Digitoxin (Crystodigin, Purodigin)
      b. Digoxin (Lanoxin)
      c. Lanatoside C (Cedilanid)
      d. Ouabain

   B. Quinidine
      1. Action
         a. Acts as a depressant to myocardium.
         b. Slows depolarization by increasing time necessary to reach action potential.
         c. Alters cardiac muscle permeability to sodium.
         d. Decreases velocity of electric impulse conduction throughout myocardium.
         e. Has curare-like side effect on skeletal muscle.
      2. Mechanism of action: Attaches to lipoproteins present in the myocardial cell membrane, altering cell membrane permeability to positive ions such as Na^+, K^+, and Ca^{+2}. Causes depression of conduction velocity and contractility.
      3. Therapeutic uses
         a. Primary use: Treatment of atrial arrhythmias
         b. Premature ventricular contractions
      4. Side effects and hazards
         a. Ventricular tachycardia
         b. Premature ventricular contractions
         c. Ventricular fibrillation
         d. Hypotension
         e. Asystole
         f. Atrial embolism
         g. Respiratory arrest in hypersensitive patients
      5. Representative drugs
         a. Quinidine gluconate
         b. Quinidine sulfate
   C. Procainamide (Pronestyl)
      1. Action
         a. Depresses myocardial excitability.
         b. Slows conduction in the atria, bundle of His, and ventricles.
      2. Mechanism of action: Attaches to lipoproteins present in the myocardial cell membrane, altering the cell membrane's permeability to positive ions such as Na^+, K^+, and Ca^{+2}.
      3. Effects: Causes depression of conduction velocity and contractility.
      4. Therapeutic uses
         a. Premature ventricular contractions
         b. Ventricular tachycardia
         c. Atrial fibrillation
         d. Paroxysmal atrial tachycardia
      5. Side effects and hazards
         a. Atrioventricular block
         b. Ventricular extrasystoles (possibly progressing to ventricular fibrillation)
   D. Lidocaine (Xylocaine)
      1. Action: Increases the threshold for electrical stimulation of the ventricle.
      2. Mechanism: Appears to act on myocardial tissue in the same manner as quinidine or procainamide.
      3. Therapeutic uses
         a. Cardiac arrhythmias, especially ventricular arrhythmias or those that appear after myocardial infarction
         b. Arrhythmias that may occur during cardiac surgery
      4. Side effects and hazards
         a. Hypotension
         b. Bradycardia

      c. Cardiovascular collapse and cardiac arrest

      d. Seizures

  E. Other agents stabilizing or depressing membrane excitability

    1. Phenytoin (Dilantin)

    2. Tocainide (Tonocard)

    3. Mexiletine (Mexitil)

    4. Flecainide (Tambocor)

    5. Encainide (Enkaid)

  F. Calcium–channel blocking agents

    1. Action: Decrease the inward current of the cardiac action potential.

    2. Mechanism of action: Prevent the influx of Ca^{+2} into cells (primarily myocardial and vascular smooth muscle) at specific membrane sites, thus inhibiting muscle contraction by decreasing the availability of Ca^{+2} for actinmyosin interaction.

    3. Effects

      a. Decrease myocardial contractility and metabolism.

      b. Decrease blood pressure.

      c. Decrease smooth muscle activity.

      d. General negative inotropic effect.

    4. Therapeutic uses

      a. Antiarrhythmic (paroxysmal supraventricular tachycardia, atrial flutter, atrial fibrillation)

      b. Antianginal

      c. Improve hemodynamics in cardiomyopathy

      d. Antihypertensive

    5. Side effects and hazards

      a. Headache

      b. Nausea

      c. Transient hypotension ⎫

      d. Bradycardia   ⎬ when used with beta blocker

      e. Ventricular asystole ⎭

    6. Representative drug: Verapamil (Calan, Isoptin)

  G. Agents that prolong repolarization, with an increase in action potential duration

    1. Bretylium (Bretylol)

    2. Amiodarone (Cordarone)

BIBLIOGRAPHY

Cherniack RM (ed): *Drugs for the Respiratory System.* Orlando, Fla, Grune & Stratton, 1986.

DeKornfeld TJ: *Pharmacology for Respiratory Therapy.* Sarasota, Fla, Glenn Educational Medical Services, 1976.

DiPalma JR: *Basic Pharmacology in Medicine.* New York, McGraw-Hill Book Co, 1976.

Egan DF: *Fundamentals of Respiratory Therapy*, ed 3. St Louis, CV Mosby Co, 1977.

Evaluations of Drug Interactions, ed 2. Washington, DC, American Pharmaceutical Association, 1976.

Flaum SF, Zelis R: *Calcium Blockers*, Baltimore, Urban & Schwarzenberg, 1982.

Goodman LS, Gilman A (eds): *The Pharmacological Basis of Therapeutics*, ed 7. New York, Macmillan Publishing Co, 1987.

Goth A: *Medical Pharmacology*, ed 10. St Louis, CV Mosby Co, 1983.

Lehnert BE, Schachter EN: *The Pharmacology of Respiratory Care.* St Louis, CV Mosby Co, 1980.

Leonard RG, Talbot RL: Calcium channel blocking agents. *Clin Pharmacol* 1982; 34:189.

Mathewson HS: *Pharmacology for Respiratory Therapists*, ed 2. St Louis, CV Mosby Co, 1981.

Meyers FH, Jawetz E, Goldfine A: *Review of Medical Pharmacology*, ed 6. Los Altos, Calif, Lange Medical Publications, 1984.

Product information, New York, Breon Laboratories.

Rau JL: Autonomic airway pharmacology. *Respir Care* 1977; 22:263.

Rau JL: *Respiratory Therapy Pharmacology*, ed 3. Chicago, Year Book Medical Publishers, 1989.

Year Book of Critical Care Medicine 1983. Chicago, Year Book Medical Publishers, 1983.

Young JA, Crocker D: *Principles and Practice of Respiratory Therapy*, ed 2. Chicago, Year Book Medical Publishers, 1976.

Chapter 41 _____

Microbiology

I. Classification of Microorganism by Cell Type
  A. Eukaryotic (Protista)
    1. Algae (except blue-green)
    2. Protozoa
    3. Fungi
    4. Slime molds
  B. Prokaryotic (lower Protista)
    1. Blue-green algae
    2. Bacteria
    3. Rickettsiae
    4. Mycoplasmas
  C. Viruses
    1. Nucleic acid chain (DNA or RNA)
    2. Protein coat
II. Eukaryotic Cell Structure (Fig 41-1)
  A. Surface layers
    1. Cell membrane: Complex lipoprotein structure.
    2. Cell wall: Rigid to moderately rigid polysaccharide structure.
  B. Nucleus
    1. Well-defined nucleus surrounded by nuclear membrane.
    2. Control center for cell growth and development.
      a. Contains chromosomes
      b. Contains RNA
      c. Nuclear membrane continuous with endoplasmic reticulum (ER)
  C. Cytoplasmic structures
    1. Endoplasmic reticulum: System of large sacs and smaller tubules responsible for macromolecular transport.
      a. Smooth ER (without attached ribosomes): Involved in lipid and steroid synthesis.
      b. Rough ER (with attached ribosomes): Involved in protein synthesis.
    2. Mitochondria: Responsible for production of ATP and aerobic metabolism (Krebs' cycle and electron transport chain). Seen in animal cells.
    3. Chloroplasts: Contain pigments, starches, and enzymes used in photosynthesis.

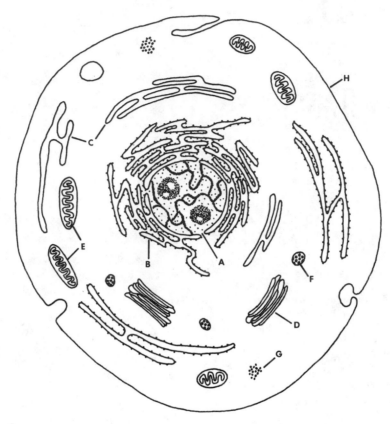

FIG 41–1.
Eukaryotic cell: **A,** nucleus; **B,** rough endoplasmic reticulum; **C,** smooth endoplasmic reticulum; **D,**
Golgi body; **E,** mitochondria; **F,** lysosome; **G,** free ribosomes; **H,** cell membrane.

            4. Ribosomes: Free or attached to endoplasmic reticulum; responsible for pro-
tein synthesis.

            5. Lysosomes: Contain proteolytic enzymes for metabolism of ingested organic
material.

       D. Motility organelles

          1. Cilia

            a. Numerous on cell exterior

            b. Move in coordinated waves

          2. Flagella

            a. Singular or present in small numbers

            b. Move in undulating motion

            c. Longer than cilia

   III. Prokaryotic Cell Structure (Fig 41–2)

       A. Surface layers

          1. Cell membrane or plasma membrane

            a. Is a lipoprotein structure.

            b. Is the inner layer beneath the cell wall.

            c. Acts as osmotic barrier and is site of some enzyme activity.

          2. Cell wall: Moderately rigid to very rigid structure

            a. Protects cell from bursting in low osmotic pressure conditions.

            b. Maintains cell shape.

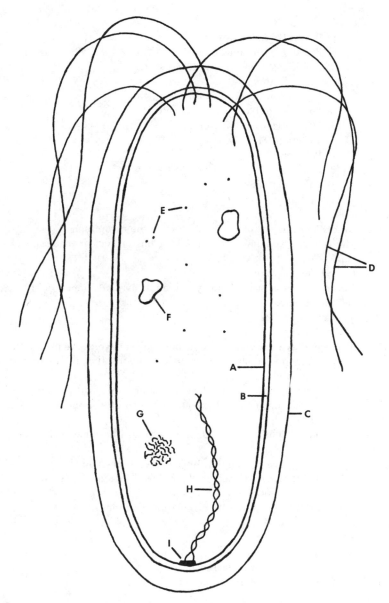

FIG 41-2.
Prokaryotic cell: **A,** cell membrane; **B,** cell wall; **C,** capsule; **D,** flagella; **E,** ribosomes; **F,** storage granule; **G,** nucleoid; **H,** DNA; **L,** mesosome.

3. Cell wall in gram-positive bacteria
   a. High lipid content
   b. Murein network: Peptide chains attached to larger polysaccharide chains
4. Cell wall in gram-negative bacteria: Three-layers
   a. The inner layer is a mucopeptide.
   b. The middle layer is lipopolysaccharide.
   c. The outer layer is a lipoprotein.
5. Capsule
   a. Layer surrounding outside of cell produced by the cell itself; common in
      pathogenic organisms.

      b. Functions
        (1) Prevents phagocytosis.
        (2) Prevents virus attachment.
        (3) Functions as external nutrient storage
      c. Causative factors
        (1) High sugar concentration
        (2) Presence of blood serum in culture
        (3) Microorganism living in a host organism
      d. Composition: Mucilaginous
        (1) Polypeptides
        (2) Dextran
        (3) Polysaccharides
        (4) Cellulose

B. Nucleus
    1. No distinct nucleus; No separation from the cytoplasm.
    2. The cell may contain one or more regions of nuclear material called *nucle-oids*.
    3. No mitotic apparatus.
    4. Chromosomes exist freely in cytoplasm; it may be circular or attached to the cell membrane.

C. Cytoplasmic structures
    1. ER is absent.
    2. Mitochondria are absent. Aerobic metabolic enzymes are present in the form of multienzyme complexes; they are attached to the cell membrane or other internal membranes.
    3. Chloroplasts are absent. Photosynthetic enzymes and pigments are present in special arrangements; these are not separated from the cytoplasm by a membrane.
    4. Ribosomes: slightly smaller than eukaryotic ribosomes; exist freely in cytoplasm.
    5. Mesosome: They are found in the cell membrane and allow for attachment of DNA in cell division. They are found chiefly in gram-positive forms.
    6. Lysosomes are absent.
    7. Cell nutrients are stored by cytoplasmic granules.

D. Motility organelles
    1. Flagella
      a. They are different from eukaryotic flagella.
      b. One or many are in each cell.
      c. They move in rotary motion.
    2. Pili
      a. They are short, fine filaments.
      b. Their function is not known; may function in specialized bacterial sexual reproduction.

E. Bacterial endospores
    1. They are the intermediate form of the organism that develops in response to adverse environmental conditions.
    2. They will regenerate to a vegetative cell when conditions improve.
    3. They are notably produced by the aerobic genus *Bacillus* and the anaerobic genus *Clostridium*, also *Sporosarcina*.
    4. They resist adverse environmental conditions of dryness, heat, and poor nutrition.
    5. A true endospore is a highly refractile body formed within the vegetative bacterial cell.

6. They function as a protective coat around nucleic material that may remain inside the cell (endospore) or extend beyond the width of the cell (exospore).
7. They are metabolically active and contain essential enzymes of Krebs' cycle.

IV. Bacterial Growth Requirements
    A. Growth medium: Needs will vary with bacteria.
        1. Simple nutrients: Water, carbon, hydrogen, nitrogen, oxygen, sulfur, phosphorus, calcium, potassium, and magnesium
        2. Complex nutrients: Sugar, amino acids, blood products
    B. Atmospheric gas requirements
        1. Obligate anaerobes reproduce only in an oxygen-free environment. Oxygen is toxic to these organisms.
        2. Aerotolerant anaerobes are organisms unaffected by exposure to oxygen.
        3. Facultative anaerobes reproduce under both aerobic or anaerobic conditions.
        4. Microaerophilic anaerobes reproduce best at low oxygen tensions. High oxygen tensions are inhibitory.
        5. Obligate aerobes require oxygen for reproduction.
        6. Chemolithotrophic and photolithotrophic bacteria use carbon dioxide as their principal source of carbon.
    C. Temperature requirements
        1. Psychrophilic: $-5°C$ to $30°C$ (optimum $10°C-20°C$)
        2. Mesophilic (pathogenic): $10°C$ to $45°C$ (optimum $20°C-40°C$)
        3. Thermophilic: $25°C$ to $80°C$ (optimum $50°C-60°C$)
    D. The osmotic pressure requirement varies with each bacterial species. Most require a 0.9% saline environment.
    E. Hydrogen ion (pH variations)
        1. Pathogens: 7.2 to 7.6 (optimum range)
        2. Acidophiles: 6.5 to 7.0
        3. Neutrophiles: 7.5 to 8.0
        4. Alkalophiles: 8.4 to 9.0
    F. Moisture: Water is essential for all bacterial growth.
    G. Light
        1. Most bacteria prefer darkness.
        2. Ultraviolet and blue light are destructive to bacteria

V. Microbial Reproduction
    A. Asexual (binary fission)
        1. This is the most common form of reproduction.
        2. Two identical daughter cells result from a single parent cell.
        3. Chromosome replication is normal.
    B. Sexual (conjugation)
        1. This is present in a few bacterial species.
        2. DNA is transferred from one bacterium to another.

VI. Growth Pattern
    • A new culture of bacteria will develop similar to the growth curve seen in Fig 41-3.
    A. Lag phase: Adaptation to new environment; little reproduction.
    B. Exponential phase: Stage of rapid cell growth.
    C. Stationary phase: Equal death and growth rates.
    D. Death phase: Depletion of culture nutrients and buildup of toxic waste; death rate exceeds growth rate.

VII. Measurement of Growth
    A. Cell concentration: Expressed as the number of viable cells.
    B. Cell density: Expressed as dry weights.

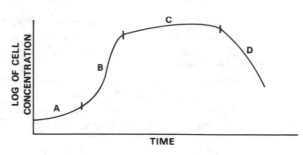

FIG 41–3.
Growth pattern of a new closed culture: **A,** lag phase; **B,** exponential phase; **C,** stationary phase; **D,** death phase.

VIII. Microbial Relationships
    A. Autotroph: An organism capable of using simple inorganic matter as nutrients (nonpathogenic).
    B. Heterotroph: An organism that requires organic matter for growth and survival (pathogenic).
    C. Symbiosis: Two dissimilar organisms existing together.
        1. Ammensalism: One organism is inhibited, and the other is not affected.
        2. Commensalism: One organism benefits, and the other is not affected.
        3. Mutualism: Each organism benefits and is unable to survive without the other.
        4. Parasitism: One organism benefits, and the other is harmed.
        5. Synnecrosis: Both organisms are harmed by the relationship.
  IX. Microbial shapes (Fig 41–4)
    A. Spherical: Coccus
    B. Rod: Bacillus
    C. Spiral: Spirillum, spirochete
    D. Comma-shaped: Vibrios
    E. Spindle-shaped: Fusiform
  X. Staining
    A. Purpose: Used to identify and categorize bacteria on the basis of cell components.

FIG 41–4.
Bacterial shapes: **A,** cocci; **B,** bacilli; **C,** vibrios; **D,** spirillum, spirochette; **E,** fusiform.

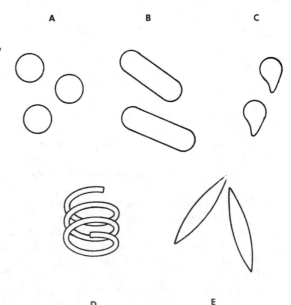

B. Gram staining
    1. Bacteria can be separated into two general categories by virtue of their staining properties: gram-positive or gram-negative.
    2. Variation in staining is determined by cell wall construction.
    3. Staining sequence
        a. Basic dye is crystal violet (all organisms take up this dye).
        b. The specimen is covered with Gram's iodine.
        c. A water rinse is done.
        d. The specimen is decolorized with acetone.
        e. A water wash is done.
        f. The specimen is counterstained with red dye (usually safranin).
        g. A final water rinse is done.
    4. Gram-positive results are blue or violet.
    5. Gram-negative results are red or pink.
C. Acid-fast (Ziehl-Neelsen) stain
    1. It identifies bacteria of the genus *Mycobacterium*.
    2. Acid-fast bacteria appear red against a blue background.
    3. Staining sequence
        a. Carbolfuchsin (red)
        b. Water rinse
        c. Destain with hydrochloric acid alcohol
        d. Counterstain with methylene blue

XI. Definitions Related to Microorganisms
    A. Contamination: Presence of a microorganism in an otherwise sterile environment.
    B. Pathogen: Any disease-producing microorganism.
    C. Virulence: Heightened ability of an organism to produce infection in its host.
    D. Aerobic: Growth only in the presence of oxygen.
    E. Anaerobic: Growth in the absence of oxygen.
    F. Toxins: Poisonous substances produced by bacteria.
        1. Exotoxin
            a. It is produced primarily by gram-positive bacteria.
            b. Composed of protein and normally excreted by bacteria into surrounding media.
            c. Some are extremely lethal.
        2. Endotoxin
            a. Produced primarily by gram-negative bacteria.
            b. Is a lipopolysaccharide and normally is released when the bacterial cell is destroyed.
    G. Vegetative cell: Metabolically active form of a bacterium in which reproduction can occur.
    H. Vector: An insect, animal or other carrier that transfers an infecting agent or pathogen from one host to another.
    I. Host: An organism that harbors or furnishes nutrition to a dissimilar organism.
    J. Bacteremia: The presence of bacteria in the blood.
    K. Septicemia: A condition in which pathogens and their associated toxins are present in the blood.
    L. Toxemia: The presence of bacterial toxins in the blood.
    M. Pyogenic: Pus producing.
    N. Pyemia: Condition in which pus-forming bacteria have entered the bloodstream.
    O. Pyrogenic: Fever producing.

XII. Definitions Related to Immunologic Response
    A. Infection: An inflammatory process resulting from the presence and growth of a pathogenic organism.

B. Inflammation: A tissue response to injury or stress that can cause local vascular dilation, fluid exudation, and/or leukocyte accumulation at site.

C. Superinfection: Infection developed primarily in the debilitated or immunosuppressed patient previously treated with antibiotics.

D. Nosocomial infection: Hospital-acquired infection.

E. Immunity: The ability of the body to resist or overcome infection or disease.

F. Plasma cell: Cells that specialize in the production of antibodies.

G. Eosinophils: White blood cells with two to three lobed nucleus and large cytoplasmic granules.
   1. They are able to phagocytize antigen-antibody complexes.
   2. Increase in number occurs with hypersensitivity and parasitic infections.

H. Lymphocyte: White blood cells formed in the lymphatic system and by the thymus gland.
   1. Have a single nucleus with no granules.
   2. Can become plasma cells that may form antibodies.
   3. Can attract and localize macrophages to an area of infection.

I. T lymphocytes: Specialized white blood cells formed by the thymus gland.

J. Macrophage: Large mononuclear phagocytic cell.
   1. Travels to sites of infection.
   2. Can phagocytize antigens or microbes.

K. Monocyte: White blood cell (leukocyte) with a single nucleus (mononuclear) that is capable of phagocytosis.

L. Polymorphonucleated leukocyte (neutrophil): White blood cell with a multilobed nucleus capable of phagocytosis.
   1. Can migrate into tissues.
   2. Acts as a defensive mechanism against bacteria.

M. Antibody: Developed in response to antigen.
   1. Produced by lymphoid tissue in response to an antigen.
   2. Antibodies can cause invading antigens or microbes to clump, rendering them easier for ingestion by macrophages and granulocytes.
   3. Can cause lysis of some microbial cells.

N. Antigen: A substance, often a protein, which gains access to the bloodstream or a body tissue.
   1. It stimulates or induces antibody formation.
   2. Certain antigens cause specific lymphocytes to gather at the site of an infection.

O. Immunoglobulins: Circulating antibodies.
   1. IgA: A surface immunoglobulin found on mucous membranes of the gastrointestinal tract and upper respiratory tract.
   2. IgE: Involved with allergic responses
   3. IgG: Most abundant of the immunoglobulins; serves to activate the complement system.
   4. IgM: Helps agglutinate antigenic matter.

XIII. Notable Gram-Positive Pathogenic Bacteria (Table 41–1)

A. *Bacillus:* Genus characteristics
   1. Is rod shaped, is arranged in chains, and is spore forming.
   2. Is gram-positive and aerobic.
   3. Secretes exotoxin.

B. Specific organisms
   1. *Bacillus anthracis*
      a. Causes skin infections, septicemia, enteritis, meningitis, anthrax, and pneumonia (Woolsorters' disease).
      b. Found in soil.

TABLE 41–1.
Commonly Encountered Bacterial Genera

Genera	Gram Stain	Shape/Configuration	Aerobic/Anaerobic	Species	Antibiotic Susceptibility
Bacillus	Positive	Rod, chain	Aerobic	*B. anthracis*	Penicillin
Bordetella	Negative	Rod	Aerobic	*B. pertussis*	Erythromycin
					Ampicillin
Clostridium	Positive	Rod, separate, chain, pairs, palisade	Anaerobic	*C. tetani, C. botulinum, C. perfringens*	Penicillin
Corynebacterium	Positive	Rod, palisade	Aerobic	*C. diphtheriae*	Penicillin
					Erythromycin
Diplococcus	Positive	Coccus, encapsulated pairs	Aerobic	*D. pneumoniae*	Penicillin
Staphylococcus	Positive	Coccus, clusters	Aerobic	*S. aureus*	Penicillin
					Tetracycline
Streptococcus	Positive	Coccus, chain	Aerobic	Groups A, B, C, & D	Penicillin
Mycobacterium	Positive	Rod, separate or "ccrds"	Aerobic	*M. tuberculosis, M. leprae*	Isoniazid
					Rifampin
					Ethambutol
					Streptomycin
Neisseria	Positive	Coccus, pairs	Aerobic	*N. meningitidis*	Penicillin
Proteus	Negative	Rod, seperate	Aerobic	*N. mirabilis, N. vulgaris*	Penicillin
					Ampicillin
					Gentamicin
					Streptomycin
Pseudomonas	Negative	Rod, separate	Aerobic	*P. aeruginosa*	Carbenicillin
					Gentamicin
					Polymyxins
					Chloramphenicol
Serratia	Negative	Rod, separate	Aerobic	*S. marcescens*	Gentamicin
Escherichia	Negative	Rod, separate	Aerobic, facultatively anaerobic	*E. coli*	Gentamicin
					Sulfonamides
					Cephalosporin
Klebsiella	Negative	Rod, separate	Aerobic	*K. pneumoniae*	Gentamicin
Haemophilus	Negative	Rod, separate	Aerobic	*H. influenzae, H. haemolyticus, H. parainfluenzae*	Ampicillin
					Chloramphenicol
Salmonella	Negative	Rod, separate	Aerobic, facultatively anaerobic	*S. typhi, S. enteritidis*	Ampicillin
					Chloramphenicol

     c. Transmitted via injured skin or inhalation.

     d. Treatment: Penicillin.

2. *Clostridium:* Genus characteristics

     a. Is a gram-positive anaerobe.

     b. Is rod shaped and is found singly, in pairs, in parallel groups (palisade), or in short chains.

     c. Is spore forming.

     d. Secretes exotoxins.

3. *Clostridium botulinum*

     a. It causes botulism—toxic food poisoning (a flaccid paralysis).

     b. The exotoxin prevents the transmission of acetylcholine at the neuromuscular junction.

     c. It is found in soil, feces, and poorly canned or preserved food.

     d. It is transmitted via ingestion of infected food or through puncture wounds.

     e. Treatment

        (1) Antitoxins

        (2) Guanidine HCl

        (3) Ventilatory support if there is respiratory failure

4. *Clostridium perfringens*

     a. Causes gas gangrene.

     b. Found in normal intestinal flora, animal feces, and soil.

     c. Transmitted via deep wounds.

     d. Treatment

        (1) Antitoxins

        (2) Surgical debridement of wound

        (3) Penicillin

        (4) Hyperbaric wound treatment

5. *Clostridium tetani*

     a. Produces tetanus—rigid descending paralysis.

     b. Found in soil and feces.

     c. Transmitted via deep wounds.

     d. Treatment

        (1) Antitoxins

        (2) Surgical debridement

        (3) Penicillin

        (4) Respiratory care

            (a) Airway management

            (b) Paralyzing agents

            (c) Sedatives

            (d) Respiratory support

C. *Streptococcus:* Genus characteristics

  1. Is a gram-positive aerobe.

  2. Is a coccus, arranged in chains.

  3. May produce capsules.

  4. Classification

     a. Group A, β-hemolytic streptococci: Septicemia tonsillitis, scarlet fever, pneumonia, nasopharyngitis, middle ear infections, rheumatic fever, endocarditis, glomerulonephritis.

     b. Group B, β-hemolytic streptococci: Female genital tract infections; possibly endocarditis, meningitis, neonatal sepsis.

     c. Group C, β-hemolytic streptococci erysipelas: throat infections and opportunistic infections.

        d. Group D, β-hemolytic streptococci: Urinary tract infections and endocarditis.

        e. Found commonly in humans, animals, and plants.

        f. Transmitted by contact with other individuals.

        g. Treatment: Penicillin.

    5. Specific organisms

        a. *Streptococcus pneumoniae* (also called *Diplococcus pneumoniae*)

           (1) Commonly found in nasopharynx.

           (2) Can cause empyema, septicemia, meningitis, and peritonitis.

           (3) Causes lobar pneumonia (most common out-of-hospital pneumonia).

           (4) Treatment: penicillin.

        b. *Streptococcus pyogenes*

           (1) Commonly found in the gastrointestinal tract and mouth.

           (2) Causes endocarditis, bronchopneumonia, urinary tract infections, glomerulonephritis, skin lesions, and septic sore throat.

           (3) Treatment: Penicillin.

D. *Staphylococcus:* Genus characteristics

    1. It is gram-positive, aerobic, and facultatively anaerobic.

    2. It is a coccus arranged in irregular (grapelike) clusters.

    3. It produces an exotoxin and enterotoxin.

    4. Specific organisms

        a. *Staphylococcus aureus*

           (1) Causes pimples, abscesses, or boils.

           (2) Can cause pneumonia, empyema, and wound infections.

           (3) Can cause nonfatal food poisoning.

           (4) Found as normal flora of skin, respiratory tract, and gastrointestinal tract (especially in hospital personnel).

           (5) Transmitted by body contact, contact with contaminated articles, and blood and lymphatic drainage from localized infections.

           (6) Treatment: Tetracycline.

E. *Corynebacterium:* Genus characteristics

    1. It is a gram-positive aerobe.

    2. It is rod shaped (often club shaped), often arranged in a palisade pattern.

    3. It secretes exotoxin.

    4. Specific organisms

        a. *Corynebacterium diphtheriae*

           (1) It is found in nasopharynx of carriers.

           (2) It causes diphtheria.

           (3) Exotoxin produces a pseudomembrane in the pharynx and larynx (results from necrosis of mucous membrane).

           (4) Treatment

               (a) Penicillin

               (b) Erythromycin

XIV. Notable gram-negative bacteria

    A. *Pseudomonas:* Genus characteristics

        1. It is a gram-negative aerobe and facultative anaerobe.

        2. It is rod shaped and found as a single organism.

        3. Specific organisms

           a. *Pseudomonas aeruginosa*

             (1) It causes up to 10% of all hospital-acquired infections.

             (2) Diseases are opportunistic.

             (3) It causes pneumonia with characteristic green odiferous sputum.

    (4) It causes wound infection, urinary tract infection, empyema, meningitis, and septicemia.

    (5) It is found in soil and water, and can be cultured from nebulizers.

    (6) It is also found in the gastrointestinal tract and on the skin.

    (7) Treatment

      (a) Carbenicillin

      (b) Gentamicin

      (c) Polymyxins

      (d) Chloramphenicol

B. *Serratia:* Genus characteristics

  1. Gram-negative, aerobe

  2. Rod shaped

  3. Specific organisms

    a. *Serratia marcescens*

    (1) Causes empyema, septicemia, and wound infections and is responsible for some hospital epidemics.

    (2) Is widely distributed in nature.

    (3) Treatment: Gentamicin.

C. *Escherichia:* Genus characteristics

  1. Gram-negative, aerobe, and facultative anaerobe

  2. Rod shaped, found as a single organism

  3. Specific organisms

    a. *Escherichia coli*

    (1) Is found as normal flora of the gastrointestinal tract.

    (2) Is responsible for about 45% of all nosocomial infections.

    (3) Causes necrotizing pneumonia, septicemia, endocarditis, meningitis, wound infections, and urinary tract infections.

    (4) Is transmitted by person-to-person contact.

    (5) Treatment

      (a) Gentamicin

      (b) Sulfonamides

      (c) Cephalosporin

D. *Klebsiella:* Genus characteristics

  1. Gram-negative, aerobe and facultative anaerobe.

  2. Short rod found as a single organism.

  3. Produces capsules.

  4. Specific organisms

    a. *Klebsiella pneumoniae* (Friedländer's bacillus)

    (1) Found as normal flora in the nose, mouth, and intestines.

    (2) Causes necrotizing pneumonia with characteristic "red currant jelly" sputum.

    (3) Causes lung abscesses, endocarditis, and septicemia.

    (4) Treatment: Gentamicin.

E. *Haemophilus:* Genus characteristics

  1. Gram-negative aerobe and facultative anaerobe

  2. Minute rod found as a single organism

  3. Specific organisms

    a. *Haemophilus influenzae* (Pfeiffer's bacillus)

    (1) Found as normal flora in the upper respiratory tract.

    (2) Most common cause of epiglottitis in children.

    (3) Causes meningitis, laryngitis, croup, and subacute bacterial endocarditis.

          (4) Treatment
            (a) Chloramphenicol
            (b) Ampicillin
      b. *Haemophilus haemolyticus*
          (1) Found as normal flora in the upper respiratory tract.
          (2) Causes pharyngitis.
          (3) Treatment
            (a) Chloramphenicol
            (b) Ampicillin
      c. *Haemophilus parainfluenzae*
          (1) Found as normal flora in the upper respiratory tract.
          (2) Causes bacterial endocarditis.
          (3) Treatment
            (a) Chloramphenicol
            (b) Ampicillin

F. *Salmonella:* Genus characteristics
   1. Is gram-negative, aerobe and facultative anaerobe.
   2. Is rod shaped, found as single organism.
   3. Forms exotoxin.
   4. Is resistant to freezing.
   5. Specific organisms
      a. *Salmonella typhi*
          (1) Found in sewage.
          (2) Causes typhus.
          (3) Transmitted through contaminated water and, less frequently, contaminated food.
          (4) Treatment
            (a) Chloramphenicol
            (b) Ampicillin
      b. *Salmonella enteritidis*
          (1) Found in animals, particularly shellfish, swine, and fowl.
          (2) Causes enteritis that may progress to meningitis, encephalitis or nephritis.
          (3) Transmitted orally via contaminated milk, turtles, eggs, undercooked chicken, fish, clams, and pork.
          (4) Treatment
            (a) Chloramphenicol
            (b) Ampicillin
            (c) Strict liquid diet

G. *Bordetella:* Genus characteristics
   1. Gram-negative
   2. Minute, nonmotile coccobacilli
   3. Specific organisms
      a. *Bordetella pertussis*
          (1) Hemolytic bacillus responsible for whooping cough
          (2) Infection transmitted via the respiratory tract
          (3) Treatment
            (a) Erythromycin
            (b) Ampicillin

H. *Neisseria:* Genus characteristics
   1. It is a gram-negative aerobe.
   2. Coccus is found as diplococci with their adjacent sides flattened.

3. Specific organisms
    a. *Neisseria meningitidis*
        (1) Causes meningococcal meningitis, bacteremia and pneumonia.
        (2) Is the normal flora of nasopharynx.
        (3) Is transmitted via lymph canal in predisposed individuals; the method of transmission of virulent strains is still unknown.
        (4) Treatment: Penicillin.

I. *Proteus:* Genus characteristics
   1. Gram-negative aerobe and facultative anaerobe.
   2. Rod shaped, found as a single organism.
   3. Specific organisms
      a. *Proteus mirablis* and *Proteus vulgaris*
         (1) It is found as normal fecal flora.
         (2) It causes chronic urinary tract infections, pneumonia, gastroenteritis, and bacteremia.
         (3) Transmission is by contact. Diseases are usually opportunistic.
         (4) Treatment
            (a) Gentamicin
            (b) Penicillin
            (c) Ampicillin
            (d) Streptomycin

XV. *Mycobacterium:* Genus characteristics
  A. It consists of acid-fast, gram-positive, aerobic rods.
  B. Inert forms are found singly; virulent strains are found in "cords"—two chains in a side-by-side parallel arrangement.
  C. Specific organisms
    1. *Myobacterium tuberculosis*
      a. It is very slow growing, requiring 3 to 6 weeks for culturing.
      b. Reaction time in newly infected individuals requires 3 to 6 weeks for a positive skin test result.
      c. It causes pulmonary tuberculosis, spinal tuberculosis, and miliary tuberculosis.
      d. Diagnosis is based on positive culture and identification of organism in sputum.
      e. It is transmitted through inhalation of droplet nuclei.
      f. Confirmation of exposure to the organism is based on a positive skin test reaction.
      g. It causes a necrotizing lesion with caseating center.
      h. Cavitation can result.
      i. Treatment is long-term therapy (18–24 months) with a combination of various agents.
      j. Effective agents
         (1) Isoniazid (INH)
         (2) Ethambutol
         (3) Rifampin
         (4) Streptomycin
         (5) Paraaminosalicylic acid.
    2. *Mycobacterium leprae* (Hansen's bacillus)
      a. It causes leprosy. It is a true parasite found in the host.
      b. Transmission is via intimate contact.
      c. It cannot be cultured on artificial media.
      d. Treatment
         (1) Isoniazid (INH)

(2) Ethambutol

(3) Rifampin

(4) Streptomycin

3. *Mycobacterium kansasii, Mycobacterium intracellulare,* and *Mycobacterium avium*

a. It causes chronic pulmonary disease.

b. It causes disseminated disease in immunocompromised individuals.

4. *Mycobacterium marium* and *Mycobacterium ulcerans:* Cause skin infections.

5. *Mycobacterium bovis*

a. Ingested in contaminated milk.

b. Causes lymphatic intestinal disease in children.

XVI. Legionellaceae

A. Family characteristics

1. It is gram-negative (difficult to stain).

2. It is motile and rod shaped.

3. It can be visualized in tissue by the Dieterle silver impregnation stain.

4. It can be visualized directly by fluorescent antibody methods.

5. Agar: Charcoal yeast extract agar buffered with N-(2-acetamido)-2-aminoethanesulfonic acid.

6. It is slow growing, 3 to 5-day incubation wih 2- to 6-hour generation.

7. Optimum temperature is 37°C.

8. It uses amino acids as the major energy source.

9. It may survive as long as 139 days at room temperature in distilled water.

10. It can survive longer than 1 year in tap water.

11. Growth can occur in tap water.

12. It is found in air-conditioning cooling towers and evaporative condensers.

13. There are approximately 21 different species in this family.

B. Specific organisms

a. *Legionella pneumophila*

(1) It is found in lakes, cooling towers, and water supplies of hospitals and hotels.

(2) It is found to cause 10% to 30% of hospital-acquired pneumonias.

(3) It causes epidemic pneumonia, sporadic pneumonia, and a mild upper respiratory illness called "Pontiac fever."

(4) It is spread by airborne water sources, such as showers, whirlpools, and nebulizers.

(5) Symptoms of Pontiac fever include fever, chills, headache, and myalgias. It is self-limiting.

(6) Legionnaire's disease varies from mild pneumonia to adult respiratory distress syndrome.

a. Incubation is 2 to 10 days.

b. There is rapid onset of high fever, nonproductive cough, chills, headache, myalgias, and diarrhea.

c. A productive cough follows in 3 to 4 days, with patchy or segmental alveolar infiltrates usually in one lobe.

d. It may be accompanied by pleural effusion, empyema, pneumothorax, hyponatremia, and respiratory failure.

b. *Legionella pneumophila* is a facultative intracellular parasite.

(1) After phagocytosis by neutrophils and pulmonary macrophage, it survives and grows intracellularly.

(2) It can lead to cell death and lysis and release of host cellular enzymes and other factors that may lead to lung tissue damage.

   c. Diagnosis
      (1) Direct demonstration of the organism in a clinical specimen.
      (2) Culture.
      (3) Detection of specific antibodies.
   d. Treatment
      (1) Erythromycin
      (2) Also sensitive to rifampin
XVII. *Mycoplasma*
   A. Structure
      1. Surface layer
         a. Three-layer membrane.
         b. No cell wall.
      2. Nucleus
         a. No distinct nucleus.
         b. Circular DNA.
      3. Cytoplasmic structures
         a. Ribosomes: Randomly distributed; occasionally seen in helical formation.
         b. Granules: Contain various enzymes.
      4. Motility organelles: None present.
   B. Genus characteristics
      1. Gram-negative.
      2. Highly pleomorphic, aerobic.
      3. Present as singular organisms.
   C. Species
      1. *Mycoplasma hominis*
         a. Diseases
            (1) Pharyngitis
            (2) Tonsillitis
            (3) Pelvic inflammatory disease
         b. Found as normal flora in the upper respiratory and genitourinary tracts.
         c. Transmitted via person-to-person contact.
         d. Treatment
            (1) Tetracycline.
            (2) Erythromycin.
            (3) Body may produce antibodies to the organisms.
      2. *Mycoplasma pneumoniae* (Eaton agent, primary atypical pneumonia, pleuropneumonia-like organism, PPLO)
         a. Causes a self-limiting respiratory syndrome that may have generalized symptoms or be asymptomatic.
         b. Found as normal flora of the upper respiratory tract.
         c. Transmitted via person-to-person contact.
         d. Treatment
            (1) Tetracycline
            (2) Erythromycin
XVIII. *Rickettsiae*
   A. Considered a true bacterium
      1. Contains DNA and RNA.
      2. Multiplies by binary fission.
      3. Has metabolic enzymes.
      4. Can be killed or controlled by antibiotics.
   B. Characteristics
      1. It is gram-positive and requires special straining techniques for identification.

2. It is a pleomorphic rod or coccus.
3. It occurs singly, paired, chained, or in filaments.
4. Diseases have clinical findings of fever, headaches, malaise, and rash.
   a. Typhoid fever
   b. Rocky Mountain spotted fever
   c. Q fever
   d. Trench fever
5. Normally it inhabits arthropods as an obligate intracellular parasite.
6. It is transmitted via a bite of an infected organism.
7. Treatment
   a. Para-aminobenzoic acid
   b. Chloramphenicol
   c. Tetracycline

XIX. *Chlamydia*
   A. It is a gram-negative bacteria.
   B. It is nonmotile and coccoidal.
   C. It is an obligate intracellular parasite
      1. Developmental cycle in cytoplasm
      2. Metabolically limited
   D. *Chlamydia psittaci* causes psittacosis (parrot fever).

XX. Viruses
   A. Structure
      1. Surface layers
         a. Simple virus: Protein coat.
         b. Complex virus: Protein coat with some polysaccharides and lipids present (lipoprotein membrane).
      2. Nucleus: No nucleus; single strand of DNA or RNA present.
      3. Cytoplasmic structure
         a. No organelles present.
         b. Contain no metabolic enzymes.
      4. Motility organelles: None present.
   B. Characteristics
      1. Do not stain by conventional means.
      2. Come in a variety of shapes and forms, all of which are very small (maximum diameters 0.1–0.3 mμ).
      3. Obligate intracellular parasite.
      4. Replication by diverting host metabolism to produce new viruses.
      5. No antibiotic susceptibility.
   C. Species
      1. Respiratory syncytial virus (RSV): Single most important agent causing infantile bronchiolitis and pneumonia.
      2. Influenza virus: Causes an acute respiratory tract infection characterized by chills, malaise, fever, muscular aches, prostration, cough, and sputum production.
      3. Parainfluenza virus: *Primary causes of croup in children and also may cause other upper respiratory problems.*
      4. Adenovirus: Commonly causes both upper and lower respiratory infections, pharyngitis, rhinitis, otitis, and laryngitis.
      5. Rhinovirus: Primary agent causing the common cold.
      6. Retrovirus: Primary etiologic agent of acquired immune deficiency syndrome (AIDS).
         a. It is also known as HTLV-III, lymphadenopathy-associated virus (LAV), and the human immunodeficiency virus (HIV).

b. It infects T4 lymphocytes that possess CD4 antigen (its receptor).

c. These are T cells with helper-induced function.

d. Other cells in which it can multiply are monocytes, macrophages and brain astrocytes, and microglia.

e. The HIV destroys these cells.

f. The result is severe and apparently irreversible immunodeficiency.

(1) Suppression of the immune response predisposes the infected person to opportunistic infections and malignancies.

(2) *Pneumocystic carinii:* Pneumonia, an opportunistic protozoal pneumonia in AIDS victims.

(3) Kaposi's sarcoma is an AIDS-associated cancer.

g. The HIV is only one of several viruses that cause or are related to viruses that cause AIDS in humans and monkeys.

XXI. Fungi (Yeasts and Molds)

A. These are primarily decomposers of dead and decaying matter (saprophytes).

1. Occasionally they result in a pulmonary infection or pneumonia.

a. Usually they are acquired through inhalation of the spore form.

b. Generally they are treated with amphotericin B.

2. Some parasitic fungi can derive their food directly from living plants or animals.

3. Diseases in humans are usually restricted to the skin or mucous membranes.

B. Structure

1. Single cells: Yeasts.

2. Tubular strands of single cells: More complex forms; hyphae, or series of branching filaments, that form mycelium.

a. Vegetative mycelium: Part of fungus feeding and growing in medium.

b. Aerial mycelium: Part of fungus protruding from medium.

C. Reproduction

1. Sexual sporulation

2. Asexual sporulation

D. Specific organisms

1. *Coccidioides immitis*

a. It is a saprophytic dimorphic fungus.

b. It is endemic in areas of South America and the southwestern United States.

c. It causes coccidioidomycosis, which has three clinical forms.

d. Primary pulmonary coccidioidomycosis is most common.

(1) Usually asymptomatic or mild respiratory infection.

(2) Self-limiting.

(3) Can be called valley fever or San Joaquin Valley fever.

e. Disseminated coccidioidomycosis is a multisystem infection.

(1) Involves organs other than the lungs.

(2) Is rare in non-Caucasians.

(3) Can be life threatening due to widespread organ system dysfunction.

(4) Frequently involves skin, meninges, central nervous system, or bone.

f. Chronic progressive pulmonary coccidioidomycosis

(1) It is a residual pulmonary disease that includes nodule and cavity formation in the lung or pulmonary abscess formation.

(2) Symptoms include fever, sweats, weight loss, and respiratory symptoms occurring from several months to years.

g. Treatment: Amphotericin B.

2. *Aspergillus fumigatus*
   a. It is a saprophytic mold commonly associated with decaying vegetative matter.
   b. It causes aspergillosis, which may take several forms.
   c. It may form a fungus ball in preexisting tuberculin cavities, resulting in mycetoma, or aspergilloma.
   d. It may induce an allergic aspergillosis with asthma-like symptoms, abnormal bronchograms, high serum IgE levels, and eosinophilia.
   e. It may cause an invasive granuloma of the lungs.
      (1) Enters the respiratory system.
      (2) Causes a severe pneumonia that may lead to hemorrhage, pulmonary infarction, or granulomas.
   f. It is found in immunosuppressed patients, those with leukemia, and those receiving corticosteroid therapy.
3. *Cryptococcus neoformans*
   a. This is a saprophytic yeast found commonly in pigeon droppings, fruits, vegetables, and soil.
   b. It causes cryptococcis, an infection acquired through the respiratory tract.
   c. The infection is acquired through inhalation of spore form.
   d. Usually it is a mild illness.
4. *Candida albicans*
   a. This is a normal saprophyte of the human gastrointestinal and upper respiratory tracts and female genital tract.
   b. It is found in immunosuppressed or debilitated patients and in individuals on excessive antibiotic therapy.
   c. It may cause septicemia, thrombophlebitis, endocarditis, and a lower respiratory tract infection (candidiasis).
5. *Histoplasma capsulatum*
   a. This is a yeast normally found in soil and bird excreta.
   b. It is especially common in the east-central and eastern United States (Ohio and Mississippi valleys).
   c. Exposure to bat excreta in caves may also result in contamination.
   d. It is an intracellular parasite and may give miliary calcification on chest x-ray films.
   e. Infection is through inhalation. The initial disease may show flu-like symptoms.
   f. Serious systemic infections can occur and may cause death.
6. *Blastomyces dermatitidis*
   a. This is a fungus that may cause a rare pulmonary infection.
   b. It is restricted primarily to the North American continent.
   c. Generally it causes a mild, self-limiting disease, blastomycosis.
   d. Respiratory infection may cause pneumonia, pleural effusion, and lymph node enlargement.

XXII. Notable Protozoan Pathogens
   A. Protozoa are eukaryotic, nonphotosynthetic animals.
   B. Some are parasitic in humans.
   C. *Pneumocystic carinii*
      1. Generally it is accepted as a protozoan, although genetic evaluation may alter this classification.
      2. It resembles a yeastlike fungus.
      3. It is widely distributed in animals in nature but is normally not pathogenic.

4. It is rarely problematic in healthy people.
   a. In most individuals it may be dormant, with no host damage.
   b. Seventy percent of healthy subjets have humoral antibody to the organism.
   c. Subclinical infection may be widespread.
5. It is an extracellular opportunist that can cause a diffuse pneumonia.
6. Assumed mode of transmission is by inhalation.
7. It adheres to the pneumocyte cell surface during a phase of its replication.
8. In an immunocompromised host, the organism occurs in massive numbers. A reported 64% of humans with AIDS have pneumocystic infections.
9. Usually there is panlobular involvement in the lungs.
10. Clinical onset is usually abrupt, with fever, tachypnea, hypoxia, cyanosis, and asphyxia in the acute stage.
11. The alveolar septum is thickened in debilitated infants, with interstitial plasma cell and lymphocyte infiltration.
12. Definitive diagnosis is made with biopsy of the involved tissue.
13. The tissue is stained with methenamine silver nitrate, toluidine blue, and Giemsa-type stains.
14. Treatment
    a. Trimethoprim-sulfamethoxazole (TMP-SMX) by intravenous or oral route.
    b. Pentamidine isethionate by intravenous, intramuscular or aerosol (experimental) route.
    c. Trimetrexate-leucovorin (experimental drug).
D. *Plasmodium ovale*, as well as *Plasmodium malariae*, *Plasmodium falciparum*, and *Plasmodium vivax* are parasitic protozoa that cause malaria.
E. *Toxoplasma gondii* causes a rare form of protozoan lung disease, toxoplasmosis.
F. *Entamoeba histolytica* causes amoebic dysentery.

XXIII. Normal Flora
A. Skin
   1. Staphylococci
   2. Streptococci
   3. Coliform bacteria
   4. Enterococci
   5. Diphtheroids (aerobic and anaerobic)
   6. *Proteus* species
   7. *Pseudomonas* species
   8. *Bacillus* species
   9. Fungi (lipophilic)
B. Respiratory tract
   1. Staphylococci
   2. Streptococci
   3. *Klebsiella*
   4. *Neisseria* species
   5. *Haemophilus* species
   6. Diplococci (pneumococci)
   7. *Mycoplasma*
   8. *Candida albicans* and other fungi
C. Gastrointestinal tract
   1. Coliform bacteria
   2. Enterococci
   3. *Clostridium* species
   4. *Proteus* species

5. Yeasts
6. *Penicillium* species
7. Enteroviruses
8. *Pseudomonas aeruginosa*
9. Streptococci
10. Staphylococci
11. *Alcaligenes faecalis*
12. *Bacteroides* species
13. *Lactobacillus* species

BIBLIOGRAPHY

Amundson DE: Hemoptysis associated with a lower-lobe mass. *Respir Care* 1988; 33:8.

Brock TD: *Biology of Microorganisms.* Englewood Cliffs, NJ, Prentice-Hall, 1970.

Corkery KJ, et al: Aerosolized pnetamidine for treatment and prophylaxis of *Pneumocystis carinii* pneumonia: An update. *Respir care* 1988; 33:8.

DeLaat NCD: *Microbiology for the Allied Health Professions,* ed 2. Philadelphia, Lea & Febiger, 1979.

Deshpande VM, Pilbeam SP, Dixon RJ: *A Comprehensive Review in Respiratory Care.* Norwalk, Conn, Appleton & Lange, 1988.

Griggs BM, Reinhardt DT: *Fundamentals of Nosocomial Infections Associated with Respiratory Therapy.* New York, Projects in Health, 1975.

Jawetz E, Melinick JL, Adelberg EA: *Review of Medical Microbiology,* ed 12. Los Altos, Calif, Lange Medical Publications, 1976.

Joklik WK, Willett HP, Amos DB, et al (eds): *Zinsser Microbiology,* 19 ed. Norwalk, Conn, Appleton and Lange, 1988.

Mikat DM, Mikat KW: *A Clinician's Guide to Bacteria,* ed 2. Indianapolis, Eli Lilly and Co, 1975.

Novikoff AB, Holtzman E: *Cells and Organelles,* ed 2. New York, Holt, Rinehart and Winston, 1976.

Shapiro BA, Harrison RA, Trout CA: *Clinical Application of Respiratory Care.* Chicago, Year Book Medical Publishers, 1975.

Smith LA: *Principles of Microbiology,* ed 7. St Louis, CV Mosby Co, 1973.

Swanson CD, Webster DL: *The Cell,* ed 4. Englewood Cliffs, NJ, Prentice-Hall, 1977.

Walton JR, et al: *Serratia* bacteremia from mean arterial pressure monitors. *Anesthesiology* 1975; 43:113.

Chapter 42

Disinfection and Sterilization

I. Definitions Related to Disinfection and Sterilization
  A. Suffixes:
    1. -cide: When a killing action is implied.
    2. -statis or -static: When the organism is only inhibited in growth or prevented from reproducing.
  B. Bactericide (bacteriocidal): Kills or destroys bacteria.
  C. Fungicide (fungicidal): Kills or destroys fungi.
  D. Virucide (virucidal): Kills or destroys viruses.
  E. Tuberculocide (tuberculocidal): Kills or destroys *Mycobacterium tuberculosis* and related mycobacterium.
  F. Sporicidal: Killing of bacterial endospores.
  G. Germicide: Chemical agent that kills vegetative cells of microorganisms.
  H. Bacteriostatic: Inhibits or retards growth of bacteria.
  I. Antiseptic: Opposes sepsis or putrefaction either by killing microorganisms or by preventing their growth; free from living organisms.
  J. Antisepsis: Preventing the growth of bacteria or stopping bacterial activity.
  K. Medical asepsis: Killing or inhibiting of pathogenic microorganisms to prevent their transmission from one person to another.
  L. Surgical asepsis: Sterilization or decontamination of items used in the operating room.
  M. Antiseptic: Free from living microorganisms; also, an agent that destroys or inhibits the growth of microorganisms.
  N. Cleaning: The removal of all foreign matter such as sputum, blood, dirt, or organic matter from an item that might provide a favorable environment for bacterial growth; precedes sterilization.
  O. Disinfectant: Germicidal agent used on inanimate objects.
  P. Sanitizer: An agent that reduces the number of bacteria to a safer level for handling of material.
  Q. Sterilization: Complete destruction or inactivation of all forms of microorganisms.
    1. The implication of this term is absolute destruction.
    2. Sterile: Free from all living microorganisms.
  R. Disinfection: A process that eliminates vegetative, pathogenic microorganisms on inanimate objects.
  S. High-level disinfectants: Germicidal agents capable of killing all microorganisms except their spores.

T. Low-level disinfectants: Germicidal agents capable of killing some, but not all, vegetative bacteria, fungi, and lipophilic viruses.

U. Decontamination: The process of removing a contaminant by chemical or physical means.

V. Sanitization: Any process that reduces total bacterial contamination to a level consistent with safety in handling.

W. Semicritical items: Objects that come in contact with mucous membranes but that do not enter tissue or the vascular system.

X. Noncritical items: Objects that do not come in contact with mucous membranes or skin that is not intact.

II. Dynamics of Disinfection and Sterilization

  A. Selection of the procedure is determined by the situation.

    1. Items used for surgery, intravascularly, or within tissues must be sterile.

    2. Media and glassware for the microbiology laboratory must be sterile.

    3. Items not in contact with mucous membranes or that touch only intact skin need only be disinfected.

  B. Death rate of microorganism

    1. Criterion of death is the irreversible loss of the ability to reproduce.

    2. Exposure of a bacterial population to a lethal agent results in a time interval in which there is a progressive reduction in the number of survivors.

      a. This reduction may be logarithmic with time when the sterilizing agent is strong.

      b. This reduction may be sigmoidal, the rate being slower at the beginning, if the agent is less potent.

    3. The larger the initial number of cells to be killed, the longer and more intense the required treatment for sterilization.

    4. The rate of disinfection is related to the concentration of the disinfecting agent.

  C. Factors affecting the potency of disinfectants

    1. Concentration and type of agent and organism involved.

    2. Amount of exposure time.

    3. Hydrogen ion concentration, which affects bactericidal action.

      a. pH changes may affect both the organism and the bacterial agent.

      b. The pH determines the degree of ionization of the agent, which can alter its level of activity and ability to penetrate the cell membrane.

      c. Generally, nonionized agents pass through cell membrane more quickly.

  D. Temperature

    1. Killing action increases with temperature.

    2. At low temperatures, a 10°C increase doubles the death rate.

  E. Nature of the organism

    1. Species and presence of special structures such as capsules or spores

    2. Growth phase of culture and previous history

    3. The number of organisms present

  F. Presence of extraneous material such as organic or foreign matter

III. Mechanisms of Action of Various Agents

  A. Agents that damage the cell membrane

    1. Surface-acting disinfectants reduce surface tension.

      a. These are notably the cationic and anionic agents.

      b. Cationic agents are the quarternary ammonium compounds such as benzalkonium chloride (Zephiran), cetyldimethylbenzl ammonium chloride (Triton K-12), and cetylpyridinium chloride (Ceepryn).

      c. Anionic detergents are soaps and fatty acids such as (Duponol LS) and Triton W-30.

      d. Used together, anionic and cationic agents neutralize each other.

2. Phenol compounds cause leakage of cell contents and irreversibly inactivate membrane-bound oxidases and dehydrogenases.
   a. Phenol is the parent compound (carbolic acid) but is fairly caustic and toxic.
   b. Cresols are alkyl phenols (e.g., Lysol and Creolin).
   c. Diphenyl compounds are halogenated diphenyls (e.g., hexachlorophene, which can be mixed with soap).
3. Alcohols disorganize the lipid structure of cell membranes.
   a. They also denature cellular proteins.
   b. Ethanol and isopropyl alcohol are examples.
B. Agents that denature proteins
   1. They cause unfolding of peptide chains.
   2. Examples are alcohols, acids, alkalies, acetone, and other organic solvents.
C. Agents that affect functional protein groups and nucleic acids
   1. They inhibit enzyme activity and inactivate functional groups of walls, membranes, and nucleic acids.
   2. Mercury or arsenic compounds combine with the sulfhydryl (SH) group of proteins and inactivate them.
   3. Heavy metals such as mercurial compounds and silver compounds poison enzyme activity.
   4. Oxidizing agents such as peroxide, iodine, and chlorine compounds inactivate enzymes by converting functional SH groups to the oxidized S-S form.
   5. Some coal-tar dyes are inhibitory in high dilutions.
   6. Alkylating agents, such as formaldehyde, ethylene oxide, and glutaraldehyde alkylate proteins, resulting in inhibition of enzyme activity.

IV. Preparation for Sterilization
   A. Equipment must be washed clean of all organic matter.
      1. An alkaline soap is used to prevent formation of curds on the equipment.
      2. Small items are hand washed with a brush.
      3. Ultrasonic washers may be used for large items.
   B. Rinsing should be complete.
   C. Equipment is air dried.
   D. Items should be packaged appropriately for the sterilization process.

V. Sterilization and Disinfection by Temperature Change
   A. Many, but not all, bacteria are killed by exposure to freezing.
      1. This process disinfects but does not sterilize.
      2. Repeated freezing and thawing are more effective.
      3. Formation of ice crystals outside the cell causes the withdrawal of water from the cell, increasing the electrolyte concentration, and denatures proteins.
      4. The cell membrane is damaged, and intracellular organic compounds leak out.
      5. When the cell is frozen rapidly to less than $-35°C$, ice crystals form inside, producing a lethal effect during thawing.
      6. Freeze-drying, however, is a method of preserving bacterial cultures.
   B. Heat is the most reliable and universally applied method of sterilization.
      1. The time required is inversely related to temperature.
      2. Heat causes denaturation of proteins and coagulation.
      3. The efficiency of heat sterilization is determined by the heat capacity of the gas involved in the sterilization process.
      4. The heat capacity of water at any temperature significantly exceeds the heat capacity of air.
      5. Steam has a heat capacity many times greater than that of water at the same temperature due to the latent heat of vaporization of water molecules.
      6. The heat capacity of steam increases logarithmically with increasing pressure.

    7. Order of efficiency of sterilization and disinfection by heat:
        a. Steam under pressure (autoclave)
        b. Steam at atmospheric pressure
        c. Boiling water
        d. Dry heat under pressure
        e. Dry heat at atmospheric pressure
        f. Water below its boiling point (pasteurization)

C. Autoclaving
    1. Steam and pressure are used to produce the most efficient method of sterilization.
    2. Sterilization occurs as a result of heat transfer from the condensation and evaporation of steam on the surface of the substance being sterilized.
    3. Equipment is packaged in material that allows steam to enter but prevents microorganisms from entering.
        a. Muslin
        b. Linen cloth
        c. Kraft paper
        d. Nylon
        e. Brown paper
        f. Crepe paper
        g. Vegetable parchment
    4. Variables involved in proper autoclaving
        a. Temperature
        b. Pressure
        c. Concentration of steam
    5. Holding time is the minimum amount of time necessary to kill spores at a specific pressure.
    6. The actual sterilization time is one and one-half times the holding time.
    7. Examples of autoclaving cycles
        a. 121°C at 15 pounds per square inch (psi) for 15 min
        b. 126°C at 20 psi for 10 min
        c. 134°C at 29.4 psi for 3 min
    8. Heat-sensitive indicators are applied to all equipment to be autoclaved.
        a. These indicate that the equipment has been exposed to conditions necessary for sterilization.
        b. They do not indicate sterilization.
    9. Biologic indicators are used to ensure that actual sterilization has been accomplished.
        a. *Bacillus stearothemophilus* spores are normally used because of their high heat resistance.
        b. Capsules containing 10^6 spores should be placed in at least one load each day and inspected for viable cells.
    10. Oil and grease must be removed from items before processing.
    11. Autoclaving is not effective for substances that cannot be penetrated by steam such as parafin or oil.
    12. It may melt some plastics and rubbers.
    13. It may be corrosive to some metals.

D. Dry heat
    1. Efficiency is considerably lower than steam heat.
    2. In general, dry heat should be used only on materials in which moist heat would be deleterious or unable to permeate the product being sterilized.
    3. Temperature-time relationships
        a. 170°C: 60 min
        b. 160°C: 120 min

      c. 150°C: 150 min

      d. 140°C: 180 min

      e. 121°C: Overnight

    4. Dry heat is limited primarily to the sterilization of glassware, and materials such as oils, powders, jellies, glass, dressings, and cutting instruments that cannot be penetrated by steam or may be damaged by the moisture.

    5. The lethal action is the result of heat conveyed from the material with which the organisms are in contact.

    6. It is important that heating is uniform.

    7. The most widely used type is the hot air oven.

    8. Another form includes incineration of disposable objects.

  E. Tyndallization

    1. This is a fractional method of sterilization that consists of three separate heatings on three consecutive days of a liquid or semisolid to be sterilized.

    2. For the sterilization of certain liquids or semisolids that are easily destroyed by heat, this provides a fractional method of sterilization.

    3. The material is heated at 80°C to 100°C for 30 min on 3 consecutive days.

    4. The rationale is that vegetative cells and some spores are killed during the first heating. More resistant spores subsequently germinate and are killed on either the second or third heating.

    5. It is used for sterilizing heat-sensitive culture media such as serum or egg.

  F. Pasteurization

    1. Pasteurization is the submergence of equipment in medium hot water for a specified period of time.

    2. It is effective only in the destruction of vegetative cells.

    3. Equipment is immersed for 10 min in water that is 75°C.

    4. When the equipment is removed from the pasteurization unit, it must be dried and packaged.

VI. High-Energy Waves for Sterilization and Disinfection

  A. Sunlight possesses some bactericidal activity.

    1. This has a disinfectant action due to ultraviolet (UV) rays.

    2. Most rays are screened by glass or ozone in atmosphere.

    3. Ultraviolet light is absorbed by bacteria and damages DNA.

    4. This effect is reversible if cells are immediately irradiated with visible light (photoreactivation).

    5. Mercury vapor lamps produce UV radiation.

    6. It is used primarily in control of airborne infection for disinfection of enclosed areas such as operating rooms.

  B. Ionizing radiation

    1. It is classified as having mass and being charged or uncharged or classified as energy only.

    2. Some is produced by radioactive decay, others by x-ray machines, and others by particle bombardment.

    3. Those with most practical value are the electromagnetic, x-rays and gamma rays, and the particulate cathode rays.

    4. Penetrating power contributes to their effectiveness.

    5. Ionizing rays collide with orbiting electrons, causing electron ejection. As the ejected electrons move through a medium, the electrons ionize, exciting other atoms.

    6. This causes ionization of water molecules, which form free hydroxl and hydrogen ions. These then react with DNA molecules, causing lysis.

    7. Spores are the most radiation-resistant microorganism known.

    C. Gamma irradiation
       1. Gamma waves are very short wavelength light waves possessing extremely high energy and having the ability to ionize a substance.
       2. Ionization of water molecules inactivate DNA molecules by increasing the rate of reaction of DNA with hydrogen and hydroxyl ions.
       3. Advantages
          a. They are high efficiency.
          b. Temperature change is negligible.
          c. Equipment may be prepackaged and sealed.
       4. Disadvantages
          a. Sterilization time is prolonged 48 to 72 hours.
          b. Polyvinyl chloride (PVC) may release chlorine gas.
          c. It is feasible on only a large-scale industrial level.
  D. Ultrasonic and sonic vibrations
       1. Sound vibrations in the ultrasonic range (20–1,000 kc/sec) are useful in disrupting cells.
       2. Passage of sound through a liquid causes alternating pressure changes.
       3. If of sufficient pressure, these cause cavity formation.
       4. Cavities are about 10 μ in diameter.
       5. These grow in size until they collapse violently.
       6. This causes high local velocities and pressures of the order of 1,000 atm.
       7. During this abrupt collapse, the cell disintegrates, and chemical and physical changes occur in the suspending medium.
          a. Hydrogen peroxide is formed when the liquid contains oxygen.
          b. It can also cause depolymerization of the macromolecules.
       8. Most susceptible are gram-negative rods.
       9. Staphylococci are most resistant.
      10. Consequently, this technique is not practical for disinfection or sterilization.
      11. It is used primarily for decontamination.
VII. Filtration
  A. Filtration is used in laboratories for disinfection of heat-sensitive materials such as serum, plasma, and trypsin.
  B. Most popular are the membrane filters made of porous discs of biologically inert cellulose esters.
  C. Available membrane pore size is 0.023 to 14 μ.
  D. Most popular is 0.22 μ since this is adequate for filtration of bacteria.
  E. Filtration cannot screen out viruses.
  F. High-efficiency particulate air filters can be used in laminar flow rooms and hoods in hospitals and laboratories.
  G. Membrane filters are used on most respiratory therapy equipment.
       1. They are composed of thin sheets of cellulose esters or other polymeric material folded many times to ensure a large surface area.
       2. Most may be autoclaved for reuse; however, some are disposable.
       3. They can be used as main-flow bacterial filters and nebulizer line filters on mechanical ventilators.
VIII. Glutaraldehydes
  A. These are a widely used disinfectant and sterilizing agent for surgical instruments and respiratory therapy equipment.
  B. They are a form of cold, liquid disinfectant that kills by the binding to SH or amino groups of proteins in microorganisms, interrupting metabolism and reproduction.
  C. Effectiveness is not diminished by protein-containing materials.

D. They are most commonly used in respiratory care for disinfection of noncritical items.

E. Material must be washed and all foreign matter removed before soaking in this liquid to expose all surfaces.

F. All surfaces must be in contact with the agent for it to be effective.

G. A variety of glutaraldehydes are available on the market.

H. In general, they are bactericidal, tuberculocidal, fungicidal, and virucidal in 10 to 30 min and sporicidal in about 10 hours.

I. Shelf life varies from about 2 to 4 weeks.

J. Glutaraldehyes in general are irritating to skin, mucous membranes, and eyes, are damaging to some rubbers and plastics, and are corrosive to carbon steel instruments.

K. Items must be rinsed thoroughly after use, dried, and packaged in a sterile or clean manner.

L. Cidex and Cidex 7 are 2% glutaraldehyde solutions.
   1. pH: 7.5 to 8.5.
   2. Shelf life: Cidex, 14 days for manual systems; Cidex 7, 28 days for manual systems and 14 days for machines (Cidomatic).
   3. Germicidal times 10 to 30 min and sporicidal time is 10 hours at room temperature.
   4. They are mixed with a buffer prior to use.
   5. Sodium nitrate is added as corrosion inhibitor.
   6. They cannot be used with heat or an ultrasonic device. Both cause rapid polymerization of the active di-aldehyde monomer.
   7. They are corrosive to carbon steel.

M. Cidex Plus
   1. pH: 7.5 to 7.8.
   2. This is 3.2% glutaraldehyde with odor inhibitor added.
   3. It is effective for 28 days after mixing it with the buffer.
   4. It has similar characteristics to Cidex.

N. Cidex Plus Machine
   1. It has an alkaline pH.
   2. It is 9.4% glutaraldehyde.
   3. It is good for 14 days in the machine after buffer activation.
   4. It can be heated to 30°C and will kill *M. tuberculosis* in 15 min at this temperature.
   5. It is very corrosive to some metals.

O. Other commercial brands similar to Cidex: Omnicide, Metricide, Steril-ize, Procide 28, Co-cide, Vitacide, Sporex, and Glutarex

P. Wavicide
   1. pH: 6.2 to 6.4.
   2. It is 2% glutaraldehyde.
   3. No activator is required.
   4. It sterilizes in 1 hour at 60°C, 5 hours at 40°C, and 10 hours at 20°C to 21°C.
   5. It is germicidal in 10 to 30 min depending on the dilution.
   6. It can be diluted to lower concentrations, but exposure time varies with dilution.
   7. It can be reused from 21 to 42 days, depending on the specific agent in use.
   8. It is corrosive to carbon steel.
   9. Wavicide-solution contains 0.25% glutaraldehyde and 1.5% triethylene-glycol. It kills *M. tuberculosis* in 30 min at room temperature and human immunodeficiency virus (HIV) in 1 min but is not sporicidal.

Q. Sporicide
   1. pH: 3.0 to 4.5.
   2. It is 2% glutaraldehyde.
   3. No activation ingredient is required.
   4. Germicidal time is 10 min.
   5. It sterilizes in 1 hour at 60°C and 20 hours at room temperature.
   6. It is good for 35 days in manual systems.
   7. It may be corrosive to some metals.
   8. It is limited to single use for sterilization and disinfection when *M. tuberculosis* is suspected.

R. Sporicidin
   1. pH after activation: 7.4.
   2. Active ingredients: 7.05% phenol, 2.35% sodium tetraborate, 2% glutaraldehyde, 1.2% sodium phenate.
   3. It is germicidal in about 10 min at room temperature and sterilizes in about 6¾ hours.
   4. Shelf life is 15 to 30 days.
   5. It can be diluted but cannot be heated or used in ultrasonic cleaners.

IX. Ethylene Oxide: $(CH_2)_2O$
   A. An alkylating agent extensively used in gas sterilization
   B. Characteristics of ethylene oxide (ETO)
      1. It is a gas at room temperature but liquefies readily under moderate pressure.
      2. It has a pleasant ethereal odor.
      3. It causes irritation of tissues, especially the mucous membranes.
      4. It is flammable and explosive at certain concentrations and temperatures.
      5. Normally it is used in 10% to 12% mixtures with carbon dioxide or halogenated hydrocarbons (e.g., dichlorodifluoromethane [Freon 12], which acts as a damping agent), making up the remainder of the gas mixture. These mixtures are nonflammable at temperatures up to 55°C.
   C. Mechanism of action
      1. Alkylation occurs at specific enzyme sites and interrupts normal metabolism and reproduction.
      2. Coordination of the following factors is necessary for proper sterilization:
         a. Gas concentration
         b. Humidity
         c. Temperature
         d. Time
      3. The addition of H_2O vapor increases sensitivity of both vegetative cells and spores to ETO.
      4. Sterilization proceeds most rapidly at relative humidities of 30% and slows progressively below or above that level.
      5. Other factors being equal, the effectiveness of ETO doubles for each 10°C rise in temperature up to 60°C.
      6. System pressure for carbon dioxide mixtures is between 20 and 30 psi and for hydrocarbon mixtures is between 5 and 7 psi.
      7. Typical systems
         a. Temperature of 54.4°C, relative humidity of 30% to 60%, and pressure of 5 to 7 psi with 450 mg of ETO/L of air for 6 hours results in sterilization.
         b. If the concentration of ETO is raised to 850 mg/L, sterilization occurs in 3 hours.

8. The packaging material used should be permeable to humidity and ETO but not to microorganisms.
   a. Wrapping paper
   b. Cloth
   c. Muslin
   d. Polyethylene
   e. Nylon film
9. The use of indicator tape identifies exposure to ETO but does not guarantee sterility of equipment.
10. A biologic indicator is used to ensure that conditions necessary for sterility have been achieved. Cultures of *Bacillus subtilis* var. *globigi* should be used daily.
11. Aeration time
    a. Most materials require at least a 24-hour aeration time in a well-ventilated area (aeration chambers can significantly decrease this time).
    b. Substances made of neoprene rubber or polyvinyl chloride require extended aeration times: up to 7 days, depending on thickness; because of their tendency to absorb ETO.
12. Ethylene oxide residues
    a. Substances that have been previously gamma irradiated, especially polyvinyl chloride, react with ETO to form ethylene chlorhydrin, which is very irritating to tissue.
    b. If the material to be sterilized is not dry, the water on it reacts with ETO to form ethylene glycol. (This usually results in a very sticky residue on the material.)
13. The ETO residues are mutagenic for bacteria.
14. Toxicity to humans includes mutagenicity and carcinogenicity.

X. Liquid Disinfectants
  A. Alcohol
    1. Alcohol disorganizes the lipid structure of membranes and also denatures cellular proteins.
    2. It is used extensively for skin cleaning prior to cutaneous injections and is also used for disinfection of thermometers.
    3. It is active against gram-positive, gram-negative, and acid-fast bacteria.
    4. It is only slightly irritating, leaves no residue, removes fats and lipids from skin surfaces, and is inexpensive.
    5. Alcohols are *not* sporicidal or virucidal to all viruses.
       a. Ethanol has been shown to be effective against HIV.
       b. Neither 70% ethanol nor isopropanol is effective against tubercle bacillus in sputum.
    6. Alcohol is very volatile and a powerful organic solvent that may damage rubber and plastic materials.
    7. The ethanol (ethyl alcohol) is used at 50% to 70% concentration.
    8. Isopropyl alcohol is used at 75% to 100% concentration.
    9. Toxic effects of isopropanol are greater and more long lasting than ethanol if ingested or inhaled in large quantities.
    10. Sometimes alcohol is used as part of the composition of other disinfecting agents such as Lysol spray (79% ethanol).
  B. Quaternary ammonium compounds
    1. These are surface-acting, cationic agents that cause a loss of membrane semipermeability and leakage of nitrogen and phosphorus containing compounds from the cell.
       a. Lysis of the cell follows by the action of the cell's own autolytic enzymes.
       b. The agent may then enter the cell and denature its proteins.

    2. Activity is greatest at an alkaline pH.

    3. These compounds are bactericidal for a wide range of organisms, but gram-positive species are more susceptible.

    4. Antibacterial activity is reduced by the presence of organic matter.

    5. They can be reused.

    6. Ineffective against tuberculosis bacillus spores, enteroviruses, hepatitis B, bacterial endospores, or some fungi and notably are not very pseudomonocidal.

    7. Examples: Zephiran, Triton K-12, Control III, Stan-Pac, Airwick A 33, 456, Barquat and Merquat.

C. Acetic acid

    1. Acetic acid has long been known as a preservative.

    2. It inhibits the growth of many bacteria and fungi.

    3. Antimicrobial activity is related to its acidity.

        a. Acidiotic pH prevents organisms from maintaining a normal pH balance as excessive hydrogen ions enter the cell and cannot be expelled rapidly enough.

        b. It can result in denaturation of cellular proteins.

        c. It has an indirect effect due to ionization of organic compounds in the medium that permits them to penetrate the cell more rapidly and disrupt cell metabolism.

    4. A 1.25% acetic acid solution seems to be sufficiently effective to disinfect equipment. (One part vinegar and two parts water is a 1.7% solution.)

    5. It is used extensively in the cleaning of respiratory care equipment, such as hand-held nebulizers, in the home.

    6. Effectiveness is significantly reduced if a solution is reused.

D. Formaldehyde

    1. It is an alkylating agent that results in denaturation of proteins by direct replacement of a hydrogen atom with a hydroxymethyl group on carboxyl, hydroxyl, and sulfhydryl groups of cellular proteins.

    2. It is available in 37% solutions commercially or as a solid polymer (paraformaldehyde) that is 91% to 99% formaldehyde.

    3. It is used extensively to inactivate viruses in vaccine preparation since it does not affect their antigenic properties (concentrations of 0.2%–0.4%).

    4. It is used as a gas to decontaminate rooms, buildings, fabrics, and instruments.

    5. It is used as a tissue preservative and as a component of embalming fluids.

    6. It is sporicidal with prolonged exposures (6–12 hours).

    7. It is toxic to tissues and has a pungent, penetrating, irritating odor.

E. Phenol and related compounds

    1. They cause leakage of cell contents and irreversible inactivation of membrane-bound enzymes.

    2. Cresols are simple alkyl phenols obtained industrially from the distillation of coal tar.

    3. The three primary types are orthocresol, metacresol and paracresol (usually employed as a mixture of tricresol).

    4. Examples are Lysol and Creolin, which are emulsified mixtures of cresols and green soap.

        a. Some have virucidal properties

        b. They are not sporicidal.

        c. They are used for cleaning instruments and general housekeeping.

    5. Other phenol-type compounds include Amerse (27.35% phenol), and Omni II.

        a. These are tuberculocidal at high dilutions (1:32).

        b. They do not kill spores at room temperatures.

      c. They may not be effective against all viruses.

      d. Amerse may be corrosive to some plastic, rubber, and fiberoptic instruments.

  6. Halogenated diphenyl compounds

      a. The most notable is hexachlorophene.

      b. They are effective against gram-positive bacteria, especially staphylococci, and streptococci.

      c. They are used in germicidal soaps and antiperspirants.

      d. Absorption through skin may cause neurotoxicity, especially in infants.

      e. One example is pHisoHex.

F. Iodine and related compounds

  1. These are oxidizing agents that inactivate bacterial cell enzymes.

  2. They are used primarily in skin preparations but may stain hands and fabrics.

  3. They have effective bactericidal, virucidal, and fungicidal activity.

  4. Some have sporicidal effects.

  5. Iodine tincture USP is 2% iodine and 2% sodium iodide in dilute alcohol.

  6. Iodophores are mixtures of iodine and various surface-acting agents.

      a. Examples include Wescodyne, Betadine, GSI, HI-Sine, Septodyne, Prepodyne, Povidine, and Neotec.

      b. They are effective at room temperatures against vegetative microorganisms, fungi, and lipophilic viruses.

      c. They are not effective against spores.

      d. Recent reports question tuberculocidal activity.

      e. They decompose rapidly with heat and are affected by water hardness and the presence of organic matter.

G. Chlorine and related compounds

  1. Like iodine, they are strong oxidizing agents that inactivate enzymes.

  2. In addition to chlorine compounds, the hypochlorites and the inorganic and organic chloramines are also oxidizing disinfectants.

  3. They are effective against most bacteria, viruses, and fungi.

  4. They are not sporicidal at room temperatures.

  5. They have no effect in the presence of organic matter.

  6. They are highly corrosive to metals and cannot be used with rubber.

  7. Chlorine is used to purify the water supply and is widely used in swimming pools (0.6–1.0 ppm).

  8. Hypochlorites are widely used in the food and dairy industries for sanitization.

      a. They are also employed as sanitizers in hospitals, households, and public buildings.

      b. A 0.2% solution of sodium hypochlorite has been recommended by the Pasteur Institute for use on inanimate objects for inactivation of HIV with a 10-min contact time.

  9. Commercial household bleach is usually bottled as a 5.25% hypochloride solution. (Storage reduces percentage and effectiveness.)

  10. Chlorhexidine gluconate solutions

      a. Examples are Hibitan (5%), Hibistat (0.5%), and Novalsan (2%).

      b. They are used as disinfectants for skin and inanimate surfaces.

  11. Alcide is a combination of sodium chlorite and lactic acid.

      a. It is very effective against all microorganisms at room temperature.

      b. It is effective after activation for 14 days.

      c. It may be harmful to silicon rubbers and tarnishing to stainless steel, aluminum, and copper.

      d. Examples are Exspor, Astracids, and An-Fa-Cide.

H. Hydrogen peroxide
1. This is a strong oxidizing agent similar to iodine and chlorine in bacterial activity.
2. The reaction of peroxide with iron may produce additional free hydroxide radicals that may account for part of its germicidal activity.
3. A 3% solution is used as a mild antiseptic for wound cleaning and as a disinfectant of inanimate materials.
4. It has seen increasing use in recent years as a disinfectant of medical-surgical devices and soft plastic contact lenses.
5. It is also used for cleaning tracheostomy tubes and the incision site.

I. Heavy metal compounds that affect protein and nucleic acids
1. Soluble salts of arsenic, mercury, and silver, in addition to other heavy metals, alter enzyme activity by forming mercaptides with the sulfhydryl groups of cysteine residues.
2. Mercurials
   a. Mercury chloride is very toxic and has limited commercial use, although once a popular disinfectant.
   b. Organic mercurials such as Merthiolate, Metaphen, and mercurochrome are less toxic but not reliable as skin disinfectants.
   c. Phenylmercury salts are effective against gram-positive and gram-negative (especially pseudomonas) fungi and algae. They are used in ophthalmic and cosmetic solutions and pharmaceutical preparations.
3. Silver compounds
   a. Soluble silver salts and colloidal preparations are used as antiseptics.
   b. The most common is silver nitrate with good bactericidal action against gonococci and prophylactically for ophthalmia neonatorum in newborn infants.
   c. Silver nitrate or silver sulfadiazine in cream is used topically for burn victims.

XI. Guidelines for Disinfection of Respiratory Care Equipment in the Home*
A. Contamination from person-to-person or person-to-inanimate objects should be avoided.
B. Hands should be washed frequently and properly before and after handling the patient or the patient's equipment.
C. Individuals with respiratory infections should avoid contact with patients in the home or extended care facility.
D. Respiratory care equipment should be routinely disinfected and dried thoroughly.
1. For simplicity it is recommended that respiratory care equipment such as ventilator circuits, nebulizers and related equipment be disinfected daily (every 24 hours).
2. Forty-eight hours may be adequate but daily may be more predictable for the patient and family members to comply with.
3. Equipment should then be thoroughly rinsed and allowed to be dried completely before storage.
4. Large equipment surfaces such as ventilators or suction equipment should be hand-wiped with a damp cloth as needed.
E. Solutions and medications used in the home should be dispensed using regularly cleaned equipment and handled and stored carefully.
F. Water used in humidifiers and nebulizers or as a diluent should be boiled and then stored in a boiled container under refrigeration for no more than 24 hours.

*Adapted from the American Respiratory Care Foundation: *Respir Care* 1988; 33:801–808.

G. It is currently being recommended that suction catheters be used only once and discarded and that sterile gloves should be used for suctioning.

H. The Centers for Disease Control *Guidelines for Handwashing and Hospital Environmental Control,* 1985, state*:

1. Suctioned fluids . . . and secretions may be carefully poured down a drain connected to a sanitary sewer.

2. Sanitary sewers may also be used for the disposal of other infectious wastes capable of being . . . flushed into the sewer.

I. The incidence of pulmonary infections in the home may be lower than in the hospital environment because of less risk of cross-contamination from hospital personnel and other patients.

J. Acetic acid solutions, quaternary ammonium compounds, and household bleach may be used for equipment disinfection.

1. However, available studies have not been performed to verify the usefulness of these agents.

K. Alcohol and hydrogen peroxide can be used for skin cleaning and disinfection.

BIBLIOGRAPHY

American Hospital Association Advisor Committee on Infections: *Infection Control in the Hospital,* ed 4. Chicago, American Hospital Association, 1979.

AMA Z-79, Subcommittee on Ethylene Oxide Sterilization: Ethylene oxide sterilization: A guide for hospital personnel. *Respir Care* 1977; 22:12.

American Respiratory Care Foundation: Guidelines for disinfection of respiratory care equipment used in the home. *Respir Care* 1988; 33:801–808.

Bageant RA, et al: In-use testing of four glutaraldehyde disinfectants in the cidematic washer. *Respir Care* 1981; 26:1255–1261.

Becker KO: Decontamination area for inhalation therapy. *J Am Hosp Assoc* 1971; 45:68.

Becker KO: Inhalation therapy department chooses ETO. *J Am Hosp Assoc* 1971; 45:68.

Block SS: *Disinfection, Sterilization and Preservation,* ed 2. Philadelphia, Lea & Febiger, 1977.

Boyd RF, Hoerl BG: *Basic Medical Microbiology,* ed 2. Boston, Little, Brown & Co, 1981.

Chatburn RL, Kalistrom RJ, Bajaksouzian S: A comparison of acetic acid with a quaternary ammonium compound for disinfection of hand-held nebulizers. *Respir Care* 1988; 33:179–186.

Deshpande VM, Pilbeam SP, Dixon RJ: *A Comprehensive Review in Respiratory Care.* Norwalk, Conn, Appleton & Lange, 1988.

Haselhuhn DH, Brason FW, Borick PM: In-use study of buffered glutaraldehyde for cold sterilization of anesthesia equipment. *Anesth Analg* 1967; 46:468.

Joklik WK, Willett HP, Amos DB, et al: *Zinsser Microbiology,* ed 19. Norwalk, Conn, Appleton & Lange, 1988.

Leach ED: A new synergized glutaraldehyde-phenate sterilizing solution and concentrated disinfectant. *Infect Control* 1981; 1:26–31.

Masferrer R, Ramguez R: Comparison of two activated glutaraldehyde solutions: Cidex solution and Sonacide. *Respir Care* 1977; 22:257.

McLaughlin AJ: *Manual of Infection Control in Respiratory Care.* Boston, Little, Brown & Co, 1983.

Nelson EJ: *Respiratory Therapy Equipment Contamination Surveillance Program: Part 1. Techniques of Infection Control in Respiratory Therapy and Anesthesia.* Seattle, Olympic Medical Corp, Series 5, 1977.

Perkins JJ: *Principles and Methods of Sterilization in Health Sciences.* Springfield, Ill, Charles C Thomas, Publisher, 1969.

*From US Department of Health and Human Services, Public Health Service, Centers for Disease Control: *Guidelines for Handwashing and Environmental Controls.* Atlanta, Centers for Disease Control, 1985.

Rendell-Baker L, Roberts RB: Safe use of ethylene oxide sterilization in hospitals. *Anesth Analg* 1972; 51:658.

Rubbo SD, Gardner JF: *A Review of Sterilization and Disinfection.* Chicago, Year Book Medical Publishers, 1965.

Starkey DH, Himmelsbach CK: On the avoidance of failures in sterilization. *Hospitals* 1974; 48:143.

Sykes G: *Disinfection and Sterilization.* London, E and EN Spon, 1958.

Sykes MK: Sterilization of ventilators. *Int Anesthesiol Clin* 1972; 10:131.

Synder JE: Infection control. *Hospitals* 1970; 44:80.

Synder RW, Cheatle EL: Alkaline glutaraldehyde, an effective disinfectant. *Am J Hosp Pharm* 1965; 22:321.

Technical Standards and Safety Committee, AART: Recommendations for respiratory therapy equipment: Processing, handling, and surveillance. *Respir Care* 1977; 22:928.

US Department of Health and Human Services, Public Health Service, Centers for Disease Control: *Guidelines for Handwashing and Environmental Control.* Atlanta, Centers for Disease Control, 1985.

Wilson RD, et al: An evaluation of the acidemic decontamination system for anesthesia equipment. *Anesth Analg* 1972; 51:658.

Index